Health Law and Policy

A Survival Guide to Medicolegal Issues for Practitioners

Bryan A. Liang, M.D., Ph.D., J.D.
*Dr. Arthur W. Grayson Distinguished Visiting
Professor of Law and Medicine, Southern
Illinois University School of Law, Carbondale*

BUTTERWORTH
HEINEMANN

Boston   Oxford   Auckland   Johannesburg   Melbourne   New Delhi

Recognizing the importance of preserving what has been written, Butterworth–Heinemann prints its books on acid-free paper whenever possible.

 Butterworth-Heinemann supports the efforts of American Forests and the Global ReLeaf program in its campaign for the betterment of trees, forests, and our environment.

Library of Congress Cataloging-in-Publication Data
Liang, Bryan A.
      Health law and policy : a survival guide to medicolegal issues
for practitioners / Bryan A. Liang.
            p.   cm.
      Includes bibliographical references and index.
      ISBN 0-7506-7107-6 (alk. paper)
      1. Medical laws and legislation — United States. 2. Medical
jurisprudence — United States.   3. Physicians — United States
Handbooks, manuals, etc. I. Title.
      KF3821.L53   2000
      344.73´041 — dc21   99-34309
                                                                                              CIP

British Library Cataloguing-in-Publication Data
A catalogue record for this book is available from the British Library.

The publisher offers special discounts on bulk orders of this book.
For information, please contact:

Manager of Special Sales
Butterworth–Heinemann
225 Wildwood Avenue
Woburn, MA 01801-2041
Tel: 781-904-2500
Fax: 781-904-2620

For information on all B–H medical publications available, contact our World Wide Web home page at:
http://www.bh.com

10 9 8 7 6 5 4 3 2 1

Printed in the United States of America

Coventry University

Health Law and Policy

This book is due to be returned not later than the date and
time stamped above. Fines are charged on overdue books

To Charles C. Liang and Anna R. Liang and Shannon M. Biggs and the Gang, who provide me with all my fulfillment.

Contents

About the Author

BRYAN A. LIANG received his undergraduate training in Chemistry, obtaining his B.S. degree from M.I.T. He also has formal training in Policy Studies, Medicine, and Law, being granted a Ph.D. degree from the Harris School of Public Policy Studies at the University of Chicago, where he was the J. Howard Pew Freedom Trust Fellow in the Program on Medicine, Arts, and the Social Sciences; an M.D. degree from Columbia University College of Physicians and Surgeons, where he was supported by the ABMAC Foundation Fellowship for International Study, the Warner-Lambert Clerkship Grant for Study in the Health Sciences, the College of Physicians and Surgeons Institutional Research Award, the National Institutes of Health Fellowship for Biomedical Research, the Medical, Educational, and Scientific Foundation Award for Medical Writing, and the Titus Munson Coan Prize for the Outstanding Paper in the Biological Sciences; and a J.D. degree from Harvard Law School, where he was the inaugural Sheldon Seevak Law and Economics Research Fellow and supported by the Edward Arthur Mellinger Foundation, the MacArthur Foundation, and the John M. Olin Foundation Program in Law and Economics. Professor Liang does not have a high school diploma. He is currently the Dr. Arthur W. Grayson Distinguished Visiting Professor of Law and Medicine at Southern Illinois University School of Law. His research interests focus upon the interface between law, health care, economic incentive structures, and patient safety. He serves on the editorial boards of *Hospital Physician*, *Journal of Clinical Anesthesia*, and *Survey of Anesthesiology*, and has published in a variety of journals, including *Harvard Journal on Legislation*, *Yale Law and Policy Review*, *Virginia Tax Review*, *Notre Dame Law Review*, *Journal of General Internal Medicine*, *Journal of Health Politics*, *Policy and Law*, and *Journal of Legal Medicine*.

Contributor

Anna V. Schlotzhauer, J.D.

Anna V. Schlotzhauer obtained her B.S. degree in Biological Sciences from the University of California at Irvine in 1993. After two years as a scientist in the biotechnology industry, she attended Pepperdine University School of Law and obtained her J.D. degree in 1998. She is currently an attorney-at-law in Los Angeles, CA, with an interest in bioethics and health law.

Preface

Many, if not most, people skip introductions and for good reason. If you are one of these persons, you certainly will lose nothing by skipping this one. If you choose to continue reading, you will discover my thoughts on the audience I perceive for this book and a broad overview of its contents.

This book is aimed at those people interested in learning about the current rules and directions of the health care enterprise in the United States. Although everyone has some exposure to the delivery system, I hope that this book can provide a foundation to understand the discussion of health care around us — in the media and professional press, in the places we give and get health care, and between our professional and personal selves.

With this audience in mind, the book's approach is explanatory, rather than prescriptive. Basic information is provided in the main text, and current issues of debate are introduced in the notes. Of course, any book that attempts to provide information on a dynamic topic (and few topics today are more dynamic than health care) is likely to be doomed to failure; as in the computer industry, it is outdated as soon as it is available. However, by providing the basic information to understand how the system works, along with its constraints and at least some current areas of debate, the reader will be able to formulate informed opinions and advocate most effectively in whatever role he or she plays in the health care system.

The book is divided into four parts. Part I describes topics usually considered "traditional" legal medicine: the legal system, malpractice, informed consent, medical records, and the provider–patient relationship. Part II represents the segue into modernity. Here, the insurance structure (i.e., paying for care) is outlined, including descriptions of public programs, such as Medicare and Medicaid, as well as private systems, particularly managed care. Of course, there is a significant move to integrate the two, and this area is explored in the chapter on managed care. Part III brings the reader squarely within the modern delivery environment, discussing important nonclinical aspects that have an impact on health care delivery. Therefore, the areas of contracting and employment, licensure and practice limitations, and the exceedingly important areas of fraud and abuse, antitrust, and alternative dispute resolution are reviewed. As might be expected, the chapters on fraud and abuse and antitrust are lengthy due to their importance and seemingly singular focus by state and federal government authorities. Finally, in Part IV, information on important aspects at the end of life are provided in chapters reviewing advance directives and definitions of death. Note that Part IV is not a bioethics primer, although certainly the information can inform bioethical discussions.

Because the book is aimed at a broad audience, sources for additional information are derived from different forums. The medical, legal, and policy literature relevant to the topics discussed are provided. As well, web sites are listed that may be helpful in supplementing and providing additional information; note, however, as in all areas of the Internet, the existence and content of web sites are a function of the person or organization creating and updating them. In any event, I would very much welcome readers to direct me to any relevant publications, web sites (and links that are dead), and other sources that may better inform future readers and myself.

Of course, the person on the title page of any book is not singularly responsible for its creation. This book is no exception. I would like to thank Steve Asciutto, Pete Gimino, Kurt Hartman, Anne Macaulay, and Kris Storti for their substantive contributions to this work. I would also like to thank Susan Pioli, Director of Medical Publishing, Butterworth–Heinemann, for her initiation and support of this project; Jana Friedman Brown, former Associate Editor of the Medical Division, and my editor at Butterworth–Heinemann, for her patience, good humor, and support; and Jodie Allen, my production editor at Butterworth–Heinemann, for her support and incredible attention to detail. A special thanks to Anna V. Schlotzhauer, coauthor of the "Definitions of Death" chapter, for her patience and tolerance under pressure.

Finally, I thank the most important persons in my life, my parents, Charles C. Liang and Anna R. Liang, and Shannon M. Biggs and the Gang, for their limitless support, understanding, patience, and ready smiles. To these very special persons, I dedicate this work.

Part I
Traditional Legal Medicine

1

Concepts of Law

The law in the United States has significant impact on medical practice, the relationships between parties, and the obligations of those within and external to the actual delivery process. Therefore, an overview of legal principles is important to allow the nonlawyer to recognize important legal issues and know when to bring in competent legal counsel. However, it should be noted that this overview is not designed to provide an exhaustive explanation of legal concepts; standard legal treatises and reference works should be used for such a detailed study.

Structure

The foundation of all law in the United States is the U.S. Constitution, which often is referred to as the supreme law of the land. All powers of lesser authority that result in and from law are derived from the Constitution.

There are two general structures for lawmaking in the United States: federal and state. Each level has its own structures, including governing constitutions and three operational divisions: legislatures, which pass laws; executives, which approve and implement law; and courts, which determine the interpretation, applicability, and validity of the law. The major sources of law are the state legislatures/Congress with the approval of the executive (governor in states, the president for the country) and state and federal courts. These sources are briefly reviewed.

Legislative Bodies

State legislatures and Congress draft bills, and if approved by both legislative bodies (all states have two legislative bodies with the exception of Nebraska, which has only one; Congress is made up of the House of Representatives and the Senate), the bill then is sent to the executive (the governor in states; the president in the federal system) for his or her consideration. If approved by the executive, the bill becomes statutory law for the state or country. If vetoed by the executive, the bill may become law only if the requisite number of legislators vote to override the veto. If a bill is passed, either through executive passage or a veto override, generally the bill is provided to the executive branch for its implementation as law. Critically, this includes having administrative agencies and bureaus write regulations to implement and enforce the law. These regulations generally have the force and effect of law similar to the statute on which they are based.

Courts

The courts serve as lawmakers in the United States by assessing and resolving disputes and interpreting the law, and whose interpretations may be used by future courts. When parties have a conflict due to some purported public or private breach, the public or private parties can set their dispute in front of a court for its determination of how the law applies to the particular facts and circumstances of the case. The initial adjudication generally is considered to be on the trial court level. Each state and territory of the United States has a separate court system and generally operates independent of the others. Trial courts on the state level can adjudicate on a wide variety of specific subject matters such as family disputes, disputes that involve less than a certain amount of money, probate disputes, and criminal actions or they can be courts of first resort for all general disputes, depending on the particular state. The trial court generally is responsible for both discovering the facts and applying the law; this is where juries sit to decide the resolution of disputes. Note, however, that jury trials in noncriminal suits are not mandatory; only if a party requests a jury trial does the case get tried as such. If no party requests a jury, then the case is tried by the judge alone. A disappointed litigant may appeal a case decision to an intermediate appeals court for review if the state has such an intermediate court (most do). This appeal generally is granted as a matter of right to the disappointed litigant. The case is reviewed only on issues of law; factual matters are assumed to be as the trial court determined. The appellate court may agree with the trial court's legal determination and affirm the trial court judgment, disagree with the trial court's legal determination and reverse the trial court judgment, or agree and disagree with different portions of the trial court and affirm in part and reverse in part the trial court's legal determinations. A disappointed litigant may appeal from the appellate court's decision to the state's highest court, usually known as the supreme court (New York is a notable exception; the supreme court is its trial court, the appellate division is its intermediate appellate court, and the Court of Appeals is its highest court). The state supreme court usually has discretion whether or not to take a case for review and generally is the final arbiter of state-based disputes. It, too, focuses on matters of law. Finally, even though the U.S. Supreme Court is a federal court, if the case involves U.S. constitutional issues, the case may be appealed to it by filing a *writ of certiorari*, a document describing the case and requesting review. The U.S. Supreme Court also takes cases on a discretionary basis.

The federal courts operate in parallel with the state system. Normally, cases flow through either the state courts or the federal courts and not between the two. In contrast with the many state trial courts, the United States has only 91 federal districts, each representing an area of responsibility for a single trial court. A state will have between one and four federal district courts. Federal district courts do not hear all cases. They are courts of specificity, generally hearing only cases involving disputes based on federal law or disputes involving parties with "diversity of citizenship" (i.e., the parties are citizens from different states), in which at least $75,000 is at issue in the dispute. The latter can involve state law, and the federal court will apply the law of the state in which it sits to resolve the dispute. Like state trial courts, federal courts determine the facts and apply the law in the case; in addition, federal district courts can involve juries, except in situations where the federal law allows adjudication only by judge. A disappointed litigant in federal court may appeal to the intermediate federal appellate court, the Circuit Court of Appeals. There are 13 such circuit courts, each with 4 to 10 states in its purview. The appeal from a federal district court to a Court of Appeals generally is a matter of right. Federal appellate courts, like state intermediate courts, focus on reviewing the trial court's assessment of the law, rather than making any determination of the facts. Finally, a disappointed litigant after Court of Appeals adjudication may file a *writ of cer-*

tiorari to the U.S. Supreme Court, which may or may not grant the writ and hear the case. The U.S. Supreme Court denies most writs.

Courts are important lawmaking entities because the resolution of disputes on the appellate court level (intermediate and supreme courts on both the state and federal levels) are given precedential value under the doctrine of *stare decisis* (i.e., to adhere to decided cases). This type of judge-made law is called *common law*. Therefore, the decisions with regard to the interpretation of law by courts of superior rank must be adhered to by courts of inferior rank. In such a way, theoretically, courts will provide consistent assessments of law. Hence, state supreme court interpretation must be adhered to by the state's appellate and trial courts; state appellate court decisions must be adhered to by the trial courts within its geographic purview; the U.S. Supreme Court's interpretations generally must be followed by all courts; and the Court of Appeals decisions must be followed by all federal district courts of the circuit.

Types of Law

Law can be divided into three basic categories: civil law, criminal law, and administrative law.

Civil Law

In the United States, *civil law* traditionally refers to the law between private parties (or public parties acting in a private capacity, such as a government contracting to purchase goods or services) and involves two major areas: contracts and torts. Civil law is a creation of both the common law and statutory law; generally, however, the principles of civil law originate from the British common law and have been statutorily adopted by legislatures. Civil law generally is the province of state law. The standard of adjudication generally is a preponderance of the evidence; that is, it is more likely than not. So, to prevail, a litigant must show it is more likely than not that his or her claim regarding the dispute is correct.

Contract Law

Contract law is the law of agreements and their enforcement. These rules govern agreements made between parties if the parties are competent, the parties agree to bind themselves to mutually understood actions, and the subject of the agreement is legal. *Competence* refers to the ability to enter validly into contracts on the basis of age and mental capacity; that is, the party must be of majority age and have the mental capability to understand the ramifications of binding him- or herself in contract. With regard to the agreement itself, the parties must pass "consideration"; that is, they each must exchange something of value, usually promises to bind themselves to do something they were previously not obligated to do. Generally, one party offers to do a particular thing and the other accepts such an offer. Both parties must understand the rights and obligations of each in the bargain for the contract to be valid, and thus enforceable by the courts. Note that contract law requires that the party promise to actually do something, even conditionally; "promises" that do not obligate one party to do anything (e.g., "I'll purchase the item *if I feel like it*") are considered illusory and not valid consideration on which to base a contract. In addition, there can be no fraud, duress, or unconscionability inducing a purported "bargain." Finally, the subject matter of the contract must be legal. Competent parties who exchange valid promises as consideration will not have the terms of their contracts enforced by the courts if the contract is for illegal means, purposes, or ends. If these three characteristics are applicable, then contract law rules will govern the agreement and provide for remedies for breach of a party's promises.

Note that, for the most part, there is no need to have contracts in writing. Oral contracts generally are enforceable. The major problem with oral agreements is that selective remembrance may cause conflicts. Further, common law contract law requires certain kinds of contracts to be in writing. According to the Statute of Frauds, contracts in consideration of marriage (not marriage itself), contracts that by their terms cannot be performed within a year of their making, contracts for the sale of land, contracts for the sale of goods over $500, and contracts for suretyship (assuming the debts of others) must be in writing.

Although much of contract law stems from the British common law and has been adopted statutorily by state legislatures, the law of contract differs depending on the state. Legislatures may have altered some of the common law rules; courts may have altered the interpretation of these rules. Therefore, it is essential, for a complete understanding of relevant contractual rights, local legal counsel be consulted *before* signing a contract.

If one party does not perform his or her part of the bargain, generally courts award monetary damages or, less frequently, use their equity powers to require that the party in breach to perform. Damages usually provide the "benefit of the bargain" (i.e., expectation damages), where the nonbreaching party is entitled to have the contract performed by someone else with the additional reasonable costs and other foreseeable damages the responsibility of the breaching party. Equitable relief, such as a court ordering specific performance, is available for certain situations such as sales of goods; however, it generally is not available for personal services contracts due to the inappropriate nature of forcing one party to work involuntarily for another. This "involuntary servitude" smacks of slavery and so generally is prohibited.

Case. Dr. A is interested in purchasing a set of blood pressure cuffs for his office. Ms. C is selling blood pressure cuffs for $20 each. Dr. A calls and indicates to Ms. C that he would like to purchase ten blood pressure cuffs and asks the price. Ms. C indicates that each cuff is $20. Dr. A then states, "I'll take 20. Please bill me." Ms. C states, "Fine. They'll be in your office tomorrow." However, Ms. C then decides not to sell the cuffs to Dr. A; she calls Dr. A the next day and says she will not deliver the cuffs. Dr. A then goes to another dealer of cuffs and pays $21 each and then sues Ms. C for breach of contract.

Legal Discussion. Here, a valid, enforceable contract has been formed. Both parties are competent. During preliminary negotiations, in response to Dr. A's request for information on price, Ms. C provides it. Then Dr. A states that he will purchase 20 (at the price of $20/cuff); this represents his offer to purchase: Dr. A promises to pay $20/cuff for 20 cuffs. Ms. C accepts this offer when she okays the purchase; she has promised to sell Dr. A the 20 cuffs at $20/cuff, delivery to be the next day. There seems to be no question as to both parties understanding the transaction. Both parties have bound themselves to do something, thus there are no illusory promises to consider. The subject matter of the transaction is a legal purchase and sale of blood pressure cuffs. Finally, this contract is not within the Statute of Frauds because it is not a sale for over $500 and therefore does not need to be in writing. Thus, the contract is binding for both parties. When Ms. C stated that she would not perform on the contract, she breached the contract. The court most likely would award damages to Dr. A on the basis of the extra costs of the cuffs ($1 extra/cuff × 20 cuffs) or $20, plus any other reasonably foreseeable costs associated with the transaction.

Tort Law

The law of torts governs civil wrongs committed by one party against another party's person, property, or interests that are not contractually based; that is, wrongs that are not due to a breach of contract. The standard division of torts is threefold: strict liability torts, intentional torts, and negligence-based torts. Strict liability torts are those in which the party causing the harm is strictly liable; simply put, if the harm occurs, the party pays. These torts are most common in the products liability sphere; for example, if there is broken glass in a can of soda and an individual drinks the soda and sustains injury, the manufacturer is strictly liable for the harm. Intentional torts, reassuringly, are intentional actions of one party that harm another; the classic examples are assault and battery. Assault in tort is the intentional and willful threat to inflict injury to another, coupled with an apparent ability to do so, with a show of force that would give the victim reason to fear or expect immediate bodily harm. Battery in tort is the actual use of the threatened force of an assault, or the intentional, unprivileged harmful or offensive touching of one by another. Finally, there are the negligence-based torts. These torts are by far the most frequently asserted torts generally as well as in health care liability situations. Negligence-based torts are those that impose liability on a party for failing to act with reasonable care. To show negligence, an aggrieved party must show that the other party had a duty to exercise reasonable care, breached that duty, and this breach foreseeably caused the aggrieved party damages. Thus, negligence encompasses a wide array of circumstances. Torts based on negligence include medical malpractice and lack of informed consent.[1] Damages in tort cases generally focus on compensation to the aggrieved party for present and future damages associated with the harm. Note also that, in contrast to contract, in tort punitive or exemplary damages are available for egregious behavior.

Case. Dr. A is an otolaryngologist. C consulted Dr. A, complaining of symptoms in his right ear. Dr. A examined the right ear and noted that C's ear had a large perforation in the caudal portion of the eardrum as well as a large polyp in the middle ear. Dr. A also examined C's left ear, but could not make a full assessment due to a considerable amount of cerumen. Dr. A appropriately suggested an operation to remove the polyp in C's right ear. After getting a second opinion, C agreed to the operation. C was not told of any problem with the left ear and believed only an operation to the right ear was necessary. Dr. A discussed the need for surgery, pointing out the benefits and risks of the surgery as well as other treatments and doing nothing. C signed the informed consent form. While C was under anesthesia, Dr. A removed the cerumen in C's left ear to make a more thorough examination. Dr. A discovered a significantly more diseased ear than on the right, with a perforation located cranially and the bone of the inner wall of the ear totally diseased and dead. Dr. A then made the decision to operate on the right ear rather than the left. Dr. A performed the surgery in a medically appropriate manner, but the treatment resulted in deafness in that ear. When C discovered that the left ear was not operated on but the right had been, C sued Dr. A for battery, due to the operation on his left ear, and lack of informed consent, indicating he would not have consented to the procedure.

Legal Discussion. Dr. A may be liable for tort injury on the basis of the case on which this illustration is based.[2] First, Dr. A's action can be considered an intentional tort. Technically, Dr. A inflicted a battery on C: Dr. A intentionally made an unauthorized touching of C because she had no permission to touch C's left ear, only

his right. By operating on his left ear, Dr. A committed battery on C. Further, Dr. A may be liable for the negligence-based tort of lack of informed consent. Dr. A had a duty to provide all information material to the operation, including the possibility of operating on the left ear, since she was in a physician–patient relationship with C; she breached that duty by not providing the information; and she caused damages associated with the ear on the basis of her lack of the consent, which resulted in C having a deaf left ear.

Criminal Law

Criminal law generally is a creation of state statute, although there are notable federal criminal statutes. Criminal law provides the rules for societal protection by specifying the boundaries of acceptable social conduct. Therefore, criminal adjudications are brought by representatives of public institutions (as denoted by *State* v. *X* or *People* v. *X*) against another party. Examples of criminal acts are the commonly understood activities such as murder, theft, as well as *criminal* assault and battery, with these latter actions being similar, but not necessarily identical, to their civil namesakes. Criminal law adjudications require that the state prove its case beyond a reasonable doubt. Note that criminal and civil actions are not mutually exclusive; the same act can result in both criminal prosecution and civil suit as well as differing determinations of liability (e.g., the O. J. Simpson trials). Criminal penalties include imprisonment, fine, or both.

Case. Dr. E was the physician for AL, a patient admitted to a nursing home after being diagnosed with renal failure. To treat AL's renal failure, a peritoneal dialysis catheter was put into place. However, Dr. E mistakened this catheter for a gastronomy feeding tube and directed that the patient be fed through the catheter. AL received numerous feedings through the catheter. Dr. E was notified of the mistake approximately 36 hours later. Dr. E then phoned a nephrologist, who advised Dr. E to admit the patient to the hospital. However, although Dr. E knew that peritonitis could be fatal if untreated, Dr. E did not order AL's transfer from the nursing home to the hospital until ten hours later. On admission, AL was diagnosed with peritonitis caused by the feedings through the peritoneal dialysis catheter. The patient died due to the peritonitis. Public Health Law in the state provides for criminal penalties for "willful violation of health laws," including willfully committing an act of neglect. *Neglect* is defined in the state statute as "failure to provide timely, consistent, safe, adequate and appropriate services, treatment, and/or care to patient."

Legal Discussion. Dr. E most likely would be criminally liable under this statute for willfully committing an

[1]See Chapters 2 and 3.
[2]Mohr v. Williams, 104 N.W. 12 (Minn. 1905).

act of neglect according to the case on which this illustration is based.[3] The evidence showed that Dr. E was aware of, and consciously disregarded the substantial risk of serious physical injury of AL by not performing the transfer from the nursing home to the hospital until ten hours after being told of the appropriate action to take. Thus, Dr. E willfully acted in a manner that failed to provide timely, consistent, safe, adequate, and appropriate treatment to AL, in violation of the Public Health Law. As such, he was subject to criminal penalties if the jury found that such actions were proved beyond a reasonable doubt by the state prosecutors.

Administrative Law

Administrative law is the creation of statute. Generally, after laws are passed by legislatures or Congress, implementation of the law passes to the executive branch. However, the complexity of the rules and subject matter may induce the legislative bodies to delegate authority to legislatively created agencies in the executive branch, who then take the legislative language in the statute and implement them by issuing regulations. These regulations and their adoption usually are subject to some public approval procedure through a state or federal administrative procedures statute, which includes a mandated period for public comment. Thus, when drafting regulations, administrative agencies have significant rule-making power akin to legislative bodies. Further, however, administrative agencies also have some judicial-like powers. When there is conflict with regard to the application and interpretation of regulations, administrative agencies often are given the power to resolve these conflicts through an administrative law process. Depending on the specific administrative agency, these conflicts are heard by a variety of quasi-judicial administrative officers, with the final determination generally subject to judicial review. Judicial review, however, occurs only after the exhaustion of administrative appeals and usually gives great deference to the administrative determinations. Examples of administrative agencies include the federal Health Care Financing Administration in the Department of Health and Human Services, the federal National Labor Relations Board in the Department of Labor, the Federal Trade Commission, the Food and Drug Administration, the Internal Revenue Service, state departments of health, state departments of insurance, state departments of corporations. Note that administrative adjudications do not require juries nor are the rules of evidence strictly applied.

Example. Medicare is a federal program administered by the Health Care Financing Administration (HCFA), an agency within the Department of Health and Human Services. HCFA, as an agency, has been granted broad powers to resolve conflicts in the Medicare program. For example, HCFA outsources to private "carriers" the responsibility to determine whether the rendered services are covered under Part B of Medicare, which provides for payment for physician services. In addition, the carriers are responsible for other administrative concerns, such as whether the Medicare beneficiary has met his or her deductible for the service, whether the services were medically necessary, whether any coinsurance amounts are due from the beneficiary, and how much should be paid by Medicare and to whom (beneficiaries can assign their benefits to providers so that providers are paid directly by the program). If a Medicare beneficiary has been provided a service by a physician, and the physician then bills the carrier for the service, the carrier may deny some or all of the claim. Assume that the claim involves an amount greater than $1000. The carrier issues an Explanation of Medical Benefits form, which is sent to the physician if benefits have been assigned or to the beneficiary if not. Challenge to this denial then goes through the administrative law process for these types of claims:

1. If the assignee physician or beneficiary is dissatisfied with the determination, he or she may request a review of the initial determination within six months.
2. A party who is dissatisfied with the review decision may request a hearing before a hearing officer appointed by the carrier if done so within six months.
3. If the party who requested the hearing is dissatisfied with the hearing and hearing officer determination, another hearing officer may be requested for another hearing or the disgruntled party may proceed to a government administrative law judge (ALJ) hearing.
4. If the party who requested the ALJ hearing is dissatisfied with the results of this hearing, the party may obtain further review by the government appeals council.
5. If the party who requested the hearing is not satisfied with the decision of the appeals council, judicial review in federal district court is the final step. However, judicial review can occur only after administrative review has been performed and is limited to issues that are not precluded by statute, to those claims that meet a minimum financial threshold, and to remedies provided by statute.

As is apparent, a significant set of procedures are mandated by administrative review of a conflict before access to a court is appropriate.

The Structure of a Civil Lawsuit

Although medical providers are subject to adjudication in civil, criminal, or administrative courts, the most common

---

[3]People v. Einaugler, 618 N.Y.S.2d (App.Div. 1994).

are those in civil disputes. A medical malpractice claim against a physician is used to illustrate the process of a civil suit.

Initiation of the Suit

A malpractice suit usually is initiated by service of process; that is, a complaint and summons from the patient-plaintiff. This notice of suit is usually sent by the plaintiff's attorney to the physician and indicates the claim against the physician, here, a tort claim for malpractice, by alleging the facts as understood by the plaintiff and requesting relief by the court. The notice also may be served by an officer of the court after being filed with the clerk of the court, including a sheriff or other person. This notice indicates the court in which the suit has been filed; generally this will be a state trial court or, less frequently, a federal district court. After receiving the complaint and summons, a provider is prudent to contact his or her malpractice insurer. Generally, the malpractice insurer has the right and power to select an attorney to defend the physician, who is now the defendant. Fees are paid by the insurer. Physicians also may have their own attorney, whom they pay from their own pocket. This may not be necessary but may be prudent if it is possible that the interests of the physician may conflict with that of the insurer. However, the insurer's attorney generally controls the litigation. Note that the suit must be initiated within the relevant state statute of limitations for the cause of action in the complaint and summons to survive.

Meeting with Attorneys

Once the complaint and summons have been served, the defendant physician and his or her attorney(s) will investigate the claim, determine a strategy, and formally respond to the complaint.

Pleadings

Pleadings are documents filed with the court for the purpose of setting forth each party's position on the case. Basic pleadings encompass the complaint by the plaintiff and the answer by the defendant. The plaintiff generally puts forward his or her understanding of the facts of the malpractice claim, the standard of care, and how that care was breached by the defendant. With respect to the plaintiff's allegations, the defendant in his or her answer can admit, deny, deny in part, or indicate he or she has no knowledge to admit or deny.

Thus, after the plaintiff has served the defendant with the complaint and summons, the defendant and his or her attorney(s) must respond to the suit, usually within 15 to 20 days (a default judgment may be entered against the defendant if he or she does not respond within this time period with no valid excuse). Also at this response stage, the defendant may file preliminary objections before answering the complaint, including potential errors that may defeat the plaintiff's case, such as improper service of process, lack of court jurisdiction, expiration of the statute of limitations, or other technical legal objections. The court may allow the plaintiff to correct these errors through a new or amended complaint or, much more rarely, may dismiss the case due to the significance of the errors.

The defendant also may bring forth a motion to dismiss the case because it does not provide for a cause of action recognized by law. If the case is dismissed by the judge, the plaintiff may obtain appellate review of this decision. But if the court refuses to dismiss the case, the defendant must answer the plaintiff's complaint. After the defendant answers, the plaintiff can file objections to the defendant's answer. The court then resolves all pleading objections at the pretrial stage.

Judgment on the Pleadings

After the pleadings are filed and are complete on both sides, many states allow for either party to move for judgment on the pleadings. The judge then assesses the case only on the basis of the pleadings to determine whether judgment can be rendered on the basis of the undisputed merits of the case in the pleadings. Usually, however, there is disagreement on the critical aspects of the case, and judgment on the pleadings cannot be accomplished. If there is no judgment on the pleadings, this point is when parties begin considering appropriate witnesses, including expert witnesses, with whom to speak, as well as what documentation will be needed to support their respective positions; that is, it sets the stage for discovery.

Discovery

In most state courts and all federal courts, both litigants have the right to discovery; that is, examination of witnesses and documents and requests for admissions before trial. Generally, for witnesses, each party presents a list of questions to the other party and his or her witnesses. These lists comprise interrogatories (i.e., questions that are answered, usually in writing, under oath) that relate to the facts of the case. Oral questions and answers provided under oath are called *depositions*. Depositions also are used to obtain testimony if a particular witness will not be present and can be used to explore the strength of the other side's case and for impeachment at trial. Physicians and others who answer interrogatories and participate in depositions therefore must be very cautious and clear regarding answers and should consult with counsel before answering. This is particularly true since the standard rules of evidence do not apply during depositions and virtually any relevant question may be asked.

Note also that discovery "examination" can include a physical or mental examination of a party if it is relevant to the case. For documents, each party may request the court to order the other to allow for examination and copying of medical records and other relevant information. Finally, a request for admission is an extremely important discovery request. The primary importance of these requests is that, if these requests are not answered within a certain prescribed time, the information therein is considered admitted for the purposes of trial; that is, both sides agree that the information is true.

Also note that some insurers require particular discovery information to be provided at certain times; it is essential that the defendant's attorney comply with these requirements.

Pretrial Conferences

Pretrial conferences are between the judge and attorneys for the parties; the parties generally are not present. During the pretrial conferences, the judge and attorneys decide technical issues, such as the deadline for discovery, date for disclosing expert and other witnesses, and the ultimate trial date.

Trial

After discovery, if either party requests one, a jury is impaneled. Generally, a pool of individuals is available for sitting on the jury; usually the attorneys for both sides question each potential juror and may reject a certain number. Eventually, a set of jurors is chosen for the case. Once sworn in, the trial may begin. This beginning is marked by each attorney giving an opening statement, usually a summary of what each side intends to show. Then witnesses, including expert witnesses who attempt to establish the standard of care, are called. Generally, the plaintiff's side begins, calls witnesses, and imparts information to the jury by asking a series of questions; when one side calls a witness and asks him or her questions, this is known as *direct examination*. When the plaintiff has finished questioning the witness, the defense may ask questions; when the opposing party questions a witness called by the other side, this is known as *cross-examination*. Generally, cross-examination is an effort to limit the effectiveness of the witness for the other party's side. Other witnesses may be called by the

plaintiff and further documents and other items can be introduced by the plaintiff in an effort to prove his or her case.

At the end of plaintiff's evidence, the defendant may move for the judge to direct the jury to render judgment in his or her favor, known as *directed verdict*. Recall that plaintiff must prove his or her side of the case by a preponderance of the evidence; if he or she has not, regardless of defendant's efforts or lack thereof, defendant is entitled to judgment. If the judge denies the motion, the case for the defendant is made as was that for the plaintiff; that is, through direct examination of witnesses (with cross-examination by plaintiff), introduction of documents, and provision of other materials.

At the end of defendant's case, either party may move for a directed verdict in its favor. If this is not granted for either party, then the attorneys for each side make closing arguments, generally focusing on what they believe has or has not been proven in the case and what verdict the jury should render. The judge then usually instructs the jury on the specific law (e.g., the plaintiff must show by a preponderance of the evidence a preexisting duty to provide nonnegligent care to the plaintiff by the physician, a breach of that duty by providing care that fell below the standard of care, that caused the plaintiff damages). The jury then retires to another room to deliberate and reach a verdict on the basis of the facts it determines are credible and the law as stated by the judge. Once a verdict is reached, the jury returns to the court and indicates to the judge what verdict was reached. The judge then renders the judgment based on the jury verdict. Note that at this point, the losing party may move for a judgment notwithstanding the verdict (also known in some courts as *judgment as a matter of law*) or for a new trial. If neither of these motions is granted, the judgment is final as to that court. The losing party then may appeal the judgment.

Appeals

Generally, a disappointed litigant may appeal once as a matter of right. The appellate court reviews a case on the basis of the trial record, written summaries, and brief oral arguments by the attorneys. The appellate court generally assesses the case on the basis of law; determinations of fact by the trial court are given great deference by the appellate court. The decision of the appellate court may be rendered by an issuance of a written opinion, which generally is published and used for stare decisis purposes. Further appeals may occur: on the state level, to the state supreme court; on the federal level, to the U.S. Supreme Court. However, acceptance of such appeals generally is discretionary and, as a matter of general concern, denied.

Notes on Concepts of Law

Attorney–Client Privilege

Generally, information communicated by the provider to his or her attorney is confidential between the two, similar to the relationship between physician and patient. Providers, to avail themselves to such privilege, should ensure adherence to two basic tenets. First, all reports and documents compiled or created by the provider that are related to the lawsuit and communicated to legal counsel must be maintained in a secure place, preferably away from the site of practice. Critically, none of these documents should be placed in the patient's chart. Second, the provider must not discuss the substantive aspects of the litigation with parties other than the provider's attorney, for this constitutes a waiver of the privilege; conversations with others are discoverable and therefore discussions with third parties vitiates the attorney–client privilege protections. Indeed, often the provider will be asked if he or she has had discussions regarding the case with anyone. By discussing that information with a third party, any information on the case including facts, issues, strategy, and the like is available to opposing counsel. The privilege generally covers the provider, the attorney, and the liability insurer's claim agent. Any other person who requests information should be referred to the attorney to determine if the information should be divulged or if it is covered by the privilege.

Additional Reading. American Bar Association Tort and Insurance Practice Section, *Attorney-Client Privilege in Civil Litigation: Protecting and Defending Confidentiality* (Chicago: American Bar Association, 1997); T. K. Byerley, "Survival of the Attorney-Client Privilege After the Death of the Client," *Michigan Bar Journal* 77 (1998), pp. 1222–23; E. S. Epstein, *Attorney Client Privilege and the Work Product Doctrine,* 2d ed. (Chicago: American Bar Association, 1989; J. H. Friedenthal et al., *Civil Procedure,* 2d ed. (St. Paul, MN: West Publishing Co., 1993), section 7.4; M. K. Kane, *Civil Procedure: In a Nutshell,* 4th ed. (St. Paul, MN: West Publishing Co., 1996), section 5-2; K. A. Kearney, "The Attorney-Client Privilege Under Siege: Health Care Lawyers Beware," *GP Solo Small Firm Law* 15, no. 4 (1998), p. 1998.

Burdensome Discovery Requests

Generally, discovery requests should not require the party receiving the request to act to obtain information he or she does not have. Hence, if a discovery request requires that the recipient to take significant steps to obtain this information or if it would take an inordinate amount of time and resources to obtain the requested information, the request may be inappropriate. Consultation with an attorney is the most appropriate avenue to take when discovery requests seem unreasonably burdensome.

Additional Reading. B. R. Anderson, *Discovery in Legal Decision Making* (Norwell, MA: Kluwer Academic Publishers, 1996); P. B. Broida, "Burdensome Discovery," in *A Guide to Merit Systems Protection Board Law and Practice* (Arlington, VA: Dewey Publishers, 1998), Chapter 2, Part IV.B; J. H. Friedenthal et al., *Civil Procedure,* 2d ed. (St. Paul, MN: West Publishing Co., 1993), section 7.15; R. S. Haydock, *Discovery: Theory Practice and Problems* (Boston: Little, Brown and Co. 1983); M. K. Kane, *Civil Procedure: In a Nutshell,* 4th ed. (St. Paul, MN: West Publishing Co., 1996), sections 3-30 and 3-34.

Damages and Equity

Generally, in civil suits in tort and contract, monetary damages are granted to the aggrieved party if the party prevails over the defendant. However, in certain circumstances, these "at law" damage remedies are inadequate or inappropriate. Under such circumstances, a court may "in equity" grant other forms of relief to the aggrieved party. This relief is discretionary with the court and may be fashioned to meet the needs of the specific facts and circumstances of the case. In addition, equitable relief also may be sought as ancillary relief to a pending suit to preserve rights or expedite the pending suit. For example, temporary restraining orders (TROs) may be granted by a court to maintain the status quo between the parties pending a hearing for a preliminary injunction. Indeed, TROs may be granted simply on affidavits of the complaining party with notice to the opposing party without a hearing. TROs therefore are not granted lightly and require the threat of irreparable harm from the delay before a hearing for a preliminary injunction can occur. Generally, TROs are limited to a very short time period (e.g., ten days).

Preliminary injunctions (also known as *temporary injunctions* or *interlocutory injunctions*) preserve the status quo until a trial on the merits of the case. Preliminary injunctions are issued only after notice and a hearing and remain in effect until the trial on the merits is finalized. Injunctions can be made permanent if, after the trial on the merits, it appears warranted as an appropriate equitable remedy. Generally, TROs and preliminary injunctions are very difficult to obtain; the court will assess whether the plaintiff is threatened with irreparable harm, the plaintiff appears likely to win on the merits, a balancing of the hardships of both parties due to the TRO or injunction weighs in the plaintiff's favor, and the interest of the general public weighs in the plaintiff's favor.

Additional Reading. P. S. Atihay, *The Damages Lottery* (Oxford, UK: Hart Publishing Co., 1997); D. B.

Dobbs, *Law of Remedies: Damages — Equity — Restitution*, 2d ed. (St. Paul, MN: West Publishing Co., 1993); J. A. Sebert, *Remedies: Damages, Equity, and Restitution*, 2d ed. (New York: Matthew Bender & Co., 1997); R. S. Thompson and D. O. Harris, *Compensation and Support for Illness and Injury* (Oxford, UK: Clarendon Press, 1984).

Executive Orders

Executive orders are unilateral presidential (or other executive) directives of policy issued to government officials or agencies in the executive branch. They often are in the area, particularly in the federal sphere, of ceremonial concern (e.g., holiday proclamations), routine administrative matters (e.g., recycling requirements for federal agencies), and national security and emergency matters of national importance (e.g., war). These executive orders are given great latitude by the courts and are virtually unchallengeable by private parties. As such, they are powerful tools outside the traditional three-branch separation of powers conception outlined in the Constitution.

Additional Reading.   J. M. Carey, *Executive Decree Authority* (Cambridge, UK: Cambridge University Press, 1998); B. A. Liang, *"A Zone of Twilight": Executive Orders in the Modern Policy State* (Washington, DC: National Legal Center for the Public Interest, 1999); R. P. Morgan, *The President and Civil Rights: Policy Making by Executive Order* (New York: University Press of America, 1987).

Jurisdiction

Jurisdiction is the power of the adjudicatory body to hear a case in front of it. Without appropriate jurisdiction, any decision made by that body is either void or of no precedential value. Thus, for example, if a standard medical malpractice case gets filed and adjudicated in federal district court without diversity jurisdiction or other federal-based foundation, the district court lacks jurisdiction to hear the case and any adjudication by it generally is considered void.

Additional Reading.   A. D. Briggs et al., *Civil Jurisdiction and Judgements,* 2d ed. (Essex, UK: LLP Ltd., 1998); R. A. Carp, *The Federal Courts,* 3d ed. (Washington, DC: Congressional Quarterly, 1998); J. H. Friedenthal et al., *Civil Procedure,* 2d ed. (St. Paul, MN: West Publishing Co., 1993), sections 2.1, 3.1, 3.2, 3.4, 3.10, 3.14, and 3.17; M. K. Kane, *Civil Procedure: In a Nutshell,* 4th ed. (St. Paul, MN: West Publishing Co., 1996), sections 2-1–2-6.

Further Reading

Structure

Alfange D. The Supreme Court and the Separation of Powers: A Welcome Return to Normalcy? *Geo Wash L Rev* 1990;58:668–761.

Gwyn WB. The Indeterminacy of the Separation of Powers and the Federal Courts. *Geo Wash L Rev* 1989;57:474–505.

Paulsen MS. The Most Dangerous Branch: Executive Power to Say What the Law Is. *Geo Wash L Rev* 1994;83:217–345.

See Also

Krotoszynski RJ. On the Danger of Wearing Two Hats: Mistretta and Morrison Revisited. *College of Wm & Mary L Rev* 1997;38:417–85.

Structure of Courts

Baughan SB et al. Judicial Precedents as Binding or Persuasive. In: *American Jurisprudence,* 2d ed. New York: Lawyers Cooperative Publishing Co., 1995;§362–406.

Padden AL. Overruling Decisions in the Supreme Court: The Role of a Decision's Vote, Age, and Subject Matter in the Application of Stare Decisis After Payne v. Tennessee. *Geo Wash L Rev* 1994;82:1689–96.

Saint-Paul N, Wierzbicki JR. Judicial Precedents as Binding or Persuasive. In: *American Jurisprudence,* 2d ed. New York: Lawyers Cooperative Publishing Co., 1995;§147–65.

Structure of Legislative Bodies

Outzs LL. A Principled Use of Congressional Floor Speeches in Statutory Interpretation. *Colum J L & Soc Probs* 1995;28:297–304.

Najarian SD. Congress; Legislative Department. In: *American Jurisprudence,* 2d ed. New York: Lawyers Cooperative Publishing Co., 1975;§11.

See Also

Gardner JA. The Uses and Abuses of Incumbency: People v. Ohrenstein and the Limits of Inherent Legislative Power. *Fordham L Rev* 1991;60:217–55.

Rotunda RD, Nowak JE. *Treatise on Constitutional Law,* 2d ed. St. Paul, MN: West Publishing Co., 1992.

Types of Law — Administrative Law

Fox WF, Jr. *Understanding Administrative Law,* 3d ed. New York: Matthew Bender, 1997.

Gellhorn E, Levin RM. *Administrative Law and Process: In a Nutshell,* 3d ed. St. Paul, MN: West Publishing Co., 1990; Introduction, Chapter 1.

Schwartz B et al. *Administrative Law,* 4th ed. Boston: Little Brown and Co., 1994.

Types of Law — Civil Law

Glannon JW. *Civil Procedure: Examples and Explanations,* 3d ed. New York: Aspen, 1997.
Kane MK. *Civil Procedure: In a Nutshell,* 4th ed. St. Paul, MN: West Publishing Co., 1996.
Perovich JD. Adoption, Modification, and Abrogation. In: *American Jurisprudence,* 2d ed. New York: Lawyers Cooperative Publishing Co., 1976;§13.

Types of Law — Contract Law

Blum BA. *Contracts: Examples and Explanations.* New York: Aspen, 1998.
Calamari JD, Perillo JM. *Contracts,* 3d ed. St. Paul, MN: West Publishing Co., 1987;§§1.1, 2.1, 2.5, 2.11, 3.10, 4.1, 4.2, 4.4, 6.1, 6.2, 8.2, 8.3, 8.10, 19.1.
Chirelstein MA. *Concepts and Case Analysis in the Law of Contracts,* 3d ed. New York: Foundation Press, 1998.
Schaber GD, Rohwer CD. *Contracts: In a Nutshell,* 3d ed. St. Paul, MN: West Publishing Co., 1990;§§1, 3, 4, 5, 7, 46, 47, 55, 59, 69, 72, 73, 95, 100, 101.

Types of Law — Criminal Law

Israel JH, LaFave WR. *Criminal Procedure: Constitutional Limitation in a Nutshell,* 5th ed. St. Paul, MN: West Publishing Co., 1993.
LaFave WR, Scott AW. *Criminal Law,* 2d ed. St. Paul, MN: West Publishing Co., 1986;§§1.1, 1.2, 1.3, 1.8, 3.1, 7.1, 7.14, 7.15, 7.16, 8.1.
Loewy AH. *Criminal Law: In a Nutshell,* 2d ed. St. Paul, MN: West Publishing Co., 1987;§§1.01, 2.01, 4.01, 4.02, 6.03, 11.02.

Types of Law — Tort Law

Glannon JW. *The Law of Torts: Examples and Explanations.* Boston: Little, Brown and Company, 1995.
Keeton WP et al. *Prosser and Keeton on Torts,* 5th ed. St. Paul, MN: West Publishing Co., 1984;§§1, 8, 9, 10, 28, 30, 37, 38, 75, 78, 79.
Kionka EJ. *Torts: In a Nutshell,* 2d ed. St. Paul, MN: West Publishing Co., 1992;§§3-1, 3-3, 3-4, 4-1, 4-3, 4-4, 4-5, 4-6, 4-7, 6-1, 6-2.

Structure of a Lawsuit — Appeals

Friedenthal JH et al. *Civil Procedure,* 2d ed. St. Paul, MN: West Publishing Co., 1993;§§13.1, 13.2.

Kane MK. *Civil Procedure: In a Nutshell,* 4th ed. St. Paul, MN: West Publishing Co., 1996;§§7-1, 7-6, 7-7.

Structure of a Civil Lawsuit — Discovery

Friedenthal JH et al. *Civil Procedure,* 2d ed. St. Paul, MN: West Publishing Co., 1993;§§7.2, 7.7, 7.8, 7.9, 7.10, 7.12.
Glannon JW. *Civil Procedure: Examples and Explanations,* 3d ed. New York: Aspen, 1997.
Kane MK. *Civil Procedure in a Nutshell.* St. Paul, MN: West Publishing Co., 1996.
Kane MK. *Civil Procedure: In a Nutshell,* 4th ed. St. Paul, MN: West Publishing Co., 1996;§§3-21, 3-23, 3-25, 3-27, 3-28.

Structure of a Civil Lawsuit — Initiation of the Suit

Friedenthal JH et al. *Civil Procedure,* 2d ed. St. Paul, MN: West Publishing Co., 1993;§5.14.
Glannon JW. *Civil Procedure: Examples and Explanations,* 3d ed. New York: Aspen, 1997.
Kane MK. *Civil Procedure: In a Nutshell,* 4th ed. St. Paul, MN: West Publishing Co., 1996;§§3-1, 3-2, 3-3, 3-4, 3-5.

Structure of a Civil Lawsuit — Judgment on the Pleadings

Glannon JW. *Civil Procedure: Examples and Explanations,* 3d ed. New York: Aspen, 1997.
Kane MK. *Civil Procedure: In a Nutshell,* 4th ed. St. Paul, MN: West Publishing Co., 1996;§3-8.

Structure of a Civil Lawsuit — Meeting with Attorneys

Friedenthal JH et al. *Civil Procedure,* 2d ed. St. Paul, MN: West Publishing Co., 1993;§5.17.
Glannon JW. *Civil Procedure: Examples and Explanations,* 3d ed. New York: Aspen, 1997.
Kane MK. *Civil Procedure: In a Nutshell,* 4th ed. St. Paul, MN: West Publishing Co., 1996;§3-6.

Structure of a Civil Lawsuit — Pleadings

Friedenthal JH et al. *Civil Procedure,* 2d ed. St. Paul, MN: West Publishing Co., 1993;§§5.1, 5.2, 5.3, 5.7.
Glannon JW. *Civil Procedure: Examples and Explanations,* 3d ed. New York: Aspen, 1997.
Kane MK. *Civil Procedure: In a Nutshell,* 4th ed. St. Paul, MN: West Publishing Co., 1996;§§3-1–8.

Structure of a Lawsuit — Pretrial Conferences

Friedenthal JH et al. *Civil Procedure,* 2d ed. St. Paul, MN: West Publishing Co., 1993;§§8.1, 8.2.
Kane MK. *Civil Procedure: In a Nutshell,* 4th ed. St. Paul, MN: West Publishing Co., 1996;§§3-35, 3-36, 3-37.

Structure of a Lawsuit — Trial

Friedenthal JH et al. *Civil Procedure,* 2d ed. St. Paul, MN: West Publishing Co., 1993;§§10.1, 10.2.
Kane MK. *Civil Procedure: In a Nutshell,* 4th ed. St. Paul, MN: West Publishing Co., 1996;§§5-1, 5-2, 5-3, 5-12.

Other Reading

Alfange D. The Supreme Court and the Separation of Powers: A Welcome Return to Normalcy? *Geo Wash L Rev* 1990;58:668–761.
Calamari JD, Perillo JM. *Contracts,* 3d ed. St. Paul, MN: West Publishing Co., 1987.
Currie DP. *Federal Jurisdiction,* 3d ed. St.. Paul, MN: West Publishing Co., 1990.
Fox WF. *Understanding Administrative Law,* 3d ed. New York: Matthew Bender, 1997.
Friedenthal JH et al. *Civil Procedure,* 2d ed. St. Paul, MN: West Publishing Co., 1993.
Gellhorn E, Levin RM. *Administrative Law and Process: In a Nutshell,* 3d ed. St. Paul, MN: West Publishing Co., 1990.
Kane MK. *Civil Procedure: In a Nutshell,* 4th ed. St. Paul, MN: West Publishing Co., 1996.
Keeton WP et al. *Prosser and Keeton on Torts,* 5th ed. St. Paul, MN: West Publishing Co., 1984.
Kionka EJ. *Torts: In a Nutshell,* 2d ed. St. Paul, MN: West Publishing Co., 1992.

LaFave WR, Scott AW. *Criminal Law,* 2d ed. St. Paul, MN: West Publishing Co., 1986.
Loewy AH. *Criminal Law: In a Nutshell,* 2d ed. St. Paul, MN: West Publishing Co., 1987.
Saint-Paul N, Wierzbicki JR. Judicial Precedents as Binding or Persuasive. In: *American Jurisprudence,* 2d ed. New York: Lawyers Cooperative Publishing Co., 1995;§147–65.
Schaber GD, Rohwer CD. *Contracts: In a Nutshell,* 3d ed. St. Paul, MN: West Publishing Co., 1990.

Web Sites

Attorney's Toolbox: *http://www.mother.com/~randy/tools.html*
Civil Procedure home page: *http://www.law.indiana.edu/cphomepg/*
Code of Federal Regulations: *http://www.access.gpo.gov/nara/cfr/index.html*
The Federal Judicial Center: *http://www.fjc.gov/*
Federal Register: *http://www.access.gpo.gov/su_docs/aces/aces140.html*
Federal Rules of Civil Procedure: *http://www.law.cornell.edu/rules/frcp/overview.htm*
Federal Rules of Evidence: *http://www.law.cornell.edu/rules/fre/overview.htm*
Findlaw: *http://www.findlaw.com*
Law Library Resource Exchange: *http://www.llrx.com*
LawGuru: *http://www.lawguru.com*
Law.Net: *http://www.law.net/*
Legal Information Institute: *http://www.law.cornell.edu/*
U.S. bills in Congress: *http://thomas.loc.gov*
The White House: *http://www.whitehouse.gov*
World Wide Web Virtual Library: Law: Criminal Law and Evidence: *http://www.law.indiana.edu/law/v-lib/criminal.html#m*

2

Medical Malpractice

Medical providers are expected to render that level of care and skill that a member of the profession in good standing and relevant specialty would provide under similar circumstances.[1] Therefore, the focus in a malpractice case theoretically is on the care rendered, not merely untoward results that may have occurred through no fault of the provider. Bad results do not de facto constitute medical malpractice.

General Considerations

Medical malpractice is adjudicated on the basis of the negligence rule in tort law. The patient-plaintiff, in order to prevail, must show by a preponderance of the evidence (i.e., it is more likely than not[2]) that the physician or other medical provider had a *duty* to the patient to render nonnegligent care (i.e., that care a practitioner in good standing would have provided), *breached* that duty by not providing such care, and this breach *caused* the patient *injury or damages*. As in all negligence claims, the plain-

tiff must show all these factors to obtain a judgment in his or her favor and monetary damages to compensate for the injury. Otherwise, the provider is entitled to judgment. Note that because the standard by which the provider will be judged is a professional one, expert witness testimony generally will be required to show what care and actions a reasonable provider would have provided and performed in the circumstances.

Concept.
To demonstrate medical malpractice, a plaintiff-patient must show that the provider had a duty to provide nonnegligent care to the patient, that the provider breached that duty by providing negligent care, and that this breach caused the patient injury or damage.

Case. Ms. H, an unmarried woman with a history of smoking, was pregnant but did not have access to prenatal care due to her socioeconomic circumstances. However, after being assisted by a church-based community service organization, in July 1985, during her 26th week of pregnancy, she became a patient of Dr. D, an obstetrician-gynecologist. In September 1985, she began to have contractions; on September 28, 29, and 30 she was admitted to a hospital but then released with a diagnosis of false labor/abdominal pain. On October 1, during her 36th week of pregnancy, Dr. D saw Ms. H as an outpatient. A physical exam showed a thinning and dilation of Ms. H's uterus. Dr. D referred her to the hospital where she was placed on Pitocin, a drug that induces uterine contractions. On October 2, Ms. H gave birth to a son, DH. After birth, DH's APGAR scores were high, indicating a healthy infant. However, after a brief stay in the nursery, DH developed respiratory distress syndrome (RDS) and was transferred to the neonatal intensive care unit (NICU). In the NICU, DH's condition worsened to the point where, on October 3, he was placed on a

---

[1]See, e.g., Nowatske v. Osterloh, 543 N.W.2d 265 (Wis. 1996); Kalsbeck v. Westview Clinic 375 N.W.2d 861 (Minn. Ct. App. 1985); Blair v. Eblen, 461 S.W.2d 370 (Ky. Ct. App. 1970); Watson v. Medical Emergency Servs., 532 N.E.2d 1191 (Ind. Ct. App. 1989); Swan v. Lamb, 584 P.2d 814 (Utah 1978); see also Morlino v. Medical Ctr. of Ocean County, 706 A.2d 721 (N.J. 1998); Centman v. Cobb, 581 N.E.2d 1286 (Ind. Ct. App. 1991); but see Helling v. Carey, 519 P.2d 981 (Wash. 1974) (rejecting provider-based standard); and Gates v. Jensen, 595 P.2d 919 (Wash. 1979).

[2]See, e.g., Bromme v. Pavitt, 7 Cal.Rptr.2d 608 (Cal. Ct. App. 1992), *rev. denied*, 1992 Cal. LEXIS 3777 (Cal. July 23, 1992); Shively v. Klein, 551 A.2d 41 (Del. 1988); Borkowski v. Sacheti, 682 A.2d 1095 (Conn. App. Ct. 1996); Volz v. Ledes, 895 S.W.2d 677 (Tenn. 1995); Fabio v. Bellomo, 489 N.W.2d 241 (Minn. Ct. App. 1992); Kilpatrick v. Bryant, 868 S.W.2d 594 (Tenn. 1993).

mechanical ventilator. Although the NICU physicians managed the RDS appropriately, DH experienced complications including sepsis (generalized infection in the blood), thrombocytopenia (a reduction in platelets), and a cerebral hemorrhage. These resulted in multiple disabilities, including blindness, cerebral palsy, diabetes insipidus, and severe retardation. DH continued to be hospitalized until January 9, when he was discharged. After his second birthday, DH died. Ms. H filed a medical malpractice suit against Dr. D, alleging that he fell below the standard of care in his management of her pregnancy that resulted in the death of DH. Dr. D countered that he provided medically appropriate care and that Ms. H's smoking contributed to the risks and subsequent complications of DH.

Legal Discussion.   The court that decided the case on which this illustration was based indicated that Ms. H could not recover on her medical malpractice claim against Dr. D.[3] Dr. D had an affirmative duty to provide Ms. H with medically appropriate care since he was her attending obstetrician-gynecologist managing her pregnancy. According to the court, he may or may not have breached his duty with regard to the type of treatment he rendered to Ms. H. However, this issue did not have to be reached because there was no causation; that is, Dr. D's activities did not cause the damages or injury that Ms. H experienced, namely, DH's death. Obstetrical expert testimony for Dr. D indicated that babies born at gestational ages of 20–37 weeks are premature and likely to develop RDS due to the immaturity of their lung surfactant, that approximately 20% of premature babies experience RDS, and that premature babies are more susceptible to infection than full-term babies. This expert indicated that, in his judgment, DH's prematurity caused the difficulties experienced; however, he would defer to the judgment of a neonatologist on the issue of RDS and its potential effects on babies. Neonatal expert testimony indicated that, although DH's prognosis was favorable on the basis of the APGAR scores, DH was premature and this may have caused his RDS difficulties. However, DH's condition was extremely uncommon, and even if DH had been born at full term (i.e., one additional week of gestation), he still could have experienced RDS and its accompanying sequelae. Indeed, this expert indicated that, other than prematurity, she could find nothing at birth to which she could attribute DH's difficulties, that the severity of DH's illness made questionable the contention that at full term DH would not have experienced complications, and that the mother's smoking, low socioeconomic status, and the unmarried state all contribute to a baby's risk of premature delivery. Thus, even if Dr. D breached the standard of care by inducing delivery prematurely, because

DH's condition most likely would have been similar a week later, Dr. D's action did not cause DH's significant disease and subsequent death. Hence, Dr. D was entitled to judgment.

Case.   Ms. W was a 21-year-old African-American woman of generally good health. However, on August 18, she experienced severe pelvic and abdominal pain. She was taken to the emergency room where she was treated and released. However, five weeks later, on September 24, she returned to the emergency room with abdominal pain, vomiting, neck pain, lethargy, and a red, pruritic (itchy) rash on her arms and thighs. The emergency room physician diagnosed a "viral illness" and prescribed aspirin, pain, and nausea medication and then discharged Ms. W. Four days later, on September 28, Ms. W experienced two grand mal seizures and again was brought to the emergency room with fever, lethargy, and headache; she also was "hot to the touch." After an initial diagnosis of encephalitis and stabilization by medical staff, Ms. W was referred to Dr. A, an internal medicine physician. He admitted her to the hospital; however, he did not take her medical, social, or family history during her five-day stay nor did he review her medical records from her August 18 and September 24 emergency room visits. On admission, Ms. W was tachycardic (elevated heart rate), and blood tests showed elevated levels of liver and heart enzymes as well as other abnormalities. Based on Ms. W's symptoms and lab tests, Dr. A diagnosed either viral encephalitis or viral meningitis. Dr. A treated Ms. W with Vibramycin, an antibiotic. However, he did not repeat any laboratory studies nor did he ask for a neurological consult to investigate her grand mal seizures. Further, on this hospitalization, Ms. W again broke out in a generalized rash, which Dr. A believed was an adverse reaction to the Vibramycin. In response, he substituted the antibiotic with erythromycin and gave Ms. W calamine lotion and Benadryl for the rash. Ms. W was discharged on October 2. However, Ms. W went to Dr. A's office the next day because the rash had gotten worse. Dr. A then treated her with an injection of Benadryl and increased her oral dosage of Benadryl. At this time, Dr. A noted that Ms. W had a swollen face and swollen lymph nodes behind the ear. Dr. A did nothing for these signs.

On October 5, Ms. A returned to the emergency room again due to the generalized rash, which was not responding to Benadryl. The emergency room physician started Ms. W on high-dose prednisone (a steroid). The next day she went to Dr. A's office; because she was feeling some relief from her symptoms, Dr. A continued her on this regimen of prednisone and Benadryl. She continued on this treatment until November 7, when Dr. A discontinued her steroids. On November 10, Ms. W went back to Dr. A's office with complaints of chest pain; however, Dr. A did not order an EKG and simply continued her on Benadryl. On November 12, Ms. W returned to Dr. A's

---

[3]Hoot v. Woman's Hosp. Foundation, 691 So.2d 786 (La. Ct. App. 1997).

office but saw Dr. A's colleague, who believed that Ms. W was suffering from "collagen vascular disease Lupus E." Although Dr. A's colleague spoke to Dr. A regarding this diagnosis, Dr. A performed no additional studies or an EKG. Ms. W returned to see Dr. A the next day with complaints of labored breathing, lethargy, and chest pains. Dr. A decided that she still had a viral infection and again treated her with Vibramycin. Dr. A did not run any tests at that time. However, later that afternoon, Ms. W experienced fever, severe chest pain, tender abdomen, an enlarged liver, and an enlarged heart surrounded by fluid. Dr. A admitted Ms. W to the hospital, and lab tests ordered on admission showed significant organ failure and tissue death. Dr. A in response treated Ms. W with Vibramycin. However, her condition deteriorated to such an extent that Dr. A called for a cardiology consult. The cardiologist ordered tests for lupus and strongly recommended steroid treatment due to the likelihood of collagen vascular disease. Dr. A did not initiate steroid therapy until ten hours later; nine hours after that, Ms. W died due to cardiac arrest. Ms. W's family sued Dr. A for medical malpractice, claiming that Dr. A's management of Ms. W's treatment was below the standard of care. Dr. A claimed that there was no malpractice because the standard of care was met and that the cause of Ms. W's death was not determined.

Legal Discussion. Dr. A was found liable for medical malpractice in the case on which this illustration is based.[4] Dr. A clearly had a duty to provide nonnegligent care to Ms. W, since he was her attending physician. The court indicated that Dr. A breached that duty by providing substandard care. On the basis of expert testimony given by Dr. M, Dr. A provided substandard care in a broad range of circumstances. Dr. M noted that Dr. A did not obtain a full medical, social, and family history; Dr. A did not properly evaluate or follow up Ms. W's grand mal seizures; Dr. A incorrectly used Vibramycin, an antibiotic, to treat a viral infection; Dr. A did not obtain follow-up liver function tests, heart studies, and other laboratory tests that were and continued to be abnormal during the time she was in Dr. A's care; Dr. A failed to note that termination of her steroid treatment was associated with Ms. W's clinical deterioration; and that Dr. A failed to obtain the appropriate consultations when faced with Ms. W's diagnostic difficulties. Further, Dr. M noted that Ms. W fell well within the standard presentation of an individual afflicted with lupus due to her race, age, gender, symptoms, medical signs, and laboratory values, a suspicion that three other physicians harbored. With regard to causation, although the cause of Ms. W's death was not known to a certainty, lupus was more probable than not to be the cause of her death, and Dr. A's improper treatment

eliminated her chance of surviving this illness. Finally, because she suffered death due to Dr. A's mismanagement of her disease (i.e., her damages and injury), Ms. W fulfilled all the requisite requirements for malpractice. Therefore, the court held that Dr. A was liable for damages in tort for medical malpractice.

Notes on Medical Malpractice

Cause of Harm

In a medical malpractice case, plaintiffs, in order to prevail, need not show that the medical provider's action was the *sole* cause of harm; further, the plaintiffs need not show that all other possibilities of harm are negated. All a plaintiff need show by the preponderance of the evidence is that he or she suffered some injury because of the provider's conduct; this claim must be supported by expert medical testimony indicating the provider's substandard care proximately caused the harm.[5] Proximate cause requires two components to be shown: first, that the harm would not have occurred but for the actions of the provider;[6] and second, that harm was reasonably foreseeable by the provider as a natural and probable result of the provider's actions.[7] A consequence of the latter is that providers will not be liable for remote and unforeseeable results.[8]

Additional Reading. C. T. Drechsler, "Malpractice Actions and Procedure," in *American Jurisprudence,* 2d ed. (New York: Lawyers Cooperative Publishing Co., 1981), section 359; D. L. Keith, "The Court's Charge in Texas Medical Malpractice Cases," *Baylor Law Review*

[4]Martin v. East Jefferson Hosp., 582 So.2d 1272 (La. 1991).

[5]Clark v. Baton Rouge Gen. Med. Ctr., 657 So.2d 741, *writs denied*, 95-1911, 95-1794 (La. Oct. 27, 1995).

[6]See, e.g., Fitzgerald v. Manning, 679 F.2d 341 (4th Cir. 1982); Delisi v. St. Luke's Episcopal-Presbyterian Hosp., Inc., 701 S.W.2d 170 (Mo. Ct. App. 1984); Zalesak v. Taylor, 888 S.W.2d 143 (Tex. App. 1994); Bramlette v. Charter-Medical-Columbia, 393 S.E.2d 914 (S.C. 1990); Volz v. Ledes, 895 S.W.2d 677 (Tenn. 1995); see also Gardner v. Pawliw, 696 A.2d 599 (N.J. 1997); Falcon v. Memorial Hosp., 443 N.W.2d 431 (Mich. Ct. App. 1989) (*reversed in part for different reasons*).

[7]See, e.g., Campos v. Ysleta Gen. Hosp. Inc., 836 S.W.2d 791 (Tex. App. 1992); Bradley v. Rogers, 879 S.W.2d 947 (Tex. App. 1994), *reh'g denied* (Tex. July 28, 1994); Wadley Research Inst. v. Beeson, 835 S.W.2d 689 (Tex. App. 1992); LaPoint v. Shirley, 409 F.Supp. 118 (W.D. Tex. 1976); see also Stevens v. Jefferson, 436 So.2d 33 (Fla. 1983); Kolosky v. Winn Dixie Stores, 472 So.2d 891 (Fla. Dist. Ct. App. 1985); Sizemore v. Montana Power Co., 803 P.2d 629 (Mont. 1990); Hart v. Van Zandt, 399 S.W.2d 791 (Tex. 1965).

[8]See, e.g., Levitt v. Lenox Hill Hosp., 585 N.Y.S.2d 401 (N.Y. App. Div. 1992).

48 (1996), pp. 675–814; R. W. Scott, *Health Care Malpractice: A Primer on Legal Issues for Professionals,* 2d ed. (New York: McGraw-Hill, 1998); F. A. Sloan, *Suing for Medical Malpractice* (Chicago: University of Chicago Press, 1993). See also J. Makdisi, "Proportional Liability: A Comprehensive Rule to Apportion Tort Damages on Probability," *North Carolina Law Review* 67 (1989), pp. 1063–1101.

Contracts to Limit Liability and Specify Forum for Adjudication

Efforts to use contracts to limit liability in tort by medical providers generally are looked on with disfavor. Courts are not receptive to providers that attempt to avoid malpractice damages by requiring patients to sign documents that purportedly waive their right to sue.[9] However, providers have been relatively successful in broadly mandating other forums, such as arbitration rather than the courts for adjudicating disputes for patient injury.[10] But some courts have limited the applicability of these clauses[11] and invalidated the application of these clauses if there is some fraud against the patient in inducing him or her to agree to the clause.[12]

Additional Reading. N. S. Blackman et al., *Liability in Medical Practice* (London: Harwood Academic Publishers, 1990); J. Gillespe, "Physician-Patient Arbitration Agreements: Procedural Safeguards May Not Be Enough," *Journal of Dispute Resolution* 1997 (1997), pp. 119–32; M. J. Mehlman, "Fiduciary Contracting Limitations on Bargaining Between Patients and the Health Care Providers," *University of Pittsburgh Law Review* 51 (1990), pp. 365–417; E. H. Morreim, "Cost Containment and the Standard of Medical Care," *California Law Review* 75 (1987), pp. 1719–63.

Criminal Prosecution for Malpractice

Generally, ordinary malpractice is not subject to criminal proceedings. However, if the negligence rises to gross lack of competency, inattention, or wanton indifference to the patient's safety, providers may face not only civil penalties but also criminal prosecution.[13] As usual in criminal law, the state's criminal statutes will define the requisite standards under which a physician's actions will be judged.

Additional Reading. C. T. Drechsler, "Criminal Responsibility," in *American Jurisprudence,* 2d ed. (New York: Lawyers Cooperative Publishing Co., 1981), section 395; C. T. Drechsler, "Nature of Act or Omission Causing Death," in *American Jurisprudence,* 2d ed. (New York: Lawyers Cooperative Publishing Co., 1968), section 99; R. W. Scott, *Health Care Malpractice: A Primer on Legal Issues for Professionals,* 2d ed. (New York: McGraw-Hill, 1998).

Experts

The concept of being an expert for legal purposes differs from that within the medical profession. Experts for legal purposes may testify on the standard of care even though that person has never treated a disease such as the one afflicting the plaintiff so long as the expert has some general experience with the clinical issue and causation.[14] Experts in malpractice cases also do not necessarily need to be in the same specialty as the defendant provider[15] nor be physicians, even when a physician is the defen-

---

[9]See, e.g., Tunkl v. Regents of the Univ. of Cal., 383 P.2d 441 (Cal. 1963); Emory Univ. v. Porubiansky, 282 S.E.2d 903 (Ga. 1981); Kozan v. Comstock, 270 F.2d 839 (5th Cir. 1959); Meiman v. Rehabilitation Ctr., 444 S.W.2d 78 (Ky. 1969); Olson v. Molzen, 558 S.W.2d 429 (Tenn. 1977); Ash v. New York Univ. Dental Ctr., 564 N.Y.S.2d 308 (N.Y. App. Div. 1990); Cudnik v. William Beaumont Hosps., 525 N.W.2d 891 (Mich. Ct. App. 1994).

[10]See, e.g., Buracczynski v. Eyring, 919 S.W.2d 314 (Tenn. 1996); Coon v. Nicola, 21 Cal.Rptr.2d 846 (Cal. Ct. App. 1993); Michaelis v. Schori, 24 Cal.Rptr.2d 380 (Cal. Ct. App. 1993); Broemmer v. Otto, 821 P.2d 204 (Ariz. 1991); Morris v. Metriyakool, 344 N.W.2d 736 (Mich. 1984); Wilson v. Kaiser Found. Hosps., 190 Cal.Rptr. 649 (Cal. Ct. App. 1983); Hawkins v. Superior Ct., 152 Cal.Rptr. 491 (Cal. Ct. App. 1979); Madden v. Kaiser Found. Hosps., 552 P.2d 1178 (Cal. 1976).

[11]See, e.g., Colorado Permanente Med. Group v. Evans, 926 P.2d 1218 (Colo. 1996); Neaman v. Kaiser Found. Hosps., 11 Cal.Rptr.2d 879 (Cal. Ct. App. 1992); Obstetrics and Gynecologists v. Pepper, 693 P.2d 1259 (Nev. 1985); Kaiser Found. Hosps. v. Superior Ct., 23 Cal.Rptr.2d 431 (Cal.), *rev. denied* (Cal. Jan. 13, 1994); Morrison v. Colorado Permanente Med. Group, 983 F.Supp. 937 (D. Colo. 1997).

[12]See, e.g., Engalla v. Permanente Med. Group, 938 P.2d 903 (Cal. 1997).

[13]See, e.g., State v. Lester, 149 N.W. 297 (Minn. 1914); State v. McFadden, 93 P. 414 (Wash. 1908); Estate of Muldoon, 275 P.2d 597 (Cal. Ct. App. 1954); Einaugler v. Supreme Court, 918 F.Supp. 619 (E.D. N.Y. 1996).

[14]Harmon v. Patel, 617 N.E.2d 183 (Ill. App. Ct. 1993).

[15]See, e.g., Weinberg v. Geary, 686 N.E.2d 1298 (Ind. Ct. App. 1997); James v. City of East Orange, 588 A.2d 412 (N.J. Super. Ct. App. Div. 1991); Guerrero v. Smith, 864 S.W.2d 797 (Tex. App. 1993); Hauser v. Bhatnager, 537 A.2d 599 (Me. 1988); Lewis v. Read, 193 A.2d 255 (N.J. Super. Ct. App. Div. 1963); Barrett v. Samaritan Health Servs., 735 P.2d 460 (Ariz. Ct. App. 1987); see also Gaston v. Hunter, 588 P.2d 236 (Ariz. Ct. App. 1978).

dant.[16] Note, however, that the standard of care indicated by experts must be appropriate for the circumstances existing at the time of the event;[17] there must be some basis other than personal anecdote supporting the standard;[18] and in any event, experts cannot claim a standard of perfection for any provider.[19]

Additional Reading. R. N. Arntz, "Competency of Medical Expert Witnesses: Standards and Qualifications," *Creighton Law Review* 24 (1991), pp. 1359–96; A. S. Klein, "Competency of General Practitioners to Testify as Expert Witness in Action Against Specialist for Medical Malpractice," in *American Law Reports,* 3d ed. (New York: Lawyers Cooperative Publishing Co., 1971), vol. 31, pp. 1163–81; H. B. Zobel et al., *Doctors and the Law: Defendants and Expert Witnesses* (New York: W.W. Norton & Co., 1993); R. W. Scott, *Health Care Malpractice: A Primer on Legal Issues for Professionals,* 2d ed. (New York: McGraw-Hill, 1998).

Failure to Refer

Failing to refer a patient when a provider lacks the expertise to appropriately treat him or her also may create malpractice liability.[20] Further, a provider that does not give the patient information about the potential results associated with not seeing a specialist may be held liable in tort.[21]

Additional Reading. J. J. Director, "Malpractice: Physician's Failure to Advise Patient to Consult Specialist or One Qualified in a Method of Treatment Which Physician Is Not Qualified to Give," in *American Law Reports,* 3d ed. (New York: Lawyers Cooperative Publishing Co., 1971), vol. 35, pp. 349–76; J. M. Zboyan and E. C. Moran, "The Physician's Duty to Refer to a Specialist," *Colorado Law* 23 (1994), pp. 79–82; R. W. Scott, *Health Care Malpractice: A Primer on Legal Issues for Professionals,* 2d ed. (New York: McGraw-Hill, 1998).

Good Samaritan Acts

Good Samaritan statutes have been enacted in virtually all states. These statutes generally immunize health care providers from tort liability if they negligently injure an individual while voluntarily rendering emergency aid. Generally, for the Good Samaritan laws to apply, the provider must not have a preexisting duty to the patient,[22] such as an existing physician–patient relationship with the party or have been called to the accident officially to treat the patient. The definition of an emergency is within the province of the court; however, in practice, this definition is broad and can encompass situations where the patient is stable.[23]

Additional Reading. C. T. Drechsler, "Special Defenses," in *American Jurisprudence,* 2d ed. (New York: Lawyers Cooperative Publishing Co., 1981), section 306; D. R. Veilleux, "Construction and Application of 'Good Samaritan' Statutes," in *American Law Reports,* 4th ed. (New York: Lawyers Cooperative Publishing Co., 1989), vol. 68, pp. 294–333.

HIV Status

Providers may be sued for exposing patients to HIV without disclosure; but it should be noted that the status of these suits remains in tremendous flux. First, patients who have been exposed to HIV through an employee of a hospital or medical organization may be able to sue that organization for negligence on the theory that the hospital or organization did not establish or enforce appropriate infection control procedures, as is possible in non-HIV cases.[24] However, with regard to HIV specifically, some courts have ruled that an HIV-negative patient cannot sue a provider or hospital simply because the patient feared

---

[16]See, e.g., Tomkins v. Bise, 910 P.2d 185 (Kan. 1996); Gooding v. St. Francis Xavier Hosp., 487 S.E.2d 596 (S.C. 1997).

[17]See, e.g., Jackson v. Huang, 514 So.2d 727 (La. Ct. App. 1987), *cert. denied,* 518 So.2d 1050 (La. 1988); Etienne v. Caputi, 679 N.E.2d 922 (Ind. Ct. App. 1997); Nicoll v. LoCoco, 701 So.2d 1062 (La. 1997); East v. United States, 745 F.Supp. 1142 (D. Md. 1990); Mackey v. Greenview Hosp., 587 S.W.2d 249 (Ky. Ct. App. 1979), *reh'g denied* (Ky. May 11, 1979); Cleary v. Group Health Ass'n, 691 A.2d 148 (D.C. 1997).

[18]See, e.g., Travers v. District of Columbia, 672 A.2d 566 (D.C. 1996); see also Bloome v. Wiseman, 664 N.E.2d 1125 (Ill. App. Ct. 1996), *reh'g denied* (Ill. May 29, 1996); Sheffler v. Arana, 950 S.W.2d 259 (Mo. Ct. App. 1997); Messina v. District of Columbia, 663 A.2d 535 (D.C. 1995).

[19]See, e.g., Shevak v. United States, 528 F.Supp. 295 (W.D. Pa. 1983); Mayhorn v. Pavey, 456 N.E.2d 1222 (Ill. App. Ct. 1985); Harwell v. Pittman, 428 So.2d 1049 (La. Ct. App. 1983), *writ denied,* 434 So.2d 1092 (La. 1983); Matthews v. Louisiana State Univ. Med. Ctr., 467 So.2d 1238 (La. Ct. App. 1985); Gage v. St. Paul Fire & Marine Ins. Co., 282 So.2d 147 (La. Ct. App. 1973); James v. Gordon, 690 So.2d 787 (La. Ct. App. 1996), *writ denied,* 693 So.2d 738 (La. 1997).

[20]Phillips v. United States, 566 F.Supp. 1 (D.S.C. 1981); Sewell v. United States, 629 F.Supp. 448 (W.D. La. 1986); Weinstock v. Ott, 444 N.E.2d 1227 (Ind. Ct. App. 1983).

[21]Morre v. Preventive Medicine Med. Group, Inc., 223 Cal.Rptr. 859 (Cal. Ct. App. 1986).

[22]Perkins v. Howard, 283 Cal.Rptr. 764 (Cal. Ct. App. 1991).

[23]Breazeal v. Henry Mayo Newhall Mem. Hosp., 286 Cal.Rptr. 207 (Cal. Ct. App. 1991).

[24]Thompson v. Methodist Hosp., 367 S.W.2d 134 (Tenn. 1962); Howard v. Alexandria Hosp., 429 S.E.2d 22 (Va. 1993).

contracting AIDS from a surgeon who died of the disease when that patient was not directly exposed to the provider.[25] Generally, claims in these suits must be supported by actual exposure, not merely fear of being exposed.[26] On the other hand, courts have ruled that an HIV-negative patient who reasonably fears possible contraction of HIV and AIDS can recover for tort injury after learning a surgical procedure was done by a surgeon who died of AIDS.[27]

Additional Reading. J. R. Adams, "Patient of HIV Positive Physician May Have Action for Fear of AIDS," *Defense Counsels' Journal* 60 (1993), pp. 603–04; C. H. Bird, *The Persecution and Trial of Gaston Naessens: The True Story of the Efforts to Suppress an Alternative Treatment for Cancer, AIDS, and Other Immunological Diseases* (Tiburon, CA: H.J. Kramer & Co., 1991); V. A. Fink, "Emotional Distress Damages for Fear of Contracting AIDS: Should Plaintiffs Have to Show Exposure to HIV?" *Dickinson Law Review* 99 (1995), pp. 779–805; I. Yip, "AIDSphobia and the 'Window of Anxiety': Enlightened Reasoning or Concession to Irrational Fear?" *Brooklyn Law Review* 60 (1994), pp. 461–90. See also K. C. Robling, "Negligent HIV Testing and False-Positive Plaintiffs: Pardoning the Traditional Prerequisites for Emotional Distress Recovery," *Cleveland State Law Review* 43 (1995), pp. 655–92.

"Loss of Chance" or "Lost Chance" Doctrine

In addition to standard medical malpractice actions, some states have recognized a "loss of chance" cause of action against a medical provider, usually in circumstances of a provider's failure to diagnose a terminal illness. The loss of chance stems from the failure to diagnose in time for the patient to have a chance at recovery. In the states that do recognize the cause of

action, generally the patient must show that the lost chance is statistically significant[28] or the patient's lost chance was at least a 50% chance[29] or substantial chance[30] of cure or survival.

Additional Reading. S. F. Brennwald, "Proving Causation in 'Loss of Chance' Cases: A Proportional Approach," *Catholic University Law Review* 34 (1985), pp. 747–90; J. D. Hodson, "Medical Malpractice: 'Loss of Chance' Casualty," in *American Law Reports,* 4th ed. (New York: Lawyers Cooperative Publishing Co., 1988), vol. 54, pp. 10–84; R. A. Reisig, "The Loss of Chance Theory in Medical Malpractice Cases: An Overview," *American Journal of Trial Advocacy* 13 (1990), pp. 1163–85.

Malpractice Insurance

Most practice sites (e.g., group practice, managed care organization, hospital) require that physicians carry a specified level of malpractice insurance coverage. Some practice sites will provide this insurance as a benefit; others require that physicians provide their own. Malpractice insurance generally is divided into two forms: occurrence and claims-made. Occurrence insurance provides malpractice coverage for any claims that arise from treatment during the covered period, regardless of when the claim is filed. In contract, claims-made insurance covers claims filed only during the specific term of the insurance. This form is more common in the malpractice insurance industry. Because of the nature of claims-made insurance, a physician who changes practice sites or insurers must purchase "tail" coverage insurance to cover the time period in which potential claims still may be filed but

---

[25]Kerins v. Hartley, 33 Cal.Rptr.2d 172 (Cal. Ct. App. 1994); Doe v. Surgicare of Joliet, 643 N.E.2d 1200 (Ill. App. Ct. 1994), *appeal denied*, 645 N.E.2d 1357 (Ill. 1994); Carroll v. Sisters of St. Francis Health Servs., 868 S.W.2d 585 (Tenn. 1993); see also Pendergist v. Pendergrass, 961 S.W.2d 919 (Mo. Ct. App. 1998); Bain v. Wells, 936 S.W.2d 618 (Tenn. 1997).

[26]See, e.g., Brzoska v. Olson, 668 A.2d 1355 (Del. 1995); Barrett v. Danbury Hosp., 654 A.2d 748 (Conn. 1995); K.A.C. v. Benson, 527 N.W.2d 553 (Minn. 1995).

[27]Faya v. Rossi, 620 A.2d 327 (Md. 1983); see also Doe v. Noe, 690 N.E.2d 1012 (Ill. App. Ct. 1997); Caldor v. Bowden, 625 A.2d 959 (Md. 1993) (*in dissent*); Williamson v. Waldman, 677 A.2d 1179 (N.J. Super. Ct. App. Div. 1996); Doe v. Northwestern Univ., 682 N.E.2d 145 (Ill. App. Ct. 1997), *reh'g denied* (Ill. July 23, 1997).

[28]See, e.g., Anderson v. Brigham Young Univ., 879 F.Supp. 1124 (D. Utah 1995), *aff'd*, 89 F.3d 849 (10th Cir. 1996); Jones v. Owings, 456 S.E.2d 371 (S.C. 1995); Bromme v. Pavitt, 7 Cal.Rptr.2d 608 (Cal. Ct. App. 1992), *rev. denied*, 1992 Cal. LEXIS 3777 (Cal. July 23, 1992); Swain v. Curry, 595 So.2d 168 (Fla. Dist. Ct. App. 1992), *rev. denied*, 601 So.2d 551 (Fla. 1992); Donnini v. Ouano, 810 P.2d 1163 (Kan. Ct. App. 1991); Hampton v. Greenfield, 576 So.2d 630 (La. Ct. App. 1991), *cert. denied*, 581 So.2d 686 (La. 1991); Falcon v. Memorial Hosp., 443 N.W.2d 431 (Mich. Ct. App. 1989), *aff'd*, 462 N.W.2d 44 (Mich. 1990).

[29]Fennell v. Southern Maryland Hosp. Ctr., 580 A.2d 206 (Md. 1990); Hurley v. United States, 923 F.2d 1091 (4th Cir. 1991); Kilpatrick v. Bryant, 868 S.W.2d 594 (Tenn. 1993); Borkowski v. Sacheti, 682 A.2d 1095 (Conn. App. Ct. 1996), *cert. denied*, 686 A.2d 120 (Conn. 1996); Pillsbury-Flood v. Portsmouth Hosp., 512 A.2d 1126 (N.H. 1986); see also Sherer v. James, 351 S.E.2d 148 (S.C. 1986).

[30]See, e.g., Delaney v. Cade, 873 P.2d 175 (Kan. 1994); Seafidi v. Seiler, 574 A.2d 398 (N.J. 1990).

before the physician has obtained new claims-made malpractice coverage. Occurrence insurance is more expensive than claims-made. This differential should be taken into account in managed care contracts if the managed care company provides the insurance coverage. Similarly, provisions for tail coverage also should be clarified between the physician and practice site at the outset of the relationship.

Additional Reading. E. R. Anderson and J. Gold, "Malpractice Insurance: Careful Choice Can Prevent Later Problems," *Medical Malpractice Law and Strategy* 13, no. 7 (1996), pp. 1–4; B. A. Liang, "General Considerations for Managed Care Contracting," *Hospital Physician* 31, no. 5 (1995), pp. 41–51; R. E. Margolis, "Coordination of Medical Malpractice Insurance Benefits: Circuits Ponder Who Pays?" *HealthSpan* 10, no. 1 (1993), pp. 16–17.

Minority Practice Doctrine

Of course, experts sometimes disagree as to the standard of care. When there are alternative schools of thought by which providers could assess the rendered care in a particular circumstance, the defendant provider is entitled to be judged by the tenets of the school he or she follows.[31] This is sometimes known as the *minority practice doctrine*. The school of thought, however, must be accepted and recognized by a respectable minority of the profession.[32] A provider who appropriately follows this minority practice is not negligent.

Additional Reading. D. R. Brown, "Panacea or Pandora's Box: The 'Two Schools of Medical Thought' Doctrine After Jones v. Chidester, 610 A.2d 964 (Pa. 1992)," *Washington University Journal of Urban and Contemporary Law* 44 (1993), pp. 223–34; J. P. Dailey, "The Two Schools of Thought and Informed Consent Doctrines in Pennsylvania: A Model for Integration," *Dickinson Law Review* 98 (1994), pp. 713–37; C. T. Drechsler, "Duty of Care; Liability for Malpractice," in *American Jurisprudence,* 2d ed. (New York: Lawyers Cooperative Publishing Co., 1981), section 213.

National Practitioner Data Bank

The National Practitioner Data Bank (NPDB) is a repository of records that includes virtually all malpractice payments in the United States. It was created in an effort to prevent unethical or incompetent practitioners from moving from state to state to avoid discovery of their low quality of care. If a physician is adjudicated negligent *or* there is a payment made to a plaintiff on behalf of the physician in settlement of a malpractice claim, this event *must* be reported to the National Practitioner Data Bank within 30 days of adjudication or payment by the party who makes the payment (e.g., insurer, hospital).[33] In addition to circumstances of malpractice adjudication or payment, other events also must be reported to the NPDB: state licensing boards must report any actions that result in revocation, suspension, or other restriction of a physician's license as well as any actions that result in censure, reprimand, probation, or surrender of the provider's license. The relevant response of the state medical boards also must be reported. In addition, an adverse action that restricts, reduces, suspends, limits, or denies a physician clinical privileges or membership in a health care entity for greater than 30 days must be reported to the NPDB. These actions are to be reported by the relevant hospital, health care entity, managed care organization, or professional review committee. Generally, for actions relating to clinical privileges, only activities related to patient care are reportable; actions based on other deficiencies such as poor staff meeting attendance or inappropriate advertising are not reportable. In addition, professional societies are obligated to report revocation of a physician's membership in the professional society after appropriate peer review if the revocation is based on clinical care considerations.

Physicians automatically receive a report if they have been reported to the NPDB. They may file factual challenges to the report with the reporting entity. If the dispute cannot be resolved at this point, the physician may appeal to the Department of Health and Human Services, which makes the final decision. Physicians also may submit a rebuttal to the report (limited to 600 words), which does not have to go through the formal review process.

---

[31]See, e.g., Force v. Gregory, 27 A. 1116 (Conn. 1893); Chumbler v. McClure, 505 F.2d 489 (6th Cir. 1974); Becker v. Hidalgo, 556 P.2d 35 (N.M. 1976); Hood v. Phillips, 554 S.W.2d 160 (Tex. 1977); Roberts v. Tardif, 417 A.2d 444 (Me. 1980); Creasey v. Hogan, 637 P.2d 114 (Or. 1981); Hersh v. Hendley, 626 S.W.2d 151 (Tex. App. 1981); Levine v. Rosen, 616 A.2d 623 (Pa. 1992); Jones v. Chidester, 610 A.2d 964 (Pa. 1992); Wemmett v. Mount, 292 P. 93 (Or. 1930); see also Clement v. United States, 772 F.Supp. 20 (D. Me. 1991); Melville v. Southward, 791 P.2d 383 (Colo. 1990); Tesavro v. Perrige, 650 A.2d 1079 (Pa. Super. Ct. 1994).

[32]Joy v. Chau, 377 N.E.2d 670 (Ind. Ct. App. 1978); Henderson v. Heyer-Shulte Corp., 600 S.W.2d 844 (Tex. Civ. App. 1980); Slais v. United States, 522 F.Supp. 989 (M.D. Pa. 1981); Chumbler v. McClure, 505 F.2d 489 (6th Cir. 1974); Clark v. Department of Prof. Reg., 463 So.2d 328 (Fla. Dist. Ct. App. 1985); Downer v. Veilleux, 322 A.2d 82 (Me. 1974).

[33]42 U.S.C.A. §§11101 *et seq.*

Filing a factual challenge does not prohibit submitting a rebuttal, and a physician may do both. Currently, the NPDB *must* be used by hospitals to evaluate applications for privileges and *must* be used every two years to evaluate current staff members. The information in a provider's NPDB file is confidential and public access is not allowed. Other groups that may access the NPDB include group practices, professional societies, state licensing boards, and managed care organizations.

Additional Reading.   B. E. Appel et al., "National Practitioner Data Bank: Fact Sheets," American Law Institute–American Bar Association SC39 (1997), pp. 123–32; M. A. Kadzielski, "The National Practitioner Data Bank: Big Brother or Paper Tiger?" *HealthSpan* 9, no. 7 (1992), pp. 8–11; B. A. Liang, "Beyond the Malpractice Suit: The National Practitioner Data Bank," *Hospital Physician* 31, no. 7 (1995), pp. 11–14; R. E. Margolis, "Dentists and Physicians Wiggling Out of National Practitioner's Data Bank?" *HealthSpan* 10, no. 9 (1993), pp. 25–26; D. J. Meiselman, "National Practitioner Data Bank," *Westchester Bar Journal* 18 (1991), pp. 125–33; J. B. Pape, "Physician Data Banks: The Public's Right to Know versus the Physician's Right to Privacy," *Fordham Law Review* 66 (1997), pp. 975–1028.

National Standard of Care

In the past, the standard of care focused on the practice of providers in the local community. However, this "locality rule" generally is inapplicable to modern malpractice cases for specialists. Because of the national nature of practice and training, with board certification examinations and other national indices of competence, national standards of care are those utilized in malpractice cases.[34] Note that for interns, residents, and some general practitioners, the local standard is more likely to be applicable.[35] Further, the vestiges of the locality rule still may exist since some courts require that the standard of care

be indicated by providers in similar communities.[36] Hospitals are subject to the locality rule only to show adequacy of services or facilities.[37]

Additional Reading.   C. T. Drechsler, "Duty of Care: Liability for Malpractice," in *American Jurisprudence,* 2d ed. (New York: Lawyers Cooperative Publishing Co., 1981), section 219; J. M. Zitter, "Standard of Care Owed to Patient by Medical Specialist as Determined by Local, 'Like Community,' State, National, and Other Standards," in *American Law Reports,* 4th ed. (New York: Lawyers Cooperative Publishing Co., 1981), vol. 18, pp. 603–22.

Practice Guidelines

Clinical practice guidelines, also known as *practice parameters,* are guides to clinical care for particular circumstances. Although useful in the context of determining what kinds of care could be appropriate under given circumstances, practice guidelines have weaknesses both as a legal tool for the standard of care and for substantive clinical care. Practice guidelines are not recognized as the standard of care in malpractice suits against physicians; therefore, adherence to them provides little protection in court. In addition, since practice guidelines conflict on the basis of the source from which they emanate, most are promulgated on the basis of consensus rather than the gold standard of double-blind study, they attempt to use population data to treat individual patients, they often are outdated, and they often are manipulated by local physicians before use; substantively they may have limited usefulness in daily practice.

Additional Reading.   G. F. Anderson, M. A. Hall, and E. P. Steinberg, "Medical Technology Assessment and Practice Guidelines: Their Day in Court," *American Journal of Public Health* 83 (1993), pp. 1635–39; T. A. Brennan, "Practice Guidelines and Malpractice Litigation: Collision or Cohesion?" *Journal of Health Politics Policy & Law* 16 (1991), pp. 67–85; D. W. Hong and B. A.

---

[34]See, e.g., Chapel v. Allison, 785 P.2d 204 (Mont. 1990); O'Neil v. Great Plains Women's Clinic, Inc., 759 F.2d 787 (10th Cir. 1985); May v. Moore, 424 So.2d 596 (Ala. 1982); Logan v. Greenwich Hosp. Ass'n, 465 A.2d 294 (Conn. 1983); Taylor v. Hill, 464 A.2d 938 (Me. 1983); Aasheim v. Humberger, 695 P.2d 824 (Mont. 1985); Bates v. Meyer, 565 So.2d 1 (Ala. 1990); Brune v. Belinkoff, 235 N.E.2d 793 (Mass. 1968).

[35]See, e.g., Cudnik v. William Beaumont Hosp., 525 N.W.2d 891 (Mich. Ct. App. 1994); Chapel v. Allison, 785 P.2d 204 (Mont. 1990); Jalaba v. Borovoy, 520 N.W.2d 349 (Mich. Ct. App. 1994); Leazer v. Kiefer, 821 P.2d 957 (Idaho 1991), *reh'g denied* (Idaho Nov. 18, 1991); see also Ott v. Weinstock, 444 N.E.2d 1227 (Ind. Ct. App. 1983); Slezak v. Girzadas, 522 N.E.2d 132 (Ill. App. Ct. 1988).

[36]See, e.g., Raines v. Lutz, 341 S.E.2d 194 (Va. 1986); DeWitt v. Brown, 669 F.2d 516 (8th Cir. 1982); Lemke v. United States, 557 F.Supp. 1205 (D.N.D. 1983); Gonzales v. United States, 600 F.Supp. 1390 (W.D. Tex. 1985); Purtill v. Hess, 489 N.E.2d 867 (Ill. 1986); Cleveland v. Wong, 701 P.2d 1301 (Kan. 1985); Hanzlik v. Paustian, 344 N.W.2d 649 (Neb. 1984), *cert. denied,* 469 U.S. 854 (1984); McPherson v. Ellis, 287 S.E.2d 892 (N.C. 1982); Plaintiff v. City of Parkersburg, 345 S.E.2d 564 (W. Va. 1986); Vassos v. Roussalis, 658 P.2d 1284 (Wy. 1983).

[37]See, e.g., Gusky v. Candler Gen. Hosp., 385 S.E.2d 698 (Ga. Ct. App. 1989); Dent v. Memorial Hosp. of Adel, 490 S.E.2d 509 (Ga. Ct. App. 1997); see also Wickliffe v. Sunrise Hosp., 706 P.2d 1383 (Nev. 1985).

Liang, "The Scope of Clinical Practice Guidelines," *Hospital Physician* 32, no. 5 (1996), pp. 46–59; B. A. Liang, "Error in Medicine: Legal Impediments to U.S. Reform," *Journal of Health Politics Policy & Law* 24 (1999), pp. 27–58; U.S. General Accounting Office, "Practice Guidelines: The Experience of Medical Specialty Societies," pub. no. GAO/PEMD-91-11 (Washington, DC: U.S. General Accounting Office, 1991).

Promising a Result

If a medical provider promises a particular result, such as guaranteeing a cure or specific result or minimal side effects, and these results do not materialize, physicians may be sued under a breach of contract theory.[38] Breach of contract liability theories generally have the advantage of a longer statute of limitations period for the patient to bring suit; specific periods depend on the state where care was rendered. Note that "therapeutic assurances" to alleviate the patient's concerns are not considered guarantees.[39] However, prudence would suggest not to make any statements that could be deemed any sort of promise or guarantee of a particular result.

Additional Reading. C. T. Drechsler, "Relation of Physician and Patient," in *American Jurisprudence,* 2d ed. (New York: Lawyers Cooperative Publishing Co., 1981), section 161; R. E. Sarnacki, "Contractual Theories of Recovery in the HMO Provider-Subscriber Relationship: Prospective Litigation for Breach of Contract," *Buffalo Law Review* 36 (1987), pp. 119–64; J. W. Shaw, "Recovery Against Physician on Basis of Breach of Contract to Achieve Particular Result of Care," in *American Law Reports,* 3d ed. (New York: Lawyers Cooperative Publishing Co., 1973), vol. 43, pp. 1221–60.

Relevance of Board Certification

Sometimes board certification is thought to be a relevant characteristic with regard to a malpractice suit. However, this belief generally is erroneous. A medical provider's ability to pass license and board certification examinations generally is *not* relevant evidence in a malpractice

case with regard to whether the provider was negligent in performing a procedure or treatment and is not admissible for this purpose.[40]

Additional Reading. J. J. Smith, "The Specialty Boards and Antitrust: A Legal Perspective," *Journal of Contemporary Health Law and Policy* 10 (1993), pp. 195–219.

Third Parties

Generally, providers have been liable for injury on the basis of the duties inherent in the patient–provider relationship. However, liability can extend outside this relationship to injured third parties. For example, providers who prescribe medications to patients that could impair the patients' ability to drive but fail to warn the patients of this fact have been held liable to the third parties if injury occurs to a third party due to this impairment.[41] In addition, providers may have a duty to warn identifiable third parties of foreseeable harm from their patients.[42] Generally, providers risk liability to third parties if (1) the harm was foreseeable to the provider and (2) the provider did not take reasonable steps to protect third parties from the harm.[43]

Additional Reading. F. R. Fahrner, "The Physician's Duty to Warn Non-Patients: AIDS Enters the Equation," *Cooley Law Review* 5 (1988), pp. 353–72; K. L. Kelley, "Negligence–Third Party Liability — Physician Owes Duty of Care to Third Party When His Negligence in Failing to Warn Patient Not to Drive Contributes to Third Party Injury," *St. Mary's Law Journal* 15 (1984), pp. 493–503; J. Taylor, "Sex Lies and Lawsuits: A New Mexico Physician's Duty to Warn Third Parties Who Unknowingly May Be at Risk of Contracting HIV from a Patient,"

[38]See, e.g., Hawkins v. McGee, 146 A. 641 (N.H. 1929); Esposito v. Jenson, 645 N.Y.S.2d 240 (N.Y. App. Div. 1996); Clevenger v. Haling, 394 N.E.2d 1119 (Mass. 1979); Tschirhart v. Pethtel, 233 N.W.2d 93 (Mich. Ct. App. 1975), *reh'g denied* (Mich. Aug. 6, 1975); see also Sullivan v. O'Conner, 296 N.E.2d 183 (Mass. 1973); Haase v. Starnes, 915 S.W.2d 675 (Ark. 1996).

[39]Rogola v. Silva, 305 N.E.2d 571 (Ill. App. Ct. 1973); Ferlito v. Cecola, 419 So.2d 102 (La. Ct. App. 1982); Sullivan v. O'Connor, 296 N.E.2d 183 (Mass. 1973).

[40]Beis v. Dias, 859 S.W.2d 835 (Mo. Ct. App. 1993).

[41]See, e.g., Welke v. Kuzilla, 375 N.W.2d 403 (Mich. Ct. App. 1985); Bader v. State, 716 P.2d 925 (Wash. Ct. App. 1986); Turner v. Jordan, 957 S.W.2d 815 (Tenn. 1997); Cram v. Howell, 680 N.E.2d 1096 (Ind. 1997); see also Harden v. Allstate Ins. Co., 883 F.Supp. 963 (D. Del. 1995); Reisner v. Regents of the Univ. of Cal., 37 Cal.Rptr.2d 518 (Cal. Ct. App. 1995).

[42]See Tarasoff v. University of Cal., 551 P.2d 334 (Cal. 1976); DiMarco v. Lynch Homes-Chester County, Inc., 559 A.2d 530 (Pa. Super. Ct. 1989), *aff'd,* 583 A.2d 422 (Pa. 1990); Wilschinsky v. Medina, 775 P.2d 713 (N.M. 1989); Troxel v. Dupont Inst., 675 A.2d 314 (Pa. Super. Ct. 1995); but see Praesel v. Johnson, 967 S.W.2d 391 (Tex. 1998) (treating physicians do not have a common law duty to third parties to warn epileptic patients not to drive); Van Horn v. Chambers, 970 S.W.2d 542 (Tex. 1998) (treating physician does not have duty to protect hospital workers from dangerous patient after transfer out of hospital critical care unit).

[43]See, e.g., Cram v. Howell, 680 N.E.2d 1096 (Ind. 1997); Freese v. Lemmon, 210 N.W.2d 576 (Iowa 1978).

New Mexico Law Review 26 (1996), pp. 481–511. See also M. R. Geske, "Statutes Limiting Mental Health Professionals' Liability for the Violent Acts of Their Patients," *Indiana Law Journal* 64 (1989), pp. 391–422.

Res Ipsa Loquitur: Changing the Burden of Proof

In a medical malpractice case, generally the plaintiff must prove the factors of duty, breach, causation, and damages. However, there are exceptional circumstances where the plaintiff may use the doctrine of *res ipsa loquitur* (the thing speaks for itself) to shift the burden of proof to the defendant physician regarding breach and causation. This doctrine is based on the superior and sometimes exclusive knowledge of what happened that led to the patient's injury being in the hands of the treating physician(s).[44] Thus, *res ipsa loquitur* is an evidentiary doctrine that establishes an inference of negligence from the surrounding circumstances of the treatment involved. Three factors must classically be shown by plaintiff to avail him- or herself to the doctrine:

1. The injury sustained was a kind that does not ordinarily occur in the absence of negligence.
2. The injury was caused by an agency or instrumentality in the exclusive control of the defendant.
3. The injury was not due to any voluntary action or contribution on the part of the plaintiff.[45]

Note that under factor 1, expert testimony is not needed to sustain this condition and it can be supported on the basis of "common knowledge," although expert testimony also can be the source of this information.[46] Thus, the doctrine acts to create a presumption of negligence without a requirement to show the standard of care; the defendant must rebut this presumption to avoid liability.

Concept.

Doctrine of res ipsa loquitur *is applicable where medical injury was probably the result of negligence (based on common knowledge or expert testimony), was caused by an agency or instrumentality in the exclusive control of the defendant, and was not due to any voluntary action or contribution on the part of the defendant.*

---

[44]Fraser v. Sprague, 76 Cal.Rptr. 37 (Cal. Ct. App. 1969).

[45]See, e.g., Ybarra v. Spangard, 154 P.2d 687 (Cal. 1944); Seneris v. Haas, 291 P.2d 915 (Cal. Ct. App. 1955); May v. Broun, 492 P.2d 776 (Or. 1972).

[46]See, e.g., Simmons v. Egwu, 662 N.E.2d 657 (Ind. Ct. App. 1996); Neary v. Charleston Area Med. Ctr., 460 S.E.2d 464 (W. Va. 1995); Fiumefreddo v. McLean, 496 N.W.2d 226 (Wis. Ct. App. 1993); Cherry v. Herques, 623 So.2d 131 (La. Ct. App. 1993).

Case. Ms. M injured her back, which caused her a great deal of discomfort. She was referred to Dr. D, a surgeon, for diagnosis and treatment. After Ms. M underwent a myelogram, Dr. D indicated that the best treatment for her condition was a laminectomy, a surgical procedure where the problematic vertebral lamina is excised. She agreed to the procedure. During the surgery, cottonoid sponges were used to retract tissues in the surgical field. Each sponge contained a radiopaque marker generally visible on X ray, and each was attached to a string that led outside the surgical field and the patient's body to allow for determination of the number and location of the sponges. Dr. D used these sponges and placed them as needed during the operation. Close to the end of the operation, one of the nurses indicated that one of the strings of the cottonoid sponge had separated from the sponge itself. Dr. D asked the circulating and scrub staff for a sponge count as well as searched the patient's incision and the entire operating room. The sponge could not be found. An intraoperative X ray was taken of the patient, but Dr. D, Dr. D's assistant, and the radiologist could not locate the marker on the X-ray film. Dr. D then closed the incision and sent Ms. M to the recovery room. However, several days later, Ms. M began experiencing severe pain, out of proportion to the surgery she had undergone. Dr. D ordered additional X-ray studies, which revealed the missing cottonoid sponge. Ms. M then underwent another surgery, and at this point, Dr. D removed the sponge from Ms. M's body. Ms. M sued Dr. D for medical malpractice indicating that Dr. D fell below the standard of care when the sponge was left in her body and that the court should apply the doctrine of *res ipsa loquitur* to the case. Dr. D indicated that expert testimony was needed to prove negligence in this case.

Legal Discussion. The court on which this case illustration was based indicated that the doctrine of *res ipsa loquitur* applied.[47] The court noted that, during the course of surgery, when a foreign object such as a cottonoid sponge is left or lost inside the patient, a presumption of negligence will be made because these events generally do not occur in the absence of negligence. No expert testimony would be needed for this conclusion since it was a matter of common knowledge. Next, it was apparent that the instrumentality in question, the cottonoid sponge, was in the exclusive control of Dr. D and his agents. Dr. D, as the surgeon in the case, placed these sponges in the locations necessary for the operation to proceed. Finally, since Ms. M was unconscious during the operation, there was not any voluntary action or contribution on her part with regard to the medical injury that she sustained. Because the factors for the

---

[47]Mudd v. Dorr, 574 P.2d 97 (Colo. Ct. App. 1977).

res ipsa loquitur doctrine were fulfilled, Ms. M was entitled to have the doctrine applied by the court and to shift the burden to Dr. D to rebut her claims regarding his negligence.

Notes on *Res Ipsa Loquitur*

Additional Applicable Situations

Some other examples of circumstances where the *res ipsa loquitur* doctrine has been applied include injuries to the patient in areas that were not under or in the area of treatment,[48] patient burns due to the use of infrared rays while the patient had ingested opiates,[49] leg burns after cardiac surgery,[50] knocking out a patient's tooth while the patient was under anesthesia for a tonsillectomy,[51] fracturing a patient's jaw when extracting a tooth,[52] patient burns by heat application post-Cesarean section while the patient was unconscious,[53] nerve injury due to hypodermic injection,[54] and urinary incontinence and impotence after removal of the prostate.[55]

Additional Reading.   C. T. Drechsler, "Malpractice Actions and Procedures," in *American Jurisprudence,* 2d ed. (New York: Lawyers Cooperative Publishing Co., 1981), section 334. See also J. W. Puryear, "Schmidt v. Gibbs: The Application of Res Ipsa Loquitur to Arkansas Medical Malpractice Litigation," *Arkansas Law Review* 46 (1993), pp. 397–431.

Extension to Other Actors

The doctrine of *res ipsa loquitur* may be used against multiple defendants. Therefore, if a patient who is unconscious suffers injuries outside the sphere of that expected by the treatment, suit may be brought against all operating and assisting physicians, medical assistants, and others who had joint control over the plaintiff's person or the instrumentalities that harmed the patient; all these defendants then must rebut the presumption of negligence.[56]

Additional Reading.   J. Teshima, "Applicability of Res Ipsa Loquitur in Case of Multiple Medical Defendants — Modern Status," in *American Law Reports,* 4th ed. (New York: Lawyers Cooperative Publishing Co., 1989), vol. 67, pp. 544–708.

Nonapplicable Situations

Generally, the doctrine will not be applicable in situations where the injury is merely an uncommon complication or an inherent risk of the operation or medical treatment.[57] And, of course, merely because injury occurs does not provide the basis for application of the doctrine.[58] This concept is founded on the premise that an injury alone usually does not indicate negligence.

Additional Reading.   C. T. Drechsler, "Circumstances Rendering Doctrine Inapplicable," in *American Jurisprudence,* 2d ed. (New York: Lawyers Cooperative Publishing Co., 1981), section 335.

Referral Responsibility

Note that simply referring a patient to another provider, such as a surgeon, does not give the referring physician such control or responsibility for the patient to render the referring physician subject to the *res ipsa loquitur* doctrine.[59]

Additional Reading.   C. T. Drechsler, "Malpractice Actions and Procedures," in *American Jurisprudence,* 2d ed. (New York: Lawyers Cooperative Publishing Co., 1981), section 333.

---

[48]See, e.g., Jackson v. Oklahoma Mem. Hosp., 909 P.2d 765 (Okla. 1995); Ybarra v. Spangard, 154 P.2d 687 (Cal. 1944); Adams v. Leidholdt, 563 P.2d 15 (Colo. Ct. App.), *aff'd*, 579 P.2d 618 (Colo. 1978); McCann v. Baton Rouge Gen. Hosp., 276 So.2d 259 (La. 1973).

[49]McCullough v. Langer, 73 P.2d 649 (Cal. Ct. App. 1937).

[50]Carranza v. Tucson Med. Ctr., 662 P.2d 455 (Ariz. Ct. App. 1983).

[51]Brown v. Shorlidge, 277 P. 134 (Cal. Ct. App. 1929).

[52]Zettler v. Reich, 11 N.Y.S.2d 85 (N.Y. App. Div.), *aff'd*, 281 N.Y. 729 (1939).

[53]Timbrell v. Suburban Hosp., Inc., 47 P.2d 737 (Cal. 1935).

[54]Bauer v. Otis, 284 P.2d 133 (Cal. Ct. App. 1955).

[55]Fehrman v. Smirl, 121 N.W.2d 255 (Wis.), *reh'g denied*, 122 N.W.2d 439 (Wis. 1963).

[56]Ybarra v. Spangard, 154 P.2d 687 (Cal. 1944).

[57]Surabian v. Lorenz, 40 Cal.Rptr. 410 (Cal. Ct. App. 1964); Tangora v. Matanky, 42 Cal.Rptr. 348 (Cal. Ct. App. 1964); Siverson v. Weber, 372 P.2d 97 (Cal. 1962); Tappe v. Iowa Methodist Med. Ctr., 477 N.W.2d 396 (Iowa 1991).

[58]Moore v. Guthrie Hosp., Inc., 403 F.2d 366 (4th Cir. 1968); Huffman v. Lindquist, 234 P.2d 34 (Cal. 1951); DiFilippo v. Preston, 173 A.2d 333 (Del. 1961); Anderson v. Gordon, 334 So.2d 107 (Fla. Dist. Ct. App. 1976); Rhodes v. De Haan, 337 P.2d 1043 (Kan. 1959); Schmidt v. Stone, 194 N.W. 917 (N.D. 1923); Eckleberry v. Kaiser Foundation Northern Hosp., 359 P.2d 1090 (Or. 1961); Danville Comm. Hosp., Inc. v. Thompson, 43 S.E.2d 882 (Va. 1947).

[59]Oldis v. La Societé Française de Bienfaisance Mutuelle, 279 P.2d 184 (Cal. Ct. App. 1955).

TRADITIONAL LEGAL MEDICINE

Spoliation

Spoliation is the destruction of evidence or significant or meaningful alteration of a document or instrument. In medical cases, this generally means absence or disappearance of medical records. In a malpractice case, if spoliation of evidence consists of missing medical records, this results in a rebuttable presumption on the main issues of medical negligence and causation against the provider[60] or even an irrebuttable, conclusive presumption of negligence.[61] Thus, as in *res ipsa loquitur*, when spoliation occurs, the burden of proof shifts to the defendant; however, unlike *res ipsa loquitur*, in some courts, that shift is irrebuttable.

Additional Reading. F. Buckner, *"Cedars-Sinai Medical Center vs. Superior Court* and the Tort of Spoliation of Evidence," *Legal Medical Perspectives* 6, no. 1 (1999), pp. 1–3; C. Casamassima, "Spoliation of Evidence and Medical Malpractice," *Pace Law Review* 14 (1994), pp. 235–99; "Jury Finds That Physician Did Not Intentionally Destroy Evidence," *Verdicts, Settlements, and Tactics* 9, no. 2 (1989), pp. 38–39.

Further Reading

Res Ipsa Loquitur

Albin KK. Res Ipsa Loquitur and Expert Opinion Evidence in Medical Malpractice Cases: Strange Bedfellows. *Va L Rev* 1996;82:325–55.

Courtade CR et al. Res Ipsa Loquitur. *American Jurisprudence,* 2d ed., New York: Lawyers Cooperative Publishing Co., 1989;§2238.

Drechsler CT. Malpractice Actions and Procedures. *American Jurisprudence,* 2d ed. New York: Lawyers Cooperative Publishing Co., 1981;§333–39.

Liang BA. Speaking for Itself: The Doctrine of *Res Ipsa Loquitur* in a Case of Pediatric Anesthesia. *J Clin Anes* 1996;8:398–401.

Liang BA. Teeth and Trauma: *Res Ipsa Loquitur* in a Case of Intubation. *J Clin Anes* 1998;10:432–34.

See Also

Eaton TA. Res Ipsa Loquitur and Medical Malpractice in Georgia: A Reassessment. *Ga L Rev* 1982;17:33–76;

Liability for Injuries. In: *American Jurisprudence,* 2d ed., New York: Lawyers Cooperative Publishing Co., 1968;§41.

Other Reading

Appel BE. Medical Malpractice Bibliography. *American Law Institute–American Bar Association* 1996;SB19:341–83.

Bovbjerg RR. Medical Malpractice: Research and Reform. *Va L Rev* 1993;79:2155–2207.

Cleckley FD, Hariharan G. A Free Market Analysis of the Effects of Medical Malpractice Damage Cap Statutes: Can We Afford to Live with Inefficient Doctors? *W Va L Rev* 1991;94:11–71.

Drechsler CT. Modern Approaches to Dealing with Malpractice Claims. In: *American Jurisprudence,* 2d ed., New York: Lawyers Cooperative Publishing Co., 1981;§372–77.

Feeder DW. When Your Doctor Says, "You Have Nothing to Worry About," Don't Be So Sure: The Effect of Fabio v. Bellomo on Medical Malpractice Actions in Minnesota. *Minn L Rev* 1994;78:943–74.

Grady MF. Better Medicine Causes More Lawsuits, and New Administrative Courts Will Not Solve This Problem. *NW U L Rev* 1992;86:1068–93.

Imershein AW, Brents AH. The Impact of Large Medical Malpractice Awards on Malpractice Awardees. *J Legal Med* 1992;13:33–49.

Keeton WP et al. Circumstantial Evidence—*Res Ipsa Loquitur.* In: *Prosser and Keeton on Torts,* 5th ed., St. Paul, MN: West Publishing Co., 1984;§39.

Keeton WP et al. Elements of a Cause of Action. *Prosser and Keeton on Torts,* 5th ed., St. Paul, MN: West Publishing Co., 1984;§30.

Kinney ED. Malpractice Reforms in the 1990's: Past Disappointments, Future Success? *J Health Pol Pol'y & L* 1995;20:99–135.

Liang BA. Beyond the Malpractice Suit: The National Practitioner Data Bank. *Hosp Phys* 1995;31(7):11–14.

Liang BA. Legal Issues in Transfusing a Jehovah's Witness Patient Following Cesarean Section. *J Clin Anes* 1995;7:522–24.

Liang BA. Medical Malpractice: Do Physicians Have Knowledge of Legal Standards and Assess Cases as Juries Do? *U Chi Law Sch Roundtable* 1996;3:59–111.

Liang BA. Assessing Medical Malpractice Jury Verdicts: A Case Study of an Anesthesiology Department. *Cornell J Law Pub Policy* 1997;7:121–64.

Liang BA. A Case of Resident Malpractice Administering Spinal Anesthesia. *J Clin Anes* 1997;9:341–44.

Liang BA. Blood, Bone, and Dura: Anesthesia Responsibility and Pediatric Neurosurgery. *J Clin Anes* 1997;9:597–601.

Liang BA. Ulnar Nerve Injury After Abdominal Surgery. *J Clin Anes* 1997;9:671–74.

Liang BA. Diabetic Silent Hearts and Anesthesia: The Duty to Assess. *J Clin Anes* 1998;10:610–12.

Liang BA. Clinical Assessment of Malpractice Case Scenarios in an Anesthesiology Department. *J Clin Anes* 1999; 11: 267–79.

Rake B, Thrasher B. Medical Malpractice Myths, Truths and Solutions. *Ariz Att'y* 1996;32(March):20–26.

---

[60]Sweet v. Sisters of Providence in Washington, 895 P.2d 484 (Alaska 1995); DeLaughter v. Lawrence County Hosp., 601 So.2d 818 (Miss. 1992).

[61]Public Health Trust of Dade County v. Valcin, 507 So.2d 596 (Fla. 1987)

Simone NM. Medical Malpractice Litigation: A Comparative Analysis of United States and Great Britain. *Suffolk Transnat'l L J* 1989;12:577–602.

Thomas WJ. The Medical Malpractice "Crisis": A Critical
Examination of a Public Debate. *Temp L Rev*
1992;65:459–527.

Web Sites

American College of Legal Medicine: *http://www.aclm.org*

Association for Responsible Medicine: *http://www.a-r-m.
org/*

Clinical Practice Guidelines/National Guideline Clearinghouse: *http://www.guidelines.gov*

Health Law Resource: *http://www.netreach.net/
~wmanning/*

Medical Malpractice and Professional Liability:
http://www.afss.com/medliab.htm

Medical Malpractice Expert, Inc.: *http://www.lawinfo.com/
biz/medi-legal/*

Medical Malpractice Law Forum: *http://www.prairielaw.
com/mm/*

Medical Malpractice, Medico-Legal Information Services:
http://www.mlis-th.com/

Medical Malpractice Resource Page: *http://www.sdtec.net/
fish/medmal.htm*

Medical Risk Management: *http://www.medrisk.com/*

3

Informed Consent

Informed consent is the process by which a medical provider communicates and discusses the material risks and benefits of each diagnostic or treatment alternative, including doing nothing, for the patient's disease state in a manner in which the patient can comprehend.[1] The basis of the concept is fundamental: Each person has the right to determine what shall and shall not be done to his or her person and only through a process of consent can an action be taken on that person. However, if the process of informed consent is followed and obtained, then the doctrine of *volenti non fit injuria* applies (to one who is willing, no wrong is done). Note, however, that a violation of informed consent is an entirely separate cause of action from malpractice; one does not rely on the other.

General Considerations

Generally, there are two basic forms of legal informed consent: a professional, provider-centered form, where the material risks and benefits of a diagnostic effort or treatment is gauged against what information a reasonable provider would have given in the circumstance; and a patient-centered form, where the material risks and benefits of the relevant diagnosis and treatment activities are gauged against what a reasonable patient in the circumstance would have desired. The specific consent standard is a function of state law where the provider practices.

Each of these informed consent standards is assessed under the legal rule of negligence: The plaintiff-patient must show that there was a *duty* to provide the informed consent under the appropriate standard just indicated, that there was a *breach* of that duty through nondisclosure of material information, and that breach *caused* the patient *injury or damage*. If all of these factors can be shown by the plaintiff by a preponderance of the evidence, there is a

lack of informed consent and the medical provider generally will be liable for tort damages; if even one of these factors cannot be satisfied, there is no liability.

Concept: Physician-Centered Standard.

Informed consent requires that the medical provider disclose to the patient the material risks and benefits associated with relevant diagnostic and treatment alternatives that a reasonable provider in similar circumstances would have given.

Case. Mr. S experienced abdominal pains. He went to his family physician, who prescribed Mylanta and a bland diet. However, the pains persisted. After the patient underwent an upper and lower gastrointestinal series, the pains were found apparently to result from a mass or tumor in his lower intestine. Mr. S consulted with his family physician and a surgeon, who recommended, as a diagnostic test, an intravenous pylogram (IVP), where dye would be injected into Mr. S to visualize the kidneys and ureters. Death or a serious allergic reaction to the dye can occur; patients with asthma or allergies have a greater risk of reaction, but there does not appear to be a higher risk of fatality between these groups. The estimated chance of reaction is 1 in 40,000. Radiologist Dr. R was scheduled to perform the procedure. One month after Mr. S began experiencing abdominal pains, he presented to Dr. R for performance of the IVP. Although he had a long history of allergies, Mr. S did not inform Dr. R about them. Dr. R did not inform Mr. S about the potential for a fatal reaction to the dye, on the basis of Dr. R's concern that Mr. S would become apprehensive and, as such, that would heighten Mr. S's potential for a reaction. However, soon after the procedure began, Mr. S had a severe allergic reaction to the contrast dye and died. Mrs. S brought suit against Dr. R for lack of informed consent on the basis of not informing Mr. S about the potential for severe reaction to the dye and death. Dr. R claimed, through expert testi-

---

[1]See, e.g., Hudson v. Parvin, 582 So.2d 403 (Miss. 1991).

mony, that the standard of disclosure by a reasonable physician would not include such a discussion of risk.

Legal Discussion. In the jurisdiction from which this illustration arises, the professional or physician-centered standard for informed consent was considered the relevant standard.[2] Therefore, to sustain an action against the physician for a violation of informed consent, plaintiff needed to show a preexisting duty on the part of the physician to provide information that a reasonable physician with similar training would do in similar circumstances, a breach of that duty by not providing that amount of information, and that breach caused the plaintiff injury or damage.

Clearly, there was a preexisting duty to provide the necessary information for the IVP by Dr. R since Dr. R was the physician who was to perform the procedure. However, according to the court, there was no breach of duty in this case. The professional standard requires that the physician disclose those risks that a reasonable practitioner of like training would have disclosed under the same or similar circumstances. Expert testimony was required to determine that amount of information. Dr. R obtained expert testimony that indicated that a similarly trained physician in Dr. R's position would not have provided the information on the potential severe reaction to the dye. Because Dr. R met the standard of disclosure that similarly situated and trained professionals in Dr. R's position would have provided, he did not breach the duty of informed consent to Mr. S and was not liable in tort for damages associated with Mr. S's death.

Concept: Patient-Centered Standard.

Informed consent requires disclosure to the patient by the medical provider of the material risks and benefits associated with relevant treatment alternatives, including doing nothing, that a reasonable patient under similar circumstances would wish to know.

Case. Ms. A was diagnosed with endometriosis and possible ovarian cysts by Dr. F. Dr. F suggested to Ms. A that the most appropriate method of treating her disorder was through laparoscopic examination to determine the sites of endometriosis and/or cysts and then fulguration (i.e., cauterization) of the endometriosis. Dr. F indicated that the procedure was a "simple" and "easy" operation and a "piece of cake." Further, Dr. F described the procedure as "ambulatory" and not very risky. Ms. A signed a preprinted hospital consent form. On the day of the procedure, Dr. F began the procedure; however, during the process of fulguration, one of Ms. A's ureters was severed. After awakening and discovering her ureter was severed, Ms. A sued for lack of informed consent on the

basis of her contention that Dr. F did not provide her with all material information regarding the procedure, including the risk of ureter injury, and that she would not have undergone the procedure had she known of the risk. Dr. F claimed that he did provide all the necessary information and obtained valid informed consent since there was only a 3–4% risk of injury in the operative area.

Legal Discussion. Here, it appears that informed consent was not obtained according to the case on which the illustration is based.[3] First, this state had a patient-centered informed consent standard; that is, the physician owed a duty to disclose to the patient all significant medical information that the physician possessed or should reasonably possess that was material to allow an intelligent decision by the patient whether to undergo the procedure.[4] Therefore, for the plaintiff-patient to prevail in this case, she had to show a preexisting duty for her physician to obtain informed consent from her for the treatment, a breach of that duty through lack of full disclosure of all material factors that caused her injury.

Plaintiff met her burden. Clearly, Dr. F had a preexisting duty to obtain informed consent under the patient-centered standard from Ms. A, as Dr. F was the physician who was to perform the procedure on Ms. A. That duty was breached, according to the court, when Dr. F did not provide information on the potential risks to organ systems within the operative field; both the plaintiff and a reasonable patient in similar circumstances would have not consented to the procedure since this was a material risk — a fact supported by Dr. F's testimony that there existed a 3–4% risk of injury in the operative field. This breach of duty to Ms. A caused her to suffer injury to her ureter. Thus, Ms. A fulfilled her burden and Dr. F was liable for tort damages stemming from this lack of informed consent.

Notes on Informed Consent

Battery

In addition to traditional informed consent actions, patients have sued providers under a theory of battery when informed consent was not obtained. Battery is a harmful or offensive contact with a person without his or her consent. Originally, before informed consent causes of action were recognized, battery was the cause of action pleaded by patients in informed consent situations. Currently, when providers are sued for battery, these causes of actions generally arise only in circumstances where the

---

[2]Hook v. Rothstein, 316 S.E.2d 690 (S.C. 1984).

[3]McMahon v. Finlayson, 632 N.E.2d 410 (Mass. App. Ct. 1994).
[4]See, e.g., Harnish v. Children's Hosp. Med. Ctr., 439 N.E.2d 240 (Mass. 1982).

provider performs unauthorized surgery or other diagnostic procedures on the patient.[5] Some courts require a total absence of efforts to obtain consent, rather than incomplete disclosure, for a patient to bring a battery claim against a provider.[6] Battery cases have become more common in circumstances where patients sue for nondisclosure of a provider's positive HIV status; courts facing these complaints often require that actual exposure to HIV be shown.[7] Battery actions are important because punitive damages are available, whereas in traditional informed consent negligence actions, punitive damages generally are excluded.

Additional Reading.   G. L. Boland, "The Doctrine of Lack of Consent and Lack of Informed Consent in Medical Procedure in Louisiana," *Louisiana Law Review* 45 (1984), pp. 1–38; E. S. Langston, "Changes in the Arkansas Law of Informed Consent: What's Up, Doc?" *University of Arkansas Little Rock Law Journal* 19 (1997), pp. 263–89; T. Lundmark, "Surgery by an Unauthorized Surgeon as a Battery," *Journal of Law & Health* 10 (1996), pp. 287–95; W. J. McNichols, "Informed Consent Liability in a 'Material Information' Jurisdiction: What Does the Future Portend?" *Oklahoma Law Review* 48 (1995), pp. 711–53; F. E. Van Oosten, *The Doctrine of Informed Consent in Medical Law* (New York: Peter Lang Publishing, 1991).

Capacity

Competent adults have an almost absolute right to make health care decisions, even if they lead to death.[8] However, difficulties with informed consent occur when the patient lacks the capacity to consent. Incapacity can exist for a variety of reasons, including intoxication and mental incompetence. The critical issue to assess is whether the individual can understand and weigh the risks and benefits of the treatment versus doing nothing; that is, "Does the patient have sufficient mind to reasonably understand the

condition, the nature and effect of the proposed treatment, attendant risks in pursuing the treatment, and not pursuing the treatment?"[9] Unfortunately, this determination must be made for each specific factual circumstance at hand on the basis of the best judgment of the medical provider — a difficult determination at best. Courts have split on this issue with regard to whether incompetent adults can refuse treatment and whether providers may render treatment without the incompetent patient's consent.[10] Of course, if the individual has a guardian or conservator over his or her person or if another individual such as a spouse may reasonably consent for the patient, then consent generally can be obtained validly from that individual.[11]

Additional Reading.   W. M. Altman, "Autonomy, Competence, and Informed Consent in Long-Term Care: Legal and Psychological Perspectives," *Villanova Law Review* 37 (1992), pp. 1671–1704; New York State Task Force on Life and Law, *When Others Must Choose: Deciding for Patients Without Capacity* (Washington, DC: Health Education Service, 1992). See also M. M. Walkow, "Informed Consent-Legal Competency Not Determinative of Person's Ability to Consent to Medical Treatment — Miller v. Rhode Island Hospital," *Suffolk University Law Review* 625 (1994), pp. 271–77.

Comatose Patients

Another difficult circumstance occurs when the patient is comatose or in a persistent vegetative state and was

---

[5]See, e.g., Fox v. Smith, 594 So.2d 596 (Miss. 1992); Daum v. Spinecare Med. Group, 61 Cal.Rptr.2d 260 (Cal. Ct. App. 1997); Espander v. Cramer, 903 P.2d 1171 (Colo. Ct. App. 1995); Bloskas v. Murray, 646 P.2d 907 (Colo. 1982); Franklin v. United States, 992 F.2d 1492 (10th Cir. 1993); Reikes v. Martin, 471 So.2d 385 (Miss. 1985).

[6]See, e.g., VanSice v. Sentany, 595 N.E.2d 264 (Ind. Ct. App. 1992); Roybal v. Bell, 778 P.2d 108 (Wy. 1989); O'Neal v. Hammer, 953 P.2d 561 (Haw. 1998); Sagala v. Tavares, 533 A.2d 165 (Pa. Super. Ct. 1987); Miller v. Kennedy, 522 P.2d 852 (Wash. Ct. App. 1974).

[7]See, e.g., Brzoska v. Olson, 668 A.2d 1355 (Del. Super. Ct. 1995); K.A.C. v. Benson, 527 N.W.2d 553 (Minn. 1995); Kerins v. Hartley, 33 Cal.Rptr.2d 172 (Cal. Ct. App. 1994); Doe v. Noe, 690 N.E.2d 1012 (Ill. App. Ct. 1997); Ashcraft v. King, 278 Cal.Rptr.2d 900 (Cal. Ct. App. 1991).

[8]See, e.g., Kirby v. Spivey, 307 S.E.2d 538 (Ga. Ct. App. 1983); Bouvia v. Superior Ct., 225 Cal.Rptr. 297 (Cal. Ct. App. 1986); In re Dubreuil, 629 So.2d 819 (Fla. 1993); Lasley v. Georgetown Univ., 842 F.Supp. 593 (D.D.C. 1994); Foy v. Greenblott, 190 Cal.Rptr. 84 (Cal. Ct. App. 1983); In the Matter of Roche, 687 A.2d 349 (N.J. Super. Ct. Ch. Div. 1996); In re Martin, 538 N.W.2d 399 (Mich. 1995); Anderson v. Hooker, 420 S.W.2d 235 (Tex. Civ. App. 1967).

[9]In the Matter of William Schiller, 372 A.2d 360, 367 (N.J. Super. Ct. Ch. Div. 1977); see also In the Matter of Edith Armstrong, 573 S.W.2d 141 (Mo. Ct. App. 1978); In re Quackenbush, 383 A.2d 785 (N.J. Prob. Div. 1978); State Dept. of Human Serv. v. Northern, 563 S.W.2d 197 (Tenn. Ct. App. 1978).

[10]See, e.g., Nolen v. Peterson, 544 So.2d 863 (Ala. 1989) (patient can refuse); Guardianship of Weedon, 565 N.E.2d 432 (Mass. 1991) (patient can refuse); In re Zuckerman, 477 N.W.2d 523 (Minn. Ct. App. 1991) (certain tests do not require informed consent); see also Rivers v. Katz, 495 N.E.2d 337 (N.Y. 1986) (patients may refuse or state may act without consent, depending on circumstances); In re Dorothy, 692 N.E.2d 388 (Ill. App. Ct. 1998) (state may act without consent, depending on circumstances).

[11]F. A. Rozovsky, *Consent to Treatment: A Practical Guide,* 2d ed. (New York: Aspen, 1990), section 1.5.1.

known to have expressed a wish to refuse treatment under such circumstances. On the one hand, the patient's wishes, through a surrogate, have led courts to allow the termination of treatment without literal informed consent from the patient so as to be in consonance with the patient's wishes.[12] However, in less dramatic circumstances, where the patient is comatose but the state may not be permanent or does not approach the level of a vegetative state, courts have allowed treatment that goes contrary to the patient's wishes.[13]

Additional Reading. A. N. Grubb, *Decision Making and Problems of Incompetence* (New York: John Wiley and Sons, 1994); D. D. King, "Where Death Begins While Life Continues," *South Texas Law Review* 31 (1990), pp. 145–90; E. A. Lyon, "The Right to Die: An Exercise of Informed Consent, Not an Extension of the Constitutional Right to Privacy," *University of Cincinnati Law Review* 58 (1990), pp. 1367–95; M. Poston, "Who Speaks for the Comatose?" *Arizona Bar Journal* 23 (1988), pp. 14–36.

Expert Witnesses

The varying standards of informed consent also raise the issue of expert witnesses and the need for them. Under the objective standard of what a reasonable physician would have disclosed to the patient, here expert witness testimony is necessary to establish the standard of relevant disclosure. Simply put, when the standard is what a reasonable medical provider would have said, one needs a medical provider to indicate what information would be disclosed under similar circumstances. On the other hand, if the standard is based on the information that a reasonable patient would desire, then no expert testimony is needed regarding what a reasonable physician would have done, since a reasonable patient's disclosure needs are at issue, which is ascertainable by a layperson, not what a reasonable physician would have indicated. However,

medical provider testimony in these latter cases is acceptable to show the relative risks of the alternative forms of treatment so that the jury can assess whether a reasonable patient would want that information.

Additional Reading. C. T. Drechsler, "Consent to Treatment," in *American Jurisprudence*, 2d ed. (New York: Lawyers Cooperative Publishing Co., 1981), section 194; D. E. Feld, "Necessity and Sufficiency of Expert Evidence to Establish Existence and Extent of Physicians' Duty to Inform Patient of Risks of Proposed Treatment," in *American Law Reports,* 3d ed. (New York: Lawyers Cooperative Publishing Co., 1974), vol. 52, pp. 1084–1105; H. B. Zobol and Stephen N. Rous, *Doctors and the Law: Defendants and Expert Witnesses* (New York: W.W. Norton & Co., 1993). See also D. L. Merideth, "The Medical Expert Witness in Mississippi: Outgunning the Opposition," *Mississippi Law Journal* 64 (1994), pp. 85–115.

Financial Arrangements

In the world of managed care, varying financial arrangements such as capitation or withhold arrangements have become extant that provide the physician incentives to minimize care.[14] However, at present, it does not appear that these financial arrangements must be disclosed to patients routinely as part of the informed consent process. However, in some circumstances, medical providers who participate in the Medicare and Medicaid programs[15] may be required to disclose this information to state and federal governments; and fiduciaries for employee benefits plans governed by the Employee Retirement Income Security Act of 1974 may have an obligation to disclose these financial arrangements.[16] Further, if a provider has research or financial interests in the tissue of the patient, the provider should disclose these interests to the patient.[17]

Additional Reading. H. T. Greely, "Direct Financial Incentives in Managed Care: Unanswered Questions," *Health Matrix* 6 (1996), pp. 53–88; D. C. McGraw, "Financial Incentives to Limit Services: Should Physicians Be Required to Disclose These to Patients?" *Georgia Law Journal* 83 (1995), pp. 1821–47; A. F. Walsh, "The Legal

---

[12]See, e.g., In re Storar, 438 N.Y.S.2d 266 (N.Y.), *cert. denied*, 454 U.S. 858 (1981); In re Gardner, 534 A.2d 947 (Me. 1987); Corbett v. D'Allessandro, 487 So.2d 368 (Fla. Dist. Ct. App. 1986), *rev. denied*, 492 So.2d 1331 (Fla. 1986); In the Matter of Eichner, 423 N.Y.S.2d 580 (N.Y. Sup. Ct. 1979); Delio v. Westchester County Med. Ctr., 129 A.2d 1 (N.Y. App. Div. 1987); In re Guardianship of Myers, 610 N.E.2d 663 (Ohio 1993); In re Martin, 538 N.W.2d 399 (Mich. 1995); Thor v. Superior Court, 855 P.2d 375 (Cal. 1993).

[13]See, e.g., In re Clark, 510 A.2d 136 (N.J. Super. Ct. Ch. Div. 1986); In re Darrell Dorone, 534 A.2d 452 (Pa. 1987); President and Director of Georgetown College, 331 F.2d 1000 (D.C. Cir. 1964); In re Dep't of Veterans Affairs Med. Ctr., 749 F.Supp 495 (D.N.Y. 1990); see also In re Martin, 538 N.W.2d 399 (Mich. 1995).

[14]B. A. Liang, "Deselection Under Harper v. Healthsource: A Blow for Maintaining the Patient-Physician Relationship in the Era of Managed Care?" *Notre Dame Law Review* 72 (1997), pp. 799–861.

[15]61 Fed. Reg. 69,034 (1996).

[16]Shea v. Esensten, 107 F.3d 625 (8th Cir.), *cert. denied*, 118 S.Ct. 297 (1997).

[17]Moore v. Regents of the Univ. of Cal., 793 P.2d 479 (Cal. 1990), *cert. denied*, 499 U.S. 936 (1991).

Attack on Cost Containment Mechanisms: The Expansion of Liability for Physicians and Managed Care Organizations," *John Marshall Law Review* 31 (1997), pp. 207–44.

"Guaranteed Results"

Providers who indicate to a patient that a particular result will occur from the treatment or otherwise "guarantee" a result, through the consent process, may establish a contract for a specific result. If that result does not occur, the patient may sue for breach of contract and the provider may be liable for damages.[18] It therefore is imperative that providers do not promise a particular result or make unsubstantiated claims regarding treatment. Otherwise, in addition to potential tort damages associated with medical malpractice, they may be subject to contractual damages. Further, even if tort damages do not arise due to lack of negligence in treatment, the provider may be independently liable for breach of contract due to the promise for a particular result if that result does not occur.

Additional Reading. D. T. Landis, "Measure and Elements of Damages in Action Against Physician for Breach of Contract to Achieve Particular Results in Care," in *American Law Reports,* 3d ed. (New York: Lawyers Cooperative Publishing Co., 1980), vol. 99, pp. 303–15; D. Peacock, "Haase v. Starnes: The Arkansas Supreme Court Refusal to Require Expert Testimony in Express Warranty Medical Malpractice Litigation," *Arkansas Law Review* 50 (1998), pp. 731–57; R. E. Sarnacki, "Contractual Theories of Recovery in the HMO Provider-Subscriber Relationship: Prospective Litigation for Breach of Contract," *Buffalo Law Review* 36 (1987), pp. 119–64.

HIV Status

Despite the very small probability of transmission of HIV from a medical provider to a patient, courts have placed a duty on medical providers to disclose their HIV-positive status if the provider is proposing an invasive procedure or treatment.[19] Further, some state licensing boards require that such status be reported to them by infected providers;[20] board publication of a physician's HIV infection after death has been held to be not actionable as an invasion of

privacy.[21] Also, depending on the state, an HIV-positive provider, or the organization for which he or she works, has an affirmative duty to notify patients who may have been exposed to the provider if no informed consent regarding this information was given.[22] Even when state statutes protect the identity of HIV-positive persons, health care organizations can require provider disclosure of such information to patients for informed consent purposes as well as restrict a provider's practice privileges.[23] While some cases based on federal statutory authority indicate that providers should not be discriminated against due to their HIV status,[24] many courts have held that the critical determination of whether the individual is "otherwise qualified" to perform their medical duties is not met in health care circumstances by HIV-positive providers.[25] Plaintiffs may win emotional injury claims if provider disclosure was not given even if they do not contract HIV.[26]

On the other hand, patients have no similar duty of disclosure of HIV-positive status to providers, nor can they be discriminated against for this status by providers or others.[27] With regard to informed consent for HIV

---

[18]See, e.g., Hawkins v. McGee, 146 A. 641 (N.H. 1929).

[19]See, e.g., Behringer v. Medical Ctr. at Princeton, 592 A.2d 1251 (N.J. Super. Ct. Law Div. 1991); Faya v. Almaraz, 620 A.2d 327 (Md. 1993); see also *Texas Health and Safety Code Annotated* (St. Paul, MN: West, 1997), section 85.201.

[20]*Louisiana Revised Statutes Annotated* (St. Paul, MN: West, 1997), section 37.1747; *Minnesota Statutes Annotated* (St. Paul, MN: West, 1997), section 214.19; Lecklet v. Board of Comm'rs of Hosp. Dist. 1, 909 F.2d 820 (5th Cir. 1990).

[21]Estate of Philip D. Benson v. Minnesota Bd. of Med. Practice, 526 N.W.2d 634 (Minn. Ct. App. 1995).

[22]410 *Illinois Compiled Statutes Annotated* 325/5.5 (St. Paul, MN: West, 1998); In re Milton S. Hershey Med. Ctr., 634 A.2d 159 (Pa. 1992); Brzoska v. Olson, 668 A.2d 1355 (Del. 1995); see also Doe v. Vanderbilt Univ., 958 S.W.2d 117 (Tenn. Ct. App. 1997); Doe v. Noe, 690 N.E.2d 1012 (Ill. App. Ct. 1997); Doe v. Northwestern Univ., 682 N.E.2d 145 (Ill. App. Ct. 1997).

[23]See, e.g., Behringer v. Medical Ctr. at Princeton, 592 A.2d 1251 (N.J. Super. Ct. Law Div. 1991).

[24]See, e.g., In re Westchester County Med. Ctr., Dec. No. 191, Docket No. 91-504-2, DHHS Departmental Appeals Bd. (Apr. 20, 1992) (pharmacist discriminated against under §504 of Rehabilitation Act, 29 U.S.C.A. §794); see also Reno v. Doe, 116 S.Ct. 2543 (1996) and Lane v. Pena, 116 S.Ct. 689 (1996) (federal violation of Rehabilitation Act not shielded by sovereign immunity).

[25]See, e.g., Doe v. Washington Univ., 780 F.Supp. 628 (E.D. Mo. 1991); Bradley v. University of Texas M.D. Anderson Cancer Ctr., 3 F.3d 922 (5th Cir.), *cert denied*, 510 U.S. 1119 (1983); Mauro v. Borgess Med. Ctr., 886 F.Supp. 1349 (W.D. Mich. 1995); John Doe v. University of Md. Med. Sys. Corp., 50 F.3d 1261 (4th Cir. 1995); see also Scoles v. Mercy Health Corp., 887 F.Supp. 765 (E.D. Pa. 1994).

[26]See, e.g., Doe v. Noe, 690 N.E.2d 1012 (Ill. App. 1997).

[27]See Bradgon v. Abbott, 118 S.Ct. 2196 (1998); Jairath v. Dyer, 972 F.Supp. 1461 (N.D. Ga. 1997); Cahill v. Rosa, 674 N.E.2d 274 (N.Y. 1996); Fiske v. Rooney, 663 N.E.2d 1014 (Ohio Ct. App. 1995); Howe v. Hull, 873 F.Supp. 72 (D. Ohio 1994); Ordway v. County of Suffolk, 583 N.Y.S.2d 1014 (N.Y. Sup. Ct. 1992); In re Marriage of Bonneau, 691 N.E.2d 123 (Ill. App. Ct. 1998); see also Gates v. Rowland, 39 F.3d 1439 (9th Cir. 1994); Harris v. Thigpen, 941 F.2d 1495 (11th Cir. 1991); Severino v. North Fort Myers Fire Control Dist., 935 F.2d 1179 (11th Cir. 1991); Doe v. Garrett, 903 F.2d 1455 (11th Cir. 1990) (HIV positive status constitutes protected disability).

screening, generally it is wise to obtain informed consent for this highly sensitive information, since many state statutes require this.[28] Note, however, that all states mandate that health care providers must report AIDS cases to the Centers for Disease Control and Prevention,[29] and many states indicate that HIV positivity is reportable as well to local or state health departments.[30] States have sued providers to compel providers to fulfill such reporting responsibilities.[31] Further, defendants in criminal cases involving rape and sexual assault may be required to undergo HIV testing, with the results provided to the victim.[32]

[28]See, e.g., *California Health and Safety Code* §199.22 (St. Paul, MN: West, 1997); *Colorado Revised Statutes* §25-4-1404 (1997); *Connecticut, General Statutes Annotated* (St. Paul, MN: West, 1997), section 19A-582; *Florida Statutes Annotated* (St. Paul, MN: West, 1997), section 381.004; *Indiana Code Annotated* §16-1-9.5-2.5 (St. Paul, MN: West, 1997), section 16-1-9.5-2.5; *Louisiana Revised Statutes Annotated* §40:1300:13 (St. Paul, MN: West, 1997), section 40:1300:13; *Maine Revised Statutes Annotated* (St. Paul, MN: West, 1997), title 5, section 19203; *Maryland Code Annotated, Health-General I* (1997), section 18-336; *Massachusetts General Laws Annotated* (St. Paul, MN: West, 1997), chapter 111, section 70F; *Montana Code Annotated* §50-16-1007 (1997); *McKinney's New York Public Health Law* §2781 (1997); *Ohio Revised Code Annotated* (St. Paul, MN: West, 1997), section 3701.242; *Wisconsin Statutes Annotated* (St. Paul, MN: West, 1997), section 146.025.

[29]See, e.g., *Iowa Code Annotated* (St. Paul, MN: West, 1997), section 141.22A(5); *Administrative Rules of South Dakota* 44:20:02:08(3) (1998); *Texas Health and Safety Code Annotated* (St. Paul, MN: West, 1997), section 162.004; *Washington Revised Code Annotated* (St. Paul, MN: West, 1997), section 70.24.105(2)(c); see also *California Health and Safety Code* (St. Paul, MN: West, 1997), section 120980(I); *Montana Code Annotated* §50-16-1013(5) (1997).

[30]See, e.g., *Colorado Revised Statutes Annotated* (St. Paul, MN: West, 1997), section 25-4-1403; *Florida Statutes Annotated* (St. Paul, MN: West, 1997), section 384.25; *Georgia Code Annotated* §31-22-9.2; *Hawaii Revised Statutes Annotated* (Charlottesville, VA: Michie, 1997), section 325-101; 20 *Illinois Compiled Statutes Annotated* (St. Paul, MN: West, 1998), section 505/22.3; *Indiana Code Annotated* (Charlottesville, VA: Michie, 1998), section §16-41-2-3; *Michigan Compiled Laws Annotated* (St. Paul, MN: West, 1998), section 333-5114; *General Statutes of North Carolina* §130A-135 (1997); *Ohio Revised Code Annotated* (St. Paul, MN: West, 1998), section 3701.24; *South Carolina Code Annotated* (New York: Lawyers Cooperative Publishing Co., 1997), section 44-29-250; *Texas Health and Safety Code Annotated* (St. Paul, MN: West, 1997), section 81.041; see also *Delaware Code Annotated* tit. 18, §7404 (1997).

[31]See, e.g., Middlebrooks v. State Bd. of Health, 710 So.2d 891 (Ala. 1998); see also Whalen v. Roe, 429 U.S. 589, 602 (1977) (disclosure of private medical information by physicians to public health agencies does not automatically amount to an impermissible invasion of privacy).

[32]See, e.g., United States v. Ward, 131 F.3d 335 (3d Cir. 1997).

Additional Reading.   J. H. Barney, "A Health Care Worker's Duty to Undergo Routine Testing for HIV/AIDS and to Disclose Positive Results to Patients," *Louisiana Law Review* 52 (1992), pp. 933–70; B. J. Belke, "Kerins v. Hartley: A Patient's Silent Cry for Mandatory Disclosure by HIV-Positive Physicians," *Southwestern University Law Review* 25 (1995), pp. 205–22; J. W. Buehler et al., "Reporting of AIDS: Tracking HIV Morbidity and Mortality," *JAMA* 262 (1989), pp. 2896–2906; L. Gostin, "Hospitals, Health Care Professionals and Aids: The 'Right to Know' the Health Status of Professionals and Patients," *Maryland Law Review* 48 (1989), pp. 12–54; S. H. Rennert, *AIDS/HIV and Confidentiality: Model Policy and Procedure* (Chicago: American Bar Association, 1991).

Implied Consent

Theoretically, there is no need for written or oral consent if, by reasonable inference, the patient's action would indicate that he or she consents to the treatment or procedure.[33] However, in the modern health care context, the scope of this inference is limited, since the basis of implied consent is that a reasonable person should be aware that the actions of providers will lead to some cognizable actions affecting the patient. Hence, although perhaps an injection would be within this implied consent, more complex procedures would not. Therefore, it is prudent to always obtain informed consent when there is any doubt regarding the extent of knowledge of or consent by the patient.

Additional Reading.   C. T. Drechsler, "Consent to Treatment," in *American Jurisprudence*, 2d ed. (New York: Lawyers Cooperative Publishing Co., 1981), section 183; M. B. Kapp, "Enforcing Patient Preferences: Linking Payment for Medical Care to Informed Consent," *JAMA* 261 (1989), pp. 1935–61.

Ineffective Consent

Further, it should be noted that consent may not be effective if the medical provider coerces the patient into consenting, the patient was mistaken in his or her understanding of the information and the provider knew or should have known of such mistake, or if the provider exceeded the consent. Basically, the idea behind these cir-

[33]See, e.g., O'Brien v. Cunard Steamship Co., 28 N.E. 266 (Mass. 1891); Jones v. Malloy, 412 N.W.2d 837 (Neb. 1987); Millard v. Nagle, 587 A.2d 10 (Pa. Super. Ct. 1991); Plutshack v. University of Minnesota Hosps., 316 N.W.2d 1 (Minn. 1982); Busalacchi v. Vogel, 429 So.2d 217 (La. Ct. App. 1983); see also Miller v. Rhode Island Hosp., 625 A.2d 778 (R.I. 1993); Beck v. Lovell, 361 So.2d 245 (La. Ct. App. 1978).

cumstances is that a medical provider must make a full and complete disclosure of the potential treatments to the patient in good faith and the patient must understand this information. Further, exculpatory clauses on consent forms that purport to waive the patient's right to sue are considered invalid,[34] and indeed, the court may invalidate the entire consent on the basis of the presence of such clauses.

Additional Reading. R. B. Axelrod, "Medical Malpractice," in *Florida Jurisprudence,* 2d ed. (New York: Lawyers Cooperative Publishing Co., 1996), section 24; C.A. Crocca, "Arbitration of Medical Malpractice Claims," in *American Law Reports,* 5th ed. (New York: Lawyers Cooperative Publishing Co., 1995), vol. 24, pp. 1–131.

Materiality

The information that need be disclosed for valid informed consent is that which is considered *material*. Unfortunately, *material* is not a well-defined term and depends on the facts and circumstances of each case. On the one hand, the standard laundry list of material factors includes the patient's diagnosis, the nature and purpose of proposed treatment, the risks of consequences of the proposed treatment, the probability that the proposed treatment will be successful, the feasible treatment alternatives, and the alternatives and prognosis if the proposed treatment is not given as a function of probability of an adverse outcome or severity of potential injury.[35] Less common disclosure requirements include a history of chronic alcoholism[36] and experience in performing the proposed procedure.[37] However, certain risks of treatment have been deemed *not* material. These include risks already known by the patient, risks that are obvious such that they may be assumed to be known by the patient,[38] remote risks of a treatment inherent in a procedure if they are generally known to be present and are low in inci-

dence,[39] and risks of which a provider could not have been aware[40] that were not foreseeable[41] and that could not be ascertained using ordinary care.[42] Note that if a patient indicates that he or she will agree to treatment without regard to risks or that he or she does not desire to know of the risks,[43] then of course there is no issue of materiality and a lack of informed consent action cannot be sustained. However, prudence dictates that this blanket agreement or blanket refusal be documented carefully.

Additional Reading. W. J. McNichols, "Informed Consent Liability in a 'Material Information' Jurisdiction: What Does the Future Portend?" *Oklahoma Law Review* 48 (1995), pp. 711–53; J. F. Merz, "On a Decision-Making Paradigm of Medical Informed Consent," *Journal of Legal Medicine* 14 (1993), pp. 231–59; D. M. Wallach et al., "Informed Consent in Texas: A Proposal for Reasonableness and Predictability," *St. Mary's Law Journal* 18 (1987), pp. 835–82.

Minors

In nonemergency circumstances, obtaining informed consent from minors as permission to treat or perform a procedure generally is considered invalid, and consent must be obtained from the appropriate parent or guardian.[44] Only if there is an emergency[45] will the minor be legally considered an adult generally or for the particular medical circumstance.[46] However, it should be noted that,

[34]See, e.g., Tatham v. Hoke, 469 F.Supp. 914, *aff'd,* 622 F.2d 584 (4th Cir. 1980); see also Vodopest v. MacGregor, 913 P.2d 779 (Wash. 1996) (exculpatory clause for injury due to research experiment invalid); Colton v. New York Hosp., 414 N.Y.S.2d 866 (N.Y. Sup. Ct. 1979) (exculpatory clause for injury associated with nonnegligent treatment valid).

[35]"Consent to Medical and Surgical Procedures," *Hospital Law Manual* (1994), section 203; Yeats v. Harms, 393 P.2d 982 (Kan. 1962); Wilson v. Scott, 412 S.W.2d 299 (Tex. 1967); see also Arato v. Avedon, 858 P.2d 598 (Cal. 1993) (physicians did not have duty to disclose life expectancy of pancreatic cancer patients nor information relevant to patient's nonmedical interests).

[36]Hidding v. Williams, 578 So.2d 1192 (La. Ct. App. 1991).

[37]Johnson v. Kokemoor, 545 N.W.2d 495 (Wis. 1996).

[38]Fleishman v. Richardson-Merrell, Inc., 226 A.2d 843 (N.J. Super. Ct. App. Div. 1967).

[39]See, e.g., Craig v. Borcicky, 557 So.2d 1253 (Ala. 1990); Smith v. Cotter, 810 P.2d 1204 (Nev. 1991); Lembke v. United States, 557 F.Supp. 1205 (D.N.D. 1983); Henderson v. Milobsky, 595 F.2d 654 (D.C. Cir. 1978); Parker v. St. Paul Fire & Marine Ins. Co., 355 So.2d 725 (La. Ct. App. 1976); Longmire v. Hoey, 512 S.W.2d 307 (Tenn. Ct. App. 1974).

[40]See, e.g., Kozup v. Georgetown Univ., 663 F.Supp. 1048 (D.D.C. 1987).

[41]Block v. McVay, 126 N.W.2d 808 (S.D. 1964).

[42]Precourt v. Frederick, 481 N.E.2d 1144 (Mass. 1985); Meeks v. Marx, 550 P.2d 1158 (Wash. Ct. App. 1976).

[43]Putensen v. Clay Adams, Inc., 91 Cal.Rptr 319 (Cal. Ct. App. 1970).

[44]Moss v. Rishworth, 222 S.W. 225 (Tex. Comm'n App. 1920); Browning v. Hoffman, 111 S.E. 492 (W. Va. 1922); Bishop v. Shurly, 211 N.W. 75 (Mich. 1926); Aoski v. Gaines, 260 N.W. 99 (Mich. 1935); Sullivan v. Montgomery, 279 N.Y.S. 575 (1935); Rogers v. Sells, 61 P.2d 1018 (Okla. 1936); Bonner v. Moran, 126 F.2d 121 (D.C. Cir. 1941); In re Hudson, 126 P.2d 765 (Wash. 1942).

[45]See the section "Emergency Treatment Exception to Informed Consent," later in this chapter.

[46]Cardwell v. E. L. Bechtol, 724 S.W.2d 739 (Tenn. 1987); Luka v. Lowrie, 136 N.W. 1106 (Mich. 1912); see also Kozup v. Georgetown Univ., 851 F.2d 437 (D.C. Cir. 1988); A.D.H. v. State Dept. of Human Resources, 640 So.2d 969 (Ala. Civ. App. 1994); Bonner v. Moran, 126 F.2d 121 (D.C. Cir. 1941).

generally, parents have no authority to refuse lifesaving medical treatment for their children if there is agreement that treatment would be beneficial and there is a good prognosis; this is true even if the parental basis for these refusals is religious.[47] On the other hand, if treatment would not be medically appropriate and generally futile, parents may refuse care for their minor children.[48]

Additional Reading. G. B. Melton, *Children's Competence to Consent* (New York: Plenum Publishing Corp., 1983); A. Popper, "Averting Malpractice by Information: Informed Consent in the Pediatric Treatment Environment," *DePaul Law Review* 47 (1998), pp. 819–36; F. E. Van Oosten, *The Doctrine of Informed Consent in Medical Law* (New York: Peter Lang Publishing, 1991); D. R. Veilleux, "Medical Practitioner's Liability for Treatment Given Child Without Parent's Consent," in *American Law Reports,* 4th ed. (New York: Lawyers Cooperative Publishing Co., 1989), vol. 67, pp. 511–34.

Option of Doing Nothing

It is critical to note that if there are significant consequences as a result of doing nothing with regard to the patient's disease state, the medical provider must indicate to the patient the potential adverse consequences of such inaction.[49] Simply restating that the patient should have the proposed treatment is not enough; an affirmative discussion regarding the potential results associated with doing nothing must be given for the provider to avoid liability. The basic rationale is that informed consent includes informed refusal of a treatment; that refusal can be informed only if its consequences are known by the patient. However, if the patient has provided an "informed refusal," it then must be honored, regardless of

its basis.[50] Of course, the provider is not liable for the disclosed (and documented) consequences of this refusal.

Additional Reading. G. L. Boland, "The Doctrine of Lack of Consent and Lack of Informed Consent in Medical Procedure in Louisiana," *Louisiana Law Review* 45 (1984), pp. 1–38; E. M. Levine, "A New Predicament for Physicians: The Concept of Medical Futility, The Physician's Obligation to Render Inappropriate Treatment and the Interplay of the Medical Standard of Care," *Journal of Law & Health* 9 (1995), pp. 69–108; E. Lu, "The Potential Effect of Managed Competition in Healthcare on Provider Liability and Patient Autonomy," *Harvard Journal on Legislation* 30 (1993), pp. 519–52.

Other Legal Standards

There are alternate forms of informed consent as well as the ones already indicated. They include a subjective standard that focuses on what the specific patient would wish to know and a standard that is a combination of the objective patient (or physician-centered) and subjective forms; for example, one that looks to what a reasonable provider would indicate to a patient but with the caveat that if the provider knows that a particular patient would want specific information, that information must be disclosed.[51] The specific informed consent standard is dictated by the state law in the jurisdiction where the patient and physician are located. However, it appears that the provider-based standard is the majority rule in the United States,[52] although more and more states are moving to the patient-based standard.

Additional Reading. L. B. Frantz, "Modern Status of Views as to General Measure of Physician's Duty to Inform Patient of Risks of Proposed Treatment," in *American Law Reports,* 3d ed. (New York: Lawyers Cooperative Publishing Co., 1978), vol. 88, pp. 1008–44; R. A. Heinemann, "Pushing the Limits of Informed Consent: Johnson v. Kokemoor and Physician-Specific Disclosure," *Wisconsin Law Review* 1997 (1997), pp. 1079–1121; J. F. Merz, "On a Decision Making Paradigm of Medical Informed Consent," *Journal of Legal Medicine* 14 (1993), pp. 231–64.

[47] See, e.g., Prince v. Mass., 321 U.S. 158, 170, *reh'g denied,* 321 U.S. 804 (1944); In re Eric B., 235 Cal.Rptr. 22 (Cal. Ct. App. 1987); In re Tara Cabrera, 552 A.2d 1114 (Pa. Super. Ct. 1989); Custody of a Minor, 393 N.E.2d 836 (Mass. 1979); State v. Perricone, 181 A.2d 751 (N.J.), *cert. denied,* 371 U.S. 890 (1962); O.G. v. Baum, 790 S.W.2d 839 (Tex. 1990); see also Hoener v. Bertinato, 67 N.J.Super. 517 (1961); Newmark v. Williams, 588 A.2d 1108 (Del. 1991); *Arizona Revised Statutes Annotated* (St. Paul, MN: West, 1997), section 36-2281; *Louisiana Civil Code Annotated* (St. Paul, MN: West, 1997), article 1554; *Maryland Code Annotated, Family Law* §50203(b)(1) (1997); *New Jersey Statutes Annotated* (St. Paul, MN: West, 1997), section 30:4C-6, 9:6-1.1; 55 *Pennsylvania Consolidated Statutes* §349.4 (1997).

[48] Newmark v. Williams, 588 A.2d 1108 (Del. 1991); M.N. v. Southern Baptist Hosp., 648 So.2d 769 (Fla. Dist. Ct. App. 1994); see also In re Green, 292 A.2d 387 (Pa. 1972).

[49] Truman v. Thomas, 611 P.2d 902 (Cal. 1980); Madsen v. Park Nicollet Med. Ctr., 419 N.W.2d 511 (Minn. Ct. App. 1988).

[50] In re Conroy, 486 A.2d 1209 (N.J. 1985); Kimmel v. Dayrit, 693 A.2d 1287 (N.J. Super. Ct. App. Div. 1997); Norwood Hosp. v. Munoz, 564 N.E.2d 1017 (Mass. 1991); see also Battenfeld v. Gregory, 589 A.2d 1059 (N.J. Super. Ct. App. Div. 1991); In re Brown, 689 N.E.2d 397 (Ill. App. Ct. 1997).

[51] Distefano v. Bell, 544 So.2d 567 (La. Ct. App.), *cert. denied,* 550 So.2d 650 (La. 1989); McKinney v. Nash, 174 Cal.Rptr. 642 (Cal. Ct. App. 1981).

[52] B. R. Furrow et al., *Health Law,* vol. 1 (St. Paul, MN: West, 1995).

Referring Physician

If a physician refers the patient to another provider who will perform a procedure or provide treatment, the latter provider must obtain all necessary informed consents. Therefore, the physician who refers the patient generally has no duty to inform the patient about the possible risks and complications of any therapeutic actions by the referred-to provider as long as the referring physician does not participate in the referred-to diagnosis or treatment.[53] If, however, the referring physician does retain some control, he or she may also have a duty to obtain informed consent from the patient.[54]

Additional Reading. P. Watter, "The Doctrine of Informed Consent: To Inform or Not to Inform?" *St. Johns Law Review* 71 (1997), pp. 543–67. See also C. T. Drechsler, "Consent to Treatment," in *American Jurisprudence,* 2d ed. (New York: Lawyers Cooperative Publishing Co., 1981), section 197.

Relation to Malpractice

It should be noted that informed consent suits are totally separate from potential negligence suits for medical malpractice. The care rendered by a medical provider to a patient may comport with all relevant standards of care, cure the patient, or alleviate all problematic symptoms, but all of these considerations are irrelevant with regard to informed consent. Indeed, regardless of negligence or lack thereof in the treatment itself, an informed consent action can be brought and won by a patient if the medical provider did not obtain the requisite informed consent before diagnosis or treatment and the other factors of a negligence action can be shown.[55]

Additional Reading. L. B. Frantz, "Modern Status of Views as to General Measure of Physician's Duty to Inform Patients of Risks of Proposed Treatment," in *American Law Reports,* 3d ed. (New York: Lawyers Cooperative Publishing Co., 1978), vol. 88, pp. 1008–44.

Research

Patient participation in research requires informed consent. Generally, however, several steps must occur before patient consent is addressed. Any medical research on humans generally is addressed by federal regulations.[56] Proposed research must be reviewed by institutional review boards (IRBs), whose composition, experience, and knowledge are subject to specific requirements. IRBs must assess all research activities to determine relative risks to patients (these risks compared to substantive benefits) as well as the relevant informed consent of the patients who may be involved.[57] In addition, any research involving drugs and devices must fulfill the requirements of the Food, Drug, and Cosmetic Act.[58] Once IRB approval is obtained, federal regulations specify that potential research subjects be given information on the research, including the purposes and duration of the patient's participation; description and identification of procedures involved; description of possible discomforts, reasonable risks, and benefits to the patient; description of possible alternative procedures that may be advantageous for the patient; indication of the confidentiality of records and the extent of such confidentiality; description of any medical treatments that may be needed for projects involving more than minimal risk; an offer to answer any questions regarding the project or elements thereof; and a clear statement that the subject may withdraw his or her consent and discontinue participation in the research at any time without consequence to the subject.[59] Note that, in the area of research, hospitals that receive federal funding from the Department of Health and Human Services also must obtain informed consent in addition to the standard physician obligation;[60] violation of this duty may subject the hospital to liability.[61]

Additional Reading. D. Derrickson, "Informed Consent to Human Subject Research: Improving the Process of Obtaining Informed Consent from Mentally Ill Persons," *Fordham Urban Law Journal* 25 (1997), pp. 143–65; D. J. Mazur, *Medical Risk and the Right to an Informed Consent in Clinical Care and Clinical Research* (Philadelphia: American College of Physicians, 1998); "Symposium: Conducting Medical Research on the Decisionally Impaired," *Journal of Health Care Law Policy* 1 (1998), pp. 1–300; K. A. Tuthill, "Human Experimentation," *Journal of Legal Medicine* 18 (1997), pp. 221–50. See also J. W. Guise, "Expansion of the Scope of Disclosure Required Under the Informed Consent Doctrine: Moore v. The Regents of the University of California,"

---

[53]Edwards v. Garcia-Gregory, 866 S.W.2d 780 (Tex. App. 1993).

[54]See, e.g., O'Neal v. Hammer, 953 P.2d 561 (Haw. 1998).

[55]See, e.g., Cooper v. Roberts, 286 A.2d 647 (Pa. Super. Ct. 1971).

[56]45 C.F.R. Part 45 (1998) *et seq.*

[57]45 C.F.R. §46.111 (1998).

[58]21 U.S.C.A. §355(i); 21 C.F.R. §312.1 (1998).

[59]45 C.F.R. 46.116(a) (1998).

[60]See 45 C.F.R. Part 46 (1998).

[61]See, e.g., Kus v. Sherman Hosp., 644 N.E.2d 1214 (Ill. App. Ct. 1995); Friter v. Iolab Corp., 607 A.2d 1111 (Pa. Super. Ct. 1992); In re Orthopedic Bone Screw, WL 107556 (D. Pa. 1996); see also Jones v. Philadelphia College of Osteopathic Med., 813 F.Supp. 1125 (D. Pa. 1993); Corrigan v. Methodist Hosp., 158 F.R.D. 70 (Pa. 1994).

San Diego Law Review 28 (1991), pp. 455–75; M. D. Miller, "The Informed Consent Policy of the International Conference on Harmonization of Technical Requirements for Registration of Pharmaceuticals for Human Use: Knowledge Is the Best Medicine," *Cornell International Law Journal* 30 (1997), 203–44.

Scope of Consent

The provider who has appropriately obtained informed consent from the patient for the treatment or procedure is permitted to provide that treatment. However, the provider who extends his or her actions *beyond* the scope of the informed consent may be subject to liability for lack of informed consent[62] or battery.[63] This scope also applies to laboratory tests; persons who consent to particular tests may not have their samples used for additional testing. Such additional testing may violate informed consent statutes, privacy statutes, civil rights acts, and the Americans with Disabilities Act.[64]

Additional Reading. L. B. Frantz, "Malpractice: Questions of Consent in Connection with Treatment of Genital or Urinary Organs," in *American Law Reports,* 3d ed. (New York: Lawyers Cooperative Publishing Co., 1978), vol. 89, pp. 32–77; L. B. Frantz, "Modern Status of Views as to General Measure of Physician's Duty to Inform Patient of Risks of Proposed Treatment," in *American Law Reports,* 3d ed. (New York: Lawyers Cooperative Publishing Co., 1978), vol. 88, pp. 1008–44. See also A. Szcygiel, "Beyond Informed Consent," *Ohio Northern University Law Review* 21 (1994), pp. 171–262.

Statutes

In addition to the common law standards for informed consent, many state legislatures have enacted statutes that describe the extent and requirements for obtaining informed consent in the state. Providers and legal counsel for health care organizations should examine these statutes to be up-to-date on what the particular state requires with regard to informed consent.[65]

Additional Reading.

N. C. Abramson, "A Right to Privacy Tour de Force into Louisiana Medical Informed Consent," *Louisiana Law Review* 51 (1991), pp. 755–86. See also J. W. Guise, "Expansion of the Scope of Disclosure Required Under the Informed Consent Doctrine: Moore v. The Regents of the University of California," *San Diego Law Review* 28 (1991), pp. 455–75.

Test Results

If a patient has consented to a particular procedure and there are suspicious results, to whom should the provider who has performed the procedure report these results? Generally, if there is a referring primary care physician, the specialist who performs the procedure has a duty to report the result to the referring provider for him or her to report to the patient.[66]

Additional Reading. J. S. Talbot, "The Conflict Between a Doctor's Duty to Warn a Patient's Sexual Partner That the Patient Has AIDS and a Doctor's Duty to Maintain Patient Confidentiality," *Washington and Lee Law Review* 45 (1988), pp. 355–80. See also J. E. Zelin, "Physician's Tort Liability for Unauthorized Disclosure of Confidential Information About Patient," in *American Law Reports,* 4th ed. (New York: Lawyers Cooperative Publishing Co., 1987), vol. 48, pp. 668–713.

"Therapeutic Privilege"

Therapeutic privilege is a legal doctrine that indicates that if disclosure of particular information would be significantly detrimental to the patient's physical or mental well-being, then it is permissible for the medical provider not to disclose it, even if deemed material otherwise.[67] The exercise of the privilege is highly fact dependent and depends on the specific patient, provider, procedure or treatment, and context.[68] As a practical matter, despite some cases that have held that providers are not liable for violations of informed consent obligations, a provider who bases his or her limited disclosure on therapeutic privilege is treading on dangerous ground. It is best to provide the patient with all relevant information, since hindsight often is all too clear when injury occurs due to an undisclosed risk. If the

[62]See, e.g., Millard v. Nagle, 587 A.2d 10 (Pa. Super. Ct. 1991), *aff'd,* 625 A.2d 641 (Pa. 1993).

[63]See, e.g., Mohr v. Williams, 104 N.W. 12 (Minn. 1905); Mink v. University of Chicago, 460 F.Supp. 713 (N.D. Ill. 1978).

[64]See, e.g., Norman-Bloodsaw v. Lawrence Berkeley Lab., 135 F.3d 1260 (9th Cir. 1998).

[65]See, e.g., Morgan v. Rose, 704 A.2d 617 (Pa. 1997) (Pennsylvania statute requires informed consent only for surgical or operative procedures and doctrine of informed consent does not apply to cases of nonsurgical administration of medication).

[66]See, e.g., Mahanna v. Hirsch, 237 Cal.Rptr. 140 (Cal. Ct. App. 1987).

[67]See, e.g., DiFilippo v. Preston, 173 A.2d 333 (Del. 1961); Wilson v. Scott, 412 S.W.2d 299 (Tex. 1967); Sard v. Hardy, 379 A.2d 1014 (Md. 1977); Canterbury v. Spence, 464 F.2d 772 (D.C. Cir. 1972).

[68]See, e.g., Nishi v. Hartwell, 473 P.2d 116 (Haw. 1970); Lee v. Lee, 517 N.Y.S.2d 183 (N.Y. App. Div. 1987).

provider chooses to rely on the therapeutic privilege, documentation of the rationale for withholding the information should be made, including why the information should have been withheld, the specific information withheld, the information disclosed to the patient, the general state of the patient at the time, and an overall statement as to the medical findings that led the provider to decide to invoke the therapeutic privilege.[69]

Additional Reading. D. A. Dickerson, "A Doctor's Duty to Disclose Life Expectancy Information to Terminally Ill Patients," *Cleveland State Law Review* 43 (1995), pp. 319–50; E. S. Fisher, "Informed Consent in Oklahoma: A Search for Reasonableness and Predictability in the Aftermath of Scott v. Bradford," *Oklahoma Law Review* 49 (1996), pp. 651–75; R. E. Shugrue and K. Linstromberg, "The Practitioner's Guide to Informed Consent," *Creighton Law Review* 24 (1991), pp. 881–908.

Waiver

At times, a patient may attempt to waive his or her right to be informed regarding treatment consent. This waiver may be effective in some cases.[70] Yet it always is preferable for the provider to encourage the patient to have some understanding of the risks and benefits of the proposed treatment or diagnostic test to avoid potential difficulties later. If the patient continues to desire to waive his or her right for informed consent, this waiver should be noted in detail in the patient's chart and witnessed. Further, it should be noted that patients do not waive their ability to change their minds after one informed consent discussion and concomitant documentation has been performed. A refusal of a physician to provide additional discussions and allow for withdrawal of consent may result in liability.[71]

Additional Reading. E. Gordon, "Multiculturalism in Medical Decision Making: The Notion of Informed Waiver," *Fordham Urban Law Journal* 23 (1996), pp. 1321–62; R. S. Saver, "Critical Care Research and Informed Consent," *North Carolina Law Review* 75 (1996), pp. 205–71; R. E. Shugrue and K. Linstromberg, "The Practitioner's Guide to Informed Consent," *Creighton Law Review* 24 (1991), pp. 881–928.

Who Obtains and Documents Consent?

The medical provider proposing the treatment or diagnostic activity *always* should be the individual who discloses and discusses the relevant information and thus obtains informed consent. Further, it should be noted that the medical provider actually performing the procedure or providing treatment is the party who should obtain consent, not any referring medical provider.[72] However, the issue as to *who* obtains consent can be distinguished with how the informed consent is *documented*; this provides the distinction that valid informed consent is not merely a signed consent form.[73] After informed consent is obtained by the provider, another person may have the consent form signed, indicating that the provider discussed the relevant treatment's risks and benefits. It should be emphasized that this avenue is fraught with potential peril because the specific details and information of the informed consent will not be as accurately indicated on the form or in the chart as when the medical provider documents the information him- or herself. Therefore, a policy of medical provider documentation of the consent process is highly preferable. Note also that the hospital or other facility generally does *not* have a duty to obtain consent;[74] unless the provider is an employee of the hospital or facility or is acting on its behalf, the provider retains all liability for not obtaining appropriate informed consent.[75] However, note

[69]F. A. Rozovsky, *Consent to Treatment: A Practical Guide,* 2d ed. (Boston: Little Brown Pub. Co., 1990), section 1.16.4; Bernard v. Char, 903 P.2d 676 (Haw. Ct. App. 1995); Cornfeldt v. Tongen, 262 N.W.2d 684 (Minn. 1977); see also Char v. Strode, 904 P.2d 489 (Haw. 1995).

[70]See, e.g., Putensen v. Clay Adams, Inc., 91 Cal.Rptr. 319 (Cal. Ct. App. 1970).

[71]See, e.g., Schreiber v. Physicians Insurance Company of Wisconsin, 588 N.W.2d 26 (Wis. 1999).

[72]See, e.g., Logan v. Greenwich Hosp. Assoc., 465 A.2d 294 (Conn. 1983).

[73]See, e.g., Keomaka v. Zakaib, 811 P.2d 478 (Haw. Ct. App.), cert. denied, 841 P.2d 1075 (Haw. 1991).

[74]See, e.g., Kelley v. Kitahama, 675 So.2d 1181 (La. Ct. App.), cert. denied, 679 So.2d 1352 (La. 1996); Kelley v. Methodist Hosp., 664 A.2d 148 (Pa. Super. Ct. 1995); Perriello v. Kalman, 576 A.2d 474 (Conn. 1990); Kershaw v. Reichert, 445 N.W.2d 16 (N.D. 1989); Johnson v. Sears, Roebuck & Co., 832 P.2d 797 (N.M. Ct. App.), cert. denied, Johnson v. St. Joseph Hosp., 832 P.2d 1223 (N.M. 1992); Mathias v. St. Catherines Hosp., 569 N.W.2d 330 (Wis. Ct. App. 1997); Prindle v. Dogali, 1991 WL 32190 (Conn. Super. Ct. Feb. 22, 1991); Krane v. St. Anthony Hosp., 738 P.2d 75 (Colo. Ct. App. 1987); but see Campbell v. Pitt County Mem. Hosp., 362 S.E.2d 902 (N.C. Ct. App.), aff'd, 362 S.E.2d 273 (N.C. 1987) (hospital has duty to ensure consent obtained); Firter v. Iolab Corp., 607 A.2d 1111 (Pa. Super. Ct. 1992) (hospital in research study can assume duty to obtain consent); Magana v. Elie, 439 N.E.2d 1319 (Ill. App. Ct. 1982).

[75]See, e.g., Fiorentino v. Wenger, 227 N.E.2d 296 (N.Y. 1967); Petriello v. Kalman, 576 A.2d 474 (Conn. 1990); Pauscher v. Iowa Methodist Med. Ctr., 408 N.W.2d 355 (Iowa 1987); Kershaw v. Reighert, 445 N.W.2d 16 (N.D. 1989); Howell v. Spokane & Inland Empire Blood Bank, 785 P.2d 815 (Wash. 1990); Pauscher v. Iowa Methodist Med. Ctr., 408 N.W.2d 355 (Iowa 1985); Roberson v. Menorah Med. Ctr., 588 S.W.2d 134 (Mo. Ct. App. 1979); Cooper v. Curry, 589 P.2d 201 (N.M. Ct. App. 1978).

also that the hospital or other organization may have some liability if the provider reasonably can be seen by a patient as an employee or if enough control is exercised by the employer organization over the providers to make the provider effectively an employee; this usually occurs in hospital-based specialties such as radiology, anesthesiology, pathology, and emergency medicine.[76]

Additional Reading. G. D. Bussey, "Keomaka v. Zakaib: The Physician's Affirmative Duty to Protect Patient Autonomy Through the Process of Informed Consent," *University of Hawaii Law Review* 14 (1992), pp. 801–28; L. B. Frantz, "Modern Status of Views as to General Measure of Physician's Duty to Inform Patient of Risks of Proposed Treatment," in *American Law Reports,* 3d ed. (New York: Lawyers Cooperative Publishing Co., 1978), vol. 88, pp. 1008–44.

Emergency Treatment Exception to Informed Consent

The precept of self-determination that applies to general informed consent also applies to emergency conditions. However, because of the exigencies of medical emergencies, emergency situations limit the general need to obtain full informed consent from patients. Almost universally it has been held that an exception to the requirement of obtaining informed consent is appropriate when a patient is unconscious or lacks capacity and needs immediate medical attention due to the threat of irreparable harm. Many lawsuits[77] and state statutes[78] support this exception.

---

[76]See, e.g., Schagrin v. Wilmington Med. Ctr., 304 A.2d 61 (Del. Super. Ct. 1973); Pamperin v. Trinity Mem'l Hosp., 423 N.W.2d 848 (Wis. 1988); Arthur v. St. Peters Hosp., 405 A.2d 443 (N.J. Super. Ct. Law Div. 1979); Elam v. College Park Hosp., 183 Cal.Rptr. 156 (Cal. Ct. App. 1982); see also Hardy v. Brantley, 471 So.2d 358 (Miss. 1985); Irving v. Doctors Hosp. of Lake Worth, 415 So.2d 55 (Fla. Dist. Ct. App.), *rev. denied*, 422 So.2d 842 (Fla. 1982); Baptist Mem'l Hosp. Sys. v. Sampson, 1998 WL 253914 (Tex. 1998).

[77]See, e.g., Kritzer v. Citron, 224 P.2d 808 (Cal. Ct. App. 1950); Crouch v. Most, 432 P.2d 250 (N.M. 1967).

[78]See, e.g., *California Business and Professions Code* (St. Paul, MN: West, 1997), section 2397; *Florida Statutes Annotated* (St. Paul, MN: West, 1997), section 401.445; *Georgia Code Annotated* §31-9-3 (1997); *Hawaii Revised Statutes Annotated* (Charlottesville, VA: Michie, 1997), section 671-3; *Vermont Statutes Annotated,* tit. 12, §1909 (1997); *Washington Revised Code Annotated* (St. Paul, MN: West, 1997), section 7.70.050. See also *Arkansas Code Annotated* (Charlottesville, VA: Michie, 1997), section 16-114-206; *Connecticut General Statutes Annotated* (St. Paul, MN: West, 1997), section 17A-543; 405 *Illinois Compiled Statutes* (St. Paul, MN: West, 1998), 5/2-111.

Concept.
When a patient is unconscious or lacks capacity, is in need of emergency medical treatment, and the probability of harm from failing to treat is greater than the potential harm of the treatment itself, the medical provider may provide the treatment without informed consent.

Case. A, a 17-year-old minor, was riding on an oil car that was part of a larger freight train. At one point, he decided that he would like to get off the train; and, while the train was moving, he jumped off the car. Unfortunately, due to the motion of the freight train, as A jumped, an iron step on the car immediately behind the one on which he was riding severely cut the plaintiff in the head, forming a deep and heavily bleeding laceration. Further, he was dragged between 50 and 80 feet before being freed from the train. Due to these activities and events, A was found to have an actively bleeding, deep scalp laceration and a crushed elbow joint. His crushed elbow represented a threat to his life unless treated surgically. Dr. Y, a surgeon, was called to see A and verified that his condition was serious. Efforts were made to contact A's parents but to no avail. Therefore, without parental consent, A was placed under anesthetic, and his scalp wound closed and his arm amputated, saving A's life. However, once A's parents could be found and notified of A's condition, they sued Dr. Y for damages associated with a lack of informed consent for the arm amputation. Dr. Y claimed that he was required to act under an emergency situation and that no informed consent was necessary.

Legal Discussion. In this case, the emergency exception obviated the need for informed consent generally required.[79] Because the patient had significant injuries that required immediate action to save his life, the providers in the case were justified in taking the medically appropriate actions to save him. It should be noted that the prudence of the medical providers in attempting to contact the individuals with the power to legally discuss and provide informed consent was exemplary. However, even without this attempt, under the severe emergency circumstances with which the providers were faced, the action to save the patient's life by immediate treatment without informed consent was appropriate.

Notes on the Emergency Treatment Exception

Children and Incompetents

If an emergency involves a minor, generally the same conditions apply for emergency medical circumstances as

---

[79]Jackovach v. Yocom, 237 N.W. 444 (Iowa 1931).

in adults. Therefore, parental informed consent for their child's diagnosis and treatment in a situation where the child's life and health are immediately and imminently threatened is obviated.[80] Further, under the "mature minor" exception, minors themselves may effectively consent to treatment if the specific minor's age, maturity, and ability to understand the risks and benefits of diagnosis and treatment under the circumstances warrant finding that they can knowingly consent to the proffered medical actions.[81] In addition, emancipated minors (i.e., those minors who live, work, and function independently) also may be able to make their own health care decisions, again depending on the facts, circumstances, and law of the state in the case.[82] Generally for incompetents, if no guardian is available, the courts virtually always favor emergency treatment without consent.[83] However, if a guardian or surrogate decision maker is available, that decision maker may be able to assert privacy rights for the incompetent patient and refuse treatment if it is futile or the patient is terminally ill.[84] It is critical in these circumstances to obtain counsel to ascertain the legal statutory and common law landscape to determine the extent of allowable treatment.

---

[80]Jockovach v. Yocom, 237 N.W. 444 (Iowa 1931).

[81]In re Interest of E.G., 515 N.E.2d 286 (Ill. App. Ct. 1987), *aff'd in part, rev'd in part*, 549 N.E.2d 322 (Ill. 1989); Younts v. St. Francis Hosp. & School of Nursing, Inc., 469 P.2d 330 (Kan. 1970).

[82]See, e.g., *Colorado Revised Statutes Annotated* (St. Paul, MN: West, 1997), section 13-22-103; *Delaware Code Annotated,* title 313, section 707(a) (1997); *Louisiana Revised Statutes Annotated* (St. Paul, MN: West, 1997), section 40:1095; *Maryland Code Annotated, Health — General I* §20-102 (1997); *Massachusetts General Laws Annotated* (St. Paul, MN: West, 1997), chapter 112, section 12f; *Michigan Compiled Laws Annotated* (St. Paul, MN: West, 1997), section 722.4; *Montana Code Annotated,* section 41-1-402 (1997); *New Mexico Statutes Annotated* (Charlottesville, VA: Michie, 1997), section 24-10-1; 35 *Pennsylvania Consolidated Statutes Annotated* (St. Paul, MN: West, 1997), section 10101; *Rhode Island Gen. Laws,* section 23-4.6-1 (1997).

[83]Hawaii v. Standard Oil Co., 405 U.S. 251 (1972); In re Darrell Dorone, 534 A.2d 452 (Pa. 1987); In re A.C., 573 A.2d 1235 (D.C. 1990); see also Miller v. Rhode Island Hosp., 625 A.2d 778 (R.I. 1993); In re Guardianship of Brandon, 677 N.E.2d 114 (Mass. 1997).

[84]See, e.g., In re Farrell, 529 A.2d 404 (N.J. 1987); In re Quinlan, 355 A.2d 647 (N.J. 1976), *cert. denied*, 492 U.S. 922 (1976); Corbett v. D'Allesandro, 487 So.2d 368 (Fla. Dist. Ct. App. 1986), *rev. denied*, 492 So.2d 1331 (Fla. 1986); Foody v. Manchester Mem. Hosp., 482 A.2d 713 (Conn. Super. Ct. 1984); Conservatorship of Drabick v. Drabick, 200 Cal.App.3d 185 (Cal. Ct. App. 1988); Severns v. Wilmington Med. Ctr., 421 A.2d 1334 (Del. 1980); see also In the Matter of Edna, 563 N.W.2d 485 (Wis. 1997); In the Matter of Spring, 405 N.E.2d 115 (Mass. 1980).

Additional Reading.   D. L. Dippel, "Someone to Watch over Me: Medical Decision-Making for Hopelessly Ill Incompetent Adult Patients," *Akron Law Review* 24 (1991), pp. 639–80; T. H. Grisso, *Assessing Competence to Consent to Treatment: A Guide for Physicians and Other Health Professionals* (Oxford: Oxford University Press, 1998); J. M. Kun, "Rejecting the Adage 'Children Should Be Seen and Not Heard' — The Mature Minor Doctrine," *Pace Law Review* 16 (1996), pp. 423–62; J. L. Rosato, "The Ultimate Test of Autonomy: Should Minors Have a Right to Make Decisions Regarding Life Sustaining Treatment?" *Rutgers Law Review* 49 (1996), pp. 1–103; D. R. Veilleux, "Medical Practitioner's Liability for Treatment Given Child Without Parent's Consent," in G. L. Bounds, ed., *American Law Reports,* 4th ed. (New York: Lawyers Cooperative Publishing Co., 1989), vol. 67, pp. 511–34.

Consent for One Treatment But Need for Additional Emergency Treatment

The general rule associated with informed consent is that the diagnostic activities or treatments specified are the only ones that may be performed by the medical providers. However, if in the course of diagnosis or treatment the medical provider faces an unanticipated emergency condition that threatens the patient's life or health, the medical provider generally is authorized to treat that condition and will not be liable under the doctrine of informed consent.[85]

Additional Reading.   C. T. Drechsler, "Consent to Treatment," in *American Jurisprudence,* 2d ed. (New York: Lawyers Cooperative Publishing Co., 1981), section 185. See also J. Duff, "Malpractice — Surgeon's Liability for Inadvertently Injuring Organ Other Than That Intended to Be Operated On," in *American Law Reports,* 3d ed. (New York: Lawyers Cooperative Publishing Co., 1972), vol. 37, pp. 464–557.

Full Versus Partial Disclosure

When a conscious patient presents to the emergency room, generally full informed consent is required. However, the relative "fullness" of consent must be measured against the harm associated with such a disclosure. Therefore, in an emergency situation, such as a poisonous snakebite, the medical provider does not have to first fully

---

[85]Douget v. Touri Infirmary, 537 So.2d 251 (La. Ct. App. 1988); Danielson v. Roche, 241 P.2d 1028 (Cal. Ct. App. 1952); Wheeler v. Barker, 208 P.2d 68 (Cal. Ct. App. 1949); Stone v. Goodman, 271 N.Y.S. 500 (N.Y. App. Div. 1934); Barnett v. Barchrach, 34 A.2d 626 (D.C. 1943).

discuss all the various available methods of treating snakebite and the possible consequences, while venom is coursing through the patient's body.[86]

Additional Reading.   G. D. Bussey, "Keomaka v. Zakaib: The Physician's Affirmative Duty to Protect Patient Autonomy Through the Process of Informed Consent," *University of Hawaii Law Review* 14 (1992), pp. 801–28; D. A. Dickerson, "Doctor's Duty to Disclose Life Expectancy Information to Terminally Ill Patients," *Cleveland State Law Review* 43 (1995), pp. 319–50; W. J. McNichols, "Informed Consent Liability in a 'Material Information' Jurisdiction: What Does the Future Portend?" *Oklahoma Law Review* 48 (1995), pp. 711–53.

Immediate and Imminent Harm

The emergency exception applies only when there is a danger of immediate and imminent harm to the patient. Therefore, during authorized diagnosis and treatment, if a physician finds additional, serious medical conditions, he or she cannot treat those conditions unless they immediately and imminently threaten the patient's life and health.[87] Even if the provider is acting in the best interests of the patient by doing additional procedures or rendering additional treatment, he or she may still be liable for lack of informed consent if the medical condition does not come within the emergency exception.[88] So, strict documentation in the patient's chart regarding the injury, the specific threat to life, the immediacy of the threat, the magnitude of the threat, and the necessary treatment that will address the injury of and threat to the patient is necessary. And, significantly, attempts at proxy informed consent that were unsuccessful should be noted in the patient's chart in these circumstances.

Additional Reading.   C. T. Drechsler, "Consent to Treatment," in *American Jurisprudence,* 2d ed. (New York: Lawyers Cooperative Publishing Co., 1981), section 185.

Injury Occurs

In the best of circumstances, at times, emergency treatment may result in harm. However, an informed consent action cannot be the basis of recovery in such situations, since the medical treatment was presumed to have been consented to under the emergency exception.[89]

Additional Reading.   C. T. Drechsler, "Consent to Treatment," in *American Jurisprudence,* 2d ed. (New York: Lawyers Cooperative Publishing Co., 1981), section 185.

Jehovah's Witnesses and Blood Transfusions

Patients have the unequivocal right to refuse lifesaving treatment on the basis of their religious beliefs.[90] Jehovah's witnesses have religious beliefs that prohibit them from receiving blood transfusions. Therefore, even in emergency situations, they may validly refuse to have such transfusions even to save their lives.[91] However, if a patient who lacks capacity to consent requires blood and family members refuse to provide consent, a majority of courts on petition by the medical facility will allow such transfusions if necessary to preserve the patient's life.[92] Courts also may consider whether minor children will be affected by the decision; however, courts have decided both to order[93] and not order[94] these transfusions. In circumstances where religious beliefs conflict with medical treatment, the provider should contact the facility's general counsel's office for guidance on the appropriate protocol to obtain judicial intervention.

---

[86]Crouch v. Most, 432 P.2d 250 (N.M. 1967).

[87]Stafford v. Louisiana State Univ., 448 So.2d 852 (La. Ct. App. 1984).

[88]Chambers v. Nottingham, 96 So.2d 716 (Fla. Dist. Ct. App. 1957); Hively v. Higgs, 523 P. 363 (Or. 1927); Rolater v. Strain, 137 P.2d 96 (Okla. 1913).

[89]Shinn v. St. James Mercy Hosp., 675 F.Supp. 94 (W.D.N.Y.), *aff'd without opinion*, 847 F.2d 836 (2d Cir. 1987).

[90]See, e.g., Holmes v. Silver Cross Hosp., 340 F.Supp. 125 (N.D. Ill. 1972); In re Estate of Brooks, 205 N.E.2d 435 (Ill. 1965); In re Eichner, 420 N.E.2d 64 (N.Y. 1981); see also Fosmire v. Nicoleau, 551 N.E.2d 77 (N.Y. 1990); Montgomery v. Board of Retirement of Kerr County, 33 Cal.App.3d 447 (Cal. Ct. App. 1973).

[91]In the Matter of Melideo, 390 N.Y.S.2d 523 (N.Y. Sup. Ct. 1976); In re Brown, 478 So.2d 1033 (Miss. 1985); Erickson v. Dilgard, 252 N.Y.S.2d 705 (N.Y. Sup. Ct. 1962); St. Mary's Hosp. v. Ramsey, 465 So.2d 666 (Fla. Dist. Ct. App. 1985).

[92]John F. Kennedy Mem. Hosp. v. Heston, 279 A.2d 670 (N.J. 1971); University of Cincinnati v. Edmond, 506 N.E.2d 299 (Ohio 1986).

[93]Crouse Irving Mem. Hosp., Inc. v. Paddock, 485 N.Y.S.2d 443 (N.Y. Sup. Ct. 1985); Satz v. Perlmutter, 362 So.2d 169 (Fla. Dist. Ct. App. 1978); In the Matter of McCauley, 565 N.E.2d 411 (Mass. 1991); In re Tara Cabrera, 522 A.2d 1114 (Pa. Super. Ct. 1989); O.G. v. Baum, 790 S.W.2d 839 (Tex. App. 1990); see also In re Sampson, 317 N.Y.S.2d 641 (N.Y. Fam. Ct. 1970).

[94]See, e.g., Stamford Hosp. v. Vega, 674 A.2d 821 (Conn. 1996); Wons v. Public Health Trust, 500 So.2d 679 (Fla. Dist. Ct. App. 1987).

Additional Reading.   J. T. Gathings, "When Rights Clash: The Conflict Between a Patient's Right to Free Exercise of Religion versus His Child's Right to Life," *Cumberland Law Review* 19 (1988), pp. 585–616; B. A. Liang, "Legal Issues in Transfusing a Jehovah's Witness Patient Following Cesarean Section," *Journal of Clinical Anesthesiology* 7 (1995), pp. 522–24; E. Mayer et al., "Constitutional Protections of Religious Freedom," in *American Jurisprudence,* 2d ed. (New York: Lawyers Cooperative Publishing Co., 1988), section 572; G. K. Russell et al., "Jehovah's Witnesses and the Refusal of Blood Transfusions: A Balance of Interests," *Catholic Lawyer* 33 (1990), pp. 361–81; C. P. Stowell, *Informed Consent for Blood Transfusions* (Bethesda, MD: American Association of Blood Banks, 1997).

Other Family Members

If a patient is unconscious or lacks capacity due to medication or trauma, yet another family member is available, that family member generally can exercise consent for the patient and should be given the opportunity to do so.[95]

Additional Reading.   R. H. Lockwood, "Mental Competency of Patient to Consent to Surgical Operation or Medical Treatment," in *American Law Reports,* 3d ed. (New York: Lawyers Cooperative Publishing Co., 1970), vol. 25, pp. 1439–60.

Further Reading

Emergency Treatment Exception

Drechsler CT. Consent to Treatment. In: *American Jurisprudence,* 2d ed. New York: Lawyers Cooperative Publishing Co., 1981;§191.

Hartman KM, Liang BA. Exceptions to Informed Consent in Emergency Medicine. *Hosp Phys* 1999;35(3):53–59.

Meisel A. The "Exceptions" to the Informed Consent Doctrine: Striking a Balance Between Competing Values in Medical Decisionmaking. *Wis L Rev* 1979;1979:413.

Shugrue RE, Linstromberg K. The Practitioner's Guide to Informed Consent. *Creighton L Rev* 1991;24:881–928.

See Also

McNichols WJ. Informed Consent Liability in a "Material Information" Jurisdiction: What Does the Future Portend? *Okla L Rev* 1995;48:729–53.

---

[95]See, e.g., King v. Our Lady of the Lake Med. Ctr., 623 So.2d 139 (La. Ct. App. 1993)

Other Reading

Boland GL. Doctrines of Lack of Consent and Lack of Informed Consent in Medical Procedure in Louisiana. *La L Rev* 1984;45:1–38.

Drechsler CT. Consent to Treatment. In: *American Jurisprudence,* 2d ed. New York: Lawyers Cooperative Publishing Co., 1981;§187.

Hall MA. A Theory of Economic Informed Consent. *Ga L Rev* 1997;31:511–86.

Heinemann RA. Pushing the Limits of Informed Consent: Johnson v. Kokemoor and Physician-Specific Disclosure. *Wis L Rev* 1997;1079–1121.

Hopper KD, TenHave TR, Tully DA, et al. The Readability of Currently Used Surgical Procedure Consent Forms in the United States. *Surgery* 1998;123:496–503.

Joujan WM. Informed Consent — Legal Competency Not Determinative of Person's Ability to Consent to Medical Treatment — Miller v. Rhode Island Hosp., 625 A.2d 778. *Suffolk U L Rev* 1994;28:271–77.

Keeton WP et al. *Prosser and Keeton on the Law of Torts,* 5th ed. St. Paul, MN: West Publishing Co., 1984;§18.

Liang BA. What Needs to Be Said? Informed Consent in the Context of Spinal Anesthesia. *J Clin Anes* 1996;8:525–27.

Liang BA. *In Initio Invadere*: Issues in Infant Informed Consent, IVs, and Intubation. *J Clin Anes* 1998;10:73–76.

Mancini MR, Gale AT. *Emergency Care and the Law*. Rockville, MD: Aspen Systems Corp., 1981;Chapter 4.

Quimby CW. *Law for the Medical Practitioner*. Washington, DC: AUPHA Press, 1979; Chapter 3.

Schuck PH. Rethinking Informed Consent. *Yale L J* 1994;103:899–959.

Shugrue RE, Linstromberg K. The Practitioner's Guide to Informed Consent. *Creighton L Rev* 1991;24:881–928.

Symposium: Conducting Medical Research on the Decisionally Impaired. *J Health Care L Pol'y* 1998;1:1–300.

Watter P. The Doctrine of Informed Consent: To Inform or Not to Inform. *St Johns L Rev* 1997;71:543–90.

Web Sites

Centers for Disease Control (CDC): *http://www.cdc.gov/ search.htm*

Disclosure forms for informed consent: *http://www. in-forms.com/*

The evolution of informed consent for health care treatment: *http://www.rmf.org/b9130.html*

The issue of informed consent: *http://www.prairienet. org/laleche/detinformed.html*

Informed consent: *http://www.informedconsent.org/*

Informed consent: *http://pw2.netcom.com/~alalli/pageone. html*

Informed consent: *http://www.ozbod.demon.co.uk/consent/ index.html*

Informed consent for genetic research: *http://www.aai.org/ genetics/ashg/policy/pol-25.htm*

Informed consent in pediatrics: *http:www.nocirc.org/ consent/*

Informed consent — the patient's right to know: *http://www. h-leelaw.com/page3.htm*

Law and ethics in medicine: *http://www.vifp.monash.edu. au/PUBLICATIONS/contents.html*

Medical negligence and informed consent in managed care: *http://www.forensic-psych.com/articles/ artmedmal.html*

4

Medical Information, Records, and Confidentiality

Patient medical records represent a history that generally spans the lifetime and experience of the patient. Each test, procedure, provider visit, consent to treatment, and medical impression is memorialized in a patient's medical record. Further, information regarding a patient's psychological state, personal beliefs, HIV status, financial status, and other relevant but private information is also collected in the medical record. Generally, hospitals have been subject to specific requirements regarding the form of medical records. Both private accrediting organizations and public law mandate these standards. For example, the Joint Commission on Accreditation of Healthcare Organizations (JCAHO) requires that the medical record be accurate; include information regarding physical exam, admitting diagnosis, results of all medical evaluations, complications, orders, and notes as well as other reports, discharge summaries, and final diagnoses; be documented in a timely manner with its information readily available and accessible for prompt retrieval; and be stored in a manner to maintain confidentiality and security.[1] Substantively, JCAHO's standards are similar to those of federal regulations for hospitals[2] serving the Medicare program and other sites for care.[3] In addition, the form for medical information (e.g., for electronic transmission and privacy purposes) is mandated by federal law.[4] State requirements range from the very general to the very detailed and once again reiterate the need to assess local conditions to determine legal obligations. Generally, a complete record of the

care provided and relevant supporting activities and discussions must be documented within the medical record and is the standard. If procedures, diagnoses, treatments, or examinations are not documented in the medical record, the provider or organization or both often will have to rebut the presumption that the event did not occur and may be held liable on such a presumption.[5] Indeed, this can extend to *criminal* liability if the omission from the medical record was committed to falsify business records or hide an event that should have been recorded.[6]

Medical records generally should be kept for ten years;[7] however, state laws may change this period of required retention[8] or dictate retention requirements as a

---

[1]JCAHO, *Accreditation Manual for Hospitals* (Oak Brook, IL: JCAHO, 1995), Indicator Measurement Standard 2.3, 7.2.

[2]42 C.F.R. §§405.1026(g), 482.24 (1998).

[3]42 C.F.R. §484.48 (1998) (home health agencies).

[4]42 U.S.C.A. §1320d-2; see also 42 U.S.C.A. §1320d-4.

[5]Collins v. Westlake Comm. Hosp., 312 N.E.2d 614 (Ill. 1974); Larrimore v. Homeopathic Hosp. Ass'n, 181 A.2d 573 (Del. 1963); Hansch v. Hackett, 66 P.2d 1129 (Wash. 1937); Public Health Trust of Dade County v. Valcin, 507 So.2d 596 (Fla. 1987); Thomas v. United States, 660 F.Supp. 216 (D.D.C. 1987); see also Butterfield v. Okubo, 831 P.2d 97 (Utah 1992).

[6]People v. Smithtown Gen. Hosp., 402 N.Y.S.2d 318 (N.Y. Sup. Ct. 1978).

[7]American Hospital Association, *Preservation of Patient Medical Records in Health Care Institutions* (Chicago: AHA, 1990).

[8]See, e.g., *Alabama Administrative Code* §420-5-7.07(a) (1997) (22 years); *Arizona Administrative Code* §R9-10-221 (1997) (3 years); *California Welfare and Institutions Code* (St. Paul, MN: West, 1997), section 14124.1 (3 years); *Regulations of Connecticut State Agencies* §19-13-D3(d) (1998) (25 years); *Hawthorn Revised Statutes Annotated* (Charlottesville, VA: Michie, 1997), section 622-58 (7 years); *Louisiana Revised Statutes Annotated* (St. Paul, MN: West, 1998), section 40:1299.96 (6 years); *Minnesota Statutes Annotated* (St. Paul, MN: West, 1997), section 145.32 (3 years).

function of the type of record.[9] Federal regulations mandate record retention requirements as a function of the specific facility.[10] Medical records generally are considered to be owned by the entity or organization that created them, such as the hospital or group practice, although patients generally have a right to the information contained in them.[11] In relative contrast, physicians and other medical providers have significant latitude in the design and structure of medical records outside their Medicare and Medicaid patients.

However, common to both private offices and hospitals and other health care organizations is the sensitive information contained in the patient's medical record. Therefore, despite some standards relating to the form and substance of the medical records and information contained in them, the critical considerations for legal purposes are the confidentiality of medical information and when this confidentiality may be breached: "there are few problems which have deserved and received more concentrated attention than the protection of the personal information which a patient remits to his [or her] physician."[12]

Confidentiality of Medical Records and Information

For the purposes of literal ownership, medical records are the property of the entity that created them,[13] for example, the hospital, managed care organization, or group practice.

However, the patient generally is considered to have some ownership interest in the information in these records.[14] Physicians and other medical providers are under an affirmative duty to keep the information within these medical records confidential, as indicated by professional ethics pronouncements,[15] formal court decisions, as well as legislative means such as licensing statutes. The policy is to encourage the patient to divulge all relevant information to the provider so that the provider can make a full clinical determination and be able to provide medically appropriate treatment. Without an assurance of confidentiality, the patient might not provide such information and the therapeutic process could be hindered.

The legal mechanisms enforcing confidentiality will generally be state specific. However, under the common law, two general tort theories have been used to delineate the obligations of providers to keep medical record information confidential. Under the first, the unauthorized disclosure by a provider of patient information in his or her medical record constitutes an invasion of privacy. Such an invasion generally consists of an unauthorized release of medical records that constitutes an unwarranted appropriation or exploitation of the patient's personality; publicizing the patient's private affairs with which the public has no legitimate concern; or wrongful intrusion into the patient's private activities that would cause outrage or mental suffering, shame, or humiliation to a person of ordinary sensibilities. The second theory by which courts hold providers liable for unauthorized release of medical records is through a common law rule of confidentiality in the physician–patient relationship. A medical provider who discloses to a third party personal information learned about the patient during the course of treatment may be liable for breach of fiduciary duty of confidentiality between provider and patient, unless such disclosure is justified when there is a danger to the patient or another person. Under this rule, all physicians have an obligation to keep confidential any information obtained during the physician–patient relationship and within the medical record; if they breach this rule, they may be liable for damages in tort.

Concept — Invasion of Privacy.

An invasion of privacy for unauthorized release of medical records requires the unwarranted appropriation or exploitation of one's personality, the publicizing of one's private affairs with which the public

---

[9]See, e.g., *Florida Administrative Code Annotated*, r. 64B1-10.001 (1998) (acupuncturists' medical records 5 years); *Louisiana Revised Statutes Annotated* (St. Paul, MN: West, 1998), section 30:2351.29 (medical surveillance records duration of employment plus 30 years); *Annotated Missouri Statutes* (St. Paul, MN: West, 1998), section 188.060 (medical report of abortion 7 years); *New Jersey Statutes Annotated* (St. Paul, MN: West, 1997), section 26:8-5 (X-ray record 5 years); *Virginia Code Annotated* (Charlottesville, VA: Michie, 1997), section 32.1-274 (birth and death medical records 10 years).

[10]42 C.F.R. §482.24(b)(1) (1998) (hospitals); 42 C.F.R. §486.161 (1998) (physical therapists); 42 C.F.R. §484.48 (1998) (home health agencies); 42 C.F.R. §485.60 (1998) (comprehensive outpatient rehabilitation facilities).

[11]Waldron v. Ball Corp., 619 N.Y.S.2d 841 (N.Y. App. Div. 1994); Pyramid Life Ins. Co. v. Masonic Hosp. Ass'n, 191 F.Supp. 51 (W.D. Okla. 1961); Connell v. Medical & Surgical Clinic, 315 N.E.2d 278 (Ill. App. Ct. 1974); Gerson v. New York Women's Med., 671 N.Y.S.2d 104 (N.Y. App. Div. 1998); Clay v. Little Co. of Mary Hosp., 660 N.E.2d 123 (Ill. App. Ct. 1995); see also Cornelio v. Stamford Hosp., 1997 WL 430619 (Conn. Super. Ct. July 21, 1997); Baker v. Alexander, 745 S.W.2d 112 (Tex. App. 1988).

[12]Hammonds v. Aetna Casualty & Surety Co., 243 F.Supp. 793, 797 (N.D. Ohio 1965).

[13]McGarry v. J.A. Mercier Co., 262 N.W. 296 (Mich. 1935).

[14]Bishop Clarkson Mem. Hosp. v. Reserve Life Ins. Co., 350 F.2d 1006 (8th Cir. 1965); Pyramid Life Ins. Co. v. Masonic Hosp. Ass'n, 191 F.Supp. 51 (W.D. Okla. 1961).

[15]American Medical Association, "Principles of Medical Ethics — Confidentiality," in *Current Opinions of the Judicial Council of the American Medical Association* (Chicago: AMA, 1984).

has no legitimate concern, or the wrongful intrusion into one's private activities in such a manner as to outrage or cause mental suffering, shame, or humiliation to a person of ordinary sensibilities.

Case. Patient BP was an inpatient in the Hospital for the treatment of alcoholism from December 1981 to January 1982. She was attended by Dr. S. Dr. S and the Hospital noted that all information regarding her hospitalization was confidential. Near the end of her stay in the Hospital, an insurance claim form was filled out by Dr. S indicating her diagnosis of "acute and chronic alcoholism detoxification." This form was sent to a colleague of BP's spouse, LD; BP obtained health benefits through the spouse's employment. LD was not authorized to receive the claim form; but on receipt, he opened the envelope and saw BP's diagnosis and treatment documentation. BP sued Dr. S, indicating that publication of personal information without permission violated BP's right to privacy. Dr. S claimed that no such violation occurred since the disclosure was unintentional.

Legal Discussion. It appears that under the common law of privacy in the jurisdiction on which this illustration is based, Dr. S may have violated BP's right to privacy in medical records.[16] In this case, there is no question that Dr. S did send the offending records to a third party, thus publicizing them. It is also unchallenged that LD, the person to which the materials were sent, was not an individual or member of the public who had a legitimate concern with the information contained in the letter. Finally, the court in this illustration indicated that it is immaterial whether the disclosure was intentional or merely negligent; both have the effect of an unwarranted intrusion on the privacy of BP. Therefore, Dr. S may be considered to have violated BP's right to privacy when he sent the information to LD and hence may be liable for damages in tort for invasion of BP's privacy.

Concept — Breach of Confidentiality.
A medical provider who discloses to a third party a patient's personal information learned during course of treatment may be liable for breach of the fiduciary duty of confidentiality between provider and patient unless such disclosure is justified, as when there is a danger to the patient or another person.

Case. VM had entered into treatment with psychiatrist Dr. C. During this physician–patient relationship, VM revealed intimate details regarding himself and his personal feelings. However, during this relationship, Dr. C revealed some of the information garnered during these

therapy sessions to VM's spouse. This disclosure resulted in an end to VM's marriage, loss of employment, financial difficulties, and psychological stress that required additional psychotherapy. VM sued Dr. C for breach of Dr. C's fiduciary duty of confidentiality in the physician–patient relationship. Dr. C claimed that VM's spouse had the right to know VM's psychological problems and it was not a breach of confidentiality to speak about VM to VM's spouse.

Legal Discussion. It appears that Dr. C violated VM's right to confidentiality in the physician–patient relationship according to the case on which this illustration is based.[17] Clearly, there was a physician–patient relationship in this case between Dr. C and VM. As well, it was undisputed that Dr. C revealed some of what was said during the therapy sessions by VM to VM's spouse. At this juncture, Dr. C violated VM's right to confidentiality in the physician–patient relationship, unless there existed some danger to the patient or another person requiring disclosure. There was no such danger extant in this case; therefore, Dr. C violated VM's right to confidentiality in the physician–patient relationship and was liable for tort damages relating to the harm VM suffered as a result.

Notes on Confidentiality of Medical Records

Altering, Appending, and Correcting Medical Records

Medical records can be altered and corrected for valid purposes, such as transcribing errors or noting new information relevant to that aspect of the patient's care. These changes should be noted clearly by making a single line through the portion of the record to be altered, corrected, or appended, with the date of the change and the person's signature noted conspicuously. Further, an explanation as to why the record is being altered, corrected, or appended should be placed in the chart.[18] The exact form by which these changes are made in the medical record is dictated by state regulation, medical bylaws, or both. Generally, the purpose of changing a medical record should be to correct erroneous data or clarify information relevant to the patient's clinical condition; allowing for view of previous notes will assist to avoid any charges that the record was altered for self-serving purposes. Changes to a medical record that are made for purposes such as fraud or

[16]Prince v. St. Francis-St. George Hosp., Inc., 484 N.E.2d 265 (Ohio Ct. App. 1985).

[17]MacDonald v. Clinger, 446 N.Y.S.2d 801 (N.Y. App. Div. 1982).

[18]See, e.g., W. H. Roach, *Medical Records and the Law,* 2d ed. (Gaithersburg, MD: Aspen, 1994), pp. 34–36; J. P. Tomes, *Healthcare Records* (Dubuque, IA: Kendall/Hunt Publishing, 1990), pp. 147–149; Uniform Health-Care Information Act, *Uniform Laws Annotated,* §4-102 (1997).

intent to deceive, in some states, are subject to criminal and civil penalties (including punitive damages), medical board sanctions for unprofessional conduct, and may result in loss of licensure and malpractice insurance.[19]

Additional Reading. L. E. Foster and S. A. Nye, *Confidentiality of Health Records: The Meeting of Law Ethics and Clinical Issues* (New York: Amereon Press, 1981); B. R. Furrow et al., *Health Law,* vol.1 (St. Paul, MN: West Publishing Co., 1995), p. 234; C. I. Hanson et al., *California Physician's Legal Handbook* (Sacramento: California Medical Association, 1991), vol. 17, p. 31; E. P. Richards and K. C. Rathbun, *Law and the Physician* (Boston: Little Brown and Co., 1993), p. 76; W. H. Roach, *Medical Records and the Law,* 2d ed. (Gaithersburg, MD: Aspen, 1994), pp. 34–36; J. P. Tomes, *Healthcare Records* (Dubuque, IA: Kendall/Hunt Publishing, 1990), pp. 147–49.

Disclosure of Identity

The scope of the confidentiality relationship between the provider and patient is broad. The patient's identity, even to his or her own kin, is also within the patient's right to confidentiality under the physician–patient relationship. Therefore, a physician who delivered a patient's daughter was held to be answerable to the patient after the physician assisted the daughter in finding out her mother's identity after the child had been put up for adoption.[20] Another concern with regard to identity is when patients are used as material for a book. This use also lies within the scope of the confidentiality relationship, and a provider who utilizes such materials without the consent of the patient once again may be liable for damages in tort even if the patient's name is not disclosed.[21] Finally, it is important to note that disclosure of confidential patient information in legal actions that do not relate to any patient cause of action may violate confidentiality laws.[22]

Additional Reading. H. P. Drummond, *Jurisprudence and Confidentiality: Index of Modern Information,* rev. ed. (Washington, DC: ABBE Publishers Association, 1991); B. Friedland, "Physician Patient Confidentiality,"

Journal of Legal Medicine 15 (1994), pp. 249–77; S. M. Gilles, "Promises Betrayed: Breach of Confidence as a Remedy for Invasions of Privacy," *Buffalo Law Review* 43 (1995), pp. 1–84; "Patient's Record Disclosure in Unrelated Suit May Violate Medical Confidentiality Statute," *BNA Health Law Reporter* 7 (1998), pp. 341–42; "Physician Not Immune from Discipline for Disclosing Patient Records in Litigation," *BNA Health Law Reporter* 7 (1998), pp. 258–59.

Disclosure to Patient's Opponents in Legal Actions

Many courts hold that providers have a duty to their patients to assist them in litigation and not to assist the patient's adversary.[23] Violation of such a principle by disclosing sensitive medical information from the patient's record may be a breach of the confidential relationship between physician and patient.[24] These considerations generally attend only in civil trials; however, in criminal trials, the testimony of the provider is not privileged and therefore is allowed.[25] On the other hand, providers may be called on to discuss the patient's health condition in actions against hospitals and other parties even when they are not parties to the action themselves. In these cases, courts generally have held that when patients bring such actions and their providers disclose information regarding the patients' condition, providers are not liable for inappropriate disclosure if patients put their physical status at issue[26] or the information would be discoverable and therefore available to the opponent regardless.[27] This split in the perspective of duty to the patient with regard to medical information in litigation thus provides hazards in assessing what information may be disclosed and what may not. It is imperative that providers from whom information is requested be cognizant of their state law with regard to this duty and seek legal counsel when information is requested. Note that even when a subpoena for the medical information is issued, providers may not rely on

---

[19]See, e.g., Mirkin v. Med. Mutual Liab. Ins. Soc'y of Maryland, 572 A.2d 1126 (Md.Spec.App. 1990); Smith v. Sup. Ct. of Los Angeles, 190 Cal.Rptr. 829 (Cal. App. 1984); *California Business and Professions Code* §2262; *California Penal Code* §471.5.

[20]Humphers v. First Interstate Bank of Oregon, 696 P.2d 527 (Or. 1985).

[21]Doe v. Roe, 400 N.Y.S.2d 668 (N.Y. Sup. Ct. 1977).

[22]See, e.g., Huhta v. State Bd. of Med., 706 A.2d 1275 (Pa.Cmwlth. 1998); Warner v. Lerner, 705 A.2d 1169 (Md. App. 1998).

[23]See, e.g., Spaulding v. Hussain, 551 A.2d 1022 (N.J. Super. Ct. App. Div. 1988); Alexander v. Knight, 177 A.2d 142 (Pa. Super. Ct. 1962); Coralluzzo v. Fass, 435 So.2d 262 (Fla. Dist. Ct. App. 1983) (*in dissent*); Hammonds v. Aetna Casualty and Surety Co., 243 F.Supp. 793 (N.D. Ohio 1965); see also Manion v. N.P.W. Med. Ctr., 676 F.Supp. 585 (M.D. Pa. 1987); Morris v. Consolidation Coal Co., 446 S.E.2d 648 (W. Va. 1994).

[24]Alexander v. Knight, 177 A.2d 142 (Pa. Super. Ct. 1962); Shafer v. Spicer, 215 N.W.2d 134 (S.D. 1974).

[25]Clark v. Grigson, 579 S.W.2d 263 (Tex. Civ. App. 1978).

[26]Fedell v. Wierzbieniec, 485 N.Y.S.2d 460 (N.Y. Sup. Ct. 1985); Glenn v. Kerlin, 248 So.2d 834 (La. Ct. App. 1971); Street v. Hedgepath, 607 A.2d 1238 (D.C. 1992); Aufrichtig v. Lowell, 609 N.Y.S.2d 214 (N.Y. App. Div. 1994).

[27]Mull v. String, 448 So.2d 952 (Ala. 1984).

this for protection, since generally no relevance determination is made when such court orders issue.[28]

Additional Reading. D. M. Allison, "Physician Retaliation: Can the Physician-Patient Relationship Be Protected?" *Dickinson Law Review* 94 (1990), pp. 975–79; C. L. Companion, "Point: Fairness Demands Equal Access," *South Carolina Law* 9 (1997), pp. 37–41; J. E. Zelin, "Physicians Tort Liability for Unauthorized Disclosure of Confidential Information About Patient," in *American Law Reports,* 4th ed. (New York: Lawyers Cooperative Publishing Co., 1987), vol. 48, pp. 668–713.

Drug and Alcohol Information

There are strict requirements to maintain confidentiality of patient records regarding alcohol and drug abuse for patients participating in any federally assisted drug or alcohol abuse program, including those at hospitals and other facilities that provide alcohol or drug abuse diagnosis, treatment, or treatment referrals.[29] The regulations for these facilities preempt any state laws that allow for purported disclosure of this information, although states may pass valid laws that are more stringent than the federal requirements. The consent for disclosure of this information will be valid only if the patient consents to disclosure to a particular party in writing and the facility provides in writing to the patient-approved party the facility's name or program name, the name or title of the person to receive the information, the patient's name, the purpose or need for the disclosure, the extent or nature of the information to be disclosed, a declaration that the consent may be revoked and the time when the consent will expire automatically, the patient's signature, and the date of the signature.[30] There are specialized requirements for minors.[31] Note, however, that it appears there is no implied private cause of action for violations of these confidentiality rules as a federal cause of action; these cases may be brought in state court as an invasion of privacy claim.[32]

Additional Reading. R. C. Boldt, "A Study in Regulatory Method, Local Political Cultures and Jurisprudential Voice: The Application of Federal Confidentiality Law to Project Head Start," *Michigan Law Review* 93 (1995), pp. 2325–76; B. E. Lype, "How to Get Patient Records from Federally-Assisted Substance Abuse Education and Reha-

bilitation Facilities," *Tennessee Bar Journal* 30 (1994), pp. 30–33; D. V. Snyder, "Disclosure of Medical Information Under Louisiana and Federal Law," *Tulane Law Review* 65 (1990), pp. 192–98; G. B. Upton, "ADAPCP Confidentiality Protections on Sentencing," *Army Law* 1989 (1989), pp. 44–49.

Health Insurance Portability and Accountability Act of 1996

This federal law created a new federal crime for wrongful disclosure of health information and carries with it a fine up to $50,000 and/or imprisonment of up to one year; this penalty increases to $100,000 and five years if the perpetrator acts under false pretenses; and the penalty increases to $250,000 and ten years if the crime occurs for commercial purposes, personal gain, or malicious harm.[33] The law prohibits inappropriate disclosure of information that could be used to identify an individual, including any information that a provider obtains with regard to the individual's physical or mental health, his or her health care, or his or her payment for health care. Exceptions are made in the law for provider referrals and research.

Additional Reading. F. Gilbert, "Privacy of Medical Records? The Health Insurance Portability and Accountability Act of 1996 Creates a Framework for the Establishment of Security Standards and the Protection of Individually Identifiable Health Information," *North Dakota Law Review* 73 (1997), pp. 93–108.

The Hippocratic Oath

Professional responsibility to keep patient–physician communications confidential is imbued within the Hippocratic oath:

> I will abstain [when treating patients] . . . from whatever is deleterious and mischievous. . . . Whatever, in connection with my professional practice, or not in connection with it, I may see or hear in the lives of men which ought not to be spoken abroad I will not divulge, as reckoning that all such should be kept secret.

Additional Reading. R. M. Gellman, "Prescribing Privacy: The Uncertain Role of the Physician in the Protection of Patient Privacy," *North Carolina Law Review* 62 (1984), pp. 267–71; C. E. Koop, "Introduction," *Duquesne Law Review* 35 (1996), pp. 1–4; B. A. Rich, "Postmodern Medicine: Deconstructing the Hippocratic Oath," *University of Colorado Law Review* 65 (1993), pp.

---

[28]Allen v. Smith, 368 S.E.2d 924 (W. Va. 1988).

[29]42 U.S.C.A. §§290 dd-3, 290 ee-3; 42 C.F.R. §2.11 (1998).

[30]42 C.F.R. Part 2 (1998).

[31]42 C.F.R. §2.14 (1998).

[32]See Kathleen "S" v. Ochsner Clinic, 1997 WL 786229 (E.D. La. Dec. 18, 1997).

---

[33]42 U.S.C.A. §1320d-6.

77–136. See also R. M. Berry, "The Genetic Revolution and the Physician's Duty of Confidentiality," *Journal of Legal Medicine* 18 (1997), pp. 401–41.

HIV Status

Generally, HIV status is strictly confidential; indeed, parties such as employers and health insurers in some states cannot mandate testing. Many states have passed statutes that specifically apply to disclosure of medical information regarding HIV[34] and impose both *criminal* and *civil* penalties (including punitive damages) against providers who violate these tenets.[35] Therefore, any time records or other information that includes any mention of a patient's HIV status is requested, the provider would be prudent to remove any mention of HIV from the report unless specifically authorized in writing by the patient. Courts stringently have attempted to minimize identification of persons with HIV or AIDS, although sometimes allowing for limited disclosure.[36] Some allowable disclosure circumstances of patient HIV status are indicated later.[37]

---

[34]See, e.g., *California Health and Safety Code* (St. Paul, MN: West, 1997), section 121075; *General Statutes of Connecticut Annotated* (St. Paul, MN: West, 1997), section §19a-583; *Hawthorn Revised Statutes Annotated* (Charlottesville, VA: Michie, 1997), section 325-101; 410 *Illinois Compiled Statutes Annotated* (St. Paul, MN: West, 1998), 305/9; *Louisiana Revised Statutes Annotated* (St. Paul, MN: West, 1997), section 40:1300.11; *Annotated Statutes of Missouri* (St. Paul, MN: West, 1997), section 191.656; *New York Public Health Law* (St. Paul, MN: West, 1997), section 2782; *Ohio Revised Code Annotated* (St. Paul, MN: West, 1998), section 3701.243; 35 *Pennsylvania Consolidated Statutes Annotated* (St. Paul, MN: West, 1997), section 7607; *Washington Revised Code Annotated* (St. Paul, MN: West, 1997), section 70.24.105.

[35]See, e.g., Doe v. Roe, 599 N.Y.S.2d 350 (N.Y. App. Div. 1993); see also *Arizona Revised Statutes Annotated* (St. Paul, MN: West, 1997), section 36-667; *California Health and Safety Code* (St. Paul, MN: West, 1997), section 121110; *California Health and Safety Code* (St. Paul, MN: West, 1997), section 20980; *Michigan Compiled Laws Annotated* (St. Paul, MN: West, 1997), section 333.513; *Annotated Missouri Statutes* (St. Paul, MN: West, 1997), section 191.656; *New York Public Health Law* (St. Paul, MN: West, 1997), section 2783; *Ohio Revised Code Annotated* (St. Paul, MN: West, 1998), section 3701.244; *Texas Health and Safety Code Annotated* (St. Paul, MN: West, 1997), section 81.63.

[36]Doe v. Shady Grove, 598 A.2d 507 (Md. Ct. Spec. App. 1991); Behringer v. Medical Ctr. at Princeton, 592 A.2d 1251, 1272 (N.J. Super. Ct. Law Div. 1991); Arnold v. American Nat'l Red Cross, 639 N.E.2d 484 (Ohio Ct. App. 1994); Rasmussen v. South Florida Blood Serv., 500 So.2d 533 (Fla. 1987); Boutte v. Blood Sys., 127 F.R.D. 122 (W.D. La. 1989); Watson v. Lowcountry Red Cross, 974 F.2d 482 (4th Cir. 1992).

[37]See the section "Notes on Allowable Disclosures."

Additional Reading. U. Colella, "HIV-Related Information and the Tension Between Confidentiality and Liberal Discovery," *Journal of Legal Medicine* 16 (1995), pp. 33–100; B. A. McDonald, "Ethical Problems for Physicians Raised by AIDS and HIV Infection: Conflicting Legal Obligations of Confidentiality and Disclosure," *University of California Davis Law Review* 22 (1989), pp. 557–92; S. Taub, "Doctors, AIDS, and Confidentiality in the 1990's," *John Marshall Law Review* 27 (1994), pp. 331–46; R. C. Turkington, "Confidentiality Policy for HIV-Related Information: An Analytical Framework for Sorting Out the Hard and Easy Cases," *Villanova Law Review* 34 (1989), pp. 871–908.

Licensing Statutes

Licensing statutes often mandate that disclosure of patient records or information is unprofessional conduct and may subject the provider to disciplinary action.[38] Similar state statutes that apply to hospitals also require confidentiality of medical records.[39]

Additional Reading. E. Mayer, "Disclosure of Professional Information or Communications," in *New York Jurisprudence,* 2d ed. (New York: Lawyers Cooperative Publishing Co., 1990), section 136; J. E. Zelin, "Physician's Tort Liability for Unauthorized Disclosure of Confidential Information About Patient," in *American Law Reports,* 4th ed. (New York: Lawyers Cooperative Publishing Co., 1987), vol. 48, pp. 668–713. See also M. R. Bower, "Discovery of Plaintiff Medical Information and Protection of Privilege in DES Litigation," *Verdicts, Settlements and Tactics* 12, no. 7 (1992), pp. 222–24.

---

[38]See, e.g., *Arizona Revised Statutes Annotated* (St. Paul, MN: West, 1997), section 36-446.07; *Delaware Code Annotated,* tit. 24, §1731(12) (1997); *Florida Statutes Annotated* (St. Paul, MN: West, 1997), section 455.667; 225 *Illinois Compiled Statutes Annotated* (St. Paul, MN: West, 1998), 60/22(30); *Kentucky Revised Statutes Annotated* (Charlottesville, VA: Michie, 1996), section 311.595(16); *Minnesota Statutes Annotated* (St. Paul, MN: West, 1997), section 147.091; *Annotated Statutes of Missouri* (St. Paul, MN: West, 1997), section 334.100(k); *North Dakota Century Code* §43-17-31(13) (1997); *Oregon Revised Statutes* §677.190(5) (1997).

[39]See, e.g., *Arizona Revised Statutes Annotated* (St. Paul, MN: West, 1997), section 12-2292; 210 *Illinois Compiled Statutes Annotated* (St. Paul, MN: West, 1998), 85/6.17(b); *Indiana Code Annotated* (St. Paul, MN: West, 1998), section 16-39-6-3; *Iowa Code Annotated* (St. Paul, MN: West, 1997), section 22.7(2); *Minnesota Statutes Annotated* (St. Paul, MN: West, 1997), section 144.651(Sub.Div. 16); *North Carolina General Statutes* §131E-97 (1997); *Tennessee Code Annotated* §10-7-504 (1997).

Medical Malpractice

Breach of confidential information also may be brought as a malpractice claim in some jurisdictions. Because the provider has a duty to maintain appropriate confidences under a professional standard, a breach of that standard can amount to negligence and malpractice.[40] Therefore, it is important to note that even when there is little or no common law or statutory authority specifically indicating that there is no duty to maintain confidences, traditional malpractice may be used to seek damages for these breaches of confidence.

Additional Reading. H. P. Rockwell, "What Patient Claims Against Doctor, Hospital, or Similar Health Care Provider Are Not Subject to Statutes Specifically Governing Actions and Damages for Medical Malpractice," in *American Law Reports,* 4th ed. (New York: Lawyers Cooperative Publishing Co., 1992), vol. 89, pp. 887–995; J. E. Zelin, "Physician's Tort Liability for Unauthorized Disclosure of Confidential Information About Patient," in *American Law Reports,* 4th ed. (New York: Lawyers Cooperative Publishing Co., 1987), vol. 48, pp. 668–713. See also C. T. Drechsler, "Relation of Physician and Patient," in *American Jurisprudence,* 2d ed. (New York: Lawyers Cooperative Publishing Co., 1981), section 172.

Other Causes of Action

Beyond the standard tort causes of action just indicated, patients have brought actions for breaches of medical record confidentiality under intentional infliction of emotional distress[41] and breach of implied contract causes of action.[42] Of importance is that the former requires extreme and outrageous conduct and the latter is amenable to the generally longer statute of limitations for breach of contract actions as opposed to general tort injuries. However, as in the standard breach of confidentiality or privacy, the plaintiff must still show inappropriate disclosure of confidential information.

Additional Reading. R. E. Harris, "The Need to Know versus the Right to Know: Privacy of Patient Medical Data in an Information-Based Society," *Suffolk University Law Review* 30 (1997), pp. 1210–13; G. M. Mowery, "A Patient's Right of Privacy in Computerized Pharmacy Records," *University of Cincinnati Law Review* 66 (1998), pp. 712–15.

Physician–Patient Privilege

A majority of states have statutes providing for a physician–patient privilege that allows the provider to *not* disclose information in circumstances where the provider is compelled to testify, including testimony at trial, depositions, or administrative hearings. These statutes focus on circumstances where the patient may not be suing or has not placed his or her condition at issue. This privilege is held by the patient, and only he or she may waive it to allow the provider to testify. However, it should be emphasized that this privilege does not apply in circumstances where the patient *is* putting his or her medical condition at issue or has waived his or her right in some other way. Note that states without such statutes generally do not have a physician–patient privilege because the common law does not recognize this form of privilege,[43] and so the provider must testify in these circumstances. However, some of these states are adopting a psychiatrist–patient privilege and a psychologist–patient privilege due to the sensitive nature of mental health therapy and communication.[44] The privilege extends only to circumstances where there is a true provider–patient relationship and only to communication between the parties;[45] hence, there is some question as to whether third parties, such as nurses, are included within the privilege.[46] This latter concern

[43]John W. Strong et al., *McCormick on Evidence,* 4th ed. (St. Paul, MN: West, 1992), section 98.

[44]See, e.g., *Alabama Code* §34-26-2 (1997); *California Evidence Code* (St. Paul, MN: West, 1997), section 1012; *General Statutes of Connecticut Annotated* (St. Paul, MN: West, 1997), section 52-146d-i; *Florida Statutes Annotated* (St. Paul, MN: West, 1997), section 90.503; *Maryland Code Annotated, Courts and Judicial Proceedings* §9-909 (1997); *Annotated Laws of Massachusetts* (New York: Lawyers Cooperative Publishing Co., 1997), chapter 112, §129A; *Michigan Compiled Laws Annotated* (St. Paul, MN: West, 1997), section 333.18237; *New Mexico Statutes Annotated* (Charlottesville, VA: Michie, 1996), section 11-504; *North Dakota Century Code* §503 (1992); 42 *Pennsylvania Consolidated Statutes Annotated* (St. Paul, MN: West, 1997), section 5944; *Tennessee Code Annotated* §24-1-207 (1997); *Wisconsin Statutes Annotated* (St. Paul, MN: West, 1997), section 905.04.

[45]See McMaster v. Board of Psychology Exam'rs., 509 N.W.2d 754, 757 (Iowa 1993), *cert. denied,* 114 S.Ct. 2165 (1994) (privilege did not bar disclosure of confidential medical records since privilege only extended to testimony).

[46]See State v. Gulleckson, 383 N.W.2d 338, 340 (Minn. Ct. App. 1986) (privilege destroyed by presence of third party unless third parties necessary and communication was confidential for diagnostic and treatment purposes); Darnell v. State of Indiana, 674 N.E.2d 19 (Ind. Ct. App. 1996); Benton v. Superior Ct., 897 P.2d 1352 (Ariz. Ct. App. 1995), *rev. denied* (Ariz. July 13, 1995); State v. LaRoche, 442 A.2d 602 (N.H. 1982); see also In the Matter of C.P., 563 N.E.2d 1275 (Ind. 1990); People v. Hanf, 611 N.Y.S.2d 85 (N.Y. Sup. Ct. 1994).

[40]Saur v. Probes, 476 N.W.2d 496 (Mich. Ct. App. 1991).

[41]Humphers v. First Interstate Bank, 684 P.2d 581 (Or. Ct. App. 1984), *aff'd in part, rev'd in part,* 696 P.2d 527 (Or. 1985).

[42]Doe v. Roe, 400 N.Y.S.2d 668, 674 (N.Y. Sup. Ct. 1977).

requires careful assessment of the wording of the state statute to determine if and when the privilege applies.

Additional Reading.   B. W. Best, "Privilege, in Judicial or Quasi-Judicial Proceedings, Arising from Relationship Between Psychiatrist or Psychologist and Patient," in *American Law Reports,* 3d ed. (New York: Lawyers Cooperative Publishing Co., 1973), vol. 44, pp. 24–162; R. M. Gellman, "Prescribing Privacy: The Uncertain Role of the Physician in the Protection of Patient Privacy," *North Carolina Law Review* 62 (1984), pp. 255–94; J. V. McHale, *Medical Confidentiality and Legal Privilege* (New York: Routledge, 1993); D. W. Shuman, "The Origins of the Physician-Patient Privilege and Professional Secret," *Southwestern Law Journal* 39 (1985), pp. 661–87; W. E. Wakefield, "Physician-Patient Privilege as Extending to Patient's Medical or Hospital Records," in *American Law Reports,* 4th ed. (New York: Lawyers Cooperative Publishing Co., 1981), vol. 10, pp. 552–88.

Pictures

Pictures and films of the patient also fall within the scope of an invasion of privacy claim and indeed can support such a claim. Therefore, a physician such as a surgeon who takes before and after pictures of or films an individual and uses them without the patient's permission can be held to have invaded the privacy of the patient, even if the patient's name is not disclosed.[47] Similarly, pictures of a deceased that are used without the family's permission may be the basis of invasion of privacy suits.[48]

Additional Reading.   J. E. Zelin, "Physician's Tort Liability for Unauthorized Disclosure of Confidential Information About Patient," in *American Law Reports,* 4th ed. (New York: Lawyers Cooperative Publishing Co., 1987), vol. 48, pp. 668–713. See also B. D. Goldstein, "Confidentiality and Dissemination of Personal Information: An Examination of State Laws Governing Data Protection," *Emory Law Journal* 41 (1992), pp. 1185–1236.

Statutes

In addition to the common law, many state licensing and professions statutes for medicine indicate specifically that physicians and other providers may not reveal confidences of patients without their consent. For example, in New York,

§4504. Physician, dentist, podiatrist, chiropractor, and nurse

(a) Confidential information privileged. Unless the patient waives the privilege, a person authorized to practice medicine, registered professional nursing, licensed practical nursing, dentistry, podiatry, or chiropractic shall not be allowed to disclose any information which he acquired in attending a patient in a professional capacity, and which was necessary to enable him to act in that capacity.[49]

Therefore, in addition to the duties under the common law of privacy and confidentiality in the physician–patient relationship, statutes also may provide the grounds for suit as well as loss of licensure for medical providers who inappropriately disclose patient information.[50]

Additional Reading.   E. Klugman, "Toward a Uniform Right to Medical Records: A Proposal for a Model Patient Access and Information Practices Statute," *UCLA Law Review* 30 (1983), pp. 1349–85; J. K. Levin and T. R. Smyth, "Freedom of Information Acts," in *American Jurisprudence,* 2d ed. (New York: Lawyers Cooperative Publishing Co., 1994), section 267; J. M. Madden, "Patient Access to Medical Records in Washington," *Washington Law Review* 57 (1982), pp. 697–713.

Allowable Disclosures

Under certain circumstances the medical provider can disclose potentially embarrassing or private information without the patient's consent. However, these disclosures are circumscribed and thus quite limited in their scope. The general duty of nondisclosure continues to attend. Namely, providers should not disclose patient records and the information in them unless given express permission by the patient; otherwise, the providers may be liable in tort for damages.

Waiver

The first method by which a provider may validly disclose medical record information is through a patient waiver. A waiver generally centers around providers rendering their opinion regarding the patient and a dispute that directly relates to the condition of the patient; that is, the patient is putting his or her very medical status in

---

[47]Vassiliades v. Garfinckel's, 492 A.2d 580 (D.C. 1985); Feeney v. Young, 181 N.Y.S. 481 (N.Y. App. Div. 1920); Griffin v. Medical Soc. of State, 11 N.Y.S.2d 109 (N.Y. Sup. Ct. 1939).

[48]See, e.g., Reid v. Pierce Cty., 961 P.2d 333 (Wash. 1998).

[49]CPLR §4504(a) in McKinney's Consolidated Laws of New York (St. Paul, MN: West, 1997).

[50]Simonsen v. Swenson, 177 N.W. 831 (Neb. 1920); Abelson's, Inc. v. New Jersey State Bd. of Optometrists, 75 A.2d 867 (N.J. 1950); Berry v. Moench, 331 P.2d 814 (Utah 1958); Felis v. Greenberg, 273 N.Y.S.2d 288 (N.Y. Sup. Ct. 1966).

question in the dispute.[51] Under these circumstances, when the focus of the conflict is on the patient's medical status, generally the provider who discloses such information is not liable for invasion of privacy or breach of confidentiality due to the qualified nature of these patient protections.

Concept.

An individual's right to privacy and confidentiality in his or her medical records is qualified when he or she has filed suit for personal injuries, and disclosure of relevant information to the suit is not actionable against the provider.

Case. PM was seen at the Hospital emergency room, where she was diagnosed by an intern as having pelvic inflammatory disease. She was given a prescription for antibiotics and then left the emergency room. However, her condition worsened to such an extent that she went to another facility, where she saw Dr. K. Due to her condition, Dr. K performed a total hysterectomy on PM. After discharge and follow-up with her primary care physician, PM brought suit against the Hospital and Dr. K. The Hospital, through its insurance company, hired attorney DM. The insurance company wrote to Dr. K and requested he speak with DM. Neither PM nor her attorney was notified of or invited to this meeting. Dr. K met with DM and, while speaking with both DM and another employee of the insurance company, provided information about the diagnosis and treatment of PM. Later, PM's attorney indicated to DM that PM would be calling Dr. K as an expert witness, at which time DM informed PM's attorney that Dr. K had spoken with DM. PM, through her attorney, immediately notified Dr. K that Dr. K's communications with DM were unauthorized; however, Dr. K continued to meet with the defense counsel, allowed DM to review and copy portions of PM's medical records, and then testified as a fact (rather than an expert) witness. PM then sued Dr. K for breach of the physician–patient duty of confidentiality. Dr. K indicated that the duty was inapplicable in this case.

Legal Discussion. It appears that Dr. K was permitted to provide such information in the suit on which this

illustration is based.[52] It is apparent that the patient in this case had instituted a medical malpractice suit and thus placed her medical condition at issue. Despite the privilege for confidentiality of patient records, filing a suit reduced that expectation of privacy, since she should have anticipated that there would be some investigation as to whether her claims were true. Indeed, when patients file malpractice actions for personal injury, they implicitly consent to disclosures by their physicians concerning their medical conditions. As well, since the physician was testifying in the normal course of a judicial proceeding and the testimony was relevant and material with regard to that proceeding, on the basis of Supreme Court precedent, it was immune from liability for its content.[53] This immunity extends to pretrial communications. However, if the disclosure by the physician were not relevant nor material to the proceedings, the physician could lose the privilege and be subject to a cause of action based on a breach of confidentiality in the physician–patient relationship. Since that was not the case here, Dr. K was not liable for any improper disclosure of PM's medical records.

Case. TJ was referred by his employer to Dr. S for neuropsychological assessment. TJ believed that, on the basis of employment, TJ had a claim for workers' compensation. Dr. S performed this assessment and prepared a report that was detrimental to TJ's efforts to obtain workers' compensation benefits. Dr. S provided TJ with a copy of the report, and at the time the report was given, TJ indicated that the contents were understood and he was not in disagreement with them. However, the next day, TJ called Dr. S and indicated that the report was incorrect and should not have been written. Although TJ had another appointment with Dr. S, it was not kept. TJ then requested that another provider, Dr. O, do the assessment. On the instruction of the insurance carrier investigating TJ's workers' compensation claim, Dr. S forwarded Dr. O all pertinent testing results and reports with regard to TJ's case as well as discussed TJ's findings. Several months later, Dr. S was served with a summons indicating that TJ was suing Dr. S for violating TJ's right to privacy by disclosing the results of Dr. S's evaluation to Dr. O. Dr. S indicated that there was no violation of TJ's rights.

Legal Discussion. Dr. S did not violate TJ's privacy interests by releasing the assessment information to Dr. O as indicated by the case on which this illustration is based.[54] The information transmitted to Dr. O was forwarded on the basis of a request from the insurance carrier

[51]See, e.g., Heller v. Norcal Mut. Ins. Co., 876 P.2d 999 (Cal.), *cert. denied*, 513 U.S. 1059 (1994); *California Civil Code Annotated* (St. Paul, MN: West, 1997), section 56.10(8)(a); *Iowa Code Annotated* (St. Paul, MN: West, 1997), section 622.10; *Louisiana Revised Statutes Annotated* (St. Paul, MN: West, 1997), section 510 (b)(2); *Maine Revised Statutes Annotated* (St. Paul, MN: West, 1997), tit. 32, section 1092-a; *Montana Code Annotated* §50-16-535 (1997); *General Laws of Rhode Island* (St. Paul, MN: West, 1997), section 9-17-24; *Texas Revised Civil Statutes Annotated* (St. Paul, MN: West, 1997), art. 4495b, section 5.08(g).

[52]Moses v. McWilliams, 549 A.2d 950 (Pa. Super. Ct. 1988).
[53]Briscoe v. Lahue, 460 U.S. 325, 330-3 (1983).
[54]Jarallah v. Schwartz, 413 S.E.2d 210 (Ga. Ct. App. 1992).

investigating TJ's workers' compensation claim. Dr. S was entitled to disclose medical information to Dr. O because this medical information was relevant to the nature and extent of TJ's injuries in the context of determining whether TJ's claim was valid. Thus, Dr. S did not violate TJ's privacy rights and was not liable in tort for any damages TJ may have suffered.

Public Duty

The second basis for allowed disclosure stems from an official, public duty. Generally, if providers are asked to render an official opinion for a court or provide information pursuant to an official government requirement or law, reporting the relevant information therein to the appropriate authority is no violation of the patient's right to privacy or confidentiality.

Concept.
A provider that, under the auspices of a formal public duty such as a court order, discloses relevant information gleaned from seeing patients is permitted to disclose that information to the appropriate authorities without liability for breach of the patient's confidentiality or privacy.

Case.   DB was divorced from JL in 1978. At that time, DB was awarded custody of their son. In 1982, DB petitioned the court to allow her to move out of state with the child; DB planned to remarry in the new state. JL responded to this petition by requesting custody of the child. To resolve this conflict, the court sought the guidance of a psychologist, CP. The court requested that CP do a "custody evaluation." On May 16, 1982, CP recommended that DB be allowed to move out of state with the child and indicated that it would not be "psychologically detrimental" for the child to be moved away from JL. Accordingly, the court on May 24 permitted DB to move with her child. However, on November 10, 1982, JL requested the court to modify the earlier order because, JL claimed, since the move, DB was trying to alienate the child from JL. DB had spoken on the phone with CP regarding certain issues associated with the purported behavior. On this basis, accompanying the request for modification was a letter written by CP, addressed to the court, that outlined DB's attempts to prevent JL from seeing the child under the visitation plan in the earlier order. CP's letter further indicated that this conduct would cause the child to "suffer emotionally" and that it indicated "a more severe emotional difficulty on DB's part than was initially evident." These conclusions were partially based on CP's discussion with DB. On learning of this information, DB sued CP for invasion of privacy and breach of confidentiality.

Legal Discussion.   CP is most likely not liable for any breach of confidentiality or privacy for the disclosures regarding DB according to the case on which this illustration is based.[55] CP was consulted by the court for the purpose of child custody proceedings and performed evaluations on that basis. All information that was relevant to this role was privileged and not subject to disclosure limitations. Therefore, the information disclosed during the custody evaluation and the subsequent letter, which went directly to the issue of DB's fitness as a parent, were immune from liability due to their relevance to the custody matter. Further, even though the letter was subsequent to the initial proceedings, this fact alone did not eliminate the privilege, since CP was under an obligation to report any relevant factors to the court so it could make an appropriate custody determination. Since CP did not disclose any other information that might have been associated with therapy but not relevant to the custody proceedings, CP stayed within the permissible scope of disclosure. Consequently, CP was not liable to DB for disclosure of the information in the letter.

Public Welfare

Disclosure without patient permission also is valid when the disclosure is necessary to protect the public interest. Public interest in this context generally includes warning of a foreseeable danger or circumstances of possible death.[56]

Concept.
Provider disclosure of information obtained from a patient–provider relationship is not actionable as a breach of a patient's confidentiality or privacy and is mandated by public policy if it benefits the public welfare by warning of a foreseeable danger or harm to an individual or identifiable class of persons or assists public authorities in investigating a crime.

Case.   PP was a mentally disturbed student who was seeing Dr. M, a psychologist. PP indicated to Dr. M that he intended to kill TT. Dr. M requested that PP be detained by the police; PP was detained but then was released after he appeared rational. Two months later, however, PP in fact did kill TT. TT's parents sued Dr. M,

[55]Bond v. Pecaut, 561 F.Supp. 1037 (N.D. Ill. 1983).
[56]See, e.g., Lundgren v. Fultz, 354 N.W.2d 25 (Minn. 1984); Hamman v. County of Maricopa, 775 P.2d 1122 (Ariz. 1989); Davis v. Puryear, 673 So.2d 1298 (La. Ct. App. 1996); Bardoni v. Kim, 390 N.W.2d 218 (Mich. Ct. App. 1986); Mavroudis v. Superior Ct., 162 Cal.Rptr. 724 (Cal. Ct. App. 1980); White v. United States, 780 F.2d 97 (D.C. 1986); Evans v. Morehead Clinic, 749 S.W.2d 696 (Ky. Ct. App. 1988); see also Hutchinson v. Patel, 637 So.2d 415 (La. 1994).

alleging that Dr. M had a duty to TT to warn of the danger posed by PP. Dr. M claimed that there was no duty.

Legal Discussion.   Dr. M most likely is liable for failing to warn TT of the harm posed by PP on the basis of the case on which this illustration is based.[57] Here, there was a patient–provider relationship between PP and Dr. M. Further, there was a direct threat to an individual, TT, revealed through PP's discussions with Dr. M. The discussions Dr. M had with PP indicated that Dr. M had knowledge of the foreseeable danger to TT's life through PP's statements that he wanted to kill TT. On this basis, even though Dr. M notified the police, Dr. M also was mandated by this identifiable danger to warn TT. Since Dr. M did not, Dr. M was liable for damages associated with TT's death.

Case.   During a rape in which DB was the perpetrator, DB was bitten by his victim on his penis. The bite was severe enough to temporarily disable DB, allowing his victim to escape. DB then attempted to obtain medical care for the injury. At first, he went to the local emergency room and obtained treatment and was discharged. However, after this initial visit, DB continued to experience pain and what appeared to be an infection on his penis. DB called the hospital and attempted to speak with the physician who treated him. However, that physician was not present. Instead, Dr. T, an associate of DB's treating physician, accepted the call. Dr. T listened to DB, assessed the relevant information, and then called in a prescription for antibiotics. However, after calling in the prescription, Dr. T heard several hospital employees speaking to each other about a request for information by the police department. The police were looking for a suspected rapist who had injuries similar to DB's. Dr. T then consulted hospital authorities, legal counsel for the state medical society, and DB's original physician regarding the propriety of speaking with the police about DB. Each party indicated that it was permissible to speak with police authorities. Dr. T then reported his discussions with DB to the police. Subsequently, DB was questioned by the police, arrested, and convicted of rape. DB then brought suit against Dr. T for breach of physician–patient confidentiality.

Legal Discussion.   It appears that Dr. T would not be liable for disclosure of DB's medical information to the police according to the case on which this illustration is based.[58] In this case, the information that Dr. T obtained through his discussion with DB arguably could be considered to fall under a physician–patient relationship.

However, Dr. T's subsequent disclosure of critical identifying information to the police enabled them to apprehend a rapist and bring him to trial. This directly assisted public authorities in their investigation of a crime and benefited the public welfare; therefore, it was within the public policy exception and not actionable as a breach of the patient's privacy or confidentiality.

Notes on Allowable Disclosures

Custody Proceedings—Variations

Generally, when mental health providers are called on by the court or by the parties in lawsuits to give information with regard to parental fitness, the disclosures made by these providers are not held to be in violation of the patient's right to confidentiality. By calling the provider to testify, patients have been held to have waived their rights;[59] disclosures from court-ordered examinations have been held to be privileged and therefore not subject to liability.[60] This latter conclusion still attends even if the party whose information is disclosed has paid for the evaluation.[61] However, the privileged disclosure of information in these custody cases is limited; additional disclosure beyond that necessary for child custody purposes or disclosure of information that would not be admissible in such a hearing can subject the provider to liability.[62] Similarly, in divorce proceedings, where a provider disclosed information regarding the divorce, this disclosure also is protected if the examination is court ordered.[63]

Additional Reading.   C. R. Courtade, "Child Abuse, Custody or Neglect Proceedings," *American Jurisprudence,* 2d ed. (New York: Lawyers Cooperative Publishing Co., 1992), section 457; D. V. Snyder, "Disclosure of Medical Information Under Louisiana and Federal Law," *Tulane Law Review* 65 (1990), pp. 169–202.

Disclosure of Information to Employer

Generally, it has been held that disclosure of information by a provider to an employer is not in violation of a

---

[57]Tarasoff v. Regents of University of Cal., 551 P.2d 334 (Cal. 1976).

[58]Bryson v. Tillinghast, 749 P.2d 110 (Okla. 1988).

[59]Jordan v. Kelly, 728 F.2d 1 (1st Cir. 1984); Werner v. Kliewer, 710 P.2d 1250 (Kan. 1985).

[60]Bond v. Pecaut, 561 F.Supp. 1037 (N.D. Ill. 1983), *aff'd without opinion*, 734 F.2d 18 (7th Cir. 1983); Anderson v. Glismann, 577 F.Supp. 1506 (D. Colo. 1984).

[61]Anderson v. Glismann, 577 F.Supp. 1506 (D. Colo. 1984).

[62]Schaffer v. Spicer, 215 N.W.2d 134 (S.D. 1974).

[63]Guity v. Kandilakis, 821 S.W.2d 595 (Tenn. Ct. App. 1991), *reh'g denied*, 1991 Tenn.App. LEXIS 652 (Tenn. 1992).

patient's right to confidentiality or privacy if that information is of direct and legitimate interest to the employer. These circumstances are similar to workers' compensation cases, and courts often will hold that employers have a right to such information. Therefore, providers who supply such information are not liable.[64] However, it is important to note that, once again, the information that legitimately can be disclosed is limited to that which is directly relevant to the employer with respect to the employee; other information, even if relevant to the present work-related injury or circumstance (such as a previous history of a similar injury), may be in violation of the patient's confidentiality and privacy if disclosed without authorization.[65] Note also that if providers obtain information regarding HIV-positive status that is not directly relevant to the patient's workers' compensation claim, it has been held that liability may attach if this information is disclosed to employers, since the disclosure by the provider in these circumstances is not privileged.[66]

Additional Reading.   B. Friedland, "Physician-Patient Confidentiality," *Journal of Legal Medicine* 15 (1994), pp. 257–59; J. E. Zelin, "Physician's Tort Liability for Unauthorized Disclosure of Confidential Information About Patient," in *American Law Reports,* 4th ed. (New York: Lawyers Cooperative Publishing Co., 1987), vol. 48, pp. 668–713. See also J. P. Lundington, "Physician's Duties and Liabilities to Person Examined Pursuant to Physician's Contract with Such Person's Prospective or Actual Employer or Insurer," in *American Law Reports,* 3d ed. (New York: Lawyers Cooperative Publishing Co., 1967), vol. 10, pp. 1071–77.

Duty to Warn in the Public Interest—Variations

Information on foreseeable harm obtained through the special relationship between providers and patients generally creates a duty to warn.[67] While some courts require

that a *specific* individual be identified,[68] others impose a more general duty.[69] Providers also may be liable if they merely warn rather than institute other precautions, including confinement.[70] Further, this liability may extend to providers not warning their patients of potential risks and harms of their medical conditions,[71] including a duty to warn children through their parents as to the ramifications of their genetic disease transmissibility.[72] In addition, this requirement to warn may be applicable to warning family members of a contagious or sexually transmissible disease,[73] including, in some states, HIV. Of course, if the warning is provided under appropriate circumstances such as these, no liability will attend the provider for such disclosures.[74]

Additional Reading.   A. L. Almason, "Personal Liability Implications of the Duty to Warn Are Hard Pills to Swallow: From Tarasoff to Hutchinson v. Patel and Beyond," *Journal of Contemporary Health Law and Policy* 13 (1997), pp. 471–96; J. C. Beck, "The Psychotherapist's Duty to Protect Third Parties from Harm," *Mental and Physical Disability Law Reporter* 11 (1987), pp. 141–47; L. J. Deftos, "Genomic Torts: The Law of the Future — The Duty of Physicians to Disclose the Presence of a Genetic Disease to the Relatives of Their Patients with the Disease," *University of San Francisco Law Review* 1997;32:105-37; J. D. Piorkowski, "Between a Rock and a Hard Place: AIDS and the Conflicting Physician's Duties of Preventing Disease Transmission and Safeguarding Confidentiality," *Georgetown Law Journal* 76 (1987), pp. 169–202.

---

[64]See, e.g., Payne v. Sherrer, 458 S.E.2d 916 (Ga. Ct. App. 1995); Childs v. Williams, 825 S.W.2d 4 (Mo. Ct. App. 1992); Clark v. Geraci, 208 N.Y.S.2d 564 (N.Y. Sup. Ct. 1960).

[65]Acosta v. Cary, 365 So.2d 4 (La. Ct. App. 1978); see also Morris v. Consolidation Coal Co., 446 S.E.2d 648 (W. Va. 1994).

[66]Urbaniak v. Newton, 277 Cal.Rptr. 354 (Cal. Ct. App. 1991).

[67]See, e.g., Tarasoff v. Regents of Univ. of Cal., 551 P.2d 334 (Cal. 1976); Williams v. Sun Valley Hosp., 723 S.W.2d 783 (Tex. App. 1987); Peck v. Counseling Serv., Inc., 499 A.2d 422 (Vt. 1985); Webb v. Jarvis, 575 N.E.2d 992 (Ind. 1991); see also Tuman v. Genesis Assoc., 894 F.Supp. 183 (E.D. Pa. 1995) (parents who contracted to have daughter treated for bulimia had both contract and tort causes of action against counselor for counselor implantation of false memories that foreseeably could harm parents).

[68]See, e.g., Brady v. Hopper, 751 F.2d 329 (10th Cir. 1984); Elis v. Peter, 627 N.Y.S.2d 707 (N.Y. App. Div. 1995); Kirk v. Michael Reese Hosp. & Med. Ctr., 513 N.E.2d 387 (Ill. 1987), *cert. denied*, 485 U.S. 905 (1988); Purdy v. Public Admin., 514 N.Y.S.2d 407 (N.Y. App. Div. 1987); Thompson v. County of Alameda, 614 P.2d 728 (Cal. 1980).

[69]See, e.g., Reisner v. Regents of the Univ. of Cal., 37 Cal.Rptr.2d 518 (Cal. Ct. App. 1995); DiMarco v. Lynch Homes-Chester Cty., 583 A.2d 422 (Pa. 1990); Wilschinsky v. Medina, 775 P.2d 713 (N.M. 1989); Shuster v. Altenberg, 424 N.W.2d 159 (Wis. 1988).

[70]Lipari v. Sears Robuck & Co., 497 F.Supp. 185 (D. Neb. 1980); Hamman v. County of Maricopa, 775 P.2d 1122 (Ariz. 1989).

[71]See, e.g., Myers v. Quesenberry, 193 Cal.Rptr. 733 (Cal. Ct. App. 1983); but see Kirk v. Michael Reese Hosp., 513 N.E.2d 387 (Ill. 1987).

[72]Pate v. Threlkel, 661 So.2d 278 (Fla. 1995).

[73]See, e.g., Marlene F. v. Psychiatric Med. Clinic, 770 P.2d 278 (Cal. 1989); DiMarco v. Lynch Homes-Chester County Inc., 583 A.2d 422 (Pa. 1990); but see Britton v. Soltes, 563 N.E.2d 910 (Ill. App. Ct. 1990).

[74]See, e.g., Oringer v. Rotkin, 556 N.Y.S.2d 67 (N.Y. App. Div. 1990); MacDonald v. Clinger, 446 N.Y.S.2d 801 (N.Y. App. Div. 1982); see also Mavroudis v. Superior Ct., 162 Cal.Rptr. 724 (Cal. Ct. App. 1980).

HIV Status

Prohibitions against reporting do not apply to circumstances when the provider is required by law to report information regarding AIDS incidence and other epidemiological factors to specific authorities (such as state or local departments of public health or the Centers for Disease Control and Prevention) *as specifically delineated by law.*[75] Sexual partners, spouses,[76] and/or needle partners in some states also are allowed to know the HIV status of a patient and, under specific circumstances, are allowed access to that information regardless of patient authorization.[77] Also, many states allow specific HIV disclosure to providers who will be diagnosing or treating the patient.[78] Disclosure also may be permitted by law to

other specified third parties, including adoption agencies,[79] coroners and funeral directors,[80] epidemiologists,[81] and facilities that procure transplant organs, semen for artificial insemination, or blood products,[82] quality assurance and accreditation committees,[83] parents of minors who have been diagnosed with HIV infection,[84] researchers,[85] and victims of sexual offenses.[86] Further, disclosure of HIV status of a physician by hospitals to individuals who may have been affected by contact with the physician has been allowed.[87] However, beyond these narrow circumstances, providers should not give this

---

[75]See, e.g., *Colorado Revised Statutes Annotated* (St. Paul, MN: West, 1997), section 25-4-1403; *Florida Statutes Annotated* (St. Paul, MN: West, 1997), section 384.25; *Georgia Code Annotated* §31-22-9.2 (1997); *Hawaii Revised Statutes Annotated* (Charlottesville, VA: Michie, 1997), section 325-101; 20 *Illinois Compiled Statutes Annotated* (St. Paul, MN: West, 1998), 505/22.3; *Michigan Compiled Laws Annotated* (St. Paul, MN: West, 1997), section 333-5114; *North Carolina General Statutes* §130A-135 (1997); *Ohio Revised Code Annotated* (St. Paul, MN: West, 1998), section 3701.24; *South Carolina Code Annotated* (New York: Lawyers Cooperative Publishing Co., 1997), section 44-29-250; *Texas Health and Safety Code Annotated* (St. Paul, MN: West, 1997), section 81.041; see also *Delaware Code Annotated* tit. 18, §7404 (1997).

[76]See, e.g., Chizmar v. Mackie, 896 P.2d 196 (Alaska 1995) (physician disclosure of mistaken HIV positive result to spouse privileged and not actionable); but see Diaz Reyes v. United States, 770 F.Supp. 58 (D.P.R. 1991) (no privilege recognized to inform spouse of patient's HIV positive status).

[77]See, e.g., *Arizona Revised Statutes Annotated* (St. Paul, MN: West, 1997), section 32-1860; *California Health and Safety Code* (St. Paul, MN: West, 1997), section 121015; *Connecticut General Statutes Annotated* (St. Paul, MN: West, 1997), section 19a-584; *Georgia Code Annotated* §24-9-47 (1997); *Kansas Statutes Annotated* §65-6004 (1996); *Annotated Code of Maryland, Health General I* §18-337 (1997); *Michigan Compiled Laws Annotated* (St. Paul, MN: West, 1997), section 333.5131; *Ohio Revised Code Annotated* (St. Paul, MN: West, 1998), section 3701.243; 35 *Pennsylvania Consolidated Statutes Annotated* (St. Paul, MN: West, 1997), section 7609; *South Carolina Code Annotated* (New York: Lawyers Cooperative Publishing Co., 1997), section 44-29-146; *West Virginia Code* §16-3c-3 (1997).

[78]See, e.g., *Arizona Revised Statutes Annotated* (St. Paul, MN: West, 1997), section 32-1457; *California Health and Safety Code* (St. Paul, MN: West, 1997), section 121015; *Kansas Statutes Annotated* §65-6004 (1997); *North Carolina General Statutes* §130A-143 (1997); *Ohio Revised Code Annotated* (St. Paul, MN: West, 1998), section 3701.243; *Texas Health and Safety Code Annotated* (St. Paul, MN: West, 1997), section 81.103.

[79]See, e.g., *Florida Statutes Annotated* (St. Paul, MN: West, 1997), section 381.004; *Louisiana Revised Statutes Annotated* (St. Paul, MN: West, 1997), section 40:1300.14; *Missouri Annotated Statutes* (St. Paul, MN: West, 1997), section 191.656; *New York Public Health Law* (St. Paul, MN: West, 1997), section 2782(1)(H); *Wisconsin Statutes Annotated* (St. Paul, MN: West, 1997), section 48.371.

[80]See, e.g., *Missouri Annotated Statutes* (St. Paul, MN: West, 1997), section 191.703; *New Jersey Statutes Annotated* (St. Paul, MN: West, 1997), section 26:6-8.2; *West Virginia Code* §16-3c-3 (1997); *Wisconsin Statutes Annotated* (St. Paul, MN: West, 1997), section 252.15.

[81]See, e.g., *North Carolina General Statutes* §130a-143(1) (1997); *Oklahoma Statutes Annotated* (St. Paul, MN: West, 1997), section 1-502.2; *Puerto Rico Laws Annotated* tit. 24, §578 (1994); *Wisconsin Statutes Annotated* (St. Paul, MN: West, 1997), section 252.15.

[82]See, e.g., *Arizona Revised Statutes Annotated* (St. Paul, MN: West, 1997), section 36-664(a)(5); 410 *Illinois Compiled Statutes Annotated* (St. Paul, MN: West, 1998), 305/9; *Louisiana Revised Statutes Annotated* (St. Paul, MN: West, 1997), section 40:1300.14(b)(4); *New York Public Health Law* (St. Paul, MN: West, 1997), section 2782; *Washington Revised Code Annotated* (St. Paul, MN: West, 1997), section 70.24.105; *West Virginia Code* §16-3C-3(a)(7) (1997).

[83]See, e.g., *Arizona Revised Statutes Annotated* (St. Paul, MN: West, 1997), section 36-664(a)(6); *Connecticut General Statutes Annotated* (St. Paul, MN: West, 1997), section 19a-583(a)(6); *Delaware Code Annotated* tit. 16, §1203(a)(7) (1997); *Louisiana Revised Statutes Annotated* (St. Paul, MN: West, 1997), section 40:1300.14(b)(5); *New York Public Health Law* (St. Paul, MN: West, 1997), section 2782(1)(f); 35 *Pennsylvania Consolidated Statutes Annotated* (St. Paul, MN: West, 1997), section 7607(a)(5).

[84]410 *Illinois Compiled Statutes Annotated* (St. Paul, MN: West, 1998), 305/9; *Colorado Revised Statutes Annotated* (St. Paul, MN: West, 1997), section 25-4-1405(6); *Georgia Code Annotated* §24-9-47(c) (1997); *Louisiana Revised Statutes Annotated* (St. Paul, MN: West, 1997), section 15:535(c); *Missouri Annotated Statutes* (St. Paul, MN: West, 1997), section 191.656(2)(f).

[85]See, e.g., *Arizona Revised Statutes Annotated* (St. Paul, MN: West, 1997), section 36-664(b)(4); *California Health and Safety Code* (St. Paul, MN: West, 1997), section 121025; *Louisiana Revised Statutes Annotated* (St. Paul, MN: West, 1997), section 40:1300.14(b)(4); *New Jersey Revised Statutes* (St. Paul, MN: West, 1997), section 26:5C-8.

information to anyone or any organization without express consent of the patient or before checking with legal counsel.[88] On another level, many states either require[89] or rely on voluntary[90] reporting of providers who are HIV positive.

Additional Reading. S. Spillane, "AIDS: Establishing a Physician's Duty to Warn," *Rutgers Law Journal* 21 (1990), pp. 645–67; J. S. Talbot, "The Conflict Between a Doctor's Duty to Warn a Patient's Sexual Partner That the Patient Has AIDS and a Doctor's Duty to Maintain Patient Confidentiality," *Washington and Lee Law Review* 45 (1988), pp. 355–80; "State Statutes or Regulations Expressly Governing Disclosure of Fact That Person Has Tested Positive for Human Immunodeficiency Virus or Acquired Immunodeficiency Syndrome," in *American Law Reports,* 5th ed. (New York: Lawyers Cooperative Publishing Co., 1993), vol. 12, pp. 149–94; M. Wiseman, "Hey Doc, Can You Keep a Secret? An Ohio Physician's Right to Warn Third Parties That They May Be at Risk of Contracting HIV," *Journal of Law and Health* 6 (1992), pp. 199–221.

Medical Providers

In general, all providers involved in care of the patient are entitled access to the patient's medical record. Generally,

regulations,[91] statutes,[92] and accreditation standards[93] allow for such disclosure to medical professionals, and even administrators may have general access for patient care purposes.[94]

Other Public Policy Exceptions

In addition to circumstances of foreseeable harm to an identifiable third party or class of potential parties, other circumstances have been held to be within the purview of allowable disclosure. Two major circumstances are when formal authorities such as the district attorney or police pursuant to a valid court order request the information[95] and, more dramatically, when another's life is being threatened.[96] In these situations, providers may disclose otherwise private and confidential medical information. Note again, however, that it is important to limit the disclosure to that which is requested and directly relevant to the situation; additional information beyond this scope may subject the provider to liability under a breach of privacy or confidentiality.

Additional Reading. J. E. Zelin, "Physician's Tort Liability for Unauthorized Disclosure of Confidential Information About Patient," in *American Law Reports,* 4th ed. (New York: Lawyers Cooperative Publishing Co., 1987), vol. 48, pp. 668–713. See also D. V. Snyder, "Disclosure of Medical Information Under Louisiana and Federal Law," *Tulane Law Review* 65 (1990), pp. 169–202.

---

[86]See, e.g., *Alaska Statutes* (Charlottesville, VA: Michie, 1997), section 18.15.310; *California Penal Code* (St. Paul, MN: West, 1997), section 1524.1; *Colorado Revised Statutes Annotated* (St. Paul, MN: West, 1997), section 18-3-415; *Florida Statutes Annotated* (St. Paul, MN: West, 1997), section 960.003; *Louisiana Revised Statutes Annotated* (St. Paul, MN: West, 1997), section 15.535; *Missouri Annotated Statutes* (St. Paul, MN: West, 1997), section 191.656(2)(g); *Rhode Island General Laws* §11-37-17 (1997); *Tennessee Code Annotated* §39-13-521 (1997); *Texas Health and Safety Code Annotated* (St. Paul, MN: West, 1997), section 81.103(b); *West Virginia Code* §16-3c-3(a)(2) (1997).

[87]See, e.g., In re Application of the Milton S. Hershey Med. Ctr., 634 A.2d 159 (Pa. 1993); see also Behringer v. Medical Ctr. at Princeton, 592 A.2d 1251 (N.J. Super. Ct. Law Div. 1997).

[88]See, e.g., Doe v. High-Tech Institute, Inc., 1998 WL 379926 (Colo. App. July 9, 1998) (plaintiff may recover for both intrusion on seclusion and unreasonable disclosure of private facts when HIV status is disclosed without permission of patient).

[89]See, e.g., *Alabama Code* §22-11A-61 (1997); *Louisiana Revised Statutes Annotated* (St. Paul, MN: West, 1997), section 37:1747; *Minnesota Statutes Annotated* (St. Paul, MN: West, 1997), section 214.19; see also *Nebraska Revised Statutes* §71-534 (1997).

[90]See, e.g., 410 *Illinois Compiled Statutes Annotated* (St. Paul, MN: West, 1998), 325/5.5; *Missouri Annotated Statutes* (St. Paul, MN: West, 1997), section 191.700; *New York Public Health Law* (St. Paul, MN: West, 1997), section 2761.

[91]See, e.g., *Indiana Administrative Code* tit. 410, r. 15-2-8 (1998); *Nevada Administrative Code* ch. 449, §61154 (1998); *New Jersey Administrative Code* tit. 8, §43G-15.1 (1997); *North Carolina Administrative Code* tit. 10, r. 3C.3905 (1997); 25 *Texas Administrative Code* (St. Paul, MN: West, 1997), section 135.9.

[92]See, e.g., *Arizona Revised Statutes Annotated* (St. Paul, MN: West, 1997), section 12-2293; *Minnesota Statutes Annotated* (St. Paul, MN: West, 1997), section 253b.0921; *Rhode Island General Laws* §5-37.3-4 (1997); see also *South Carolina Code Annotated* §44-22-110 (1997).

[93]Joint Commission for Accreditation of Healthcare Organizations, *Accreditation Manual for Hospitals* (Oak Brook, IL: JCAHO, 1995).

[94]Hyman v. Jewish Chronic Disease Hosp., 258 N.Y.S.2d 397 (N.Y. 1965).

[95]Arnett v. Baskous, 856 P.2d 790 (Alaska 1993); In re Search Warrant, 810 F.2d 67 (3d Cir. 1987); Commonwealth v. Kobrin, 479 N.E.2d 674 (Mass. 1985); Chidester v. Needles, 353 N.W.2d 849 (Iowa 1984); People v. Florendo, 420 N.E.2d 506 (Ill. App. Ct. 1981); In re Brink, 42 Ohio Misc.2d 5 (1988).

[96]Viviano v. Moan, 645 So.2d 1301 (La. Ct. App.), *cert. denied,* 650 S.2d 254 (La. 1995).

Other Legal Disclosures

Beyond public policy exceptions to the general privacy and confidentiality obligations for medical information and records, practical disclosures are allowed as dictated by state law. For example, medical records may be released when transferring the patient to another facility[97] or when requested by state medical examiners[98] or department of health officials.[99] Further, information regarding patients with communicable diseases[100] and records of births and deaths[101] generally can be legally disclosed without patient permission. Even abortions are valid subjects for such state reporting requirements,[102] as is the diagnosis of cancer to cancer reporting registries.[103] Other areas of valid disclosure include suspected child abuse,[104] wounds inflicted by sharp instruments that could cause death and all gunshot wounds,[105] or simply all wounds that were a result of a criminal act.[106] In other circumstances, disclosure may be deemed permissible after a balancing test is performed by the court regarding the patient's privacy interest versus public need.[107]

Additional Reading. W. E. Wakefield, "Physician–Patient Privilege as Extending to Patient's Medical or Hospital Records," in *American Law Reports,* 4th ed. (New York: Lawyers Cooperative Publishing Co., 1981), vol. 10, pp. 552–88.

Patient Consent and Access

Of course, if a patient consents to have his or her records released to a particular party, then the provider must release the specific records to that party,[108] and there should be no

[97]See, e.g., *Minnesota Statutes Annotated* (St. Paul, MN: West, 1997), section 144.335(3); *Mississippi Code Annotated* §41-9-79 (1997); *Nevada Revised Statutes Annotated* (Charlottesville, VA: Michie, 1997), section 433.332; *Oregon Revised Statutes* §179.505(6) (1997); *Rhode Island General Laws* §5-37-22(c) (1997); *South Carolina Code Annotated* (New York: Lawyers Cooperative Publishing Co., 1997), section 44-115-30; *Virginia Code Annotated* (Charlottesville, VA: Michie, 1997), section 65.2-604.

[98]See, e.g., *Nevada Revised Statutes Annotated* (Charlottesville, VA: Michie, 1997), section 629.061; *New Hampshire Revised Statutes Annotated* §611-A:10 (1997); *North Carolina General Statutes* §130a-385 (1997); *Rhode Island General Laws* §5-37.3-4(b)(9,10) (1997); see also *Arizona Revised Statutes Annotated* (St. Paul, MN: West, 1997), section 36-445.01.

[99]See, e.g., *New York Mental Hygiene Law* §31.09 (1997).

[100]See, e.g., *Arizona Revised Statutes Annotated* (St. Paul, MN: West, 1997), section 36-665; *Colorado Revised Statutes Annotated* (St. Paul, MN: West, 1997), section 25-1-122; *Connecticut General Statutes* §19a-215 (1997); *Georgia Code Annotated* §31-21-3 (1997); 210 *Illinois Compiled Statutes Annotated* (St. Paul, MN: West, 1997), 85/6.08; *Maine Revised Statutes Annotated* (St. Paul, MN: West, 1997), tit. 22, section 822; *Nevada Revised Statutes Annotated* (Charlottesville, VA: Michie, 1997), section 441A.150; *New York Public Health Law* (St. Paul, MN: West, 1997), section 2101; *Texas Health and Safety Code Annotated* (St. Paul, MN: West, 1997), section 81.046. See Jones v. Stanko, 160 N.E. 456 (Ohio 1928); Derrick v. Ontario Comm. Hosp., 120 Cal.Rptr. 566 (Cal. Ct. App. 1975).

[101]*Idaho Code* §39-1005 (1997); *Maine Revised Statutes Annotated* (St. Paul, MN: West, 1997), tit. 22, section 2706; *Massachusetts General Laws Annotated* (St. Paul, MN: West, 1997), ch. 46, section 3; *New York Public Health Law* (St. Paul, MN: West, 1997), section 4171; *Texas Health and Safety Code Annotated* (St. Paul, MN: West, 1997), section 191.022. See Robinson v. Hamilton, 14 N.W. 202 (Iowa 1882).

[102] 720 *Illinois Compiled Statutes Annotated* (St. Paul, MN: West, 1997), 510/10.1; *Louisiana Revised Statutes Annotated* (St. Paul, MN: West, 1997), section 40:1299.35.10; *Minnesota Statutes Annotated* (St. Paul, MN: West, 1997), section 145.413; *Missouri Annotated Statutes* (St. Paul, MN: West, 1997), section 188.052; *Montana Code Annotated* §50-20-110 (1997); 18 *Pennsylvania Consolidated Statutes Annotated* (St. Paul, MN: West, 1997), section 3214; *South Carolina Code Annotated* (New York: Lawyers Cooperative Publishing Co., 1997), section 44-41-60. See also Planned Parenthood v. Danforth, 428 U.S. 52 (1976); Schulman v. New York City Health & Hosp. Corp., 342 N.E.2d 501 (N.Y. 1975).

[103]See, e.g., *Indiana Code Annotated* (St. Paul, MN: West, 1997), section 16-38-2-3; *Missouri Annotated Statutes* (St. Paul, MN: West, 1997), section 192.655; *Minnesota Statutes Annotated* (St. Paul, MN: West, 1997), section 144.68; *New York Public Health Law* (St. Paul, MN: West, 1997), section 2401; *Ohio Revised Code Annotated* (St. Paul, MN: West, 1997), section 3701.262(c); *Wisconsin Statutes Annotated* (St. Paul, MN: West, 1997), section 255.04.

[104]See, e.g., *California Penal Code* (St. Paul, MN: West, 1997), sections 11166 and 11172; *Ohio Revised Code Annotated* (St. Paul, MN: West, 1997), section 2151.421; *Virginia Code Annotated* (Charlottesville, VA: Michie, 1997), section 63.1-248.3 (Michie 1997); see also Ferraro v. Chadwick, 270 Cal.Rptr. 379 (Cal. Ct. App. 1990).

[105]See, e.g., *New York Penal Law* (St. Paul, MN: West, 1997), section 266.25.

[106]*Iowa Code Annotated* (St. Paul, MN: West, 1997), section 147.111.

[107]See Whalen v. Roe, 429 U.S. 589 (1977); McMaster v. Board of Psychology Exam'rs., 509 N.W.2d 754, 759 (Iowa 1993), *cert. denied*, 114 S.Ct. 2165 (1994); In re Krynicki, 1993 U.S. App. LEXIS 21759 (7th Cir.), *cert. denied*, 510 U.S. 1118 (1994); In re Search Warrant (Sealed), 810 F.2d 67 (3d Cir. 1987), *cert. denied*, 115 S.Ct. 75 (1994); Dr. K. v. State Bd., 632 A.2d 453 (Md. Ct. Spec. App. 1993).

[108]Pyramid Life Ins. Co. v. Masonic Hosp. Ass'n, 191 F.Supp. 51 (W.D. Okla. 1961).

liability for such disclosure.[109] This implies that, in law, patients have a right of access to their medical records,[110] although payment may be required by the provider to have copies made.[111] With regard to minor patients, parents generally have the right of access to a minor child's medical records,[112] but in specific circumstances the parent may not have unfettered access if a provider determines that access is detrimental to the child.[113] Similarly, guardians of mentally incompetent patients generally have access to medical records, but again, there may be a limit on the disclosure if the information sought contains sensitive family information or if full disclosure would be detrimental to the patient's well-being.[114]

Additional Reading. R. E. Harris, "The Need to Know versus the Right to Know: Privacy of Patient Medical Data in an Information-Based Society," *Suffolk University Law Review* 30 (1997), pp. 1183–1218; E. Klugman, "Toward a Uniform Right to Medical Records: A Proposal for a Model Patient Access and Information Practices Statute," *UCLA Law Review* 30 (1983), pp. 1349–85; J. M. Madden, "Patient Access to Medical Records in Washington," *Washington and Lee Law Review* 57 (1982), pp. 697–713.

---

[109]See, e.g., Doe v. North Greenville Hosp., 458 S.E.2d 439 (S.C. Ct. App. 1995).

[110]Wallace v. University Hosps., 170 N.E.2d 261 (Ohio Ct. App. 1960); Hutchins v. Texas Rehab. Comm'n, 544 S.W.2d 802 (Tex. Civ. App. 1976); Clay v. Little Co. of Mary Hosp., 660 N.E.2d 123 (Ill. App. Ct. 1995); Wheeler v. Commissioner of Social Servs. of the City of N.Y., 662 N.Y.S.2d 550 (N.Y. App. Div. 1997); Pyramid Life Ins. Co. v. Masonic Hosp. Ass'n, 191 F.Supp. 51 (W.D. Okla. 1961); see also Doe v. Stincer, 990 F.Supp. 1427 (S.D. Fla. 1997); Gerson v. New York Women's Med., 671 N.Y.S.2d 104 (N.Y. App. Div. 1998); Mitchell v. Subramanya, 538 N.E.2d 319 (Mass. App. Ct. 1989).

[111]Rabens v. Jackson Park Hosp. Found., 351 N.E.2d 276 (Ill. App. Ct. 1976); Clay v. Little Co. of Mary Hosp., 660 N.E.2d 123 (Ill. App. Ct. 1995); Ventura v. Long Island Jewish Hillside Med. Ctr., 492 N.Y.S.2d 96 (N.Y. App. Div. 1985); Hospital Correspondence Corp. v. McRae, 682 So.2d 1177 (Fla. Dist. Ct. App. 1996); see also Graham v. Thompson, 421 N.W.2d 694 (Mich. Ct. App. 1988); Boltja v. Southside Hosp., 582 N.Y.S.2d 635 (N.Y. Sup. Ct. 1992).

[112]McDougal v. McDougal, 422 S.E.2d 636 (W. Va. 1992); see also Leaf v. Iowa Methodist Med. Ctr., 460 N.W.2d 892 (Iowa Ct. App. 1990); *California Family Code* (St. Paul, MN: West, 1997), section 3025; *Maine Revised Statutes Annotated* (St. Paul, MN: West, 1997), tit. 19, section 1653(4); *South Carolina Code Annotated* (New York: Lawyers Cooperative Publishing Co., 1997), section 20-7-100; *Vermont Statutes Annotated* tit. 15, §670 (1997).

[113]In re Daniel C.H., 269 Cal.Rptr. 624 (Cal. Ct. App. 1990); L.E.B. v. Birker, 566 So.2d 907 (Fla. Dist. Ct. App. 1990); L.C.S. v. S.A.S., 453 S.E.2d 580 (Va. Ct. App. 1995).

[114]Gaertner v. State, 187 N.W.2d 429 (Mich. 1971); see also Cynthia v. New Rochelle Hosp. Med. Ctr., 470 N.Y.S.2d 122 (N.Y. 1983).

Public Program Beneficiaries

With the increase in government efforts to prosecute fraud and abuse in the Medicare and Medicaid programs, often investigators seize patient records from providers suspected of such illegal activities. Although it appears that providers may not assert any confidentiality privilege against public investigators, it also appears that the patients themselves have a lower privacy right when they participate in these public health insurance programs. Therefore, it has been held that beneficiaries of the Medicaid program have given up a portion of their privacy interest in their medical records by their participation in the program and that the state when investigating fraud has a compelling interest in the medical records so as to be allowed to seize and use them without patient permission.[115] Indeed, hospitals participating in the Medicaid and Medicare programs are mandated to submit medical record information to the state's Medicaid agency or to the Secretary of Health and Human Services on request, again absent patient consent.[116]

Additional Reading. R. J. Conroy and M. D. Brylski, "Access to Medical Records vs. Patients' Privacy Interests," *New Jersey Law* 173 (1995), pp. 25–28. See also M. Templeton, "The Psychotherapist-Patient Privilege: Are Patients Victims in the Investigation of Medicaid Fraud?" *Indiana Law Review* 19 (1986), pp. 831–51.

Research

Medical records and the information in them may be disclosed to researchers if the institution's IRB[117] evaluates the research project and finds it will be beneficial. These records may be released to the medical investigators with the caveat that the information is to be treated as confidential by the investigators, will be transmitted only to qualified investigators on the basis of an improved research program that is beneficial to the health of the community, and the results of the study will be presented so as to prevent identification of the individual subjects.[118]

Additional Reading. W. E. Parmet, "Public Health Protection and the Privacy of Medical Records," *Harvard Civil Rights–Civil Liberties Law Review* 16 (1981), pp. 265–304.

---

[115]Brillantes v. Superior Ct., 58 Cal.Rptr.2d 770 (Cal. Ct. App. 1997); Chidester v. Needles, 353 N.W.2d 849 (Iowa 1984); Gabor v. Hyland, 399 A.2d 993 (N.J. Super. Ct. App. Div. 1979).

[116]42 C.F.R. §431.107 (1998).

[117]See Research in the Chapter 3 section "Emergency Treatment Exception to Informed Consent."

[118] See 45 C.F.R. Part 46 (1998); 45 C.F.R. § 2.52 (1998).

Spouses

There is significant disagreement with regard to whether providers may disclose medical information to a spouse. On the one hand, although some courts indicate that disclosure by a provider to a spouse of information obtained in a physician–patient relationship sometimes is warranted and so allowed,[119] others have indicated that such a disclosure to a spouse is actionable as a breach of confidentiality.[120] Indeed, some courts have noted that even when the spouse is in divorce proceedings against the patient, disclosure by the provider is permitted.[121] The path of greatest prudence would indicate that all potential disclosures be discussed with the patient first and should occur only with the patient's express, written consent.

Additional Reading. J. E. Zelin, "Physician Tort Liability for Unauthorized Disclosure of Confidential Information About Patient," in *American Law Reports,* 4th ed. (New York: Lawyers Cooperative Publishing Co., 1987), vol. 48, pp. 668–713. See also L. J. Deftos, "Genomic Torts: The Law of the Future—The Duty of Physicians to Disclose the Presence of a Genetic Disease to the Relatives of Their Patients with the Disease," *University of San Francisco Law Review* 32 (1997), pp. 105–37; P. E. DeLaTorre, "Resurrecting a Sunken Ship: An Analysis of Current Judicial Attitudes Toward Public Disclosure Claims," *Southwestern Law Journal* 38 (1985), pp. 1151–85.

Workers' Compensation and Third-Party Examinations

In addition to the common law rule that workers who place their medical state at issue have a lower privacy and confidentiality interest in their medical records, state statutes also may provide for a similar result.[122]

Further Reading

Allowable Disclosures—Public Duty

Parmet WE. Public Health Protection and the Privacy of Medical Records. *Harv CR-CL L Rev* 1981;16:265–304.

---

[119] Pennison v. Provident Life & Accident Ins. Co., 154 So. 2d 617 (La. Ct. App.), *cert denied*, 156 So.2d 226 (La. 1963).

[120] MacDonald v. Clinger, 446 N.Y.S.2d 801 (N.Y. App. Div. 1982).

[121] Mikel v. Abrams, 541 F.Supp. 591, *aff'd without opinion*, 716 F.2d 907 (8th Cir. 1982).

[122] See, e.g., *California Civil Code* (St. Paul, MN: West, 1997), section 56.10(c)(8)(a); 740 *Illinois Comprehensive Statutes Annotated* (St. Paul, MN: West, 1998), 110/10; *Iowa Code Annotated* (St. Paul, MN: West, 1997), section 85.27; *Rhode Island General Laws* (St. Paul, MN: West, 1997), section 9-17-24; *Texas Health and Safety Code* (St. Paul, MN: West, 1997), section 5.08(g).

See Also

Gellman RM. Prescribing Privacy: The Uncertain Role of the Physician in the Protection of Patient Privacy. *NC L Rev* 1984;62:255–94.

Harris RE. The Need to Know versus the Right to Know: Privacy of Patient Medical Data in an Information-Based Society. *Suffolk U L Rev* 1997;30:1183–1218.

Allowable Disclosures—Public Welfare

Andrews LB. Torts and the Double Helix: Malpractice Liability for Failure to Warn of Genetic Risks. *Hous L Rev* 1992;29:149–84.

Bernstein B. Solving the Physician's Dilemma: An HIV Partner-Notification Plan. *Stan L & Pol'y Rev* 1995;6:127–33.

Jones JT. Battered Spouses' Damage Actions Against Non-Reporting Physicians. *DePaul L Rev* 1996;45:191–262.

Neisser J. Disclosing Adolescent Suicidal Impulses to Parents: Protecting the Child or the Confidence? *Ind L Rev* 1993;26:433–68.

Allowable Disclosures—Waiver

Kemper JR. Commencing Action Involving Physical Condition of Plaintiff or Defendant as Waiving Physician-Patient Privilege as to Discovery Proceedings. In: *American Law Reports,* 3d ed. New York: Lawyers Cooperative Publishing Co., 1969;21:912–25.

Wade RA. The Ohio Physician-Patient Privilege: Modified, Revised and Defined. *Ohio St L J* 1989;49:1147–74.

Alteration of Medical Records

Buckner F. Medical Records and Physician Disciplinary Actions. *Med Prac Mgmt* 1996;May–June:284–90.

Buckner F. The Uniform Health-Care Information Act: A Physician's Guide to Record and Health Care Information Management. *J Med Prac Mgmt* 1990;5:207–12.

Roach WH. *Medical Records and the Law,* 2d ed. Gaithersburg, MD: Aspen, 1994;34–36.

Tomes JP. *Healthcare Records.* Dubuque, IA: Kendall/Hunt Publishing, 1990;147–49.

Confidentiality of Medical Records and Information

Andrews BW. Medical Records Liability. *Health Law* 1992;6:11–16.

Drechsler CT. Relation of Physician and Patient. *American Jurisprudence,* 2d ed. New York: Lawyers Cooperative Publishing Co., 1981;§165.

Klugman E. Toward a Uniform Right to Medical Records: A Proposal for a Model Patient Access and Information Practices Statute. *UCLA L Rev* 1983;30:1349–85.

Rosenman H. Patients' Right to Access Their Medical Records: An Argument for Uniform Recognition of a Right of Access in the United States and Australia. *Fordham Int'l L J* 1998;21:1500–57.

Other Reading

Cepelewicz BB. Telemedicine's Licensing and Record-Keeping Risks. *Med Malpractice L & Strategy* 1998;15(3):3–5.

Conroy RJ, Brylski MD. Access to Medical Records vs. Patient's Privacy Interests. *NJ Law* 1995;173:25–28.

Corsey SE. The American Health Security Act and Privacy: What Does It Really Cost? *J Marshall J Computer & Info L* 1994;12:585–602.

Friedland B. Physician–Patient Confidentiality. *J Legal Med* 1994;15:249–77.

Gellman RM. Prescribing Privacy: The Uncertain Role of the Physician in the Protection of Patient Privacy. *NC L Rev* 1984;62:255–94.

Goldstein BD. Confidentiality and Dissemination of Personal Information: An Examination of State Laws Governing Data Protection. *Emory L J* 1992;41:1185–1236.

Harris RE. The Need to Know versus the Right to Know: Privacy of Patient Medical Data in an Information-Based Society. *Suffolk U L Rev* 1997;30:1183–1218.

Parmet WE. Public Health Protection and the Privacy of Medical Records. *Harv CR-CL L Rev* 1981;16:265–304.

Roach WH. *Medical Records and the Law*. New York: Aspen, 1994.

Schuchman H, ed. *Confidentiality of Health Records — The Meeting of Law, Ethics, and Clinical Issues*. New York: Gardner Press, 1982.

Tomes JP. *Healthcare Records Management, Disclosure and Retention*. Chicago: Probus Publishing Co., 1993.

Zelin JE. Physician's Tort Liability for Unauthorized Disclosure of Confidential Information About Patient. In: *American Law Reports,* 4th ed. New York: Lawyers Cooperative Publishing Co., 1987;48:668–713.

Web Sites

The controversy over medical records privacy: *http://www. cptech.org/privacy*

Ethics and the computerization of medicine: *http:// ccme-mac4.bsd.uchicago.edu/CCMEDocs/info*

Exposed — medical privacy: *http://www.washington post.com/wp-srv/national/longterm/exposed/ exposed1.htm*

Health Law Resource on Privacy: *http://www.netreach. net/~wmanning/privacy*

How private is my medical information?: *http://www. privacyrights.org/fs/fs8-med.htm*

Law and Ethics (Chapter 9, "Medical Records, Medical Certificates and Confidentiality"): *http://www.vifp. monash.edu.au/PUBLICATIONS/contents.html*

Medical records and privacy (Electronic Privacy Information Center): *http://www.epic.org/privacy/medical/*

Privacy — medical and psychiatric records and drug testing: *http://www.eff.org/pub/Privacy/Medical/*

The Women's Law Center of Maryland Inc., medical privacy in the information age: access, ethics and accountability — whose right to know?: *http://www. wlcmd.org/*

5

The Provider–Patient Relationship and the Obligation to Treat

In contrast to public accommodations (such as inns) and common carriers, both of which must serve all parties who seek their resources, physicians and other providers are generally under no legal obligation in their professional capacity to practice medicine or render services to all patients.[1] This is true even under emergency circumstances.[2] However, once a provider renders professional services to a patient at the request of the patient, a consensual provider–patient relationship is created,[3] generating certain duties and obligations on the part of the provider. This rela-

tionship generally is founded on principles of contract.[4] For the purposes of this chapter, the key duty and obligation for the provider is to provide nonnegligent care to the patient and to not abandon the patient. Critically, establishing a provider–patient relationship is a necessary condition for all malpractice claims; without such a relationship, the provider owes no duty to the person and cannot be held liable for these claims.[5] In addition, claims of abandonment or obligations regarding notice of terminating patient treatment relationships also based are on a valid provider–patient relationship and the attendant obligations are not extant if no such relationship exists.

Provider–Patient Relationship

For the purposes of simplicity, the physician–patient relationship will be described; however, the principles generally apply to other providers. The existence of a physician–patient relationship is a matter of fact, which focuses on whether the person requested the physician to provide medically appropriate care to him or her and whether the physician accepted the person as his or her patient.

---

[1]See, e.g., St. John v. Pope, 901 S.W.2d 420 (Tex. 1995); Childs v. Weis, 440 S.W.2d 104 (Tex. Civ. App. 1969); Agnew v. Parks, 343 P.2d 118 (Cal. Ct. App. 1959); Hurley v. Eddingfield, 59 N.E. 1058 (Ind. 1901); Rice v. Rinaldo, 119 N.E.2d 657 (Ohio Ct. App. 1951); Weaver v. University of Michigan Bd. of Regents, 506 N.W.2d 264 (Mich. Ct. App. 1993); Watson v. Sharp Air Freight Services, 788 F.Supp. 722 (E.D.N.Y. 1992); Lyons v. Grether, 239 S.E.2d 103 (Va. 1977) but see Bragdon v. Abbott, 118 S.Ct. 2196 (1998) (providers under the Americans with Disabilities Act are public accomodations and cannot discrimate against HIV patients in treatment).

[2]See, e.g., Childs v. Weis, 440 S.W.2d 104 (Tex. Civ. App. 1969); Hiser v. Randolph, 617 P.2d 774 (Ariz. Ct. App. 1980), *overruled on other grounds*, 688 P.2d 647 (Ariz. Ct. App. 1983).

[3]See, e.g., Travelers' Ins. Co. v. Bergeron, 25 F.2d 680 (8th Cir. 1928), *cert. denied*, 278 U.S. 638 (1928); Findlay v. Board of Supervisors, 230 P.2d 526 (Ariz. 1951); Kennedy v. Parrott, 90 S.E.2d 754 (N.C. 1956); Hull v. Enid Gen. Hosp. Found., 152 P.2d 693 (Okla. 1944); Hill v. Kokosky, 463 N.W.2d 265 (Mich. Ct. App. 1990); Weaver v. University of Michigan Bd. of Regents, 506 N.W.2d 264 (Mich. Ct. App. 1993); Pokorny v. Shafer, 1994 WL 65213 (Conn. Super. Ct. Feb. 24, 1994); Miller v. Sullivan, 625 N.Y.S.2d 102 (N.Y. App. Div. 1995).

[4]See, e.g., St. John v. Pope, 901 S.W.2d 420 (Tex. 1995); Spencer v. West, 126 So.2d 423 (La. Ct. App. 1960); Osborne v. Frazor, 425 S.W.2d 768 (Tenn. Ct. App. 1968); Hill v. Kokosky, 463 N.W.2d 265 (Mich. Ct. App. 1990); Walters v. Rinker, 520 N.E.2d 468 (Ind. Ct. App. 1988); Amer v. Akron City Hosp., 351 N.E.2d 479 (Ohio 1976); Green v. Walker, 910 F.2d 291 (5th Cir. 1990).

[5]See, e.g., Easter v. Lexington Mem. Hosp., 278 S.E.2d 253 (N.C. 1981); LoDico v. Caputi, 517 N.Y.S.2d 640 (N.Y. App. Div.), *lv. denied*, 528 N.Y.S.2d 829 (N.Y. 1988); Rand v. Miller, 408 S.E.2d 655 (W.Va. 1991); Hale v. State of New York, 386 N.Y.S.2d 151 (N.Y. App. Div. 1976); Ornelas v. Fry, 727 P.2d 819 (Ariz. 1986); Lee v. City of New York, 560 N.Y.S.2d 700 (N.Y. App. Div. 1991), *lv. denied*, 578 N.Y.S.2d 878 (N.Y. 1991); Hickey v. Travelers' Ins. Co., 558 N.Y.S.2d 554 (N.Y. App. Div. 1990); Twitchell v. MacKay, 434 N.Y.S.2d 516 (N.Y. App. Div. 1980); Anderson v. Glismann, 577 F.Supp. 1506 (D. Colo. 1984); Ortiz v. Shah, 905 S.W.2d 609 (Tex. App. 1995); Willoughby v. Wilkins, 310 S.E.2d 90 (N.C. Ct. App. 1983); Peace v. Weisman, 368 S.E.2d 319 (Ga. Ct. App. 1988).

Concept.

If a person presents to a physician for the purposes of obtaining medical treatment and the physician accepts the person as a patient by undertaking to diagnose or treat him or her, a physician–patient relationship is established.

Case.   JD was a student in the Central School District. JD was a problematic student and teachers and other students frequently complained of his aggressive and disruptive behavior. JD also was a poor achiever scholastically. JD's parents indicated that the difficulties stemmed from developmental problems. In response, JD was given special tutoring and placed in a nonclassroom environment for study and instruction for a portion of the school day. However, even with these efforts, JD's behavioral and learning difficulties continued; therefore, the Committee on the Handicapped for the Central School District determined that JD was "emotionally handicapped" and was transferred out of the school to another educational institution. JD's parents challenged this assessment and sought reconsideration by the Committee. The Committee then hired Dr. T, a psychiatrist, to examine JD and advise the Committee. Dr. T met with JD and JD's parents three times and reported the results of these interviews by letter to the Committee. Only a copy of the first letter was sent to JD's parents. Dr. T then met with the Committee, JD, and JD's parents, where the Committee considered Dr. T's assessments as well as other materials, including reports by JD's teachers. At the end of the meeting, the Committee once again determined that JD should be classified as "emotionally handicapped." JD's parents once again objected to this classification and appealed to an impartial hearing officer. Dr. T testified at that hearing and again indicated the professional opinion that JD was emotionally handicapped. JD's parents presented evidence from other experts contradicting Dr. T's assessment. However, the hearing officer upheld the Committee's and Dr. T's determination. Further, after JD's parents appealed again, the Commissioner of Education affirmed the hearing officer's decision. JD's parents then sued Dr. T for medical malpractice, indicating that Dr. T did not fully investigate JD's background and behavior problems. Dr. T indicated that no malpractice claim could lie because there was no physician–patient relationship.

Legal Discussion.   It appears that Dr. T cannot be held liable for medical malpractice due to a lack of a physician–patient relationship according to the case on which this illustration is based.[6] Damages for medical malpractice can be considered only if there is a physician–patient relationship. However, in this case, no physician–patient relationship was formed between Dr. T and JD or JD's parents. Dr. T was not retained by JD's parents but by the

Committee to provide it a professional opinion regarding JD's potential classification as emotionally handicapped rather than for any diagnostic or treatment reasons. As such, Dr. T was simply employed by the third-party Committee on its behalf for its own purposes. Thus, JD or JD's parents did not present to Dr. T to obtain medical treatment and Dr. T did not accept JD or JD's parents for the purpose of undertaking to diagnose or treat JD as a patient. Therefore, there was no physician–patient relationship and no sustainable medical malpractice claim against Dr. T.

Notes on the Provider–Patient Relationship

Charity Care

A physician–patient relationship may be established even though the care is not for financial remuneration.[7] As long as the requisite provider acceptance of a requesting patient is met, the parties have entered into a relationship that the law recognizes with its attendant duties and obligations.

Additional Reading.   C. T. Drechsler, "Relation of Physician and Patient," in *American Jurisprudence,* 2d ed. (New York: Lawyers Cooperative Publishing Co., 1981), section 159.

Minors

Although the patient–provider relationship is generally considered to be contractual in nature between parties of the age of majority, minors may also enter into a valid relationship with a medical provider, and that medical provider, if accepting the minor as a patient, must treat that minor as he or she would an adult patient.[8]

[6]Davis v. Tirrell, 443 N.Y.S.2d 136 (N.Y. Sup. Ct. 1981); see also Mrachek v. Sunshine Biscuit, 123 N.E.2d 801 (N.Y. 1954); Chiasera v. Employers Ins. Co., 422 N.Y.S.2d 341 (N.Y. Sup. Ct. 1979); In re Hoppe, 289 N.W.2d 613 (Iowa 1980); Day v. Harkins, 961 S.W.2d 278 (Tex. App. 1997); Webb v. T.D., 951 P.2d 1008 (Mont. 1997).

[7] See, e.g., DuBois v. Decker, 29 N.E. 313 (N.Y. 1891); Rule v. Cheeseman, 317 P.2d 472 (Kan. 1957); Greenstein v. Fornell, 257 N.Y.S. 673 (N.Y. Sup. Ct. 1932); see also Madden v. Kuehn, 372 N.E.2d 1131 (Ill. App. Ct. 1978); Vita v. Dolan, 155 N.W. 1077 (Minn. 1916).

[8]See, e.g., Luka v. Lowrie, 136 N.W. 1106 (Mich. 1912); Sullivan v. Montgomery, 279 N.Y.S. 575 (N.Y. Sup. Ct. 1935); Bakker v. Welsh, 108 N.W. 94 (Mich. 1906); Cardwell v. Bechtol, 724 S.W.2d 739 (Tenn. 1987); see also Bishop v. Shurly, 211 N.W. 75 (Mich. 1926).

Additional Reading. S. D. Hawkins, "Protecting the Rights and Interests of Competent Minors in Litigated Medical Treatment Disputes," *Fordham Law Review* 64 (1996), pp. 2075–2132. See also A. Popper, "Averting Malpractice by Information: Informed Consent in the Pediatric Treatment Environment," *DePaul Law Review* 47 (1998), pp. 819–36.

No Direct Request by Patient

Note that the patient requesting medical care need not approach the provider him- or herself to establish a provider–patient relationship. As long as the provider is requested to render care to a person or set of persons by a third party for the purpose of creating a therapeutic relationship and the provider agrees to do so, a provider–patient relationship is established when care is rendered to the actual patient.[9]

Additional Reading. C. T. Drechsler, "Relation of Physician and Patient," in *American Jurisprudence,* 2d ed. (New York: Lawyers Cooperative Publishing Co., 1981), p. 159; J. P. Ludington, "Physician's Duties and Liabilities to Person Examined Pursuant to Physician's Contract with Such Person's Prospective or Actual Employer or Insurer," in *American Law Reports,* 3d ed. (New York: Lawyers Cooperative Publishing Co., 1967), vol. 10, pp. 1071–77; M. A. Meyn, "The Liability of Physicians Who Examine for Third Parties," *Northern Kentucky Law Review* 19 (1992), pp. 333–50.

No Examination or Treatment

Generally, if a physician or other provider has not examined, treated, or rendered services to an individual, no provider–patient relationship is established.[10]

This concept has been held to extend to residents being supervised by attendings: If the attending has no relationship with the resident's patient other than being a supervisor of the resident, the supervising physician has not entered into a physician–patient relationship with the resident's patient.[11] Of course if there is contact, then there is a relationship notwithstanding the supervisory role.[12] Similarly, simply because a physician's name appears on a chart also does not establish a physician–patient relationship;[13] again, care generally must be requested and the physician must accept the patient and provide care to him or her for the relationship to arise. This concept also generally applies to on-call physicians who refuse to see patients,[14] although some courts extend liability in cases where the on-call physician is contractually obligated to provide care.[15] But note that, in the managed care context, a provider who is responsible for making gatekeeper decisions regarding hospital admission or other forms for care of a patient most likely has entered into a provider–patient relationship.[16] And further, in nondirect patient care specialties such as pathology and radiology or consultative specialties such as oncology, provider–patient relationships do exist notwithstanding no direct patient contact when others, such as referring physicians, have contracted with the pathologist, radiologist, or oncologist on the patient's behalf for these specialists'

---

[9]See, e.g., DuBois v. Decker, 29 N.E. 313 (N.Y. 1891); Hand v. Tavera, 864 S.W.2d 678 (Tex. App. 1993); Walters v. Rinker, 520 N.E.2d 468 (Ind. Ct. App. 1988); see also Garay v. County of Bexar, 810 S.W.2d 760 (Tex. App. 1991); McKinney v. Schlatter, 692 N.E.2d 1045 (Ohio Ct. App. 1997).

[10]See, e.g., Dodd-Anderson v. Henderson, 107 F.3d 20 (10th Cir. 1997); Roberts v. Hunter, 426 S.E.2d 797 (S.C. 1993); Saari v. Litman, 486 N.W.2d 813 (Minn. Ct. App. 1992); Hill v. Kokosky, 463 N.W.2d 265 (Mich. Ct. App. 1990); Ervin v. American Guardian Assurance Co., 545 A.2d 354 (Pa. Super. Ct. 1988); Sullenger v. Setco Northwest, 702 P.2d 1139 (Or. Ct. App. 1985); Oliver v. Brock, 342 So.2d 1 (Ala. 1977); Keene v. Wiggins, 138 Cal.Rptr. 3 (Cal. Ct. App. 1977); Miller v. Sullivan, 625 N.Y.S.2d 102 (N.Y. App. Div. 1995); but see McGulpin v. Bessmer, 43 N.W.2d 121 (Iowa 1950) (finding physician–patient relationship when physician told patient he would perform surgery); and O'Neil v. Montefiore Hosp., 202 N.Y.S.2d 436 (N.Y. App. Div. 1960) (holding relationship created when physician listened to patient's symptoms over the phone).

---

[11]See, e.g., Mozingo v. Memorial Hosp., 400 S.E.2d 747 (N.C. Ct. App.), *rev. denied*, 407 S.E.2d 537 (N.C. 1991), *aff'd*, 415 S.E.2d 341 (N.C. 1992).

[12]See, e.g., Rule v. Cheeseman, 317 P.2d 472 (Kan. 1957); Rivera v. Prince George's County Health Dep't, 649 A.2d 1212 (Md. Ct. Spec. App. 1994); see also Dodd-Anderson v. Henderson, 107 F.3d 20 (10th Cir. 1997); Klein v. Boyle, 776 F.Supp. 285 (W.D. Va. 1991).

[13]See, e.g., Mixon v. Cason, 622 So.2d 918 (Ala. 1993); Latiff v. Wyckoff Heights Hosp., 535 N.Y.S.2d 2 (N.Y. App. Div. 1988); Thomas v. Good Samaritan Hosp., 640 N.Y.S.2d 398 (N.Y. Sup. Ct. 1996); Dixon v. Siwy, 661 N.E.2d 600 (Ind. Ct. App. 1996).

[14]See, e.g., Fought v. Solce, 821 S.W.2d 218 (Tex. Civ. App. 1991); Fabian v. Matzko, 344 A.2d 569 (Pa. Super. Ct. 1975); Childs v. Weis, 440 S.W.2d 104 (Tex. Civ. App. 1969); St. John v. Pope, 901 S.W.2d 420 (Tex. 1995); see also Lazzara v. Dreyer Med. Clinic, 458 N.E.2d 958 (Ill. App. Ct. 1983).

[15]See, e.g., Hiser v. Randolph, 617 P.2d 774 (Ariz. Ct. App. 1980), *overruled on other grounds*, 688 P.2d 647 (Ariz. Ct. App. 1983); Mozingo v. Pitt County Mem'l Hosp., 415 S.E.2d 341 (N.C. 1992); Dillon v. Silver, 520 N.Y.S.2d 751 (N.Y. App. Div. 1987); Schendel v. Hennepin County Med. Ctr., 484 N.W.2d 803 (Minn. Ct. App. 1992); Hand v. Tavera, 864 S.W.2d 678 (Tex. App. 1993); see also Rivera v. Prince George's County Health Dep't, 649 A.2d 1212 (Md. Ct. Spec. App. 1994).

[16]See, e.g., Hand v. Tavera, 864 S.W.2d 678 (Tex. App. 1993).

services and with the express or implied consent of the patient.[17]

Additional Reading. A. S. Christakis, "Emergency Room Gatekeeping: A New Twist on Patient Dumping," *Wisconsin Law Review* 1997 (1997), pp. 295–320; C. T. Drechsler, "Relation of Physician and Patient," in *American Jurisprudence,* 2d ed. (New York: Lawyers Cooperative Publishing Co., 1981), section 158; S. M. Glenn, "Liability in the Absence of a Traditional Physician-Patient Relationship: What Every "On-Call" Doctor Should Know: Mozingo v. Pitt County Hospital," *Wake Forest Law Review* 28 (1993), pp. 747–74.

Simple Negligence

Even in circumstances where a physician or other provider is not in a provider–patient relationship with a person, the provider has a general duty not to inflict injury on the person negligently. Therefore, a provider who is employed by another to examine a person must exercise due care in that examination. If injury occurs, the person can sue the provider for simple or ordinary negligence; that is, the provider did not exercise the general duty of all persons to take care in their actions and not injure others.[18] This theory has been extended to referrals from the provider to other practitioners to ensure that foreseeable injuries are not incurred by the examinee.[19] Note that in the typical situation of a third party employing the provider to make an examination of a person for the third party's purposes and injury occurs to the patient, the third party also may be liable for actions or omissions of the provider.[20]

Additional Reading. S. J. Bagley, "Enough Is Enough! Congress and the Courts React to Employers' Medical Screening and Surveillance Procedures," *Dickinson Law*

Review 99 (1995), pp. 723–52; M. A. Meyn, "The Liability of Physicians Who Examine for Third Parties," *Northern Kentucky Law Review* 19 (1992), pp. 333–50.

Telephone Conversations

Generally, mere phone conversations between a treating physician and another physician do not bring the other physician into a physician–patient relationship with the treating physician's patient.[21] However, a physician or other provider who gives medical advice over the phone to a patient, regardless of whether there was physical contact between the parties, has an implied obligation that arises between the provider and patient, since the patient has been accepted by the provider after being engaged for professional services. Therefore, in general, a provider–patient relationship is established by telephone contact.[22] Courts are in conflict over the question as to whether a telephone call made by an individual to set up an appointment is enough to establish a provider–patient relationship: Some courts indicate that this may be enough if the condition is specified;[23] others, however, expressly indicate that a mere call for an appointment does not establish such a relationship.[24] Patients in managed care organizations have been

---

[17]See, e.g., Dougherty v. Gifford, 826 S.W.2d 668 (Tex. App. 1992); Walters v. Rinker, 520 N.E.2d 468 (Ind. Ct. App. 1988); Peterson v. St. Cloud Hosp., 460 N.W.2d 635 (Minn. Ct. App. 1990); Niccoli v. Thompson, 713 S.W.2d 579 (Mo. Ct. App. 1986); Salazar v. United States, 1990 WL 47442 (D. Kan. Mar. 9, 1990); see also Gilinsky v. Indelicato, 894 F.Supp. 86 (E.D.N.Y. 1995).

[18]See, e.g., Pope v. St. John, 862 S.W.2d 657 (Tex. App. 1993); Mrachek v. Sunshine Biscuit, 123 N.E.2d 801 (N.Y. 1954); Daly v. United States, 946 F.2d 1467 (9th Cir. 1991); Green v. Walker, 910 F.2d 291 (5th Cir. 1990); Felton v. Schaeffer, 279 Cal.Rptr. 713 (Cal. Ct. App. 1991); Chiasera v. Employers Ins. Co., 422 N.Y.S.2d 341 (N.Y. Sup. Ct. 1979); Meinze v. Holmes, 532 N.E.2d 170 (Ohio Ct. App. 1987); Gilinsky v. Indelicato, 894 F.Supp. 86 (E.D. N.Y. 1995); Rainer v. Frieman, 682 A.2d 1220 (N.J. Super. Ct. App. Div. 1996).

[19]See, e.g., Greenberg v. Perkins, 845 P.2d 530 (Colo. 1993).

[20]See, e.g., McKinney v. Bellevue Hosp., 584 N.Y.S.2d 538 (N.Y. App. Div. 1992); Daly v. United States, 946 F.2d 1467 (9th Cir. 1991); Knox v. Ingalls Ship Building Corp., 158 F.2d 973 (5th Cir. 1947); see also Caracci v. State, 611 N.Y.S.2d 344 (N.Y. App. Div. 1994); Hill v. Ohio Univ., 62 Ohio Misc.2d 659 (1988); but see Green v. Walker, 910 F.2d 291 (5th Cir. 1990) (holding physician–patient relationship extends to employment physicals).

[21]See, e.g., Reynolds v. Decatur Mem. Hosp., 660 N.E.2d 235 (Ill. App. Ct. 1996) (mere phone conversation between treating pediatrician and neurosurgeon did not create physician–patient relationship between neurosurgeon and patient); Hill v. Kokosky, 463 N.W.2d 265 (Mich. Ct. App. 1990); St. John v. Pope, 901 S.W.2d 420 (Tex. 1995); NBD Bank v. Barry, 566 N.W.2d 47 (Mich. Ct. App. 1997); Flynn v. Bausch, 469 N.W.2d 125 (Neb. 1991); Lopez v. Aziz, 852 S.W.2d 303 (Tex. App. 1993).

[22]See, e.g., Bienz v. Central Suffolk Hosp., 557 N.Y.S.2d 139 (N.Y. App. Div. 1990); Clanton v. Von Hamm, 340 S.E.2d 627 (Ga. Ct. App. 1986); Lyons v. Grether, 239 S.E.2d 103 (Va. 1977); Cogswell v. Chapman, 672 N.Y.S.2d 460 (N.Y. App. Div. 1998); see also Miller v. Sullivan, 625 N.Y.S.2d 102 (N.Y. App. Div. 1995).

[23]See, e.g., Lyons v. Grether, 239 S.E.2d 103 (Va. 1977); O'Neil v. Montefiore Hosp., 202 N.Y.S.2d 436 (N.Y. App. Div. 1960); see also Weaver v. University of Michigan Bd. of Regents, 506 N.W.2d 264 (Mich. Ct. App. 1993); Bienz v. Central Suffolk Hosp., 557 N.Y.S.2d 139 (N.Y. App. Div. 1990).

[24]See, e.g., Weaver v. University of Michigan Bd. of Regents, 506 N.W.2d 264 (Mich. Ct. App. 1993); Giles v. Sanford Mem. Hosp., 371 N.W.2d 635 (Minn. Ct. App. 1985); see also Miller v. Sullivan, 625 N.Y.S.2d 102 (N.Y. App. Div. 1995); Clanton v. Von Haam, 340 S.E.2d 627 (Ga. Ct. App. 1986).

allowed to sue HMOs based on the purported failures of nurses staffing a medical advice telephone line to provide reasonable advice.[25]

Additional Reading. P. F. Granade, "Medical Malpractice Issues Related to the Use of Telemedicine: An Analysis of the Ways in Which Telecommunications Affects the Principles of Medical Malpractice," *North Dakota Law Review* 73 (1997), pp. 65–91; P. F. Granade and J. H. Sander, "Implementing Telemedicine Nationwide: Analyzing the Legal Issues," *Defense Counsel Journal* 63 (1996), pp. 67–73; J. L. Rigelhaupt, "What Constitutes Physician-Patient Relationship for Malpractice Purposes," in *American Law Reports,* 4th ed. (New York: Lawyers Cooperative Publishing Co., 1981), vol. 17, pp. 132–60.

Unconceived Children

A difficult question of whether there is a physician–patient relationship arises regarding unborn, unconceived children. Can a provider be sued for injuries that occur to a subsequently born child while unequivocally being in a physician–patient relationship with the mother before the child is born or conceived? This question boils down to whether the provider reasonably could foresee that the mother would become pregnant. If the provider's relationship with the mother provides no basis for foreseeing that the mother will become pregnant, there generally will be no duty to the unborn, unconceived child.[26] However, if there is some circumstance where it is reasonably foreseeable that the mother will become pregnant, there arises a duty to the unborn, unconceived child such that the physician or other provider must act, such as recommend appropriate immunization screening.[27]

Additional Reading. M. L. Sklan, "Medicine and Law: Recent Developments," *Torts and Insurance Law Journal* 29 (1994), pp. 342–53. See also A. J. Belsky, "Injury as a Matter of Law: Is This the Answer to the Wrongful Life Dilemma?" *University of Baltimore Law Review* 22 (1993), pp. 205–15; A. Enneking, "The Missouri Supreme Court Recognizes Preconception Tort Liability: Lough v. Rolla Women's Clinic Inc.," *UMKC Law Review* 63 (1994), pp. 184–85.

Workers' Compensation and Nontherapeutic Examinations

Generally, workers' compensation and other nontherapeutic examinations are for evaluating the individual for the employer or third party, such as an insurance company, rather than for treating the patient. As such, they do not establish a provider–patient relationship, and so there is no duty on the part of the provider toward the patient.[28] However, some courts have held that if the examination unearths facts that would assist the patient if disclosed, there may be a duty to disclose these facts to the individual.[29] Further, if the provider during the examination offers medical advice or treats the person, a provider–patient relationship has been established with all its attendant duties and obligations.[30]

Additional Reading. S. J. Bagley, "Enough Is Enough! Congress and the Courts React to Employers' Medical Screening and Surveillance Procedures," *Dickinson Law Review* 99 (1995), pp. 723–52; H. E. Greenwald, "What You Don't Know Could Save Your Life: A Case for Federal Insurance Disclosure Legislation," *Dickinson Law Review* 102 (1997), pp. 131–67; J. P. Lundington, "Physician's Duties and Liabilities to Person Examined Pursuant to Physician's Contract with Such Person's Prospective or Actual Employer or Insurer," in *American Law Reports,* 3d ed. (New York: Lawyers Cooperative Publishing Co., 1967), vol. 10, pp. 1071–77.

Severing the Provider–Patient Relationship and Patient Abandonment

Once a provider–patient relationship is established, the provider has the obligation and duty to provide medically appropriate, nonnegligent care to the patient for his or her relevant patient needs. These responsibilities fall within a spectrum of "continuing attention"[31] to which the provider must adhere. However, accompanying this con-

---

[25]Shannon v. McNulty, 718 A.2d 828 (Pa. Super. Ct. 1998).

[26]McNulty v. McDowell, 613 N.E.2d 904 (Mass. 1993).

[27]Monusko v. Postle, 437 N.W.2d 367 (Mich. Ct. App. 1989).

[28]See, e.g., Deramus v. Jackson Nat'l Life Ins. Co., 92 F.3d 274 (5th Cir. 1996); Payne v. Sherrer, 458 S.E.2d 916 (Ga. Ct. App. 1995); Saari v. Litman, 486 N.W.2d 813 (Minn. Ct. App. 1992); Felton v. Schaeffer, 279 Cal.Rptr. 713 (Cal. Ct. App. 1991); Rogers v. Horvath, 237 N.W.2d 595 (Mich. Ct. App. 1975); Doe v. Jackson Nat'l Life Ins. Co., 944 F.Supp. 488 (S.D. Miss. 1995); see also Rand v. Miller, 408 S.E.2d 655 (W. Va. 1991).

[29]See, e.g., Dornak v. Lafayette Gen. Hosp., 399 So.2d 168 (La. 1981); Doe v. Prudential Life Ins. Co., 860 F.Supp. 243 (D. Md. 1993); Armstrong v. Morgan, 545 S.W.2d 45 (Tex. Civ. App. 1976); see also Meinze v. Holmes, 532 N.E.2d 170 (Ohio Ct. App. 1987); Wojick v. Aluminum Co. of America, 183 N.Y.S.2d 351 (N.Y. Sup. Ct. 1959).

[30]See, e.g., Lee v. City of New York, 560 N.Y.S.2d 700 (N.Y. App. Div. 1990); Keene v. Methodist Hosp., 324 F.Supp. 233 (N.D. Ind. 1974); Phillips v. Good Samaritan Hosp., 416 N.E.2d 646 (Ohio Ct. App. 1979); Heller v. Peekskill Community Hosp., 603 N.Y.S.2d 548 (N.Y. App. Div. 1993); Pokorny v. Shafer, 1994 WL 65213 (Conn. Super. Ct. Feb. 24, 1994).

[31]See Ricks v. Budge, 64 P.2d 208 (Utah 1937); see also Johnson v. Vaughn, 370 S.W.2d 591 (Ky. 1963).

cept of "continuing attention" are particular requirements that the provider must fulfill to effectively sever the provider–patient relationship. Termination of relationships with patients may occur on the basis of mutual consent, dismissal by the patient, or when the provider can do no more to help the patient.[32] But, in circumstances where the provider unilaterally wishes to leave the relationship, generally the provider is under a duty to continue medical care until he or she gives the patient proper and adequate notice before withdrawing from the relationship *and* gives the patient time to find other medical service providers.[33] Otherwise, the provider may be liable for abandonment of the patient under a negligence theory of malpractice if the patient is injured due to this withdrawal.

Concept.

A provider who unilaterally severs his or her professional relationship with the patient without reasonable notice and ample opportunity to obtain alternative care at a time when the patient is in critical condition or requires lifesaving treatment may be liable in tort for abandoning the patient if the patient suffers injury from the abandonment.

Case.   BS had pain in the hip and leg. She went to surgeon Dr. H, who ordered several diagnostic tests including an MRI. Because the MRI suggested that BS had a herniated disk, Dr. H believed that surgery was the appropriate treatment. However, Dr. H desired to confirm the diagnosis and have a medical workup to determine if BS was a suitable candidate for surgery because of BS's history of smoking, hypertension, coronary artery disease, angina pectoris, and chronic obstructive pulmonary disease. To confirm the diagnosis, Dr. H ordered a myelogram. This test confirmed the diagnosis of a herniated

disk and appropriate treatment by surgery. BS requested a second opinion, and the second surgeon also indicated that surgery was the medically appropriate alternative. The surgery was scheduled for August 7. To assess BS's surgical risks, Dr. H referred BS to Dr. B, an internist. Dr. B examined BS on August 6 and found a total occlusion of BS's right internal carotid artery as well as a 50% occlusion of BS's left carotid. However, on August 7, when it was time for BS's surgery, Dr. H had not yet received Dr. B's report on BS. Because Dr. H did not have the report by Dr. B, Dr. H canceled the surgery and began the process of discharging BS from the hospital and rescheduling the surgery for the next week. However, when BS's son heard of the cancellation, he became angry and confronted one of Dr. H's nurses, threatening to call BS's attorney. Because Dr. H felt that mutual trust between the physician and patient was necessary for an effective physician–patient relationship and this was destroyed by the threats, Dr. H refused to treat BS any further. Dr. H then gave her the name of several physicians, including Dr. JC, who could perform the surgery and notified these physicians that BS could be calling them. In the medical chart, a nursing note dated August 7 indicated that "Pt. requested [Dr. JC's] office phone number. States she was instructed to follow up [with] him in the future." After discharge, BS sued Dr. H for abandonment. Dr. H indicated that no abandonment occurred and that all responsible actions were taken to transfer BS's care to another physician.

Legal Discussion.   It appears that Dr. H did not abandon BS according to the case on which this illustration is based.[34] First, there was a physician–patient relationship between Dr. H and BS. BS presented herself to Dr. H, and Dr. H accepted her as a patient; therefore, there was a duty on the part of Dr. H to treat BS unless the relationship was terminated by BS, was terminated by mutual consent, evolved to circumstances where Dr. H could do no more for the patient's condition, or was terminated by valid, unilateral severance of the physician–patient relationship by Dr. H. In this situation, only the last possibility is relevant. Here, Dr. H indeed unilaterally attempted to sever the relationship after threats from BS's son. As well, Dr. H gave reasonable notice to BS when he indicated to her that he would no longer treat her on August 7. Further, Dr. H gave BS the names of suitable alternate surgeons who could treat her, as evidenced by the nursing notes of August 7; indeed, Dr. H also contacted them for her. There was no evidence that BS was in a critical stage or circumstance or that her condition was life-threatening, since the surgery could be postponed for a week. Therefore, Dr. H did not abandon BS and was not liable for the tort of abandonment.

[32]See, e.g., Manno v. McIntosh, 519 N.W.2d 815 (Iowa Ct. App. 1994); Capps v. Valk, 369 P.2d 238 (Kan. 1962); Groce v. Meyers, 29 S.E.2d 553 (N.C. 1944); Gray v. Davidson, 130 P.2d 341 (Wash. 1942); Ricks v. Budge, 64 P.2d 208 (Utah 1937); Lawson v. Conaway, 16 S.E. 564 (W. Va. 1892); Bixler v. Bowman, 614 P.2d 1290 (Wash. 1980) (*in dissent*); see also Collins v. Meeker, 424 P.2d 488 (Kan. 1967).

[33]See, e.g., Surgical Consultants v. Ball, 447 N.W.2d 676 (Iowa Ct. App. 1989); Mayer v. Baisier, 497 N.E.2d 827 (Ill. App. Ct. 1986); Miller v. Greater Southeast Comm. Hosp., 508 A.2d 927 (D.C. 1986); Overstreet v. Nickelsen, 317 S.E.2d 583 (Ga. Ct. App. 1984); Payton v. Weaver, 182 Cal.Rptr. 225 (Cal. Ct. App. 1982); Tripp v. Pate, 271 S.E.2d 407 (N.C. Ct. App. 1980); McManus v. Donlin, 127 N.W.2d 22 (Wis. 1964); Lee v. Dewbre, 362 S.W.2d 900 (Tex. Civ. App. 1962); Norton v. Hamilton, 89 S.E.2d 809 (Ga. Ct. App. 1955); McGulpin v. Bessmer, 43 N.W.2d 121 (Iowa 1950); Ricks v. Budge, 64 P.2d 208 (Utah 1937); Dicke v. Graves, 668 P.2d 189 (Kan. Ct. App. 1983).

[34]Sparks v. Hicks, 912 P.2d 331 (Okla. 1996).

Case. AH incurred a simple fracture of his leg with slight comminution in a football game on October 19; the fracture was located between the knee and ankle. His father was notified, and he immediately contacted orthopedic surgeon Dr. V to attend his son at General Hospital. Dr. V went to General Hospital, reduced the fracture, and set the leg appropriately in a cast. On October 20, Dr. V visited AH at General Hospital. On this visit, AH's father indicated to Dr. V that AH was experiencing excruciating pain in the leg with no feeling in the toes. Dr. V examined the cast but did nothing else. On October 21, Dr. V once again visited AH with his father present. The same complaints were made to Dr. V, with AH's father suggesting the cast was too tight. Dr. V strongly indicated that it was not; however, Dr. V did not examine the cast or leg and did nothing for the pain. On October 22, Dr. V left for a week without advising AH or his parents of this absence. Dr. V made no provision for AH nor did Dr. V leave instructions with another physician to assume responsibility for the cast during the absence. AH's temperature during this period was noted in the chart to be between 100.8° and 103°F; his white cell count was 16K on October 21, with 77% neutrophils, indicating an active infection. Because of AH's continuing excruciating pain, AH's father attempted to contact Dr. V on October 22 but to no avail; he also attempted to contact other physicians but also met with no success. On October 23, AH's father discovered that Dr. V had left for the week. Late that day, he obtained the services of Dr. S, who, on examination of AH, immediately cut away part of the cast near the ankle, relieving the pressure and showing significant swelling of the foot. AH also was sent for a chest X ray to determine if his apparent infection was pneumonia; the results were negative. On October 30, Dr. V returned, and again AH and his father requested that Dr. V examine the cast and patient. Dr. V refused to do so and, instead, discharged AH. AH was driven home and confined to bed. AH's temperature continued to be elevated, and the significant pain in his ankle continued. On November 7, AH's father called Dr. V and requested Dr. V to see AH. Dr. V refused and indicated there was nothing wrong with AH's leg. Dr. V suggested that AH go to see a family practitioner, Dr. C. Instead, AH's father contacted Dr. S and reported AH's symptoms. Dr. S then saw AH and removed the top portion of the cast, relieving the pressure and revealing a completely swollen leg with necrotic areas on both sides of the ankle. AH remained in bed until November 27, when he was brought to Dr. S's office and the balance of the cast removed. The entire leg and ankle continued to be swollen and drainage exuded from the ankle. The condition of the leg and ankle were so serious that AH was brought back to the hospital as an inpatient for physiotherapy until December 25. At that point, the leg became even more swollen and AH's temperature continued to rise. AH was given antibiotics. However, on December 29, Dr. S diagnosed cellulitis and surgery was performed in an effort to drain AH's leg. The leg continued to drain. Two more surgeries the next year, on August 27 and October 23, did not improve AH's condition, and necrotic tissue continued to increase. Dr. F was consulted. However, because of the nature and extent of the disease in AH's leg and ankle, Dr. F was required to amputate the leg above the knee. AH and his parents brought suit against Dr. V for abandonment and the injuries sustained by AH.

Legal Discussion. It appears that Dr. V abandoned AH according to the case on which this illustration is based.[35] Here, there was a physician–patient relationship between Dr. V and AH: AH, through his father, sought Dr. V's medical services and Dr. V agreed to and did render services to AH. Therefore, Dr. V had a duty to treat AH unless the relationship was terminated by AH, was terminated by mutual assent, evolved to circumstances where Dr. V could do no more for AH's condition, or was terminated by valid, unilateral severance of the physician–patient relationship. In this situation, only the last possibility is relevant. Here, Dr. V, during a time where AH was in critical condition as evidenced by his pain, the nature of his injury, physical signs and symptoms, and highly elevated white count, left for nine days without notice to AH or his family and with no provision for alternate care during the absence. Further, AH's father's continued entreaties to Dr. V to see AH were refused by Dr. V at all relevant junctures. The action was unilateral on Dr. V's part. Hence, Dr. V breached his duty of continued treatment and nonabandonment to AH. AH, due to this breach, suffered the damages of significant pain and immobility as well as lack of treatment to his leg, resulting ultimately in its amputation. Therefore, Dr. V abandoned AH and was liable for the injuries sustained by AH due to this abandonment.

Notes on Severing the Provider–Patient Relationship and Patient Abandonment

Actions Considered Abandonment

Although each case must stand on its own facts and specific court assessment, some actions have been specifically considered abandonment. For example, an express statement of withdrawal from the case,[36] total refusal to

[35]Vann v. Harden, 47 S.E.2d 314 (Va. 1948).
[36]See, e.g., Norton v. Hamilton, 89 S.E.2d 809 (Ga. Ct. App. 1955); Gillette v. Tucker, 65 N.E. 865 (Ohio. 1902); Pritchard v. Neal, 229 S.E.2d 18 (Ga. Ct. App. 1976); Groce v. Myers, 29 S.E.2d 553 (N.C. 1944); see also Wyatt v. Ford, 363 S.E.2d 866 (Ga. Ct. App. 1987).

attend the patient,[37] leaving the patient intraoperatively or postoperatively,[38] failing to treat the patient after expressly promising to,[39] unexcused or unexplained failure to continue treating the patient,[40] premature discharge of the patient from treatment when disease state still requires attention,[41] and failure to provide proper instructions to the patient[42] all have been held to be actions considered abandonment.

Additional Reading. C. T. Drechsler, "Duty of Care; Liability for Malpractice," in *American Jurisprudence,* 2d ed. (New York: Lawyers Cooperative Publishing Co., 1981), section 237.

Critical Stage and Expert Testimony

Physicians and other providers cannot sever the provider–patient relationship at a critical stage. What constitutes a "critical stage" must generally be provided by expert testimony; "just as expert evidence is generally necessary to establish medical negligence, so it is also necessary to demonstrate by expert evidence that a patient was at a 'critical stage' of medical care when his [or her] physician withdrew from his [or her] medical care."[43] However, a minority of courts disagree and indicate that expert testimony is not always necessary, depending on the circumstances.[44]

Additional Reading. C. T. Drechsler, "Duty of Care; Liability for Malpractice," in *American Jurisprudence,* 2d ed. (New York: Lawyers Cooperative Publishing Co., 1981), section 236; B. R. Furrow, "Forcing Rescue: The Landscape of Health Care Provider Obligations to Treat Patients," *Health Matrix* 3 (1993), pp. 31–87.

The Causal Connection Between Abandonment and Injury

Like medical malpractice, the breach of duty (here, abandonment) must cause the injury sued on. Therefore, if the purported abandonment does *not* cause the injury sued on, the patient-plaintiff has no viable cause of action for abandonment.[45] Of course, the patient may have a viable malpractice action if the requisite injury was a result of negligent care.

Additional Reading. C. T. Drechsler, "Duty of Care; Liability for Malpractice," in *American Jurisprudence,* 2d ed. (New York: Lawyers Cooperative Publishing Co., 1981), section 236; J. K. Levin, "Malpractice by Particular Professions," in *New York Jurisprudence,* 2d ed. (New York: Lawyers Cooperative Publishing Co., 1989), section 313.

Disruptive or Uncooperative Patients

Disruptive patients have the same obligations and duties owed them as other patients. Therefore, providers who wish

---

[37]See, e.g., Cazzell v. Schofield, 8 S.W.2d 580 (Mo. 1928); Vann v. Harden, 47 S.E.2d 314 (Va. 1948); Blackburn's Adm'r v. Curd, 106 S.W. 1186 (Ky. Ct. App. 1908); Hongsathavij v. Queen of Angels/Hollywood Presbyterian Med. Ctr., 73 Cal.Rptr.2d 695 (Cal. Ct. App. 1998); see also Johnson v. Vaughn, 370 S.W.2d 591 (Ky. Ct. App. 1963); Murray v. United States, 329 F.2d 270 (4th Cir. 1964); Brandt v. Grubin, 329 A.2d 82 (N.J. Super. Ct. Law Div. 1974).

[38]See, e.g., Burnett v. Layman, 181 S.W. 157 (Tenn. 1915); Longman v. Jasiek, 414 N.E.2d 520 (Ill. App. Ct. 1980); see also Magana v. Elie, 439 N.E.2d 1319 (Ill. App. Ct. 1982).

[39]See, e.g., Fortner v. Kock, 261 N.W. 762 (Mich. 1935); Ritchey v. West, 23 Ill. 329 (1860); see also McGulpin v. Bessmer, 43 N.W.2d 121 (Iowa 1950).

[40]See, e.g., McGulpin v. Bessmer, 43 N.W.2d 121 (Iowa 1950); Baird v. National Health Found., 144 S.W.2d 850 (Mo. Ct. App. 1940); Bellou v. Prescott, 64 Me. 305 (1876); Barbour v. Martin, 62 Me. 536 (1875); Stohlman v. Davis, 220 N.W. 247 (Neb. 1928); Young v. Jordan, 145 S.E. 41 (W. Va. 1928); see also Miller v. Dore, 148 A.2d 692 (Me. 1959).

[41]See, e.g., Boyd v. Andrae, 44 S.W.2d 891 (Mo. Ct. App. 1932); Baldor v. Rogers, 81 So.2d 658 (Fla. 1954); Meiselman v. Crown Heights Hosp., 285 N.Y. 389 (N.Y. 1941); Gross v. Partlow, 68 P.2d 1034 (Wash. 1937); Reed v. Laughlin, 58 S.W.2d 440 (Mo. 1933); Brooks v. Herd, 257 P. 238 (Wash. 1927).

[42]See, e.g., Beck v. German Klinik, 43 N.W. 617 (Iowa 1889); Manno v. McIntosh, 519 N.W.2d 815 (Iowa Ct. App. 1994); Vann v. Harden, 47 S.E.2d 314 (Va. 1948); see also Christy v. Saliterman, 179 N.W.2d 288 (Minn. 1970); Barnes v. Bovenmyer, 122 N.W.2d 312 (Iowa 1963).

[43]Surgical Consultants v. Ball, 447 N.W.2d 676, 682 (Iowa Ct. App. 1989); see also Cox v. Jones, 470 N.W.2d 23 (Iowa 1991); Overstreet v. Nickelsen, 317 S.E.2d 583 (Ga. Ct. App. 1984); Carroll v. Griffin, 101 S.E.2d 764 (Ga. Ct. App. 1958); Manno v. McIntosh, 519 N.W.2d 815 (Iowa Ct. App. 1994); Woodfolk v. Group Health Ass'n, 644 A.2d 1367 (D.C. 1994).

[44]See, e.g., Levy v. Kirk, 187 So.2d 401 (Fla. Dist. Ct. App. 1966); Lynch v. Bryant, 985 F.2d 560 (6th Cir. 1993); Maltempo v. Cuthbert, 504 F.2d 325 (5th Cir. 1974); see also Therrell v. Fonde, 495 So.2d 1046 (Ala. 1986); Mehigan v. Sheehan, 51 A.2d 632 (N.H. 1947); Bateman v. Rosenberg, 525 S.W.2d 753 (Mo. Ct. App. 1975).

[45]See, e.g., McAllister v. Weirton Hosp. Co., 312 S.E.2d 738 (W. Va. 1983); Baulsir v. Sugar, 293 A.2d 253 (Md. 1972); Lee v. Dewbre, 362 S.W.2d 900 (Tex. Civ. App. 1962); Childers v. Frye, 158 S.E. 744 (N.C. 1931); Skodje v. Hardy, 288 P.2d 471 (Wash. 1955); see also Baldor v. Rogers, 81 So.2d 658 (Fla. 1954); Wilson v. Martin Mem. Hosp., 61 S.E.2d 102 (N.C. 1950); Clements v. Hendi, 354 S.E.2d 700 (Ga. Ct. App. 1987); Meeks v. Coan, 302 S.E.2d 418 (Ga. Ct. App. 1983); Harlow v. Chin, 545 N.E.2d 602 (Mass. 1989); see also Sutherlin v. Fenenga, 810 P.2d 353 (N.M. Ct. App. 1991).

to sever their relationship with disruptive patients must provide the requisite notice and provide for opportunities for the patient to find alternative sources of treatment. However, if a patient is disruptive, a warning, then termination of the relationship with a provision of a list of alternative providers has been held to be enough to validly sever the patient–physician relationship, even when none of the alternative providers would take the patient and the patient had a continuing, chronic disease state that required continuous treatment.[46] In addition, when patients fail to follow directions and return for follow-up visits, this, too, has been held to block abandonment claims by the patient.[47]

Additional Reading. J. F. Daar, "A Clash at the Bedside: Patient Autonomy v. a Physician's Professional Conscience," *Hastings Law Journal* 44 (1993), pp. 1241–67; C. T. Drechsler, "Duty of Care; Liability for Malpractice," in *American Jurisprudence,* 2d ed. (New York: Lawyers Cooperative Publishing Co., 1981), section 238.

Liability to Third Parties

Generally, a provider–patient relationship is necessary for any liability for abandonment to attach; that liability therefore is limited to harm suffered by the patient. However, in certain circumstances, the foreseeability of harm to a third party by abandonment may allow that third party also to sue the provider who abandoned the patient; for example, a patient's spouse may be able to sue a provider in tort for the injuries to the patient due to abandonment.[48]

Additional Reading. C. T. Drechsler, "Malpractice Actions and Procedures," in *American Jurisprudence,* 2d ed. (New York: Lawyers Cooperative Publishing Co., 1981), section 369; B. I. McDaniel, "Recovery for Mental or Emotional Distress Resulting from Injury to, or Death of, Member of Plaintiff's Family Arising from Physician's or Hospital's Wrongful Conduct," in *American Law Reports,* 3d ed. (New York: Lawyers Cooperative Publishing Co., 1977), vol. 77, pp. 447–93.

Patient Voluntarily Goes to Another Provider

If a patient voluntarily switches from one physician or provider to another and that switch is not induced by the original provider, there can be no abandonment.[49] Since the patient is unilaterally terminating the relationship, effectively the patient has abandoned the original provider. In this situation, the provider is under no obligation to find a suitable replacement for the patient.

Provider Can Do No More for the Patient

Generally, it has been held that a provider's obligations of continuing attention cease when the provider no longer can provide beneficial services to the patient.[50] However, this does not mean that, for example, a surgeon is not obligated to provide care to his or her patient after surgery: If postoperative follow-up care is reasonably necessary, the surgeon must provide it and cannot assume that his or her obligations are terminated.[51]

Additional Reading. C. T. Drechsler, "Duty of Care; Liability for Malpractice," in *American Jurisprudence,* 2d ed. (New York: Lawyers Cooperative Publishing Co., 1981), section 241; J. K. Levin, "Malpractice by Particular Professionals," in *Ohio Jurisprudence,* 3d ed. (New York: Lawyers Cooperative Publishing Co., 1986), section 32.

Temporary Absence

The concept of continuous treatment does not mean that physicians and other providers cannot temporarily suspend access to themselves due to vacations, conferences, sickness, weekends, and the like. As long as the provider has arranged for a reasonable and competent substitute to take care of patient needs, informed the patient of the temporary unavailability in a timely fashion, and not left during a period where the patient is in a critical medical circumstance or condition, there is no abandonment by the provider.[52]

---

[46]Payton v. Weaver, 182 Cal.Rptr. 225 (Cal. Ct. App. 1982).

[47]See, e.g., Roberts v. Wood, 206 F.Supp. 579 (S.D. Ala. 1962); see also McManus v. Donlin, 127 N.W.2d 22 (Wis. 1964); Knapp v. Eppright, 783 S.W.2d 293 (Tex. App. 1989); Ried v. Johnson, 851 S.W.2d 120 (Mo. Ct. App. 1993).

[48]See, e.g., Grimsby v. Samson, 530 P.2d 291 (Wash. 1975).

[49]See, e.g., Reid v. Johnson, 851 S.W.2d 120 (Mo. Ct. App. 1993); Antal v. Porretta, 418 N.W.2d 395 (Mich. Ct. App. 1987); Knapp v. Eppright, 783 S.W.2d 293 (Tex. App. 1989); see also Weaver v. University of Michigan Bd. of Regents, 506 N.W.2d 264 (Mich. Ct. App. 1993).

[50]See, e.g., Jewson v. Mayo Clinic, 691 F.2d 405 (8th Cir. 1982); Wells v. Billars, 391 N.W.2d 668 (S.D. 1986); see also Schmit v. Esser, 236 N.W. 622 (Minn. 1931).

[51]See, e.g., Shirk v. Kelsey, 617 N.E.2d 152 (Ill. App. Ct. 1993); Longman v. Jasiek, 414 N.E.2d 520 (Ill. App. Ct. 1980); see also Hall v. Hilbun, 466 So.2d 856 (Miss. 1985); Wooten v. Curry, 362 S.W.2d 820 (Tenn. Ct. App. 1961); Thiele v. Ortiz, 520 N.E.2d 881 (Ill. App. Ct. 1988).

[52] See, e.g., Kenney v. Piedmont Hosp., 222 S.E.2d 162 (Ga. Ct. App. 1975); Miller v. Dore, 148 A.2d 692 (Me. 1959); Warwick v. Bliss, 195 N.W. 501 (S.D. 1923); Lee v. Dewbre, 362 S.W.2d 900 (Tex. Civ. App. 1962); see also Manno v. McIntosh, 519 N.W.2d 815 (Iowa Ct. App. 1994); Reed v. Gershweir, 772 P.2d 26 (Ariz. Ct. App. 1989); Skodje v. Hardy, 288 P.2d 471 (Wash. 1955).

Further Reading

Severing the Provider–Patient Relationship

Drechsler CT. Duty of Care; Liability for Malpractice. In: *American Jurisprudence,* 2d ed. New York: Lawyers Cooperative Publishing Co., 1981;§§234, 235.

See Also

Drechsler CT. Duty of Care; Liability for Malpractice. In: *American Jurisprudence,* 2d ed. New York: Lawyers Cooperative Publishing Co., 1981;§§236, 238.

Other Reading

Drechsler CT. Relation of Physician and Patient. In: *American Jurisprudence,* 2d ed. New York: Lawyers Cooperative Publishing Co., 1981;§158.

Furrow BR. Forcing Rescue: The Landscape of Health Care Provider Obligations to Treat Patients. *Health Matrix* 1993;3:31–87.

Glenn SM. Liability in the Absence of a Traditional Physician–Patient Relationship: What Every "On-Call" Doctor Should Know: Mozingo v. Pitt County Memorial Hospital. *Wake Forest L Rev* 1993;28:747–74.

Kinney ED, Selby MC. History and Jurisprudence of the Physician-Patient Relationship in Indiana. *Ind L Rev* 1997;30:263–78.

Leffler CS. Sexual Conduct Within the Physician-Patient Relationship: A Statutory Framework for Disciplining the Branch of Fiduciary Duty. *SPG Widener L Symp J* 1996;1:501–45.

Litwin JL. Relation of Practitioner and Patient. In: *Texas Jurisprudence,* 3d ed. New York: Lawyers Cooperative Publishing Co., 1997;§155.

Meyn MA. The Liability of Physicians Who Examine for Third Parties. *N Ky L Rev* 1992;19:333-50.

Rigelhaupt JL. What Constitutes Physician-Patient Relationship for Malpractice Purposes. In: *American Law Reports,* 4th ed. New York: Lawyers Cooperative Publishing Co., 1997;17:132–60.

Web Sites

The legal limits of the doctor–patient relationship: *http://ccme-mac4.bsd.uchicago.edu/CCMEFaculty/ADG/ADG1*

Patient bill of rights — summary: *http://www.igc.org/cna/pbor/*

Patient–doctor — Phase I: *http://www.mcg.edu/som/FamMed/patient.htm*

Patient–practitioner relationships: *http://www.psych.bangor.ac.uk/deptpsych/courses/p3h01/navigation/Linear/Linear.html*

Managed competition and the patient–physician relationship: *http://www.nejm.org/content/1994/0330/0009/0639.asp*

Provider-to-patient HIV transmission: *http://www.acponline.org/journals/annals/5jan99/ptophiv.htm*

PART II

The Health Care Insurance Structure

6

Private Insurance

Individuals in the United States usually finance their health care through the use of insurance rather than paying out of pocket for medical costs. However, the structures of the current health insurance programs in relationship to providers and patients can be somewhat Byzantine. This chapter will provide an overview of private insurance and its predominant regulatory structures in the United States. Additional details may be found in the reading list at the end of the chapter.

The nature of health insurance can be determined by answering a seemingly simple question: Suppose a patient requires medical care and seeks it by going to a physician or other provider; how will the patient pay for that care? This chapter will cover the private insurance market considerations; the public insurance programs Medicare and Medicaid will be covered in subsequent chapters.

Out of Pocket

One method by which patients pay for their care is simply out of pocket. Similar to paying for other goods and services, a bill is provided and the patient transfers a cash payment to the providers. This is the methodology by which approximately 15% of the U.S. population without health insurance pays for its care.[1] Since health care is an expensive commodity, this methodology most likely is undesirable for a vast portion of the population.

Private Insurance

Private, or commercial, insurance plans are those most familiar to employed, working-age individuals in the United States because health insurance generally is linked to employment. Private insurance includes standard health care plans offered by major insurance companies as well as those plans offered by Blue Cross/Blue Shield. The "Blues" at one time were given preferential tax status; however, federal tax exemption for the Blues ended with the Tax Reform Act of 1986.[2] Although some distinctions continue between the Blues and general commercial insurance plans, these differences quickly are becoming extinct due to the highly competitive health delivery markets.

The standard contractual arrangement that governs private health insurance is threefold: It involves the employee, employer, and insurer offering the coverage. Generally, employers offer a variety of options for health care insurance to employees. The employees may pay some amount to the employer to defray some of the costs of the health insurance; the employer also contributes a significant amount (75–100% of the costs) toward paying for the health insurance of its employees.[3] Either employers use the earmarked funds to purchase insurance from a commercial carrier, which covers the costs and indicates the providers to be used for health care, or employers use the money itself to cover the costs and arrange for services. These typical circumstances are reviewed here. Managed care arrangements will be covered in Chapter 9.

[1]M. A. Bobinski, "Unhealthy Federalism: Barriers to Increasing Health Care Access for the Uninsured," *University of California Davis Law Review* 24 (1990), p. 262; L. D. Brown, "The Medically Uninsured: Problems, Policies, and Politics," *Journal of Health, Political Policy, and Law* 15 (1990), p. 413; L. O. Gostin, "Securing Health or Just Health Care? The Effect of the Health Care System on the Health of America," *St Louis University Law Journal* 39 (1994), p. 20.

[2]100 Stat. 2085 (1986).

[3]Employee Benefits Research Institute, "Sources of Health Insurance and Characteristics of the Uninsured: Analysis of the March 1996 Current Population Survey," Issue Brief No. 179, 5-9 (November 1996).

Traditional Indemnity

If employers offer and employees choose traditional indemnity insurance, the employer–employee amounts paid to the insurance company represent premiums. In exchange, the insurer agrees to pay for specified health care services for the employees who chose that insurance plan. This arrangement is the classic "third-party payer" methodology for paying for medical care services. This contractual relationship can have limitations, of course; for example, the insurer may pay only for services rendered using a fee schedule, require second opinions, and/or exclude certain treatments. With regard to the patient and physician or other provider, traditional indemnity generally allows the patient to self-refer to any provider he or she wants. However, there usually are cost-sharing mechanisms such as coinsurance (the individual is responsible for a certain percentage of the provider charge, e.g., 20%) and deductibles (the individual is responsible for a certain floor amount of charges before indemnity insurance begins coverage, e.g., $500) and an annual out-of-pocket limit on expenditures for the covered individual (e.g., $1000) over which the indemnity insurance will pay all amounts. Physicians and other providers who render care for the individual usually bill the insurance company for services. The insurance company then reimburses the provider for care, subject to the deductible and coinsurance amounts, which are the responsibility of the patient. Traditional indemnity insurance is becoming increasingly rare. Because providers are paid on the basis of the services rendered, there is an incentive to provide as many services as possible and leave no stone unturned for diagnostic and treatment purposes. Due to concerns regarding escalating costs and limited ability to minimize costs before services are provided, insurers have placed significant restrictions on these types of plans, such as higher-level cost sharing for the patient; in addition, employers and employees are eschewing traditional indemnity because of its high cost relative to other forms of insurance, particularly managed care.

Self-Funded Employee Benefits Plans

Instead of taking employee contributions, adding employer amounts, and paying these amounts to an insurance company for health insurance coverage, a majority of employers are now self-insuring;[4] that is, they are fund-ing and purchasing health insurance for their employees themselves. The reason for this significant change is that employers choosing to self-fund their employee benefits plans, including employee health benefits, to a great extent are exempted from state benefits laws by the federal Employee Retirement Income Security Act.[5] Because of this exemption, the cost of regulation to the employer is significantly reduced. Employers thus are subject only to federal regulations regarding employee health benefits. When employers take this option to self-fund, they are responsible for arranging for the provision of health care services for their employees. Generally, this entails the employer contracting with one or several health care provider organizations directly to provide care to employees or outsourcing the administration of the plan to a managed care organization, which in turn arranges for health care services under the plan using its contracted providers.

Federal Regulation: ERISA

ERISA is the abbreviation for the Employee Retirement Income Security Act of 1974.[6] ERISA is a federal statute enacted in response to widely divergent state regulation of employee benefits plans (EBPs).[7] Because of extensive, conflicting, and costly state regulation (including state-imposed premium taxes) and its perceived impact on domestic industry's global competitiveness, Congress created a uniform federal regulatory structure for EBPs offered by employers engaged in interstate commerce.[8] ERISA governs participation, funding, and vesting requirements on EBPs and sets uniform standards regarding reporting, disclosure, and fiduciary responsibilities, rather than regulating the content of EBPs.[9] The federal Department of Labor (DOL) has the authority to administer the requirements of the statute and its regulations. ERISA does not govern EBPs where no contribution is made by the employer or employee organization, program participation is voluntary for employees or members, the sole functions of the employer or employee organization are to permit the insurer to publicize the program to employees or members or collect premiums through payroll deductions or dues checkoffs and then remit them to the insurer, or the employer or employee organization receives no legal consideration in connection with the program except for administrative services

---

[4]L. J. Schacht, "The Health Care Crisis: Improving Access for Employees Covered by Self-Insured Health Plans Under ERISA and the Americans With Disabilities Act, *Washington University Journal of Urban and Contemporary Law* 45 (1994), p. 311; D. A. Sullivan, "ERISA, the ADA, and AIDS: Fixing Self-Insured Health Plans with Carparts," *Maryland Journal of Contemporary Legal Issues* 7 (1994), p. 424.

[5]29 U.S.C.A. §§1001 *et seq.* See also the section "Federal Regulation: ERISA" in this chapter.

[6]29 U.S.C.A. §§1001 *et seq.*

[7]See FMC Corp. v. Holliday, 498 U.S. 52, 56-60 (1990).

[8]See 29 U.S.C.A. §1003(a)(1); and H. Rep. 93-533 (Education and Labor Committee), 93d Cong., 2d Sess., reprinted in 1974 U.S. Code Congressional and Administrative News, 4369-4670.

[9]Shaw v. Delta Air Lines, Inc., 463 U.S. 85 (1983).

charges in connection with payroll deductions or dues checkoffs.[10] An ERISA EBP is not established if the employer simply purchases insurance for the employee without assuming ownership or controlling, administering, or assuming responsibility for the plan.[11]

Three major clauses in ERISA govern much of the debate regarding the statute and health care plans: The preemption (or "relate[s] to") clause preempts all state laws that relate to EBPs;[12] the savings clause indicates that ERISA does not preempt state laws that regulate insurance, banking, or securities;[13] and although at first blush, obtaining health insurance for employees or administrating a plan as a third-party administrator seemingly is the business of insurance,[14] the "deemer" clause indicates that EBPs are not to be deemed an insurer for the purposes of the statute, thus removing health plan regulation from the states. Regulatory authority over self-funded ERISA EBPs is important because virtually all working persons are in them: ERISA regulates EBPs that cover approximately 88% of private, nonelderly employees in the United States.[15] Thus, the scope of ERISA's legal coverage and effects is enormous. EBPs that provide health care or health insurance benefits are within the purview of ERISA.[16]

Plan Document

ERISA-governed plans must indicate in writing the terms and benefits of the EBP,[17] although there have been examples of plans not in writing being treated as valid ERISA plans for the purposes of coverage.[18] The major parties to whom the plan document dictates rights and responsibilities are the plan sponsor (generally, the employer that establishes and maintains the EBP), the plan (as a promise of the employer and a separate legal entity), the participants (generally the employees and other beneficiaries such as family members of the employees), the service providers (persons or entities that provide services to the plan participants), and the plan administrator (the person or entity responsible for carrying out the terms of the plan). ERISA requires that the plan sponsor (usually, the employer or union) name at least one fiduciary in the plan document.[19] Assuming there is a written, formal plan document, it is important to note that oral statements or promises generally do not modify the written plan.[20] Thus, the formal written plan document generally indicates those benefits that are available and those that are not. However, if there is a conflict between the plan document and the summary plan description (SPD; see later), it has been held that the document that favors the employee controls.[21] EBP participants generally have the right to obtain statements of accrued benefits, the plan instrument, the plan's annual report, any trust agreement, and any document through which the EBP was established, although copying fees may apply.[22] The plan administrator may be penalized for failing to provide these documents to beneficiaries.[23] The plan administrator also is responsible for filing the appropriate documents with the DOL or IRS annually unless the plan is exempt from such a filing.[24]

---

[10]29 C.F.R. §2510.3-1(j) (1998).

[11]See, e.g., Taggart Corp. v. Life & Health Benefits Admin., Inc., 617 F.2d 1208 (5th Cir. 1980), *cert. denied* 450 U.S. 1030 (1981).

[12]29 U.S.C.A. §1144.

[13]29 U.S.C.A. §1144(b)(2)(A).

[14]See, e.g., Powell v. Chesapeake & Potomac Tel. Co., 780 F.2d 419 (4th Cir. 1985), *cert. denied* 476 U.S. 1170 (1986) (third-party administrator is not engaged in business of insurance); NGS American, Inc. v. Barnes, 998 F.2d 296 (5th Cir. 1993) (same); Insurance Bd. of Bethlehem Steel Corp. v. Muir, 819 F.2d 408 (3d Cir. 1987) (same); see also O'Reilly v. Ceuleers, 912 F.2d 1383 (11th Cir. 1990) (HMO merely acting as third-party administrator cannot invoke protection of savings clause); Aetna Life Ins. Co. v. State Bd. of Equalization, 15 Cal.Rptr.2d 26 (Cal. Ct. App. 1992) (state premiums tax is not applicable to fees collected by insurance company acting as third-party administrator); Benefax Corp. v. Wright, 757 F.Supp. 800 (W.D. Ky. 1990) (state administrator licensing statutes are applicable to third-party administrators of ERISA plans).

[15]T. Einhorn, "Note: Reigning in ERISA Preemption? Any Willing Provider Statutes After New York Blue Cross Plans v. Travelers Insurance Co.," *Journal of Contemporary Health Law Policy* 13 (1996), pp. 265–317.

[16]29 U.S.C.A. §1002.

[17]29 U.S.C.A. §1102(b).

[18]See, e.g., Donovan v. Dillingham, 688 F.2d 1367 (11th Cir. 1982); Moeller v. Bertrung, 801 F.Supp. 291 (D. S.D. 1992); Wright v. Williams, 927 F.2d 1540 (11th Cir. 1991); Scott v. Gulf Oil Corp., 754 F.2d 1499 (9th Cir. 1985); Suggs v. Pan American Life Ins. Co., 847 F.Supp. 1324 (S.D. Miss. 1994); see also Cinelli v. Security Pacific Corp., 61 F.3d 1437 (9th Cir. 1995).

[19]29 U.S.C.A. §1102(a).

[20]See, e.g., Lister v. Stark, 890 F.2d 941 (7th Cir. 1989), *cert. denied* 498 U.S. 1011 (1990); Gordon v. Barnes Pumps, Inc., 999 F.2d 133 (6th Cir. 1993); Cefalu v. B.F. Goodrich Co., 871 F.2d 1290 (5th Cir. 1989); see also Gupta v. Freixenet, 908 F.Supp. 557 (N.D. Ill. 1995); Wise v. Harris Info. Sys., 1995 WL 548742 (N.D. Ill. 1995); Haggard v. Armstrong Rubber Co., 767 F.Supp. 119 (M.D. La. 1991).

[21]See, e.g., Pierce v. Security Trust Life Ins. Co., 979 F.2d 23 (4th Cir. 1992) (if SPD favors employees in presence of disclaimer on SPD, SPD can be relied on despite disclaimer); Glocker v. W.R. Grace & Co., 974 F.2d 540 (4th Cir. 1992) (if SPD favors employer in presence of disclaimer on SPD, disclaimer will be relied on).

[22]Department of Labor Regulation §2520-104b-30.

[23]29 U.S.C.A. §§1001(b), 1132(a)(1)(b); see also Howard v. Gleason Corp., 901 F.2d 1154 (2d Cir. 1990) (discussing plan administrator liability for nonprovision of documents).

[24]29 U.S.C.A. §1024.

Table 6–1. ERISA SDP Requirements

Name and type of plan administration
Name and address of organization through which benefits are provided
Name and address of insurance company, insurance service, or insurance organization financing or administrating plan and extent to which benefits guaranteed, and nature of administrative services provided*
Name and address of plan administrator
Date plan year ends
Plan name and number
Employer's name and address
Employer Identification Number assigned by IRS to employer
Type of plan (e.g., pension, defined benefit, money purchase, profit sharing, hospitalization, disability, maternity benefits)
Sources of contribution to plan (employer, employee, employee organization) and method by which contribution is calculated
Name and address of designated agent for service of legal process
Names, titles, and addresses of all trustees if different from the administrator
Claims procedures
ERISA rights
Eligibility and participation requirements
Circumstances that can result in loss of benefits

---

*For years beginning on or after June 30, 1997. Financing includes support in whole or in part.
Source: 29 C.F.R. §2520.102-3.

Summary Plan Description

The EBP administrator is mandated by ERISA to prepare and distribute to all plan beneficiaries an SPD.[25] The SPD is a document that provides information regarding the plan in language that can be understood by an ordinary plan beneficiary.[26] Where a proportion of employees do not read English and do read the same language, a notice that assistance is available to explain the SPD must be given.[27] The DOL has issued regulations that indicate what specific information must be included in the SPD.[28] Note, however, that although generally the plan document governs what the EBP specifically provides, there has been some debate in the courts as to whether the SPD can be relied on instead.[29]

The administrator of the EBP has full responsibility for preparing the SPD. An administrator for ERISA purposes is a person designated by the EBP or, if no person is identified, the plan sponsor.[30] Generally, the plan sponsor is the employer.

The administrator must provide an employee with the SPD within 90 days after the employee becomes a participant in the EBP or 120 days after the plan is established, whichever is later.[31] As well, any substantive, material modifications in the EBP or changes in the information required to be included in the SPD must be summarized by the administrator and provided to all participants within 210 days after the end of the plan year in which the modifications to the EBP are adopted.[32] In any event, the SPD should be updated at least every five years.[33] Copies of the SPD and all modifications must be filed with the DOL.[34] There are extensive requirements for SPDs;[35] these are summarized in Table 6–1. Items on

---

[25]29 U.S.C.A. §1021(a).

[26]29 U.S.C.A. §1022(a).

[27]29 U.S.C.A. §1024(b)(1); Department of Labor Regulation §§2520.102-2(c)(1), 2520.102-2(c)(2).

[28]29 C.F.R. §§2520.102-2 (1998), 2520.102-3 (1998).

[29]See, e.g., Gridley v. Cleveland Pneumatic Co., 924 F.2d 1310 (3d Cir.), *cert. denied* 501 U.S. 1232 (1991) (plan document governs disputes over benefits); Heidgert v. Olin Corp., 906 F.2d 903 (2d Cir. 1990); Kreutzer v. A.O. Smith Corp., 951 F.2d 739 (7th Cir. 1991); Hansen v. Continental Ins. Co., 940 F.2d 971 (5th Cir. 1991) (SPD governs); Whiteman v. Graphic Comm. Int'l Union Supp. Retirement & Disability Fund, 871 F.Supp. 465 (D.D.C. 1994); Lancaster v. U.S. Shoe Corp., 934 F.Supp. 1137 (N.D.Cal. 1996); Stiltner v. Beretta USA Corp., 74 F.3d 1473 (4th Cir.), *cert. denied* 117 S.Ct. 54 (1996); Andersen v. Chrysler Corp., 99 F.3d 846 (7th Cir. 1996) (SPD may control benefits determinations); McNight v. Southern Life & Health Ins. Co., 758 F.2d 1566 (11th Cir. 1985); see also Pierce v. Security Trust Life Ins., 979 F.2d 23 (4th Cir. 1992); Springs Valley Bank & Trust Co. v. Carpenter, 885 F.Supp. 1131 (S.D. Ind. 1993).

[30]29 U.S.C.A. §1002(16)(A).

[31]29 U.S.C.A. §1024(b)(1)(A)-(B).

[32]29 U.S.C.A. §1024(b)(1)(B).

[33]29 U.S.C.A. §1024(b)(1)(B).

[34]29 U.S.C.A. §1024(a)(1)(D).

[35]29 U.S.C.A. §1022; 29 C.F.R. §2520.102-3 (1998).

the list that are not applicable for the plan are not required to be included in the SPD. Note that beneficiary reliance on a faulty or incorrect plan document as a source for ERISA claims has generated a conflict in the courts.[36] Therefore, it is important to check the local jurisdiction to determine what the applicable legal interpretation is for a specific plan.

Plan Amendments

Plans may be amended by an employer or insurer. Participants and beneficiaries generally are notified of material changes to the plan or its administration through a Summary of Material Modifications. This summary must be distributed within 60 days of the adoption of a modification or change that is material in its reduction of covered services or benefits. Materiality is governed by regulation.[37] A summary must be distributed within 210 days of the plan year close in any year in which other material modifications are adopted.[38]

 Because amending a plan is not considered within the purview of a fiduciary duty, plans may be amended that adversely affect some employees.[39] Therefore, plan design and amendments are not subject to a fiduciary duty to the beneficiary or participant; only the administration of the plan must fall within such fiduciary boundaries.[40] However, note that although the plan sponsor can reserve the right to modify and amend the EBP, it must do so following the process enumerated within the plan document. If the procedure taken by the plan sponsor is improper, a beneficiary may challenge the amendment's validity.[41]

Fiduciary Duties

In general, employers have no fiduciary duty to their employees.[42] However, for ERISA EBPs, this may be altered; therefore, it is critical to identify who the fiduciary is for an EBP, since there are legal implications for this designation.[43]

 ERISA indicates that a person or entity is a fiduciary with respect to an EBP if that person or entity

1. exercises any discretionary authority or control regarding management of the plan or disposition of its assets;
2. provides investment advice for compensation; or
3. has discretionary authority or responsibility in the administration of the plan.[44]

DOL regulations focus on whether the person's or entity's functions are discretionary or ministerial (i.e., involving only adherence to instructions without discretion) in assessing fiduciary status.[45] Further, DOL indicates that the party with authority to review and decide on whether to deny claims is a named fiduciary for purposes of ERISA claims review requirements.[46] Courts have assessed this issue on a fact-specific basis, with titles being unimportant but discretionary authority or control over part or all of the plan, its operations, or its administration the relevant factors for consideration.[47]

 Fiduciaries have certain specific responsibilities to the EBP. These responsibilities generally follow the law of trusts. A person or entity that is considered a plan fiduciary (voluntarily or involuntarily) has the following obligations to the plan:

1. the fiduciary must always act solely in the interest of the plan participants and beneficiaries;

---

[36]See, e.g., McKnight v. Southern Life & Health Ins. Co., 758 F.2d 1566 (11th Cir. 1985) (requiring reliance); Govoni v. Bricklayers, Masons & Plasterers Int'l Union, 732 F.2d 250 (1st Cir. 1984) (requiring reliance); Andersen v. Chrysler Corp., 99 F.3d 846 (7th Cir. 1996) (requiring reliance); Panaras v. Liquid Carbonic Indus. Corp., 74 F.3d 786 (7th Cir. 1996) (requiring reliance); Edwards v. State Farm Mut. Auto Ins. Co., 851 F.2d 134 (6th Cir. 1988) (not requiring reliance).

[37]See 62 Fed. Reg. 16894 (1997).

[38]29 U.S.C.A. §1024(b)(1)(B); Department of Labor Regulation 2520.104b-3.

[39]See, e.g., McGann v. H & H Music Co., 946 F.2d 401 (5th Cir. 1991), cert. denied sub nom. Greenberg v. H & H Music, 506 U.S. 981 (1992); Ownes v. Storehouse, Inc., 984 F.2d 394 (11th Cir. 1993).

[40]Lockheed Corp. v. Spink, 517 U.S. 882 (1996); but see Varity Corp. v. Howe, 516 U.S. 489 (1996) (employer a fiduciary when it knowingly and significantly deceived a plan's beneficiaries).

[41]See, e.g., Curtiss-Wright Corp. v. Schoonejongen, 514 U.S. 73 (1995); Inter-Modal Rail Employees Ass'n v. Atchison, Topeka and Santa Fe Railway, 520 U.S. 510 (1997).

[42]See, e.g., Barnes v. Lacy, 927 F.2d 539 (11th Cir.), cert. denied 502 U.S. 510 (1991).

[43]See, e.g., Gelardi v. Pertec Computer Corp., 761 F.2d 1323 (9th Cir. 1985) (corporation is plan fiduciaries with duty to select other fiduciaries with due care); Brock v. Robbins, 830 F.2d 640 (7th Cir. 1987) (trustees are fiduciaries and breached their duty by entering into contract with claims processor without exercising due care).

[44]29 U.S.C.A. §1002(21)(A).

[45]29 C.F.R. §2509.75-8 Question D-2 (1998).

[46]29 C.F.R. §2560.503-1(g) (1998); see also Simmons v. Prudential Ins. Co., 641 F.Supp. 675 (D. Colo. 1986) (claims administrator with discretionary authority to review denied claims and determine whether charges are customary and reasonable is considered a fiduciary).

[47]See, e.g., Fulk v. Bagley, 88 F.R.D. 153 (M.D. N.C. 1980); Eaves v. Penn, 587 F.2d 453 (10th Cir. 1978); Zuniga v. Blue Cross & Blue Shield, 52 F.3d 1395 (6th Cir. 1995); see also Salley v. E.I. DuPont De Nemours & Co., 966 F.2d 1011 (5th Cir. 1992) (employer liable for improper termination of payment under ERISA due to abuse of discretion when it provided only limited information to utilization reviewer).

2. the fiduciary must act for the exclusive purpose of providing benefits to participants and their beneficiaries and defraying the reasonable costs of administering the plan;

3. the fiduciary must act with the care, skill, prudence, and diligence that a prudent person acting in a like capacity and familiar with such matters would use in the conduct of an enterprise of like character and aims;

4. the fiduciary must diversify investments of the plan to minimize the risk of large losses unless it is clearly prudent not to do so; and

5. the fiduciary must act in accordance with the documents and instruments governing the plan so far as they are consistent with ERISA.[48]

In addition, plan fiduciaries must not enter into a relationship with the plan where there is a conflict of interest,[49] regardless of whether the fiduciary's conduct is on fair terms with the plan. However, providing services under contract that are reasonable, obtaining payment of no more than reasonable compensation, and providing services that are necessary for establishing or operating the plan by the fiduciary are permitted.[50]

Under ERISA, fiduciaries are subject to *personal* liability to the plan due to a fiduciary breach and will be responsible to pay any losses to the plan resulting from the breach as well as disgorge any profits made by the fiduciary through use of the assets of the plan. Courts also may order any other equitable or remedial relief they deem appropriate, including removing the fiduciary.[51] Indeed, one fiduciary may be liable for another's fiduciary breach if the first participates knowingly in another's breach or acts to conceal an act or omission of the other when it is known that the act or omission is a breach; if the first fiduciary enables the other fiduciary to commit a breach by failing to fulfill his or her fiduciary responsibilities; or if the first has knowledge of the breach by the other fiduciary and does not make reasonable efforts to remedy that breach.[52] Violation of fiduciary obligations can also subject the fiduciary and parties involved to excise taxes, civil penalties, and equitable sanctions.[53]

Denial of Benefits Standard of Review

If a beneficiary has been denied ERISA EBP benefits such as health care services and wishes to challenge this denial in court, judicial assessment of the denial is reviewed de novo by the courts unless the EBP gives the plan administrator discretionary authority to determine the eligibility for benefits or interpretation of the terms of the plan. In the latter case, the standard for review is simply abuse of discretion by the administrator, with the burden of proof placed on the plaintiff-beneficiary to show this abuse.[54] Most plans give the administrator discretion; therefore, the prevailing standard is the abuse of discretion standard, which has been articulated as whether the plan administrator acted arbitrarily or capriciously in denying an EBP benefit.[55] Note, however, that when the entity with discretion both administers and is the insurer of the EBP, courts have departed from the simple abuse of discretion standard. Some courts have adopted a "sliding scale" approach, where the court applies an abuse of discretion standard but reduces the amount of discretion in proportion to the seriousness of the issue.[56] Others have adopted a "presumptively void" test, where decision of plan administrator is presumed to be abuse of discretion unless the administrator can show under de novo review that the action was correct or that the decision was not made to serve the administrator's interest over the beneficiary's.[57] Finally, some courts have simply adopted a de novo standard of review in these circumstances.[58] Once again, it is important to review local court assessments to determine specific rights and responsibilities.

[48]29 U.S.C.A. §1104(a)(1); see also Eddy v. Colonial Life Ins. Co. of America, 919 F.2d 747 (D.C. Cir. 1990) (group health insurer HMO is liable under ERISA for failing in fiduciary duty to provide beneficiary information on options when group policy terminated).

[49]29 U.S.C.A. §§1106(a), 1106(b); see also McConocha v. Blue Cross and Blue Shield of Ohio, 898 F.Supp. 545 (N.D. Ohio 1995) (failure to inform and pass on negotiated discounts by fiduciary is a breach of fiduciary duty to the plan).

[50]29 U.S.C.A. §1108(b)(2); 29 C.F.R. §2550.408b-2(a) (1998).

[51]29 U.S.C.A. §1109(a).

[52]29 U.S.C.A. §1105(a).

[53]29 U.S.C.A. §§1132, 1111; but see Mertens v. Hewitt Assocs., 508 U.S. 248 (1993) (ERISA plan participants are not entitled to monetary damages against EBP's nonfiduciary service provider); Reich v. Rowe, 20 F.3d 25 (1st Cir. 1994) (equitable relief is not available against nonfiduciary service provider).

[54]See, e.g., Firestone Tire & Rubber v. Bruch, 489 U.S. 101, 115 (1989).

[55]See, e.g., Bellaire Gen. Hosp. v. Blue Cross Blue Shield, 97 F.3d 822, 828-9 (5th Cir. 1996).

[56]See, e.g., Doe v. Group Hospitalization & Med. Servs., 3 F.3d 80, 87 (4th Cir. 1993); Wildbur v. ARCO Chem. Co., 974 F.2d 631, 638-42 (5th Cir. 1992); Van Boxel v. Journal Co. Employees' Pension Trust, 836 F.2d 1048, 1052-53 (7th Cir. 1987); Chambers v. Family Health Plan Corp., 100 F.3d 818, 824-27 (10th Cir. 1996).

[57]See, e.g., Atwood v. Newmont Gold Co., 45 F.3d 1317, 1323 (9th Cir. 1995); citing GEORGE T. BOGERT, TRUSTS §95 (6th ed. 1987); Brown v. Blue Cross & Blue Shield, 898 F.2d 1556, 1666-67 (11th Cir. 1990), *cert. denied* 498 U.S. 1040 (1991).

[58]See, e.g., Armstrong v. Aetna Life Ins. Co., 128 F.3d 1263 (8th Cir. 1997).

ERISA Remedies

Remedies under the statute are limited. First, those who can bring suits under ERISA generally are confined to EBP participants and beneficiaries and the Secretary of Labor.[59] Second, due to the statute's detailed provisions, only suits to recover benefits, enforce rights, clarify rights, or for breach of fiduciary duty are allowed; common law tort and contract claims generally are preempted.[60] Third, the statute provides for a specific statute of limitations for breach of fiduciary duty claims. These suits must be brought within six years from the time of the last action that constituted a breach of fiduciary duty, or three years from the time of actual knowledge of a fiduciary duty breach.[61] However, there does not appear to be any statute of limitations in ERISA for other causes of action, and courts generally apply state statute of limitations periods.[62] Also note that ERISA suits generally do not provide for jury trials,[63] although some courts have attempted to recharacterize these suits and allow for such.[64]

The enumerated remedies in the statute for aggrieved participants or beneficiaries of ERISA EBPs are specifically limited to the following situations:

1. The participant or beneficiary may obtain relief from an administrator's unlawful refusal to provide information to which the participant or beneficiary is entitled.[65]
2. The participant or beneficiary may recover benefits due under the terms of the plan, enforce rights under the terms of the plan, or clarify rights to future benefits under the terms of the plan.[66]
3. The participant or beneficiary may obtain relief for breaches of fiduciary duty.[67]
4. The participant or beneficiary may enjoin any act or practice that violates ERISA or the terms of the plan or may obtain other appropriate equitable relief to redress violation or enforce ERISA provisions or plan terms.[68]
5. The participant or beneficiary may sue for interference with ERISA-protected rights.[69]

Punitive and extracontractual damage claims are *not* available under ERISA (discussed next).[70]

Preemption and Remedies

ERISA extensively regulates all self-funded EBPs and preempts all state laws that "relate to" the EBP, broadly construed.[71] State laws covered by this preemption include regulation, legislation, and common law.[72] Note that laws which are preempted include not only those that directly attempt to affect ERISA EBPs but also laws of general application and those that in fact are consistent with the statute.[73] Further, ERISA EBP beneficiaries are limited to the remedies as enumerated in the statute; that is, recovery of benefits due under the plan, enforcement of rights under the terms of the plan, and clarification of rights to future

[59]29 U.S.C.A. §1132(a).

[60]29 U.S.C.A. §1144; Pilot Life Ins. Co. v. Dedeaux, 481 U.S. 41 (1987).

[61]29 U.S.C.A. §1113.

[62]See, e.g., Pane v. RCA Corp., 868 F.2d 631 (3d Cir. 1989); Dameron v. Sinai Hosp., Inc., 815 F.2d 975 (4th Cir. 1987); Jenkins v. Local 705 Int'l Bd. of Teamsters Pension Plan, 713 F.2d 247 (7th Cir. 1983); Meade v. Pension Appeals and Review Comm., 966 F.2d 190 (6th Cir. 1992); Koonan v. Blue Cross & Blue Shield, 802 F.Supp. 1424 (E.D. Va. 1992); see also Tolle v. Carroll Touch, Inc., 977 F.2d 1129 (7th Cir. 1992); Ladzinski v. Meba Pension Trust, 951 F.Supp. 570 (D. Md. 1997).

[63]See, e.g., Pane v. RCA Corp., 868 F.2d 631 (3d Cir. 1989); Daniel v. Eaton Corp., 839 F.2d 263 (6th Cir.), *cert. denied* 488 U.S. 826 (1988); Crews v. Central States, S.E. & S.W. Areas Pension Fund, 788 F.2d 332 (6th Cir. 1986); Berry v. Ciba-Geigy Corp., 761 F.2d 1003 (4th Cir. 1985); Turner v. CF & I Steel Corp., 770 F.2d 43 (3d Cir. 1985), *cert. denied* 474 U.S. 1058 (1986); Katsaros v. Cody, 744 F.2d 270 (2d Cir.), *cert. denied* 469 U.S. 1072 (1984); Wardle v. Central States Pension Fund, 627 F.2d 820 (7th Cir. 1980), *cert. denied* 449 U.S. 1112 (1981); Calamia v. Spivey, 632 F.2d 1235 (5th Cir. 1980); In re Vorpahl, 695 F.2d 318 (8th Cir. 1982); Chilton v. Savannah Foods & Indus., Inc., 814 F.2d 620 (11th Cir. 1987).

[64]See, e.g., Padilla de Higginbotham v. Worth Publishers, Inc., 820 F.Supp. 48 (D. P.R. 1993); McDonald v. Artcraft Elec. Supply Co., 774 F.Supp. 29 (D. D.C. 1991); Gangitano v. NN Investors Life Ins. Co., 733 F.Supp. 342 (S.D. Fla. 1990); Vicinanzo v. Brunschwig Fils, Inc., 739 F.Supp. 882 (S.D. N.Y. 1990).

[65]29 U.S.C.A. §1132(a)(1)(A); see also Rakoczy v. Travelers Ins. Co., 914 F.Supp. 166 (E.D. Mich. 1996) (defective notice remedy is to remand claim for review of claim denial).

[66]29 U.S.C.A. §1132(a)(1)(B).

[67]29 U.S.C.A. §1132(a)(2).

[68]29 U.S.C.A §1132(a)(3).

[69]29 U.S.C.A. §1140.

[70]See, e.g., Massachusetts Mut. Life Ins. Co. v. Russell, 473 U.S. 134 (1985); Drinkwater v. Metropolitan Life Ins. Co., 846 F.2d 821 (1st Cir.), *cert. denied* 488 U.S. 909 (1988); Mertens v. Hewitt Associates, 508 U.S. 248 (1993).

[71]29 U.S.C.A. §1144; Shaw v. Delta Air Lines, 463 U.S. 85 (1983); Ingersoll-Rand Co. v. McClendon, 498 U.S. 133 (1990).

[72]29 U.S.C.A. §1144(c)(1); Ingersoll-Rand v. McClendon, 498 U.S. 133 (1990).

[73]See, e.g., FMC Corp. v. Holliday, 498 U.S. 52, 58 (1990); Tybout v. Karr Barth Pension Admin., Inc., 819 F.Supp. 371 (D. Del. 1993); see also District of Columbia v. Greater Washington Board of Trade, 506 U.S. 125 (1992) (ERISA preempts state laws approved in ERISA if state law relates to another EBP covered under ERISA).

benefits under the terms of the plan.[74] No punitive or extracontractual damages are allowed;[75] hence, suits for wrongful death, personal injury, or other claims for consequential damages caused by improper refusal of care or coverage by an insurer or utilization reviewer are preempted because they pray for relief not enumerated in the statute.[76] Note that ERISA does authorize a plan participant or beneficiary to obtain "appropriate" relief for breach of fiduciary duty; however, any extracontractual damages recovered pursuant to these provisions inure to the plan itself, not the individual beneficiary.[77]

Despite the apparent significant difficulties with beneficiary access to the courts to obtain what might be thought as expected remedies, ERISA was originally passed to protect plan participants.[78] The difficulty lies in the fact that courts have interpreted ERISA broadly and so have limited claims against ERISA EBPs that invoke state law, including tort and contract law. Four general categories of state law have been preempted by ERISA: laws regulating benefits or terms of ERISA plans; laws mandating reporting, disclosure, funding, or vesting requirements for ERISA plans; laws mandating benefits calculations; and laws providing remedies for misconduct arising out of ERISA administration, such as tort and contract law.[79] Even if plaintiffs are left without a remedy because ERISA itself does not provide one (e.g., personal injury damages), courts still have held that plaintiffs' non-ERISA claims are preempted.[80] Challenges by providers for exclusion from networks and plans also have been preempted.[81] However, the ERISA shield is being penetrated by other courts, which have held that quality concerns (rather than the amount of benefits) are not within the preemption provisions of ERISA,[82] and the U.S. Supreme Court, which has held

that state hospital surcharge mandates were not preempted by ERISA.[83] Yet courts continue to find that claims that arise from the manner by which benefits are administered or claims based on the type or extent of benefits promised or provided are preempted.[84] Note, however, that the negligent misrepresentation of the scope of EBP coverage has been held not to be preempted.[85] Many other areas of the law have been held to be both preempted and not preempted,[86] including direct and vicarious liability claims against managed care organizations.[87] Therefore, ERISA, preemption, and the common law will continue to be debated until a resolution of the incentives created by it is provided by Congress.[88] Meanwhile, very close attention to the extent of EBP benefits and rights is warranted to avoid the preemptive effects on injury suits by ERISA.

---

[74]29 U.S.C.A. §1132(a).

[75]Massachusetts Mut. Life Ins. Co. v. Russell, 473 U.S. 134 (1985); Drinkwater v. Metropolitan Life Ins. Co., 846 F.2d 821, 825 (1st Cir.), *cert. denied* 488 U.S. 909 (1988); Sokol v. Bernstein, 803 F.2d 532 (9th Cir. 1986); Powell v. Chesapeake & Potomac Tel. Co., 780 F.2d 419 (4th Cir. 1985).

[76]29 U.S.C.A.§§1132(a)(1)(B), 1132(a)(3).

[77]29 U.S.C.A. §§1109(a)–1132(a)(1); Massachusetts Mutual Life Ins. Co. v. Russell, 473 U.S. 134, 140-4 (1985).

[78]Fort Halifax Packing Co., Inc. v. Coyne, 482 U.S. 1 (1987).

[79]Pacificare of Oklahoma, Inc. v. Burrage, 59 F.3d 151, 154 (10th Cir. 1995).

[80]See, e.g., Corcoran v. United Healthcare, Inc., 965 F.2d 1321 (5th Cir.), *cert. denied* 506 U.S. 1033 (1992); Tolton v. American Biodyne, Inc., 48 F.3d 937 (6th Cir. 1995); Cannon v. Group Health Serv., 77 F.3d 1270 (10th Cir. 1996).

[81]See, e.g., Zuniga v. Blue Cross and Blue Shield, 52 F.3d 1395 (6th Cir. 1995).

[82]See, e.g., Dukes v. U.S. Healthcare, Inc., 57 F.3d 350 (3d Cir. 1995), *cert. denied* 516 U.S. 1009 (1995).

[83]New York State Conference of Blue Cross/Blue Shield Plans v. Travelers Ins. Co., 514 U.S. 645 (1995); see also De Buono v. NYSA-ILA Medical and Clinical Services Fund, 117 S.Ct. 1747 (1997) (New York state tax of medical centers' gross receipts are not preempted by ERISA).

[84]See, e.g., Kearney v. U.S. Healthcare, Inc., 859 F.Supp. 182 (E.D. Pa. 1994); Kuhl v. Lincoln Nat. Health Plan, 999 F.2d 298 (8th Cir. 1993), *cert. denied* 510 U.S. 1045 (1994); Elsesser v. Hospital of Phil. College, 802 F.Supp. 1286 (E.D. Pa 1992); Altieri v. CIGNA Dental Health, Inc., 753 F.Supp. 61 (D. Conn. 1990).

[85]Wilson v. Zoellner, 114 F.3d 713 (8th Cir. 1997).

[86]See, e.g., Hubbard v. Blue Cross and Blue Shield Ass'n, 42 F.3d 942 (5th Cir.), *cert. denied* 115 S.Ct. 2276 (1995) (fraud claim preempted); Anderson v. Humana, 24 F.3d 889 (7th Cir. 1994) (fraud claim preempted); Muller v. Maron, 1995 WL 605483 (E.D. Pa. Oct. 13, 1995) (fraud claim not preempted); Stuart Circle Hosp. Corp. v. Aetna Health Management, 995 F.2d 500 (4th Cir.), *cert. denied* 114 S.Ct. 579 (1993) (any willing provider law not preempted); CIGNA Healthplan v. Louisiana, 82 F.3d 642 (5th Cir. 1995), *cert. denied* 117 S.Ct. 387 (1996) (any willing provider law preempted); Warran v. Society Nat'l Bank, 905 F.2d 975 (6th Cir. 1990), *cert. denied* 500 U.S. 952 (1991) (compensatory damages available under ERISA); Harch v. Eisenberg, 956 F.2d 651 (7th Cir.), *cert. denied* 506 U.S. 818 (1992) (compensatory damages unavailable under ERISA).

[87]See, e.g., Dukes v. U.S. Healthcare, Inc., 57 F.3d 350 (3d Cir.), *cert. denied* 516 U.S. 1009 (1995) (not preempted); Rice v. Panchal, 65 F.3d 637 (7th Cir. 1995) (not preempted); Pacificare of Okla., Inc. v. Burrage, 59 F.3d 151 (10th Cir. 1995) (not preempted); Jass v. Prudential Health Care Plan, 88 F.3d 1482 (7th Cir. 1996) (preempted); Clark v. Humana Kansas City, Inc., 975 F.Supp. 1283 (D. Kan. 1997) (preempted).

[88]B. A. Liang, "Patient Injury Incentives in Law," *Yale Law and Policy Review* 17 (1998), pp. 1–93, describes how ERISA, jurisdictional error made by courts, and independent contractor tort and contract law interact to provide significant negative patient injury incentives in law that must be resolved legislatively by Congress.

COBRA and HIPAA

The Consolidated Omnibus Budget Reconciliation Act of 1985 (COBRA)[89] and Health Insurance Portability and Accountability Act (HIPAA)[90] both have amended ERISA and govern insurance coverage and its continuity for employees. Each has its own provisions, but they interact in several key areas.

COBRA

COBRA generally mandates that private employers with 20 employees or greater[91] offer employees and certain immediate family members (the "qualified beneficiaries") an opportunity to continue their group health plan coverage ("continuation coverage") after certain events such as employment termination ("qualifying events").[92] The qualifying event must cause the qualified beneficiary to lose group plan coverage for COBRA provisions to be triggered.[93] Group health plans are those plans that provide health care to participants and beneficiaries that have been set up and to which employers contribute.[94] Government plans and church plans are not subject to the requirements of COBRA.[95]

This continuation of coverage after a qualifying event must be identical to the coverage of persons who have not experienced the qualifying event.[96] The length of continuation coverage depends on the particular qualifying event that has transpired. If an employee's employment has been terminated for reasons other than gross misconduct[97] or if the employee's hours have been reduced, continuation coverage may be for 18 months after the date of the qualifying event.[98] COBRA applies regardless of whether the employee was fired or left voluntarily.[99] COBRA continuation coverage lasts for 36 months if one of the following qualifying events occur:

1. death of the employee;
2. divorce of the employee from the employee's spouse;
3. Chapter 11 bankruptcy proceedings of the employer from whom a retired employee obtained coverage;
4. employee becomes entitled to Medicare; or
5. a dependent child of the employee ceases to be a dependent child.[100]

Note that if, within 18 months of a termination of employment or reduction of the employee's hours, any of the events 1–5 occur, then the employee's continuation coverage generally will continue for 36 months from the date of the original termination or reduction in hours.[101] Employees who are disabled at the time of a termination or reduction in hours are eligible for continuation coverage for 29 months, which represents an 11-month extension from the occurrence of these qualifying events absent disability.[102]

Qualified beneficiaries must elect to accept COBRA continuation coverage. Qualified beneficiaries for the purposes of employment termination and reduction of hours include the employee, his or her spouse, and any dependents;[103] for all other qualifying events, only the spouse and dependents are qualified beneficiaries.[104] Note that an employer may not deny COBRA continuation coverage to an otherwise eligible beneficiary because the beneficiary

---

[89]Pub. L. No. 99-272, 100 Stat. 82 (1986).

[90]Pub. L. No. 104-191, 110 Stat. 1936 (1996).

[91]See 29 U.S.C.A. §1161(b).

[92]26 U.S.C.A. §4980B; 29 U.S.C.A. §§1161–1168.

[93]26 U.S.C.A. §4980B(f)(1); 29 U.S.C.A. §1161(a), Proposed Treasury Regulation §1.162-26, Q & A 18.

[94]26 U.S.C.A. §§4980B(g)(2), 5000(b)(1); 29 U.S.C.A. §1167(1).

[95]26 U.S.C.A. §4980B(d).

[96]26 U.S.C.A. §4980B(f)(2)(A); 29 U.S.C.A. §1162(1); see also Proposed Treasury Regulations §1.162-26, Q & A 10 (describing definition of health plans).

[97]See, e.g., Mlsna v. Unitel Communications Inc., 41 F.3d 1124 (7th Cir. 1994) (resignation without request from employer not termination due to gross misconduct); Paris v. F. Korbel & Bros., Inc., 751 F.Supp. 834 (N.D. Cal. 1990) (breach of company confidence not gross misconduct for COBRA purposes); Conery v. Bath Assocs., 803 F.Supp. 1388 (N.D. Ind. 1992) (employee allowed to resign to avoid being terminated for gross misconduct may not be denied COBRA benefits).

[98]26 U.S.C.A. §4980B(f)(2)(B)(i)(I); 29 U.S.C.A. §1162(2)(A)(i); see also Burgess v. Adams Tool & Engineering, 908 F.Supp. 473 (W.D. Mich. 1995) (termination of employment after reduction in hours does not constitute a second qualifying event).

[99]Proposed Treasury Regulation §1.162-26, Q & A 19.

[100]26 U.S.C.A. §4980B(f)(2)(B)(i)(IV); 29 U.S.C.A. §1162(2)(A)(iv).

[101]26 U.S.C.A. §4980B(f)(2)(B)(i)(II); 29 U.S.C.A. §1162(2)(A)(ii); but see 26 U.S.C.A. §4980B(f)(2)(B)(iv) (indicating that an employee who becomes eligible for Medicare has COBRA benefits terminated, but spouse and/or dependent child continue COBRA benefits); 26 U.S.C.A. 4980B(f)(2)(B)(i)(V) (indicating that if an employee becomes entitled to Medicare, coverage shall not terminate before 36 months after employee becomes so entitled).

[102]26 U.S.C.A. §4980B(f)(2)(B)(i); 29 U.S.C.A. §1162(2); see also 26 U.S.C.A. §4980B(f)(6)(C), 29 U.S.C.A. 1166(a)(3) (requiring the disabled employee to notify plan administrator within 60 days of determination of disability and 18 months of qualifying event); 26 U.S.C.A. §4980B(f)(2)(C); 29 U.S.C.A. §1162(3) (allowing greater premium charges for the disabled after 18th month of continuation coverage).

[103]26 U.S.C.A. §4980B(g)(1)(B); 29 U.S.C.A. §1167(3)(B).

[104]26 U.S.C.A. §4980B(g)(1)(A); 29 U.S.C.A. §1167(3)(A).

is covered under another group health plan at the time the beneficiary elects COBRA coverage.[105] The election period begins no later than the date on which coverage terminates and ends no earlier than 60 days after the time the notice is sent to the qualified beneficiary of his or her rights to continuation coverage or the time COBRA coverage terminates due to the qualifying event.[106] The qualified beneficiary has 45 days to pay the COBRA premiums after election.[107]

The group health plan most likely will require payment of premiums for continuation coverage.[108] This premium must not be greater than 102% of the "applicable premium" paid by the employer.[109] Note that this virtually always will be greater than what the employee generally pays because the employer no longer provides its contribution to subsidize the employee's health plan costs. The applicable premium is defined as the cost to the plan for similarly situated beneficiaries to whom the qualifying event has not occurred for a similar period of coverage.[110] Self-insured plans may estimate the applicable premium on the basis of cost estimates adjusted for inflation.[111] COBRA premiums may be paid on monthly installments,[112] but no plan may require payment of premiums before 45 days after the initial election is made by the beneficiary.[113] Once COBRA coverage begins, the group health plan must provide written notice to each covered employee and his or her spouse regarding the rights they have under COBRA.[114]

Employers and employees have notice obligations. Employers must notify the group health plan administrators within 30 days of a qualifying event if that event is a termination or reduction of employment, death of the employee, employee entitlement to Medicare, or the commencement of bankruptcy proceedings by the employer.[115] The beneficiary or covered employee must notify the group health plan administrator within 60 days of a qualifying event if that event is a divorce or child's loss of dependency.[116] Once the plan administrator is noti-

fied of the qualifying event, the administrator must notify each qualified beneficiary within 14 days as to the beneficiary's rights under COBRA with respect to the particular qualifying event.[117] The penalty for noncompliance with COBRA is $100/day in the form of an excise tax.[118]

In addition to lapse of the coverage time, COBRA coverage may be terminated if the employer ceases to provide any group health plan for any employee[119] or if the beneficiary does not make appropriate premium payments within 30 days after they are due (or a longer time if the plan provides for a longer grace period).[120] The coverage also can be terminated when the beneficiary becomes covered under another group health plan if the new plan does not have preexisting condition exclusions.[121]

COBRA coverage may be waived during the election period; however, this waiver may be revoked if it occurs before the end of the election period.[122] In addition, a beneficiary may exchange COBRA rights for employer-paid coverage for a lesser period if the employer is amenable.[123]

HIPAA

HIPAA provides additional rules governing group health plans, generally focusing on individual coverage portability, availability, and renewability for plan years after June 30, 1997. HIPAA expands portability of health insurance by limiting the preexisting condition exclusions. Group health plans may exclude coverage on the basis of preexisting conditions for 12 months; this period is 18 months if the employee enrolls late into the plan. However, the preexisting conditions that can be excluded are only those that relate to a physical or mental condition for which advice, diagnosis, care, or treatment was recommended or received within 6 months before enrollment into the new plan.[124] Further, children cannot be excluded if they were covered within 30 days of their birth or adoption; and pregnancy cannot be a basis for a preexisting exclusion.[125]

The 12- or 18-month exclusion is reduced by the amount of time of prior coverage.[126] Therefore, any

[105]See Geissal v. Moore Med. Corp., 524 U.S. 74 (1998).

[106]26 U.S.C.A. §4980B(f)(5)(A); 29 U.S.C.A. §1165(1).

[107]26 U.S.C.A. §4980B(f)(2)(C)(ii); 29 U.S.C.A. §1162(3)(B).

[108]See, e.g., Nichols v. Carpenters Health and Welfare Trust Fund for Calif., 19 F.3d 1440 (9th Cir. 1994) (employer coverage payment can count toward 18-month COBRA coverage period).

[109]26 U.S.C.A. §4980B(f)(2)(B)(i); 29 U.S.C.A. §1162(3)(A).

[110]26 U.S.C.A. §4980B(f)(4)(A); 29 U.S.C.A. §1164(1); see also Draper v. Baker Hughes, Inc., 892 F.Supp. 1287 (E.D. Cal. 1995) (indicating calculation methods for COBRA beneficiaries).

[111]26 U.S.C.A. §4980B(f)(4)(B); 29 U.S.C.A. §1164(2).

[112]26 U.S.C.A. §4980B(f)(2)(C)(ii); 29 U.S.C.A. §1162(3)(B).

[113]26 U.S.C.A. §4980B(f)(2)(C)(ii); 29 U.S.C.A. §1162(3)(B).

[114]26 U.S.C.A. §4980B(f)(6)(A); 29 U.S.C.A. §1166(a)(1).

[115]26 U.S.C.A. §4980B(f)(6)(B); 29 U.S.C.A. §1166(a)(2).

[116]26 U.S.C.A. §4980B(f)(6)(C); 29 U.S.C.A. §1166(a)(3).

[117]26 U.S.C.A. §4980B(f)(6)(D); 29 U.S.C.A. §1166(a)(4).

[118]26 U.S.C.A. §4980B(b)(1).

[119]26 U.S.C.A. §4980B(f)(2)(B)(ii); 29 U.S.C.A. §1162(2)(B).

[120]26 U.S.C.A. §4980B(f)(2)(B)(iii); 29 U.S.C.A. §1162(2)(C).

[121]26 U.S.C.A. §4980B(f)(2)(B)(iv)(I); 29 U.S.C.A. §1162(2)(D).

[122]See Proposed Treasury Regulation §1.162-26, Q & A 35.

[123]See Proposed Treasury Regulation §1.162-26, Q & A 32.

[124]26 U.S.C.A. §9801(a)(1); 29 U.S.C.A. §1181(a)(1).

[125]26 U.S.C.A. §9801(d); 29 U.S.C.A. §1181(d)(2)-(3).

[126]26 U.S.C.A. §9801(a)(3); 29 U.S.C.A. §1181(a)(3).

"credited coverage" under group health plans, health insurance coverage, Medicaid, Medicare, military health insurance, and other health benefits programs or plans reduces the exclusion period month for month.[127] Hence, an individual with 12 or 18 months of *previous* coverage may enroll into a new health plan without exclusions; however, any break in coverage longer than 63 days renders the coverage before that break ineligible for credited coverage.[128] Prior plans must certify the period of creditable coverage when coverage ceases, at the time of becoming covered or ceasing to be covered under COBRA provision, or on request by the individual.[129]

HIPAA also expands the availability of health coverage by instituting a broad antidiscrimination mandate. Group health plans cannot discriminate in eligibility for coverage or premiums on the basis of claims experience, genetic information, evidence of insurability or disability of the individual or dependents, health status, medical condition, or medical history; however, plans are permitted to limit their coverage for specific procedures or at specific benefits levels as long as there is no discrimination against similarly situated employees, and plans may use financial incentives for health promotion and disease prevention compliance.[130] HIPAA also mandates that if any material reduction of covered services or benefits under the health plan occurs, the employer must provide the employee with notice within 60 days after adoption of such a limitation unless the employer provides such a description of the plan at least every 90 days.[131]

HIPAA rules do not apply to government health plans; plans covering fewer than two current employees; other types of insurance in which medical care is secondary or incidental; limited dental, vision, long-term care, nursing home, or home health care insurance; disease-specific insurance under a separate policy; or Medicare supplemental insurance under a separate policy.[132]

Penalties for noncompliance mirror COBRA: $100/day tax for each adversely affected individual.[133] However, this tax is not imposed if failure to comply is not discovered in the exercise of reasonable diligence or if failure is due to a reasonable cause and corrected within 30 days after it should have been discovered.[134] The penalty can rise if the noncompliance is not corrected after notification.[135] For unintentional failures, there are other provisions for penalties that are more limited;[136] the IRS also can waive penalties.[137] Employers with 50 or fewer employees are not subject to penalties for failures in the provision of services.[138]

COBRA–HIPAA Interface

HIPAA modifies COBRA in several important ways. First, HIPAA modifies the individual's rights with regard to COBRA coverage. Originally, COBRA continuation coverage could not be terminated, even if the qualified beneficiary was covered by another plan, if the new plan imposed preexisting condition exclusions. However, HIPAA changes this by indicating that if the preexisting exclusion of the new plan does not affect the qualified beneficiary, COBRA coverage may be terminated.[139]

Second, HIPAA mandates special open enrollment rules for group health plan coverage years after June 30, 1997. Originally, an employee who did not enroll into a health plan when he or she was first eligible often had to wait until the next open enrollment period to obtain coverage. However, HIPAA modifies this rule by indicating that if an individual does not join a health plan when first eligible because that person wishes to keep other health coverage, including COBRA coverage, the employer health plan must let the person join the plan within 30 days of the date the other coverage is exhausted.[140]

Third, the definition of *qualified beneficiary* has been altered. Originally, COBRA deemed individuals qualified beneficiaries only if they had such status at the time of the qualifying event. However, HIPAA now has included as a qualified beneficiary a child born to or placed for adoption with a qualified beneficiary during the period of COBRA coverage.[141]

Fourth, the disability rules for COBRA continuation coverage have been changed. Instead of requiring that the qualifying beneficiary be disabled at the time of the qualifying event to be eligible for the disabled extension, a qualified beneficiary can be disabled within the first 60 days of COBRA coverage to qualify for the 11-month extension.[142]

Fifth, HIPAA allows for individuals who have received unemployment compensation for at least 12 weeks to use individual retirement account funds to pay for medical insurance, including COBRA continuation coverage.[143]

[127]26 U.S.C.A. §9801(c)(1); 29 U.S.C.A. §1181(c)(1).
[128]26 U.S.C.A. §9801(c)(2)(A); 29 U.S.C.A. §1181(c)(2)(A).
[129]26 U.S.C.A. §9801(e); 29 U.S.C.A. §1181(d).
[130]26 U.S.C.A. §9802.
[131]29 U.S.C.A. §1024(b)(1); 42 U.S.C.A. §300gg-12(c)(1).
[132]26 U.S.C.A. §§9831, 9834(c).
[133]26 U.S.C.A. §4980D(b)(1).
[134]26 U.S.C.A. §4980D(c)(1).
[135]26 U.S.C.A. §4980D(b)(3).
[136]26 U.S.C.A. §4980D(c)(3).
[137]26 U.S.C.A. §4980D(c)(4).
[138]26 U.S.C.A. §4980D(d)(2)(A).
[139]26 U.S.C.A. §9801.
[140]26 U.S.C.A. §9801(f)(1).
[141]42 U.S.C.A. §300bb-8(3)(A).
[142]26 U.S.C.A. §§4980B(f)(2)(B)(i), 4980B(f)(6)(C).
[143]26 U.S.C.A. §72(t)(2)(D)(i)(I).

Sixth, medical savings accounts authorized by HIPAA, although prohibited for use to pay for health insurance, can be used to pay for COBRA coverage.[144] Medical savings accounts are tax-advantaged accounts coupled with high deductible health insurance plans, the latter of which are used to cover catastrophic health care costs.[145] The cash in the medical savings accounts may be withdrawn tax free to pay for noncatastrophic care.

Seventh, individual insurance coverage is now mandated by HIPAA. As of July 1, 1997, if an individual has completed at least 18 months of previous group health plan coverage; is ineligible for Medicare, Medicaid, or group health coverage; has not been terminated from the most recent prior coverage due to nonpayment of premiums or fraud; and is eligible, has elected, paid, and exhausted COBRA or similar coverage required by state law, then the individual insurance market must make available individual health insurance coverage with no preexisting condition exclusions.[146]

Other Statutes

Balanced Budget Act of 1997

The Balanced Budget Act of 1997 (BBA)[147] is a federal statute that provides significant expansion of health care insurance coverage for children by funding state child health insurance programs. The federal government has devoted approximately $40 billion through 2007 for this initiative,[148] allocated on the basis of a geographic cost factor and the number of low-income children in the state.[149] Under the BBA, states may expand Medicaid benefits to previously ineligible children, create a new state child insurance health plan, or formulate programs that are a combination of both.[150] Significant flexibility is provided states under the BBA as to design eligibility,[151] benefits,[152] and cost-sharing[153] requirements as well as procedures for amending[154] their programs. States are permitted to allocate up to 10% of federal funds for administration, outreach, and direct purchase of insurance coverage.[155] An important provision of the BBA allows

for states to implement mandatory managed care programs without waiver authority from the Department of Health and Human Services.[156]

Family and Medical Leave Act

The Family and Medical Leave Act (FMLA)[157] is a federal statute that mandates that employers with at least 50 employees (including joint employers[158]) working 20 or more weeks in the current or previous calendar year[159] grant those employees up to 12 weeks' leave to: care for a child following birth or placement of a child with the employee; care for a child, spouse, or parent who has a serious health condition; or care for him- or herself if the employee has a serious health condition.[160] The employer must post the information regarding FMLA rights and remedies for employer violations conspicuously.[161] The employer may require medical certification for employee leave requests because of an eligible serious health condition.[162] The employer also may institute a requirement that the employee certify that he or she is fit to work after the leave has been taken if the FMLA leave was for the employee's own serious health condition, and such a requirement is uniform across employees taking such leave.[163]

Leave periods may be intermittent,[164] although if the leave is requested for planned medical treatment or recovery from a serious health condition, the employer may transfer the employee temporarily to another position.[165] Further, spouses employed by the same employer are limited to a combined 12-week leave period if the leave is for: birth or care after the birth of their child; placement with the spouses of a child for foster or adoption care or care after such placement; or care for a parent with a serious health condition.[166]

FMLA leave can be unpaid or paid, with the former more common. An employee may be able to use paid leave instead if authorized by the employer's family leave plan,[167]

---

[144]26 U.S.C.A. §220(d)(2)(B).

[145]26 U.S.C.A. §§106, 220.

[146]Pub. L. No. 104-191, 110 Stat. 1936 (1996).

[147]Pub. L. No. 105-33, 111 Stat. 251 (1997).

[148]42 U.S.C.A. §1397dd(a).

[149]42 U.S.C.A. §1397dd(b).

[150]42 U.S.C.A. §1397aa(a).

[151]42 U.S.C.A. §1397bb(b)(1).

[152]42 U.S.C.A. §1397cc.

[153]42 U.S.C.A. §1397cc(e).

[154]42 U.S.C.A. §1397ff(b)(1).

[155]42 U.S.C.A. §1397ee(c)(2)(A).

[156]42 U.S.C.A. 1397ff(b)(1).

[157]29 U.S.C.A. §§2601 *et seq.*; 29 C.F.R. §825.100 (1998).

[158]29 C.F.R. §§825.104(c)(2) (1998), 825.106 (1998).

[159]29 C.F.R. §§825.104(a) (1998), 825.105(e) (1998); see Clark v. Allegheny Univ. Hosp., 1998 WL 94803 (E.D.Pa. Mar. 4, 1998) (paid leave does not count toward hours worked calculation).

[160]29 U.S.C.A. §§2612(a)(1), 2611(11).

[161]29 U.S.C.A. §2619(a).

[162]29 U.S.C.A. §2613(a)–(e).

[163]29 U.S.C.A. §2614(a)(4); see also 29 C.F.R. 825.310(c) (1998) (employer cannot require multiple fitness for work certifications).

[164]29 U.S.C.A. §2612(b); 29 C.F.R. §825.203 (1998).

[165]29 U.S.C.A. §2612(b)(2).

[166]29 C.F.R. §825.202 (1998).

[167]29 C.F.R. §825.208 (1998).

and employers may choose to require that employees use paid leave.[168] Health care benefits must be maintained on the same level prior to taking the leave if the employee appropriately requests and pays for such benefits.[169] However, if the employee's payments are more than 30 days late, the employer's obligation to maintain health coverage ends so long as the employer has provided appropriate notice to the employee. The employer must provide equivalent benefits and health coverage on the employee's return from FMLA leave.[170] Note, though, that employees are not entitled to accrue any seniority or other similar benefits during their leave.[171]

To be eligible for FMLA leave, the employee must have been employed for at least 12 months and must have at least 1250 hours of service with the employer during that period.[172] An employee must give the employer 30 days' notice that he or she intends to take the leave or other notice if it is not practicable to give 30 days.[173] When an employee provides notice to the employer of intent to exercise the leave, the employer must provide the employee with a notice, which includes information regarding the employee's potential responsibility for any premium payments to maintain health benefits and the employee's potential liability for payment of health insurance premiums by the employer in the event the employee does not return to work.[174] An employer under these circumstances must continue to provide the employee with health insurance during this time and generally is required to provide the employee with his or her original position or a substantially equivalent position at the end of the leave granted by the FMLA.[175]

Employers must maintain FMLA records for three years.[176] An employer is prohibited from interfering with employee exercise of rights under the FMLA.[177] Employer violations are remedied through damages or equitable relief; attorneys' fees and other litigation costs are also available.[178] Employees must bring suit within

two years after the date of the last event that constituted a violation[179] or within three years for willful violations by the employer;[180] the Department of Labor also can bring suit against the employer.[181] Suit for violations of the FMLA can also be brought against persons in their individual capacity who act in the interest of the employer.[182]

FMLA interacts with COBRA. Under IRS notices,[183] a qualifying event in the context of FMLA that creates COBRA rights is the end of the employer's obligation to continue to provide coverage under FMLA. This occurs on the date the employee states to the employer that he or she is not returning to work, on the last day of the leave, or at the end of the employee's FMLA leave entitlement, whichever is *earliest*. COBRA coverage begins at the time of the qualifying event or on the date coverage actually ends, whichever is later. Employees who take FMLA leave and do not return to employment can elect COBRA at the time of the qualifying event, even though their health coverage might have lapsed during the leave period. In the event that employees do not return from unpaid leave, FMLA allows an employer to recover health premiums paid during the leave period; however, COBRA rights cannot be premised on the employee's payment of these premiums. Note that COBRA notice rules apply when an employee has experienced the FMLA-based qualifying event; therefore, the employer must notify the plan administrator of the qualifying event within 30 days of the date of the qualifying event. Employers cannot recover premiums from an employee if the employee uses other benefits, including workers' compensation or other disability benefit payments, for FMLA leave.[184] In addition, an employer cannot recover premiums if continuation, reoccurrence, or onset of a serious health condition would entitle the employee to further leave[185] or if circumstances beyond the employee's control occur, including an employee who chooses to stay home with a newborn child with a serious health condition, spousal transfer unexpectedly to another job location greater than 75 miles from the employee's work site, an employee's relative is afflicted with a serious health condition and the employee is needed to provide care for him or her, or a key employee does not return to work on being notified of the employer's intent to deny the employee's job restoration due to substantial and grievous economic injury to the employer's operations arising from the job restoration.[186]

[168]29 U.S.C.A. §2612(d)(2).

[169]29 C.F.R. §825.209 (1998).

[170]29 C.F.R. §825.212 (1998).

[171]29 U.S.C.A. §2614(a)(3)(A).

[172]29 C.F.R. §§825.110(c) (1998); 825.200(b) (1998).

[173]29 U.S.C.A. §2612(e); see also Brannon v. Oshkosh B'gosh, Inc., 897 F.Supp. 1028 (M.D. Tenn. 1995) (if leave unforeseeable, one to two days' notice is adequate); Miller v. Defiance Metal Products, 989 F.Supp. 945 (N.D. Ohio 1997); Satterfield v. Wal-Mart Stores, 135 F.3d 973 (5th Cir. 1998); Johnson v. Primerea, 1996 WL 34148 (S.D. N.Y. 1996); see also Dey v. County of Hennepin, 1997 WL 10878 (Minn. Ct. App. 1997).

[174]29 C.F.R. §825.301(b)(1) (1998).

[175]29 U.S.C.A. §2614(a)(1).

[176]29 U.S.C.A. §2616.

[177]29 U.S.C.A. §2615(a)(1).

[178]29 U.S.C.A. §2617(a).

[179]29 U.S.C.A. §255(a).

[180]29 U.S.C.A. §255(a).

[181]29 U.S.C.A. §2617.

[182]29 C.F.R. §825.104 (1998).

[183]Internal Revenue Service Notice 94-103, 1994-2 C.B. 569, I.R.B. 1994-51 (Dec. 6, 1994).

[184]29 C.F.R. §825.213(e) (1998).

[185]29 C.F.R. §825.213(a)(1) (1998).

[186]29 C.F.R. §825.213(a)(2) (1998).

States

Despite significant governance of insurance on the federal level, states under the McCarran–Ferguson Act are the traditional sites of insurance regulatory activity.[187] States have promulgated regulations that encompass health plans for those plans not subject to ERISA and drafted rules in the broad areas of allowable policy types, price and premium calculations, appropriate marketing, and solvency requirements. The National Association of Insurance Commissioners, a group with representatives from all state departments of insurance, has developed model laws in these areas and others for state guidance. With widely diverging insurance laws, specific statutes and regulations for the state of interest should be assessed to determine the rules and requirements for insurance that are relevant to the individual's interest. However, states have been given authority under HIPAA to institute more liberal standards with regard to provisions of the statute, including altering the 6-month preexisting condition period, limiting the 12- and 18-month maximum preexisting condition exclusions, increasing the 63-day break in coverage period, expanding prohibitions on conditions and persons to whom preexisting condition exclusion may be applied, and requiring additional special enrollment periods.[188]

Further Reading

ERISA Denial of Benefits Standard of Review

Capps NC. Firestone Tire and Rubber Co. v. Bruch: Are Lower Courts Following the United States Supreme Court Decision in ERISA Benefit Determinations? *Washburn L J* 1992;31:280–313.
ERISA: The Law and Code 1998 (serial) Washington, DC: BNA Books, 1998.
Jorden JF, Pflepsen WJ. *Handbook on ERISA Litigation,* 2d ed. Gaithersburg, MD: Aspen Publishers, 1997.
Russ LR. Rights upon Benefit Denial. In: *Couch on Insurance,* 3d ed. St. Paul, MN: West Publishing Co., 1997;§7:48.

ERISA Federal Regulations

Borzi PC. *ERISA Basics: A Primer of ERISA Issues — Key Requirements of the New Health Care Legislation Enacted by Congress in 1996.* Pub. no. N97EBAB ABA-LGLED V-1. Chicago: American Bar Association, 1997.
Davidson DS. Balancing the Interests of State Healthcare Reform and Uniform Employee Benefit Laws Under

---

[187]15 U.S.C.A. §1012.
[188]See 62 Fed. Reg. 16894 (1997); 42 U.S.C.A. §300gg-23(b)(2).

ERISA: A "Uniform Patient Protection Act." *Wash U J Urb & Contemp L* 1998;53:203–41.
ERISA: The Law and Code 1998 (serial) Washington, DC: BNA Books, 1998.
Harshbarger LH. ERISA Preemption Meets the Age of Managed Care: Toward a Comprehensive Social Policy. *Syracuse L Rev* 1996;47:191–224.
Kushner MG: *ERISA Regulations: Including Final, Temporary, and Proposed Rulemaking from DOL, PBGC, IRS, SEC, and Other Agencies,* Washington, DC: BNA Books, 1997.
Liang BA. Patient Injury Incentives in Law. *Yale L & Pol'y Rev* 1998;17:1–93.
Mikasen JL et al. Scope of ERISA's Preemption Provision. In: *American Jurisprudence,* 2d ed. New York: Lawyers Cooperative Publishing Co., 1988;§115.
Shah SR. Loosening ERISA's Preemptive Grip on HMO Medical Malpractice Claims: A Response to PacifiCare of Oklahoma v. Burrage. *Minn L Rev* 1996;80:1545–77.

ERISA Fiduciary Duty

Bintz EE. Fiduciary Responsibility Under ERISA: Is There Ever a Fiduciary Duty to Disclose? *U Pitt L Rev* 1993;54:979–1018.
Bortz WK, Brodie FA, et al. *ERISA Fiduciary Law.* Washington, DC: BNA Books, 1995.
Clark SJ, Wellman LL. An Overview of Pension Benefit and Fiduciary Litigation Under ERISA. *Williamette L Rev* 1990;26:665–710.
Gertner MA, Folk VC. *Annotated Fiduciary: Materials on Fiduciary Responsibility and Prohibited Transactions Under ERISA,* 3d ed. Brookfield, WI: IFEBP, 1989.
Rotenberg MS. ERISA — Fischer v. Philadelphia Electric Co.: The Third Circuit "Seriously Considers" the Fiduciary Duty to Disclose Potential Change to an Employee Benefit Plan Under ERISA. *Vill L Rev* 1997;42:1915–47.

ERISA Plan Amendments

Holloway JE. The ERISA Amendment Provision as a Disclosure Function: Including Workable Termination Procedures in the Functional Purpose of Section 402(B)(3). *Drake L Rev* 1998;46:795.
Perdue PD. *ERISA Section 204(H) Notices.* Pub. no. Q244. Chicago: American Law Institute–American Bar Association, 1996.

ERISA Plan Document

Brodie FA, Weiner SA. *ERISA. Business and Commercial Litigation in Federal Courts.* New York: Lawyers Cooperative Publishing Co., 1998;§§68.2, 68.9.

ERISA Preemption

Bulter PA. *Roadblock to Reform: ERISA Implications for State Health Care Initiative.* Washington, DC: National Governors Association, 1994.

Fellman-Caldwell RS. New York State Conference of Blue Cross & Blue Shield Plans v. Travelers Insurance Co. The Supreme Court Clarifies ERISA Preemption. *Cath U L Rev* 1996;45:1309–50.

Flint GL. ERISA Nonwaivability of Preemption. *U Kan L Rev* 1991;39:297–354.

Shah SR. Loosening ERISA's Preemptive Grip on HMO Medical Malpractice Claims: A Response to PacifiCare of Oklahoma v. Burrage. *Minn L Rev* 1996;80:1545–77.

Weisenborn N. ERISA Preemption and Its Efforts on State Health Reform. *Kan J L & Pub Pol'y* 1995;5:147–57.

ERISA Remedies

Jorden JF, Pflepsen WJ. *Handbook on ERISA Litigation,* 2d ed. Gaithersburg, MD: Aspen Publishers, 1997.

Knox JJ. Nieto v. Ecker: Incorporation of Nonfiduciary Liability Under ERISA. *Minn L Rev* 1989;73:1303–35.

Muir DM. ERISA Remedies: Chimera a Congressional Compromise? *Iowa L Rev* 1995;81:1–53.

Stoecker KJ. ERISA Remedies After Variety Corp. v. Howe. *DePaul Bus L J* 1997;9:237–58.

ERISA Self-Funded Employee Benefits Plans

Caster K. The Future of Self-Funded Health Plans. *Iowa L Rev* 1994;79:413–38.

Edwards MA. Protections for ERISA Self-Insured Employees Welfare Benefit Plan Participants: New Possibilities for State Action in the Event of Plan Failure. *Wis L Rev* 1997:351–73.

Schacht LJ. The Health Care Crisis: Improving Access for Employees Covered by Self-Insured Health Plans Under ERISA and the Americans with Disabilities Act. *Wash U J Urb & Contemp L* 1994;45:303–52.

Slivinska D. Health Care Cost Containment and Small Businesses: The Self-Insurance Option. *J L & Com* 1993;12:333–65.

Swedback JK. The Deemer Clause: A Legislative Savior for Self-Funded Health Insurance Plans Under the Employee Retirement Income Security Act of 1974. *Wm Mitchell L Rev* 1992;18:757–93.

ERISA Summary Plan Description

ERISA: The Law and Code 1998 (serial). Washington, DC: BNA Books, 1998.

Link RJ. What Documents Constitute "Summary Plan Descriptions" Under ERISA. In: *American Law Reports, Federal.* New York: Lawyers Cooperative Publishing Co., 1995;355–80.

Mertens J. Summary Plan Description. In: *Mertens Law of Federal Income Taxation.* Washington, DC: Thompson Legal Publishing, 1988;§25B.

Mikasen JL et al. Summary Plan Description. In: *American Jurisprudence,* 2d ed. New York: Lawyers Cooperative Publishing Co., 1988;§783.

Out-of-Pocket Costs

Bobinski MA. Unhealthy Federalism: Barriers to Increasing Health Care Access for the Uninsured. *U C Davis L Rev* 1990;24:255–348.

Brown LD. The Medically Uninsured: Problems, Policies, and Politics. *J Health Pol Pol'y & L* 1990;15:413–26.

Gostin LO. Securing Health or Just Health Care? The Effect of the Health Care System on the Health of America. *St Louis U L J* 1994;39:7–43.

Private Insurance

Leffler KB. Arizona v. Maricopa County Medical Society: Maximum Price Agreements in Markets with Insurance Buyers. *Sup Ct Econ Rev* 1983;2:187–212.

U.S. General Accounting Office. *Private Health Insurance: Continued Erosion of Coverage Linked to Cost Pressures.* Pub. no. GAO/HEHS-97-122. Washington, DC: U.S. General Accounting Office, 1997.

U.S. General Accounting Office. *Retiree Health Insurance: Erosion in Employer-Based Health Benefits for Early Retirees.* Pub. no. GAO/HEHS-97-150. Washington, DC: U.S. General Accounting Office, 1997.

Whitted G. Private Health Insurance and Employee Benefits. In: Williams SJ, Torrens PR. *Introduction to Health Services,* 5th ed. Albany, NY: Delmar Publishing, 1993.

Statutes

Balanced Budget Act of 1997

Wermuth A. Kidcare and the Uninsured Child: Options to an Illinois Health Insurance Plan. *Loy U Chi L J* 1998; 29:465–526.

COBRA

Donaldson RG. Construction and Application of ERISA Provisions Governing Continuation Coverage Under Group Health Plans. In: *American Law Reports, Federal.* New York: Lawyers Cooperative Publishing Co., 1997;§97.

Harris JW. Health Benefit Continuation Coverage Under COBRA. *Prob & Prop* 1991;5:11–14.

Helitzer JB. HMO's and COBRA. *Practising Law Institute* 1988;471:27–166.

Watson RC et al. *COBRA Health Continuation Benefits*. Pub. no. SC07. Chicago: American Law Institute–American Bar Association, 1997.

COBRA–HIPAA Interface

Dechene JC. Employer Obligations Under 1996 Health Insurance Act. *Law Firm Partnership & Ben Rep* 1997;3(6):1–4.

Shupe CL. *Developments Under the Health Insurance Portability and Accountability Act, COBRA, and Mental Health Parity Act*. Pub. no. SC62 ALI-ABA. Chicago: American Law Institute–American Bar Association, 1998.

Family and Medical Leave Act

Aalberts RJ, Seidman LH. The Family and Medical Leave Act: Does It Make Unreasonable Demands on Employers? *Marq L Rev* 1996;80:135–60.

Blair D, Keegan JO et. al. *The FMLA Guide: Practical Solutions to Administration and Management (Alexander Consulting Group Series on Employee Benefits)*. New York: Richard Irwin Publishing, 1995.

Cockey RR, Jeon DA. The Family and Medical Leave Act at Work: Getting Employers to Value Families. *Va J Soc Pol'y & L* 1996;4:225–34.

Duston RL, Robbins S. *FMLA: A Practical Guide to Implementing the FMLA*. Washington, DC: College and University Personnel Association, 1994.

Gitnik LJ. Will the Interaction of the Family and Medical Leave Act and the Americans with Disabilities Act Leave Employers with an "Undue Hardship"? *Wash U L Q* 1996;74:283–315.

Rogers B. Individual Liability Under the Family and Medical Leave Act of 1993: A Senseless Detour on the Road to a Flexible Workplace. *Brook L Rev* 1997;63:1299–1340.

Shannon JT. The Family and Medical Leave Act of 1993. *Ark Law* 1993;27(Sum):9–11.

Tysse GJ, Japinga KL. The Federal Family and Medical Leave Act: Easily Conceived, Difficult Birth, Enigmatic Child. *Creighton L Rev* 1994;27:361–80.

HIPAA

Dechene JC. Employers' Obligations Under 1996 Health Insurance Act. *Law Firm Partnership & Ben Rep* 1997;3(6):1–4.

Ford GM et al. *Enforcement of the Health Insurance Portability and Accountability Act*. Pub. no. SB86 ALI-ABA. Chicago: American Law Institute–American Bar Association, 1997.

Rutkowski AD, Rutkowski BL. Health Insurance Portability and Accountability Act of 1996: Are You in Compliance with the Law? *Employment L Update* 1997;12(7):1–8.

Wildman ML. New Fraud and Abuse Provisions of the Health Insurance Portability and Accountability Act of 1996. *Colo Law* 1997;26(Mar):81–84.

Traditional Indemnity Insurance

Rogers AL, Trotter JO et al. *Liability of Lawyers and Indemnity Insurance*. (International Bar Association Series. Norwell, MA: Kluwer Law International, 1995.

Herdman FT. Doctors, Insurers, and the Antitrust Laws. *Buff L Rev* 1989;37:817–20.

Other Reading

Anderson OA. *Health Services as a Growth Enterprise in the United States Since 1875*. Ann Arbor, MI: Health Administration Press, 1990.

Dees DS, Dunbar P. *Basic Law of Pensions: COBRA and Other Health Care Issues*. Pub. no. SC06 ALI-ABA 795. Chicago: American Law Institute–American Bar Association, 1997.

Jaffe AH. Health Insurance Litigation. *J Health Hosp Law* 1991;24:233–49.

Liang BA. Patient Injury Incentives in Law. *Yale Law & Pol'y Rev* 1998;17:1–93.

Steele CJ, Saue JM. Insurance Payment for Healthcare. In: National Health Lawyers Association, *Health Law Practice Guide*. Deerfield, IL: West Group, 1997.

Web Sites

Balanced Budget Act of 1997: *http://speakernews.house.gov/budgtxt2.htm*

Balanced Budget Act of 1997: *http://www.nsclc.org/bba.html*

Beneath the surface of the Balanced Budget Act of 1997: *http://www.personalhomecare.com/health.htm#anchor177260*

Complaint data solutions: General information concerning HIPAA and COBRA: *http://www.complaintdata.com/*

Compliance guide to the Family and Medical Leave Act of 1993: *http://www.nscee.edu/univ/Human_Resources/Benefits/fmguide.html*

ERISA analyzer — employee health and retirement plans: *http://www.edata-online.com*

ERISA Industry Committee: *http://www.eric.org/*

ERISA lawyers web site: *http://www.erisa-lawyers.com*

ERISA litigation review, June 1997: http://www.mwe.com/news/eris0697.htm

Family Medical Leave Act: *http://www.doli.state.mn.us/fmla.html*

FMLA Pro: Department of Labor FMLA hotline: *http://www.fmla.com/fmlalink.html*

Health insurance — HIPAA: *http://www.ipma-hr.org/govtaffairs/health.html*

HIPAA and local government health plans: *http://www.mwbb.com/services/press32.htm*

HIPAA wizard: *http://www.hipaawizard.com*

HIPAA, the employee reference sheet: *http://humanresources.miningco.com/library/weekly/aa063097.htm*

National Health Policy Forum: *http://www.nhpf.org/*

Socialized medicine vs. private health care: *http://www.free-market.org/features/spotlight/9803.html*

What is ERISA?: *http://www.consumerwatchdog.org/public_hts/medical/erisa2.htm*

Will health plans keep their ERISA shield?: *http://www.managedcaremag.com/archiveMC/9705/9705.erisa.shtml*

7

Public Insurance: Medicare

Health Insurance for the Aged and Disabled, Title XVIII of the Social Security Act, is known as *Medicare*. Medicare is the health insurance program for the elderly as well as select nonelderly (e.g., certain disabled persons and patients with end-stage renal disease, ESRD[1]). The Medicare program as originally passed comprised two parts: Part A (Hospital Insurance Program) and Part B (Supplemental Medical Insurance). Those individuals over the age of 65 who are eligible for Social Security benefits are eligible for Medicare, as are their spouses.[2] Medicare represents the largest health insurance program in the United States and, therefore, has a tremendous impact on health care finance and policy in this country.

The Medicare program is administered primarily by the Health Care Financing Administration (HCFA), an agency in the Department of Health and Human Services, with the assistance of the Social Security Administration, the agency that coordinates with HCFA to enroll beneficiaries and collect premiums. HCFA also contracts with private "fiscal intermediaries" such as Blue Shield to administer Part A on a day-to-day basis[3] and similarly contracts with "private carriers" to administer Part B.[4] Intermediaries are responsible for determining costs and reimbursement amounts, maintaining records, establishing controls, protecting against fraud and abuse or excess use of services, conducting reviews and audits, making payments to providers, assisting beneficiaries and providers, and coordinating initial beneficiary and provider appeals for Part A services. Carriers are responsible for determining charges allowed by Medicare, maintaining quality of performance records, participating in fraud and abuse investigations, assisting providers and

beneficiaries, making payments to providers and suppliers covered under Part B, and coordinating initial appeals by beneficiaries and providers for Part B services. There are approximately 40 Medicare intermediaries and approximately 30 Medicare carriers. In addition, Medicare works with peer review organizations (PROs). PROs are groups of practicing physicians and other health care professionals who contract with the federal government to review the general care provided to Medicare beneficiaries in each state and assist in improving the quality of services so rendered. The financing of Part A and Part B services and administration is through separate trust funds set up in the Treasury for Part A (Federal Hospital Insurance Trust Fund) and Part B (Supplemental Medical Insurance Trust Fund).[5] The Medicare statute also authorizes the use of state health agencies to perform certain survey and certification actions on behalf of the federal government.[6]

This chapter provides an overview of some of the fundamental aspects of the extensive Medicare program. However, the program and its associated rules and regulations are in continuous flux; publicly available materials should be accessed to obtain the most current information about the program.

Enrollment

Enrollment in Parts A and B is automatic for select persons. At age 65, individuals who already receive Social Security or Railroad Retirement benefits are enrolled automatically in Part A and Part B, with an enrollment card sent to the beneficiary about three months prior to the beneficiary's 65th birthday. Part B may be declined

---

[1]42 U.S.C.A. §426-1; 42 C.F.R. §405.2102 (1998).

[2]42 U.S.C.A. §§426, 1395c.

[3]42 U.S.C.A. §1395h; 42 C.F.R. part 421 (1998).

[4]42 U.S.C.A. §1395u; 42 C.F.R. part 421 (1998).

[5]42 U.S.C.A. §1395t.

[6]42 U.S.C.A. §1395aa; 42 C.F.R. part 488 (1998).

by following the instructions on the Medicare card. Disabled individuals automatically are enrolled in both Part A and B beginning on their 25th month of disability, again with the Medicare card mailed to the individual about three months prior to eligibility.[7]

Other individuals must apply for Medicare. Persons who are not receiving Social Security or Railroad Retirement benefits three months prior to when they would be eligible for Medicare and individuals with renal disease must apply. There is a seven-month initial enrollment period in which to apply, with the seven months beginning three months before age 65. The application process is handled through the Social Security Administration office, or Railroad Retirement Board if the individual or his or her spouse worked for the railroad. An individual who does not apply during this seven-month enrollment period must wait until the next general enrollment period, which is January 1 to March 31 of each year, with Part B coverage beginning in July.[8]

Coverage

Generally, individuals are eligible for Medicare Part A if they are 65 years old or older, have worked for 10 years in Medicare-covered employment, and are citizens or permanent residents of the United States. Spouses of these individuals are eligible as well. Medicare Part A is funded by FICA payroll taxes paid by employers and employees (1.45% of earnings paid by each, or 2.90% paid by self-employed individuals) and by law cannot be funded by general revenues.[9] Part A insurance reimburses medical costs associated with inpatient hospitalization,[10] home health services,[11] hospice care,[12] and some skilled nursing home services of limited duration after discharge from a hospital (i.e., not nursing home care).[13] Inpatient hospitalization is covered for a "benefit period" up to 90 days annually for each "spell of illness" as well as for 60 "lifetime reserve days."[14] Individuals younger than 65 are eligible for Medicare Part A if they are a kidney dialysis or kidney transplant patient (i.e., have ESRD).[15]

Individuals are eligible for Medicare Part B if they are eligible for Part A or if they are at least 65 years old and a citizen or permanent resident.[16] Part B is funded by premiums paid by individuals;[17] these premiums are heavily subsidized by general revenue funds, which now pay for approximately 75% of the Part B beneficiary's costs.[18] Part B generally reimburses approximately 80% of the charges associated with physician and other provider services.[19] Part B also extends to outpatient hospital services incident to physician services,[20] physician extender and paraprofessional services,[21] outpatient diagnostic services,[22] renal dialysis,[23] outpatient physical and occupational therapy and speech pathology services,[24] home health services,[25] durable medical equipment (DME),[26] comprehensive outpatient rehabilitation facility (CORF) services,[27] rural health clinic services,[28] screening mammography[29] and Pap smears,[30] flu vaccinations,[31] cancer drugs and prescription drugs that cannot be self-administered,[32] ambulance services,[33] ambulatory surgical center (ASC) facility services,[34]

---

[7]Health Care Financing Administration. *What Is Medicare?* Available at: http://www.medicare.gov/whatis.html.

[8]Ibid.

[9]42 U.S.C.A. §1395i; 26 U.S.C.A. §§1401(b), 3101(b), 3111(b).

[10]42 U.S.C.A. §§1395d(a);1395x(b); 42 C.F.R. §§409.10–409.19 (1998).

[11]42 U.S.C.A. §1395x(m); 42 C.F.R. §§409.40–409.47 (1998).

[12]42 U.S.C.A. §§1395d(a)(4), 1395d(d); 1395x(dd); 42 C.F.R. §§418.200–418.204 (1998).

[13]42 U.S.C.A. §§1395d(a)(2), 1395d(f); 1395x(i).

[14]42 U.S.C.A. §§1395d(a), 1395x(a).

[15]42 U.S.C.A. §426-1; 42 C.F.R. §405.2102 (1998).

[16]42 U.S.C.A. §1395o.

[17]42 U.S.C.A. §1395j.

[18]42 U.S.C.A. §1395r(e) (indicates the methodology for setting the monthly premium; in 1997, the Part B premium was only $43.80/month).

[19]42 U.S.C.A. §§1395x(q), 1395x(s)(1); 42 C.F.R. §§410.20 (1998), 410.22–410.26 (1998).

[20]42 U.S.C.A. §§1395x(s)(2), 1395x(ff); 42 C.F.R. §410.27 (1998).

[21]42 U.S.C.A. §§1395x(s)(2)(K), 1395x(s)(2)(L), 1395x(s)(11), 1395x(aa)(5), 1395x(bb), 1395x(gg); 42 C.F.R. §410.69 (1998)

[22]42 U.S.C.A. §§1395x(s)(2)(C), 1395x(s)(3); 42 C.F.R. §§410.28 (1998), 410.32 (1998).

[23]42 U.S.C.A. §§1395x(s)(2)(F), 1395x(s)(2)(P); 42 C.F.R. §§410.50 (1998), 410.52 (1998).

[24]42 U.S.C.A. §§1395x(g), 1305x(p), 1395x(s)(2)(D); 42 C.F.R. §§410.60 (1998), 410.62 (1998).

[25]42 U.S.C.A. §1395x(m); 42 C.F.R. §§409.40–409.46 (1998), 410.80 (1998).

[26]42 U.S.C.A. §§1395f(k), 1395x(n), 1395x(s)(6); 42 C.F.R. §410.38 (1998).

[27]42 U.S.C.A. §1395x(cc)(2); 42 C.F.R. §§410.100 (1998), 410.105 (1998).

[28]42 U.S.C.A. §§1395x(s)(2)(E), 1395x(aa); 42 C.F.R. §410.45 (1998).

[29]42 U.S.C.A. §§1395x(s)(13), 1395x(jj); 42 C.F.R. §410.34 (1998).

[30]42 U.S.C.A. §§1395x(s)(14), 1395x(nn).

[31]42 U.S.C.A. §§1395l(a)(1), 1395l(b)(1).

[32]42 U.S.C.A. §1395x(s)(2)(A).

[33]42 U.S.C.A. §1395x(s)(7); 42 C.F.R. §410.40 (1998).

[34]42 U.S.C.A. §§1395k(a)(2)(F)(i), 1395l(i)(2)(A); 42 C.F.R. §§416.2 (1998), 416.25 (1998), 416.26 (1998), 416.40–416.49 (1998), 416.65 (1998), 416.125 (1998).

clinical laboratory testing,[35] portable X-ray services,[36] and some diagnostic testing.[37]

Beneficiary Cost Sharing

There is cost sharing in both Part A and Part B insurance. In Part A, for each hospitalization up to 60 days, generally the Medicare beneficiary is responsible for a deductible that approximates the cost of the first day of hospitalization.[38] If hospitalization lasts 60 to 90 days, the beneficiary is responsible for a coinsurance payment equal to 25% of the deductible amount per day. If hospitalization lasts longer than 90 days and the beneficiary uses his or her lifetime reserve days from the 91st to the 150th day, the beneficiary has an additional coinsurance amount of half the deductible amount per day.[39] Other cost sharing in Part A includes coinsurance payments for skilled nursing facility care (one-eighth of the deductible amount per day during the 21st through 100th day),[40] drugs, biologicals and respite care in a hospice,[41] and blood products provided in a hospital or skilled nursing facility.[42]

In Part B, monthly premiums represent the general cost sharing required in the program. In addition, a $100 deductible is generally imposed before Part B benefits are covered.[43] After this $100 deductible requirement has been met, Part B generally reimburses 80% of the reasonable cost or charge for the service with the beneficiary paying the remaining 20% plus any additional amount the provider may charge.[44] In addition, beneficiaries under Part B are subject to a deductible for certain blood products before the program's benefits are available.[45] Services for which there is no cost sharing under Part B include diagnostic laboratory tests,[46] home health services,[47] kidney donations,[48] pneumococcal vaccines,[49] second opinions

from peer review organizations,[50] and services from federally qualified health centers.[51]

Medicare Exclusions from Payment

Medicare expressly excludes certain payments from program coverage. First, the program does not provide payment for services provided by a family member.[52] In addition, the program does not pay for services for which the beneficiary is not liable[53] or that are covered by another payment source, which usually includes other federal programs,[54] employer-based insurance, auto insurance, or workers' compensation.[55] Generally, under the Medicare as Secondary Payer Program, if the beneficiary is covered by any other insurance, the provider must look to that insurance first before attempting to collect from Medicare.[56] If the primary insurance does not cover all payment and Medicare otherwise would pay the reasonable charge, Medicare as the secondary payer will pay the lowest of the difference between the actual service charge and amount paid by the primary insurer, the amount Medicare otherwise would pay, the higher of the amount Medicare would pay net the amount already paid by the primary insurer, or the amount the primary payer allows net the amount already paid by the primary insurer.[57]

Medicare also excludes certain medical services and products, including routine checkups, eye examinations and glasses, hearing examinations and aids, some immunizations,[58] foot care, orthopedic shoes and support devices,[59] cosmetic surgery,[60] most dental services,[61] and some nonprofessional services provided in hospitals.[62]

Finally, Medicare excludes from payment and coverage those services that are "not reasonably necessary" for diagnosis and treatment of the beneficiary,[63] including treatments considered experimental[64]

[35]42 U.S.C.A. §§263a, 1395x(s)(3); 42 C.F.R. §§410.32(d)(5) (1998), 493.1–493.2001 (1998).

[36]42 U.S.C.A. §1395x(s)(3); 42 C.F.R. §§486.100 (1998), 486.102 (1998), 486.104 (1998), 486.106 (1998).

[37]42 U.S.C.A. §1395k; 42 C.F.R. §410.3 (1998).

[38]42 U.S.C.A. §1395e(a)(1).

[39]42 U.S.C.A. §1395e(a)(1).

[40]42 U.S.C.A. §1395e(a)(3).

[41]42 U.S.C.A. §1395e(a)(4).

[42]42 U.S.C.A. §1395e(a)(2).

[43]42 U.S.C.A. §1395l(b); 42 C.F.R. §410.160 (1998).

[44]42 U.S.C.A. §1395l(a).

[45]42 U.S.C.A. §1395l(b).

[46]42 U.S.C.A. §§1395l(a)(1)(D), 1395l(a)(2)(D), 1395l(b)(3).

[47]42 U.S.C.A. §§1395l(a)(2)(A), 1395l(b)(2).

[48]42 C.F.R. §410.163 (1998).

[49]42 U.S.C.A. §§1395l(a)(1)(B), 1395x(s)(10)(A), 1395l (b)(1).

[50]42 U.S.C.A. §§1395l(a)(1), 1395l(a)(2)(A), 1395l(b)(4).

[51]42 U.S.C.A. §1395l(b).

[52]42 U.S.C.A. §1395y(a)(11); 42 C.F.R. §411.12 (1998).

[53]42 U.S.C.A. §1395y(a)(2); 42 C.F.R. §411.4 (1998).

[54]42 U.S.C.A. §1395y(a)(3); 42 C.F.R. §§411.6–411.8 (1998).

[55]42 U.S.C.A. §1395y(b)(2)(A); 42 C.F.R. §§411.20–411.75 (1998).

[56]42 U.S.C.A. §1395y(b); 42 C.F.R. §§411.20–411.75 (1998).

[57]42 C.F.R. §411.33(a) (1998).

[58]42 U.S.C.A. §1395y(a)(7); 42 C.F.R. §411.15(a)–(e) (1998).

[59]42 U.S.C.A. §§1395y(a)(8), 1395y(a)(13); 42 C.F.R. §§411.15(f) (1998), 411.15(l) (1998).

[60]42 U.S.C.A. §1395y(a)(10); 42 C.F.R. §411.15(h) (1998).

[61]42 U.S.C.A. §1395y(a)(12).

[62]42 U.S.C.A. §1395y(a)(14); 42 C.F.R. §411.15(m) (1998).

[63]42 U.S.C.A. §1395y(a)(1); 42 C.F.R. §411.15(k) (1998).

[64]See, e.g., Goodman v. Sullivan, 891 F.2d 449 (2d Cir. 1989) (upholding denial of coverage for MRI as diagnostic tool for speech impediment when MRI still was listed as experimental).

or custodial.[65] These services may be paid for if the provider and the beneficiary could not know or reasonably have been expected to know that these services were excluded from coverage.[66] Finally, no services are covered that are due to war,[67] rendered outside the United States,[68] or provided by an excluded provider.

Provider Participation Requirements

To provide services in the Medicare program, Part A providers (e.g., hospitals, skilled nursing facilities) must meet specific Medicare conditions of participation and execute a participation agreement with HCFA;[69] some Part B providers also must enter into participation agreements. These latter providers generally are institutional Part B providers, such as ambulatory surgery centers, rural health clinics, freestanding renal dialysis centers, organ procurement agencies and histocompatibility laboratories, some managed care organizations, and some independent laboratories. Professional Part B providers such as physicians are not required to enter into these agreements with Medicare.

Generally, provider participation agreements require that the Medicare provider comply with civil rights legislation and anti–patient dumping legislation (the Emergency Medical Treatment and Active Labor Act[70]), limit Medicare beneficiary charges to copayments and deductibles, refund any excess reimbursements, disclose the hiring of any person who was responsible for payment decisions as an intermediary or carrier for the program, provide all covered services, participate in other federal health programs, provide beneficiaries with Medicare publications indicating their rights as beneficiaries, provide beneficiaries with a list of Medicare providers, indicate whether the hospital participates in the Medicaid program, comply with the Medicare as Secondary Payer Program, and agree not to condition admission and treatment on the basis of ability to pay.[71]

Specific conditions of participation for providers to the Medicare program are a function of the specific type of provider involved.[72] These conditions generally relate to minimum standards of the particular facility's quality and services. Compliance is monitored either by state survey authorities or appropriate accrediting organizations. Specifically for hospitals, Joint Commission on Accreditation of Healthcare Organizations accreditation is deemed to meet the hospital conditions of participation if the institution authorizes JCAHO to release the hospital's accreditation report to HCFA, and HCFA has found no significant deficiencies at the hospital. A vast majority of hospitals use this mechanism to obtain the necessary documentation to serve the Medicare program.[73] State survey and certification requirements for compliance are published as regulations for providers.[74] Prior to initial certification for participation, the state must survey the facility and make recommendations to HCFA.[75] If initial certification is given, then the state may periodically review compliance with the conditions of participation, generally on a yearly basis.[76] If the state survey finds the facility out of compliance, the state can indicate to HCFA that the facility does not qualify for Medicare participation if the noncompliance substantially affects the health and safety of patients,[77] or the state can recertify the facility subject to a correction plan if the noncompliance does not rise to this level.[78]

Part A Payment

Part A providers generally are paid under the prospective payment system (PPS)[79] using the diagnosis-related group (DRG) methodology (discussed next).[80] This DRG

---

[72]Part A providers: 42 U.S.C.A. §§1395x(p) (clinics, rehabilitation agencies, and public health agencies as providers of outpatient physical therapy or speech pathology services); 1395x(cc); 42 C.F.R. §§485.50–485.74 (1998) (comprehensive outpatient rehabilitation facilities); 42 U.S.C.A. §1395x(m), 42 C.F.R. §§484.1–484.52 (1998) (home health agencies); 42 U.S.C.A. §1395x(dd), 42 C.F.R. §§418.50–418.100 (1998) (hospice programs); 42 U.S.C.A. §1395x(e), 42 C.F.R. Part 482 (1998) (hospitals); 42 U.S.C.A. §1395i-3(a)-(d), 42 C.F.R. §§483.1-483.80 (1998) (skilled nursing facilities). Part B providers: 42 U.S.C.A. §1395k(a)(2)(F), 42 C.F.R. §§416.25–416.49 (1998) (ambulatory surgical centers); 42 U.S.C.A. §1395rr(b), 42 C.F.R. §§405.2100–405.2171 (1998) (end-stage renal disease facilities); 42 U.S.C.A. §§1395x(s)(3), 1395x(s)(15), 1395x(s)(16), 42 C.F.R. §§493.1–493.2001 (1998) (independent clinical laboratories); 42 U.S.C.A. §1320b-8(b), 42 C.F.R. §§485.301–485.308 (1998) (organ procurement organizations); 42 U.S.C.A. §1395x(p) (outpatient physical therapy services furnished by physical therapists in independent practice); 42 U.S.C.A. §1395x(s)(3) (portable X-ray services).

[73]42 U.S.C.A. §1395bb; 42 C.F.R. §§488.5, 488.6 (1998).

[74]42 C.F.R. Part 488 (1998).

[75]42 U.S.C.A. §1395aa; 42 C.F.R. §§488.11–488.12 (1998).

[76]42 C.F.R. §488.20 (1998).

[77]42 C.F.R. §488.24 (1998).

[78]42 C.F.R. §488.28 (1998).

[79]42 U.S.C.A. §1395ww(d).

[80]42 C.F.R. Parts 412–413 (1998).

---

[65]42 U.S.C.A. §1395y(a)(9); 42 C.F.R. §411.15(g) (1998).

[66]42 C.F.R. §411.400(a)(2) (1998).

[67]42 U.S.C.A. §1395y(a)(5); 42 C.F.R. §411.10 (1998).

[68]42 U.S.C.A. §§1395y(a)(4), 1395f(f); 42 C.F.R. §411.9 (1998).

[69]42 U.S.C.A. §§1395aa, 1395f(a); 42 C.F.R. Parts 482–485 (1998).

[70]See Chapter 12.

[71]42 U.S.C.A. §1395cc; 42 C.F.R. §§489.10–489.22 (1998).

PPS methodology generally applies to short-term, acute care inpatient hospitalizations. Providers not subject to the DRG PPS include psychiatric hospitals, rehabilitation hospitals, children's hospitals, long-term care hospitals, cancer hospitals, home health care, hospice care, skilled nursing care after hospitalization, some territory hospitals outside the continental United States,[81] and distinct psychiatric and rehabilitation units in acute care hospitals.[82] These latter facilities generally are reimbursed on a cost basis by Medicare.[83] Direct medical education and capital costs payments also are excluded from the DRG PPS system.[84]

There are approximately 490 DRGs.[85] DRG categories are based on those in the *International Classification of Diseases*, 9th edition, Clinical Modification Coding System (ICD-9-CM). DRG PPS reimburse providers a flat rate for each patient prospectively on the basis of diagnosis. The rates cover a broad range of services, including room and board, routine nursing services, ancillary medical services such as radiology and laboratory testing, operating costs, diagnostic and other services related to admission provided by the hospital or a subsidiary three days prior to admission, and malpractice insurance costs.[86]

The concept behind reimbursement in this manner is simple: By providing payment on a flat-rate basis by diagnosis, providers will have an incentive to minimize costs; those who do so will be efficient providers and reap a surplus from Medicare business; those providers who do not minimize costs will be "inefficient" and have a strong incentive to cut costs to become efficient. The theory is that, overall, all patients with the same diagnosis will average out to approximately the same amount as the payment rate, thus allowing efficient hospitals to make a profit. Although diagnosis is the most important factor in calculating the reimbursement scale, other factors such as labor costs, urban versus rural location, medical education participation, and degree of uncompensated care are also taken into account.

The PPS payment amount is determined by the following method:

1. At discharge, the Medicare patient's physician records the principal diagnosis that accounted for hospital admission, as well as any additional diagnoses and performed procedures.

2. The hospital takes this information and, incorporating the patient's age, gender, complications, comorbidities, and discharge status, lists the services and procedures provided on the patient's bill using the ICD-9-CM coding system.

3. The bill is submitted to the Medicare fiscal intermediary, the private organization such as Blue Cross Blue Shield that contracts with the Secretary of Health and Human Services to provide administrative services for Medicare Part A claims payment and coverage determinations.[87] Each intermediary is responsible for claims within a particular geographic region. The intermediary screens the bill to ensure proper coding and assigns the patient to a DRG using a computer system.[88] Note that if an incorrect DRG is assigned, the hospital can request a review within 60 days of such assignment.[89] Note that if the intermediary decides that a higher-weighted DRG is applicable and should be assigned, the intermediary must request that the appropriate PRO verify the change in assignment.[90]

4. The DRG then is assigned a "weight." The weight ideally represents the average amount of resources necessary to care for a patient in the DRG as compared to the average resources necessary to care for all Medicare hospital discharges nationally. DRG weights are recalibrated each year to take into account changes in technology and medical practice.[91]

5. The weight is multiplied by the "standardized amount." This standardized amount represents the cost in dollars for treating the average Medicare patient during the year of discharge. This amount has two components: a labor portion (adjusted by a wage-index factor to take into account wage variations across the United States[92]) and a nonlabor portion (adjusted to take into account status of the hospital operating in a "rural," "urban," or "large-urban" locale[93]).

6. After the amount in step 5 is calculated, adjustments may be made depending on the specific costs and hospital. If the patient's costs are extremely high, the hospital may apply for a "cost outlier" reimbursement.[94] HCFA publishes the outlier criteria each year in the *Federal Register*.[95] In addition, indirect medical

---

[81]42 C.F.R. §412.23 (1998).

[82]42 U.S.C.A. §1395ww(d)(1); 42 C.F.R. §§412.22 (1998), 412.25 (1998), 412.27 (1998), 412.29 (1998), 412.30 (1998).

[83]42 C.F.R. §412.22(b) (1998).

[84]42 U.S.C.A. §1395ww(a)(4).

[85]42 C.F.R. Parts 412–413 (1998).

[86]42 U.S.C.A. §1395ww(a)(4); 42 C.F.R. §§412.2(b) (1998), 412.2(c) (1998).

[87]42 U.S.C.A. §1395h.

[88]57 Fed. Reg. 39,746 (1992).

[89]42 C.F.R. §412.60(d) (1998).

[90]42 C.F.R. §§412.60(d)(2) (1998), 466.71(c)(2) (1998).

[91]42 U.S.C.A. §1395ww(d)(4)(C)(i); 42 C.F.R. §412.60(e) (1998).

[92]42 U.S.C.A. §1395ww(d)(3)(E).

[93]42 U.S.C.A. §§1395ww(d)(1)–1395ww(d)(3); 42 C.F.R. §412.63(c)(6) (1998).

[94]42 U.S.C.A. §1395ww(d)(5)(A)(ii); 42 C.F.R. §§412.80 (1998), 412.84 (1998).

[95]42 C.F.R. §412.80(c) (1998).

education costs may be reimbursed. Although direct graduate medical education (GME) costs are reimbursed on a cost basis,[96] for indirect medical education (IME) costs, such as additional tests and procedures ordered by residents, increased need for teaching hospitals to maintain detailed records, and sicker patients, PPS allows for an upward adjustment in reimbursement rates.[97] Finally, adjustments for disproportionate share hospitals (DSHs, which provide a greater proportion of uncompensated care),[98] sole community hospitals (which are isolated due to geography, weather, and time considerations),[99] rural referral centers (which are large rural hospitals with large urban hospital characteristics),[100] renal transplant centers,[101] Medicare-dependent small rural hospitals (MDHs),[102] essential access community hospitals (EACHs),[103] hospitals with a high percentage of end-stage renal disease discharges,[104] and hospitals in Alaska and Hawaii[105] are subject to additional PPS adjustments.

Part B Payment

Part B physician providers generally are paid under the resource-based relative value scale (RBRVS) mandated by federal law in 1989.[106] The RBRVS generally was seen as an effort to reward primary care practice and shift services away from procedure-based and specialty practice. Part B administration is performed by private carriers,[107] who administer Part B of the program similar to the fiscal intermediaries that perform the same function for Part A of the program.

The RBRVS fee schedule is based on assigning a relative weight (relative value units, RVUs) for each physician service and multiplying that RVU by the conversion factor to arrive at a dollar amount. The components taken into account in determining the RVU of the service are the relative work of the service (the skill, effort, and time spent in providing a service from preservice review, to service provision, to follow-up care and monitoring), the practice expense[108] for the physician (cost of office, office personnel, and supplies), and malpractice costs (cost of premiums and risk differentials for different specialties). These components are adjusted for geographic variation (the geographical adjustment factor, GAF).[109] Each component is assigned an RVU; the total of these components represents the RVU for the service. After multiplying by the conversion factor, the Medicare program pays 80% of this amount. The conversion factor is updated annually. Generally, if HCFA does not recommend to Congress a conversion factor update percentage, the update figure is calculated by first assessing the general increase in costs (the Medicare economic index, MEI). Second, the amount services would expect to rise due to increases in beneficiaries and other factors is assessed (the Medicare volume performance standard, MVPS). Third, the actual amount that services increased from one year to the next is calculated. The annual increase is determined to be the MEI taking into account whether the actual expenditures for services were above or below the MVPS. If above, then that percentage of the MVPS is deducted from the MEI; if below, then that percentage is added to the MEI.[110] Note that, beyond the Medicare program, the RBRVS RVUs have been adopted by other payers for reimbursement purposes.

Payment for physician services is based on two coding systems. The patient's diagnosis is coded using the ICD-9-CM system. Physician services are coded using the AMA's *Physician's Current Procedural Terminology*, now in its fourth edition (CPT-4). CPT-4 has been integrated into the HCFA common procedure coding system (HCPCS) for Part B payment purposes. There are three levels of codes. Level I, national, codes contain only CPT-4 (five-digit) codes except for anesthesia, which is updated annually. Level II codes are national HCPCS codes created by the Medicare program with the input of Blue Cross/Blue Shield Association and the Health Insurance Association of America. Level II (letter and four-digit) codes are used for physician and nonphysician services not included in CPT-4 (e.g., durable medical equipment, ambulance services). Finally, Level III, or local, codes are administrative codes provided by individual carrier or state agencies to process Medicare (and Medicaid) claims. Level III codes use the letters X, Y, and Z followed by a four-digit number. Thus, HCPCS provides codes for all or almost all medical and medically related services that Medicare patients may be provided.

[96]42 C.F.R. §§413.85 (1998), 413.86 (1998).

[97]42 U.S.C.A. §1395ww(d)(5)(B); 42 C.F.R. §412.105 (1998).

[98]42 U.S.C.A. §§1395ww(d)(5)(F)(i)–(v), 1395ww(d)(5)(F)(vii); 42 C.F.R. §412.106 (1998).

[99]42 U.S.C.A. §1395ww(d)(5)(C); 42 C.F.R. §412.92 (1998); 55 Fed. Reg. 36,051 (1990).

[100]42 U.S.C.A. §1395ww(d)(5)(C); 42 C.F.R. §412.96 (1998).

[101]42 C.F.R. §412.100 (1998).

[102]42 U.S.C.A. §1395ww(d)(5)(G); 42 C.F.R. §412.108 (1998).

[103]42 C.F.R. §412.109 (1998); 58 Fed. Reg. 30,630 (1993); 58 Fed. Reg. 45,812 (1995).

[104]42 C.F.R. §412.104 (1998).

[105]42 U.S.C.A. §1395ww(d)(5)(H).

[106]42 U.S.C.A. §§1395w-4(a)–(j).

[107]42 U.S.C.A. §§1395u(a)–(f).

[108]See 63 Fed. Reg. 58,814 (1998), 42 C.F.R. §414.22 (1998) (changing practice expense calculation methodology).

[109]42 U.S.C.A. §§1395w-4(c)(2), 1395w-4(e); 42 C.F.R. §§414.22 (1998), 414.26 (1998).

[110]42 U.S.C.A. §§1395w-4(d)(3), 1395w-4(f)(1).

Once diagnoses and services are documented, these are submitted to the Part B carrier, who assesses the coding, checks for medical appropriateness, and issues payment for the services. Claims under Part B for services provided during the first nine months of the calendar year must be submitted to carriers by the end of the following calendar year; claims for services rendered during the last three months of the calendar year must be submitted by the end of the second following year.[111] After submission, carriers send beneficiaries an explanation of medical benefits notice, indicating the amount of payment made by the program for each assigned and nonassigned claim. Assignment is covered next.

Assignment

Although professional providers such as physicians need not execute participation agreements with Medicare, they often execute assignment agreements. In Part B of the program, payments may be made either to the Medicare beneficiary or to the physician or supplier on behalf of the patient; that is, the patient has assigned the benefit payment to the provider.[112] These assignment agreements generally indicate that the provider will accept assignment for all services provided during the year to Medicare beneficiaries.[113] Assignment agreements are renewed annually unless canceled. Note that a physician or supplier who does not become a "participating provider" (i.e., who accepts assignment for all claims) still may accept assignment on a case-by-case basis.

However, a physician or other provider who accepts assignment must accept the Medicare fee schedule amount as payment in full for the particular service or item;[114] the beneficiary can be billed for only the allowable coinsurance or deductible amount. Note also that several states have indicated that physicians, as a condition of licensure, may not "balance bill"; that is, bill the patient for amounts greater than the Medicare fee schedule. This limitation effectively forces physicians to accept assignment, and courts have upheld these legal prescriptions.[115] Physicians who do not accept assign-

ment may charge a higher fee if the jurisdiction in which they practice allows it; however, this amount is limited to 115% of the fee schedule amount for participating providers,[116] and nonparticipating providers only receive 95% of the cash amounts provided by the Medicare program to participating providers.[117] This limitation also successfully has weathered legal challenge.[118] In addition, nonparticipating physicians who propose to perform elective surgery for which the charge will exceed $500 must disclose the cost beforehand in writing to the beneficiary, the estimated Medicare payment for the service, and the difference between the two or else refund any payment collected above the Medicare reasonable charge.[119] Violations of these conditions subject the provider to civil penalties and Medicare program exclusion.[120]

Accepting assignment has some advantages. First, Medicare claims that are not the subject of challenge or question are paid within 17 days by the carrier for participating physicians while nonparticipating physicians must wait up to 24 days.[121] Second, there may be marketing benefits. The Department of Health and Human Services annually publishes a directory of local participating physicians that is available at carrier offices, Social Security offices, hospitals, and senior citizen organization offices.[122] As well, carriers are required to mail this directory to beneficiaries who request it;[123] in addition, carriers must maintain a toll-free phone number through which beneficiaries may obtain the names, addresses, phone numbers, and specialties of participating physicians.[124] Further, hospital personnel who refer Medicare beneficiaries to nonparticipating providers are mandated to inform the beneficiaries of the provider's nonparticipation status and, if possible, identify a participating provider who would supply the service.[125] Beneficiaries are reminded about participating provider status, the toll-free number, and the directory each year as well as when they receive an explanation of benefits form concerning nonassigned claims.[126]

Finally, note that although beneficiaries can assign claims to providers, generally providers cannot reassign claims to others nor may patients assign claims to non-

---

[111]42 C.F.R. §424.44 (1998).

[112]42 U.S.C.A. §1395u(b)(3); 42 C.F.R. §§424.53 (1998), 424.55 (1998).

[113]42 U.S.C.A. §1395u(h).

[114]42 U.S.C.A. §1395u(b)(3)(B)(ii); 42 C.F.R. §424.55(b) (1998).

[115]See, e.g., Massachusetts Med. Soc'y v. Dukakis, 815 F.2d 790 (1st Cir.), *cert. denied* 484 U.S. 896 (1987); Pennsylvania Med. Soc'y v. Marconis, 942 F.2d 842 (3d Cir. 1991); Medical Soc'y of N.Y. v. Cuomo, 976 F.2d 812 (2d Cir. 1992); Medical Soc'y of N.Y. v. New York Dep't. of Health, 611 N.Y.S.2d 114 (App.Div. 1993), *aff'd* 633 N.E.2d 468 (N.Y. 1994).

[116]42 U.S.C.A. §1395w-4(g).

[117]42 U.S.C.A. §1395u(b)(4)(A)(iv).

[118]Garelick v. Sullivan, 987 F.2d 913 (2d Cir.), *cert. denied* 510 U.S. 821 (1993).

[119]42 U.S.C.A. §1395u(m).

[120]42 U.S.C.A. §§1395u(j)(1)–(2), 1395w-4(g)(1).

[121]42 U.S.C.A. §1395u(c)(2)(B)(iv)–(v).

[122]42 U.S.C.A. §§1395u(h)(5), 1395u(h)(6).

[123]42 U.S.C.A. §1395u(h)(2)

[124]42 U.S.C.A. §1395u(h)(2).

[125]42 U.S.C.A. §1395cc(a)(1)(N).

[126]42 U.S.C.A. §§1395u(h)(5), 1395u(h)(7).

physicians or non–Part B suppliers.[127] There are exceptions to this reassignment, allowing for reassignment to a physician or supplier's employer, to specific public and private entities where the service was rendered, pursuant to court orders, to billing agents whose compensation is independent of amounts billed or collected, and to a bank account controlled by the provider where the bank has lent money to the provider.[128]

Appeals in Medicare

Appeals regarding Medicare, including those from patients, physicians, and other providers, generally are governed by administrative processes. Only after this administrative process is completed will aggrieved parties have access to judicial review.

Individuals challenging the right to receive either Part A or B Medicare benefits must engage in an administrative process that begins with the Social Security Administration. Reconsideration of a decision rendered there is through a Social Security Administration's administrative law judge (ALJ). The ALJ decision may be reviewed by the department's Appeals Council, whose decision in turn may be reviewed judicially in federal court.[129]

A beneficiary who is in a hospital and believes he or she is being discharged too early has the right to an immediate review by a peer review organization (PRO). During this immediate review, the beneficiary has the right to stay in the hospital at no charge and the hospital cannot discharge the patient before the PRO makes its decision.[130] In a similar vein, if a Medicare beneficiary is enrolled in a managed care organization and care is requested due to a health status that could seriously jeopardize the life or health of the beneficiary, he or she may obtain expedited review for the proposed treatment within 72 hours.[131]

Qualification and termination decisions regarding provider participation in Medicare are made by the HCFA;[132] a provider whose assignment has been terminated may request a reconsideration.[133] The Department

of Health and Human Services Office of Inspector General may also place sanctions on providers, including exclusion, termination, and suspension.[134] Those providers who wish to appeal a reconsidered assessment or whose assignment has been terminated or suspended may appeal to an ALJ within the department; if resolution is not to their liking there, they may appeal to the Appeals Council.[135] Note, however, that excluded providers or excluded providers who are subject to civil monetary penalties may appeal to the ALJ and then to the Departmental Appeals Board.[136]

Part A beneficiaries who are denied benefits will receive a partial or total denial or disallowance notice from the intermediary. This initial determination is subject to administrative review.[137] A beneficiary who is not satisfied with the intermediary's initial determination of his or her Part A benefits may request a reconsideration by HCFA within 60 days, regardless of the amount being challenged; this request usually entails a letter with additional documentation for the case.[138] Note that a provider may request reconsideration only if the beneficiary states in writing that he or she does not intend to request reconsideration from HCFA or if the intermediary has waived any beneficiary liability.[139] If the reconsideration is not satisfactory, then appeal before an ALJ may be made within 60 days, as long as the amount in dispute is $100 or more.[140] If the ALJ decision is unsatisfactory, then the aggrieved party may request a review by the Appeals Council.[141] If the Appeals Council denies review or issues a review unsatisfactory to the aggrieved party, the party may obtain judicial review, but only if the case involves eligibility or benefits worth more than $1000 under Part A.[142] Only if all parties to the decision, including the Secretary of Health and Human Services, agree that the only issue impeding a favorable review for the aggrieved party is a statutory provision that is alleged as unconstitutional can the aggrieved party forgo the administrative process.[143]

A special administrative review body considers hospitals and other institutional provider claims under Part A: the Provider Reimbursement Review Board (PRRB).

[127]42 U.S.C.A. §1395u(b)(6); 42 C.F.R. §§424.80 (1998), 424.82 (1998).

[128]42 U.S.C.A. §1395u(b)(6); 42 C.F.R. §424.80 (1998).

[129]20 C.F.R. §404.900 (1998).

[130]Health Care Financing Administration, *Your Medicare Handbook 1997* (Washington, DC: U.S. Government Printing Office, 1997).

[131]See 62 Fed. Reg. 23,368, 23,375 (1997); Grijalva v. Shalala, 946 F.Supp. 747 (D. Ariz. 1996), *judgement ordered* 1997 WL 155392 (D.Ariz. Mar. 3, 1997), *aff'd* 152 F.3d 1115 (9th Cir. 1998).

[132]42 C.F.R. §§489.53 (1998), 498.3(b) (1998).

[133]42 C.F.R. §498.5(a) (1998).

[134]42 C.F.R. §§489.54 (1998), 498.3(c) (1998), 1001.1–1001.221 (1998).

[135]42 C.F.R. §498.5 (1998).

[136]42 C.F.R. §§1005.2 (1998), 1005.21 (1998).

[137]42 C.F.R. §405.704 (1998).

[138]42 C.F.R. §405.710(a) (1998).

[139]42 C.F.R. §405.710(b) (1998).

[140]42 C.F.R. §§405.720 (1998), 405.722 (1998).

[141]42 C.F.R. §405.724 (1998); 20 C.F.R. §§404.967–404.982 (1998).

[142]42 U.S.C.A. §§1395ff(b)(1), 1395ff(b)(2).

[143]42 C.F.R. §405.718e (1998).

The PRRB is appointed by the Secretary of the Department of Health and Human Services and has at least two provider members and one CPA.[144] An institutional provider that is dissatisfied with the intermediary's final determination of payment due under Medicare (known as *notice of amount of program reimbursement*, NPR) may request review by PRRB within 180 days.[145] When the intermediary indicates to a PPS hospital its PPS rates, most courts have held that the hospital may appeal immediately and wait until the end of the year for the final NPR.[146] Note that PRRB review is only allowed for disputed amounts of $10,000 or greater for a single provider or $50,000 in aggregate for multiple providers if the controversy involves common issues of fact or interpretation of law.[147] Controversies of between $1,000 and $10,000 are heard by a hearing officer or panel appointed by the intermediary;[148] this decision may be appealed to the HCFA administrator.[149]

All decisions of the PRRB must be made and supported by substantial evidence.[150] PRRB decisions can be reviewed by the administrator of HCFA, who can delegate this duty at his or her discretion to the deputy administrator,[151] if this request is made within 15 days of the PRRB decision; the administrator has the choice to affirm, modify, reverse, or remand the decision.[152] Judicial review is available for aggrieved parties; the case is heard and decision is made by a federal district court where the provider is located or in the District of Columbia and requests must be made within 60 days.[153]

For Part B services, carriers determine whether the services are covered under Part B, whether the beneficiary deductible has been met, whether proof of payment by the beneficiary is acceptable, what coinsurance amounts may be due, whether the services were medically necessary, and how much the program should pay and to whom.[154] An explanation of medical benefits form then is sent to the beneficiary as well as to the physician or other provider to whom benefits were assigned, if any. This, too, is an initial determination of benefits and may be reviewed by the carrier on request by the beneficiary or assignee of benefits within six months if benefits are denied or not covered in the desired manner. If the aggrieved party is not satisfied with the review decision and the amount in dispute is $100 or greater, the aggrieved party may request a fair hearing in front of a hearing officer appointed by the carrier.[155] If requested, the hearing officer may provide an "on-the-record" decision with no oral testimony, which may be rendered preliminarily even if an oral hearing has been requested. An aggrieved party who is not satisfied with the on-the-record review may request another on-the-record review in front of a different hearing officer or, if $500 or greater is at stake, can go directly to an ALJ hearing.[156] A party that is dissatisfied with the ALJ determination may request review by the Appeals Council, as with Part A challenges. Finally, like Part A, judicial review is available after administrative process exhaustion, as long as the controversy is worth $1000 or greater.

Note that the intermediary, carrier, hearing officer, ALJ, and Appeals Council decisions all are subject to reopening within 12 months of the case's resolution and up to 4 years after such resolution for good cause shown. PRRB and administrator decisions can be reopened for up to 3 years.[157] Administrative decisions obtained by provider fraud have no time limit to be reopened.[158]

Medigap Insurance

As seen already, Medicare imposes significant cost sharing on its beneficiaries, including deductibles, coinsurance, and premiums, as well as lack of coverage for particular items such as prescription drugs and eyeglasses. To fill this gap, a market of insurance has arisen: the Medigap market. The federal government mandates that Medigap insurance be available to beneficiaries 65 years or older for the immediate six months after they enroll in Part B, regardless of health status (the "open enrollment" period). Beneficiaries are informed of this six-month open enrollment period when they enroll in Medicare. If beneficiaries are not yet 65 years old, the six-month open enrollment period begins

[144]42 U.S.C.A. §1395oo(h).

[145]42 U.S.C.A. §1395oo(a); 42 C.F.R. §§405.1835–405.1841 (1998).

[146]See, e.g., Doctors Hosp. v. Bowen, 811 F.2d 1448 (11th Cir. 1987); Sunshine Health Systems v. Bowen, 809 F.2d 1390 (9th Cir. 1987); St. Francis Hosp. v. Bowen, 802 F.2d 697 (4th Cir. 1986); see also Washington Hosp. Ctr. v. Bowen, 795 F.2d 139 (D.C. Cir. 1986); Community Hosp. of Chandler, Inc. v. Sullivan, 963 F.2d 1206 (9th Cir. 1992).

[147]42 U.S.C.A. §1395oo(b); 42 C.F.R. §§405.1837 (1998), 405.1839 (1998).

[148]42 C.F.R. §§405.1809–405.1833 (1998).

[149]U.S. Department of Health and Human Services, Health Care Financing Administration, HIM-15, *Medicare Carrier's Manual*, Part I, §2917.

[150]42 U.S.C.A. §1395oo(d); 42 C.F.R. §405.1871(a) (1998).

[151]42 U.S.C.A. §1395oo(f)(1); 42 C.F.R. §405.1875 (1998).

[152]42 C.F.R. §§405.1875(g) (1998), 405.1875(h) (1998).

[153]42 U.S.C.A. §1395oo(f)(1); 42 C.F.R. §405.1877 (1998).

[154]42 C.F.R. §405.803 (1998).

[155]42 C.F.R. §405.820 (1998).

[156] Department of Health and Human Services, *Medicare Carrier's Manual*, Part 3, §12017.

[157]42 C.F.R. §§405.1885(a) (1998), 405.841 (1998), 405.750 (1998).

[158]42 C.F.R. §405.1885(d) (1998).

when they turn 65. Some states allow for limited open enrollment for Medigap insurance before the beneficiary turns 65 (e.g., Connecticut, Maine, Massachusetts, Minnesota, New Jersey, New York, Oklahoma, Pennsylvania, Virginia, Washington, and Wisconsin[159]).

Although the regulation of insurance traditionally is a state function under the McCarran–Ferguson Act,[160] Medigap insurance (or Medicare supplemental insurance) is heavily regulated by the federal government due to past abuses in the industry.[161] Medigap policies may not be issued in a particular state unless that state provides for a regulatory and enforcement program that follows federal requirements, such policy has been approved by the state, or such policy has been certified by the Department of Health and Human Services.[162] Generally these policies are governed by federal law, which uses National Association for Insurance Commissioner (NAIC) standards. Therefore, only a limited number of policies are available for beneficiaries in the Medigap market, allowing for some comparison shopping and competition.[163] Currently, there are ten standardized plans, referred to as plan A through J. Medigap policies must also be renewable and can only be canceled or terminated for nonpayment or "material misrepresentation" (i.e., fraud); it cannot be canceled or terminated because of health status.[164] Medicare Select is a special program that allows for Medicare beneficiaries to elect to use a managed care or preferred provider organization for their Medigap policy.[165] This program originally was limited to 15 states; however, federal legislation has expanded availability to Medicare beneficiaries in all states.[166]

Further Reading

Appeals in Medicare

Furrow BR et al. Administrative Appeals and Judicial Review of Medicare Determinations. In: *Health Law.* St. Paul, MN: West Publishing Co., 1995;§13-31–13-32.

Assignment

Furrow BR et al. Billing and Claims. In: *Health Law.* St. Paul, MN: West Publishing Co., 1995;§13-26–13-28.

---

[159]U.S. General Accounting Office, *Medigap Insurance: Alternatives for Medicare Beneficiaries to Avoid Medical Underwriting* (Washington, DC: General Accounting Office, 1996).
[160]15 U.S.C.A. §§1011, 1012, 1015.
[161]See Pub. L. No. 101-508, §§4351–4361, 104 Stat. 1388 (1990).
[162]42 U.S.C.A. §1395ss(a)(1)–(2).
[163]42 U.S.C.A. §1395ss(p).
[164]42 U.S.C.A. §1395ss(q)(1).
[165]See Pub. L. No. 104-18, 109 Stat. 192 (1995).
[166]See Pub. L. No. 104-18, 109 Stat. 192 (1995).

Beneficiary Cost Sharing

Jimenez CS. Medicare HMO's: A Consumer Prospective. *Seton Hall L Rev* 1996;26:1195–1212.
Kinney ED. Medicare Managed Care from the Beneficiary's Perspective. *Seton Hall L Rev* 1996;26:1163–94.
Kuritz MA. *The Beneficiary Book.* New York: Viking Press, 1996.

Coverage

Furrow BR et al. Covered and Excluded Services. In: *Health Law.* St. Paul, MN: West Publishing Co., 1995;§13-5–13-7.
Himelfarb RI. *Catastrophic Politics: The Rise and Fall of the Medicare Coverage Act of 1998.* University Park: Pennsylvania State University Press, 1995.
Kraus DL. *The Medicare Coverage Issues Manual.* New York: McGraw-Hill Book Co., 1992.
Szczygiel A. What Every Lawyer Should Know About Medicare Coverage of Long-Term Care. *NY St BJ* 1992;64(Dec):40–44.
Weimer SR. Medicare — After the Medicare Catastrophic Coverage Act. *Del Law* 1989;7:20–21.

CPT Coding

American Medical Association. *CPT 1992: Physicians' Current Procedural Terminology.* Chicago: American Medical Association, 1991.
Brett AS. New Guidelines for Coding Physicians' Services — a Step Backward. *N Engl J Med* 1998;339:1705–8.
Kassirer JP, Angell M. Evaluation and Management Guidelines — Fatally Flawed. *N Engl J Med* 1998; 339:1697–98.
O'Donohue WJ Jr. CPT Coding and Medicare Reimbursement: From Beans to Bullets. *Chest* 1998; 113:1431–32.

Enrollment

Inlander CB, Donio MA. *Medicare Made Easy* (Serial), 9th ed. Allentown, PA: People Medical Society, 1999.
Levin JK. Automatic Enrollees. In: *American Jurisprudence,* 2d ed. New York: Lawyers Cooperative Publishing Co., 1987;§503.
Levin JK. Automatic Enrollment. In: *American Jurisprudence,* 2d ed. New York: Lawyers Cooperative Publishing Co., 1987;§496.
Levin JK. Enrollment Generally. In: *American Jurisprudence,* 2d ed. New York: Lawyers Cooperative Publishing Co., 1987;§488.
Levin JK. Increased Premium for Late Enrollment. In: *American Jurisprudence,* 2d ed. New York: Lawyers Cooperative Publishing Co., 1987;§512.

Levin JK. Special Enrollment Period. In: *American Jurisprudence,* 2d ed. New York: Lawyers Cooperative Publishing Co., 1987;§490.

Medicare Exclusions from Payment

Furrow BR et al. Covered and Excluded Services. In: *Health Law.* St. Paul, MN: West Publishing Co., 1995;§13–17.

Levin JK. Routine Items or Services. In: *American Jurisprudence,* 2d ed. New York: Lawyers Cooperative Publishing Co., 1987;§1201.

Medigap Insurance

Medicare/Medigap, rev. ed. New York: St. Martin's Press, 1994.

U.S. General Accounting Office. *Medigap Insurance: Compliance with Federal Standards Has Increased. Pub. no.* GAO/HEHS-98-66. Washington, DC: General Accounting Office, 1998.

U.S. General Accounting Office. *Medigap Insurance: Alternatives for Medicare Beneficiaries to Avoid Medical Underwriting.* Pub. no. GAO/HEHS-96-180. Washington, DC: General Accounting Office, 1996.

Part A Payment

Furrow BR et al. Medicare Prospective Payment Under Diagnosis-Related Groups. In: *Health Law.* St. Paul, MN: West Publishing Co., 1995;§13-10–13-16.

Part B Payment

Blanchard TP. "Medical Necessity" Denials as a Medicare Part B Cost-Containment Strategy: Two Wrongs Don't Make It Right. *St Louis U L J* 1990;34:939–1040.

Furrow BR et al. Medicare Part B Payment. In: *Health Law.* St. Paul, MN: West Publishing Co., 1995;§13-21–13-25.

Provider Participation Requirements

Furrow BR et al. Provider Participation. In: *Health Law.* St. Paul, MN: West Publishing Co., 1995;§13-8.

Other Reading

Barry DM. Chapter 15 Medicare Part A Payment: Cost-Based Payments. In: National Health Lawyers Association, *Health Law Practice Guide.* Deerfield, IL: West Group, 1997.

Fox PD, Rice T, Alecxih L. Medigap Regulation: Lessons for Health Care Reform. *J Health Pol Pol'y & L* 1995;20:31–48.

Frankford D. The Complexity of Medicare's Hospital Reimbursement System: The Paradoxes of Averaging. *Iowa L Rev* 1993;78:517–668.

Frankford D. The Medicare DRGs: Efficiency and Organizational Rationality. *Yale J Reg* 1993;10:273–346.

Gosfield AG. Private Contracting by Medicare Physicians: The Pit and the Pendulum. *Health Law Digest* 1998;26(1):3–9.

Inglehart JK. The American Health Care System: Medicare. *N Engl J Med* 1992;327:1467–72.

Kelley NM. Note, Dollars and Sense: An Introduction to Medicare Part B Appeals. *New Engl L Rev* 1990;25:617–51.

Kinney ED. The Role of Judicial Review Regarding Medicare and Medicaid Program Policy: Past Experience and Future Expectations. *St. Louis Univ L J* 1991;35:759–92.

Liang BA. Analysis of the Resource-Based Relative Value Scale for Medicare Reimbursements to Academic and Community Hospital Radiology Departments. *Radiology* 1991;179:751–58.

Meyers RJ, Detlefs DA. *1999 Mercer Guide to Social Security and Medicare,* 27th ed. New York: William M. Mercer, 1999.

Reischauer RD et al. *Medicare: Preparing for the Challenges of the 21st Century.* Washington, DC: Brookings Institute, 1998.

Reiss JB. Coding, Documenting and Billing Physician Services: A Growing Target for Government Enforcement Agencies? *The Health Lawyer* 1997;9(4):9–13.

Sutter RN, Philip MS. Medicare Prospective Payment System for Inpatient Operating Costs. In: National Health Lawyers Association, *Health Law Practice Guide.* Deerfield, IL: West Group, 1997.

Wieland JB. Medicare Part B Payment for Physician Services. In: National Health Lawyers Association, *Health Law Practice Guide.* Deerfield, IL: West Group, 1997.

Web Sites

Center for Medicare Advocacy: *http://www.medicare advocacy.org/*

Electronic Policy Network: Facts on Medicare: *http://epn.org/library/agmedi.html*

Empire Medicare Services: *http://www.empiremedicare.com/*

Free Medigap info: *http://www.freemedigapinfo.com/*

Group Health Incorporated, Medicare Division: *http://www.ghi-medicare.com/*

Health Care Financing Administration: *http://www.hcfa.gov*

HealthCare Medicare Administration: *http://www.cigna medicare.com/*

Medicare and Medicaid statistics and data: *http://www.hcfa.gov/stats/stats.htm*

Medicare of Florida, beneficiary education and outreach: *http://www.medicarefla.com*

Medicare overview: *http://www.hcfa.gov/pubforms/98guide1.htm*

Medicare Payment Advisory Commission: *http://www.pprc.gov/*

Medicare Rights Center: *http://www.medicarerights.org/*

Medicare Summary for Nursing Home Care: *http://members.tripod.com/~volfangary/Medicare.html*

Medicare and you: Helpful information for Medicare beneficiaries: *http://www.medicareinfo.com/*

Medigap coverage: *http://www.hcfa.gov/pubforms/98guide4.htm#Medigap*

National Medicare Education Program: *http://www.nmep.org/*

Nationwide health plans, Medicare Part B carrier web site: *http://www.nationwide-medicare.com/*

The official U.S. government site for Medicare information: *http://www.medicare.gov/*

Xact Medicare Services: *http://www.xact.org/*

8

Public Insurance: Medicaid

Title XIX of the Social Security Act, passed in 1965 with the Medicare statute, created the Medicaid program.[1] Medicaid is the health insurance program for individuals and their families who have low incomes and resources. The program is administered and financed jointly by the states and the federal government.[2] HCFA is the responsible federal agency that administers the plan, although state agencies also administer the plan on a day-to-day basis. Therefore, Medicaid actually is a series of 50-plus separate programs, due to state variation in the populations included and services covered. States promulgate requirements for eligibility and services above a baseline federal set of requirements and also set payment rates. The federal government funds between 50% and 83% of the state's Medicaid program costs (the *federal medical assistance percentage*, FMAP, sometimes known as the *federal financial participation*, FFP) and administrative costs, depending on the per capita income of the state.[3] There is no set limit or cap on FMAP funds provided states; however, state governments must fund at least 40% of the state share of expenses (rather than local government units).[4] Further, FFP cannot be allocated to cover services for inmates at public institutions other than medical institutions,[5] care or services for mental institutional patients under age 65,[6] or for inpatient psychiatric services for individuals over age 21.[7]

This chapter presents an overview of this public insurance program. However, like Medicare, this program and its state variants are in a continuous state of flux and publicly available sources should be reviewed to obtain the most current information about the program.

Covered Groups and Eligibility

Several groups must be covered by state Medicaid programs to be eligible for FMAP. These groups, known as the *categorically needy*,[8] include recipients of Aid to Families with Dependent Children (AFDC);[9] recipients of Supplemental Security Income (SSI) benefits;[10] certain qualified Medicare beneficiaries (i.e., those who cannot afford to pay their Part A and B cost sharing with Medicaid paying for this cost sharing);[11] pregnant and postpartum women with family incomes at or under 133% of the federal poverty level and their children under 6 years of age;[12] children under age 19 born after September 30,

---

[1] 42 U.S.C.A. §§1396 *et seq.*; 42 C.F.R. parts 430–456 (1998).

[2] 42 U.S.C.A. §1396a(a)(2); 42 C.F.R. part 431, subpart A (1998).

[3] 42 U.S.C.A. §§1396b(a), 1396d(b), 1396b(a)(7); 42 C.F.R. §433.10(b) (1998).

[4] 42 U.S.C.A. §1396a(a)(2).

[5] 42 U.S.C.A. §1396d(a)(24)(A); 42 C.F.R. §§435.1008 (1998), 436.1004 (1998).

[6] 42 U.S.C.A. §§1396d(a)(24)(B), 1396d(i); 42 C.F.R. §§1008 (1998), 436.1004 (1998).

[7] 42 U.S.C.A. §§1396d(a)(16), 1396d(h); 42 C.F.R. §§435.1008 (1998), 436.1004 (1998); see also Connecticut Dept. of Income Maintenance v. Heckler, 471 U.S. 524 (1985) (differentiating nursing and intermediate care facilities from mental institutions).

[8] 42 U.S.C.A. §1396a(a)(10)(A); 42 C.F.R. §§435.2–435.170 (1998).

[9] 42 U.S.C.A. §1396a(a)(10)(A)(i)(I); 42 C.F.R. §§435.4(b) (1998), 435.110 (1998), 435.401 (1998), 436.110 (1998), 436.401 (1998).

[10] 42 U.S.C.A. §§1396a(a)(10)(A)(i)(II), 1396a(f); 42 C.F.R. §§435.120 (1998), 435.121 (1998).

[11] 42 U.S.C.A. §§1396a(a)(10)(E), 1396a(a)(10)(E)(iii), 1396d(p).

[12] 42 U.S.C.A. §§1396a(a)(10)(A)(i)(III), 1396a(a)(10)(A)(i)(IV), 1396a(a)(10)(A)(i)(VI), 1396a(l)(1)(A), 1396a(l)(1)(B), 1396a(l)(1)(C), 1396a(l)(2)(A)(ii)(II), 1396a(l)(2)(B), 1396d(n)(1).

1983, in families with incomes at or under 100% of the federal poverty level (this requirement is being phased out and will be completely eliminated by 2002);[13] recipients of adoption assistance and foster care under Title IV-E of Social Security;[14] undocumented aliens for emergency care;[15] and Pickle amendment beneficiaries (recipients of both SSI and Social Security who have lost SSI benefits due to Social Security cost-of-living adjustments).[16]

Beyond the categorically needy, a state may decide to cover optional groups and still remain eligible for FMAP. These groups include infants up to 1 year of age and pregnant women not covered under the preceding categorically needy rules but with a family income of no more than 185% of poverty;[17] selected aged or disabled beneficiaries with incomes above the SSI cutoff level but below federal poverty levels;[18] "Ribicoff" children under the age of 21, 20, 19, or 18 (at the state's option) who meet income and resource requirements for AFDC but are not otherwise eligible for the program;[19] caretaker relatives of covered children who meet income and resource standards of AFDC;[20] aged, blind, or disabled individuals who receive state-funded supplementary payments;[21] individuals who would be eligible if institutionalized but who are receiving care under home- and community-based service waivers; institutionalized individuals eligible under a special income level (set by the state, up to 300% of the SSI federal benefits rate); certain individuals infected by tuberculosis; and the "medically needy" (aged, blind, or disabled persons or families with dependent children who exceed income or asset eligibility levels as categorically needy).[22] The state cannot condition Medicaid eligibility on a state residential require-ment that excludes any person who otherwise would be eligible and intends to remain in the state, regardless of how long the individual has been in the state or whether the person was formally a resident of the state.[23] Consistent with this provision, states must make outreach efforts to enroll eligible homeless persons into Medicaid.[24] States must also provide for Medicaid services for eligible persons who temporarily are outside the state.[25] States also cannot impose an age requirement of more than 65 years old.[26]

Note that the Personal Responsibility and Work Opportunity Reconciliation Act of 1996[27] has had a significant impact on Medicaid coverage. First, some individuals who would have been eligible for the SSI program will not be due to changes in federal eligibility standards. Further, Medicaid availability will be limited for legal aliens: For legal resident aliens and other qualified aliens who entered the United States on or after August 22, 1996, whose coverage is not mandatory in the program, Medicaid is barred for five years (except for emergency services). Medicaid for aliens entering before this date and after the five-year ban is optional, as determined by the states. The open-ended cash assistance AFDC program has now been replaced with the Temporary Assistance for Needy Families (TANF) program, which provides grants to states for limited cash assistance to these families. TANF has a family lifetime limit of five years. However, persons who would have been eligible for Medicaid (i.e., they meet the requirements that were in effect on July 16, 1996) generally are still eligible, although the law does not require this result.

Also note that because each state has differing requirements and eligibility standards, there will be significant variation across states in terms of service coverage. However, determination of eligibility generally must be made within 90 days for disabled applicants and 45 days for all others.[28] Once a person is found eligible for Medicaid, coverage for services is retroactive to the third month prior to application to the program if the person would have been eligible if he or she applied during that period.[29] Medicaid coverage generally terminates at the end of the month in which the individual is no longer eli-

---

[13]42 U.S.C.A. §§1396a(a)(10)(E), 1396d(p).

[14]42 U.S.C.A. §1396a(a)(10)(A)(ii)(VIII).

[15]42 U.S.C.A. §§1396a(a)(10), 1396b(v).

[16]42 C.F.R. §§435.135 (1998), 435.136 (1998).

[17]42 U.S.C.A. §§1396a(a)(10)A)(ii)(IX), 1396a(l), 1396o(c).

[18]42 U.S.C.A. §§1396a(a)(10)(A)(ii)(X), 1396a(m).

[19]42 U.S.C.A. §§1396a(a)(10)(A)(ii), 1396d(a)(i); 42 C.F.R. §§435.222 (1998), 436.222 (1998).

[20]42 U.S.C.A. §1396a(a)(10).

[21]42 U.S.C.A. §1396a(a)(10)(A)(ii)(XI); 42 C.F.R. §§435.232 (1998), 435.234 (1998), 435.1006 (1998).

[22]42 U.S.C.A. §1396a(a)(10)(C); 42 C.F.R. §§435.300–435.350 (1998), 435.4; specifically, 42 U.S.C.A. §§1396a(a)(10)(C)(ii), 1396a(e)(4), 42 C.F.R. §435.301(b)(1) (1998) (pregnant women and children); 42 C.F.R. §435.340 (1998) (aged, blind, and disabled beneficiaries); 42 C.F.R. §§435.308 (1998), 436.308 (1998) (18–21-year-old children); 42 C.F.R. §§435.310 (1998), 436.310 (1998) (caretaker relatives of 18–21-year-old children); 42 C.F.R. §§435.320 (1998), 435.330 (1998), 436.320 (1998) (individuals over age 65); 42 C.F.R. §§ 435.322 (1998), 435.330 (1998), 436.321 (1998) (blind individuals); 42 C.F.R. §§435.324 (1998), 435.330 (1998), 436.322 (1998) (disabled individuals); 42 U.S.C.A. §§1396a(a)(47), 1396r-1 (presumptively eligible pregnant women); 42 C.F.R. §435.326 (1998) (individuals in Medicaid HMOs who lose eligibility).

[23]42 U.S.C.A. §1396a(b); 42 C.F.R. §§435.403 (1998), 436.403 (1998).

[24]42 U.S.C.A. §1396a(a)(48).

[25]42 U.S.C.A. §1396a(a)(16); 42 C.F.R. §§435.403(e) (1998), 435.403(j)(3) (1998), 436.403(e) (1998), 436.403(i)(3) (1998).

[26]42 U.S.C.A. §1396a(b)(1); 42 C.F.R. §§435.520 (1998), 436.520 (1998), 435.522 (1998).

[27]Pub. L. No. 104-193, 110 Stat. 2105 (1996).

[28]42 U.S.C.A. §1396a(a)(8); 42 C.F.R. § 435.911 (1998).

[29]42 U.S.C.A. §1396a(a)(34); 42 C.F.R. §435.914 (1998); see also Cohen v. Quern, 608 F.Supp. 1324 (N.D. Ill. 1984) (Medicaid applicant who paid for services during three-month period may receive reimbursement from provider, who then must collect from Medicaid program).

gible. However, eligibility may continue for a longer period if the person has been terminated from the SSI program,[30] loses AFDC eligibility due to employment,[31] is overcoming a disability but is still eligible for cash assistance,[32] or requests a hearing to protest termination or potential termination from the program.[33] Program benefits continue until the person is deemed ineligible.[34] Some states provide Medicaid to individuals who do not meet standard eligibility requirements; however, these state-only programs are not eligible for FMAP.

Services

Certain basic services must, by law, be offered in the Medicaid program. These include inpatient and outpatient hospital services, prenatal care, vaccines for children, physician services, medical services by a dentist, nursing facility services for persons 21 or older, family planning services and supplies (except abortion), rural health clinic services, home health care for persons eligible for skilled-nursing services, laboratory and X-ray services, pediatric and family nurse practitioner services, nurse-midwife services, federally qualified health center services, and early periodic screening, diagnostic, and treatment (EPSDT) services for children under age 21.[35] Note that mandatory services may not be denied or decreased in amount, scope, or duration solely because of the recipient's diagnosis, illness, or condition. Further, a state Medicaid program can cover certain optional services for which FMAP cost sharing is available. Of the 30 or so eligible optional services, some of the more common include diagnostic services, clinic services, intermediate care facilities for the mentally retarded (ICFs/MR), prescription drugs and prosthetics, optometrist services, eyeglasses, nursing facility services for children under age 21, transportation services, and rehabilitation and physical therapy services.[36]

The extent to which services are covered by states in their Medicaid programs is generally limited only by comparability; states must provide comparable coverage for all those categorically needy and categorically related eligible individuals. Note that medically necessary services under EPSDT that are not within the scope of mandatory or optional services under federal law still must be covered, even if those services are not included as part of the covered services of that state's plan; and states may request waivers to pay for otherwise-uncovered home- and community-based services for persons eligible for Medicaid who might otherwise be institutionalized.[37]

Payment

Medicaid pays participating providers in the program directly, using a state-based fee schedule created under federal regulatory rules.[38] Providers that participate in the Medicaid program must accept the state Medicaid program payment as payment in full except for nominal cost sharing. However, these deductibles or coinsurance provisions cannot be extended to pregnant women, children under age 18, hospital or nursing home patients who are expected to contribute most of their income to institutional care, and categorically needy individuals enrolled in HMOs. In addition, emergency and family planning services are exempted from copayments. Other than these limitations, states have broad discretion in setting payment rates for providers in the Medicaid program.

Note that the Boren amendment, which formerly mandated adequate payment levels by the states, was repealed by the Balanced Budget Act of 1997.[39] At one time, the Medicaid regulation known as the *Boren amendment* required that reimbursement rates in the Medicaid program be "reasonable and adequate to meet the costs which must be incurred by efficiently and economically operated facilities . . . to assure that individuals eligible for medical assistance have reasonable access."[40] However, the Balanced Budget Act of 1997 repealed the Boren amendment; now, states must meet less stringent payment conditions, such as utilizing a public notice-and-comment process.[41] It remains to be seen whether additional challenges and appeals to Medicaid will result from this change in the law.

---

[30]42 C.F.R. §435.1003 (1998).

[31]See 42 U.S.C.A. §§1396a(a)(10)(A)(ii), 1396d(a)(i); 42 C.F.R. §§435.222 (1998), 436.222 (1998).

[32]42 U.S.C.A. §435.1004.

[33]42 C.F.R. §§431.230 (1998), 435.1003(a)(3) (1998).

[34]42 C.F.R. §435.930 (1998).

[35]42 U.S.C.A. §§1396d, 1396d(a)(xi)(1)-(2), 1396d(a)(xi)(4), 1396d(a)(xi)(5), 1396d(a)(xi)(7), 1396d(a)(xi)(10), 1396d(a)(xi)(17).

[36]42 U.S.C.A. §1396(d).

[37]See, e.g., *Florida Statutes Annotated* (St. Paul, MN: West, 1997), section 409.9126; 305 *Illinois Compiled Statutes Annotated* (St. Paul, MN: West, 1997), 5/5-5c; *Minnesota Statutes Annotated* (St. Paul, MN: West, 1997), section 256B.0915; see also *Colorado Revised Statutes Annotated* (St. Paul, MN: West, 1997), sections 26-4-684 and 26-4-675; *Minnesota Statutes Annotated* (St. Paul, MN: West, 1997), section 256B.49.

[38]42 U.S.C.A. §1396a(a)(3); 42 C.F.R. §§447.204 (1998), 447.252 (1998), 447.253 (1998).

[39]Pub. L. No. 105-33; see also Campbell Hall v. Sullivan, 129 F.3d 113 (2nd Cir. 1997); Exeter Mem. Hosp. Ass'n v. Belshe, 145 F.3d 1106 (9th Cir. 1998); Concourse Rehab. & Nursing Ctr. v. Wing, 1998 WL 406040 (2nd Cir. 1998).

[40]42 U.S.C.A. §1396a(a)(13)(A).

[41]42 U.S.C.A. §1396a(a)(30)(A).

Appeals

The state Medicaid program must provide some form of fair hearing to beneficiaries before the state agency may deny or revoke eligibility or fail to act on eligibility in a reasonable time.[42] In general, the state agency responsible must indicate to the beneficiary the specific action it intends to take, provide its specific reasons for doing so, as well as provide the individual with information regarding his or her right to a hearing and the circumstances under which services will be continued if a hearing is requested by the individual.[43] For eligibility determination and coverage disputes, federal regulation governs the minimum requirements for a hearing, including time in which notice must be provided (usually ten days before the proposed agency action),[44] who will adjudicate the hearing (impartial person or persons not involved in initial determination),[45] when a hearing is required, the mechanics of requesting a hearing, the circumstances when group hearings are allowed, the circumstances where denial or dismissal of a request for a hearing is allowed, procedures for maintaining services, procedures for reinstatement of services, rights when an adverse decision is made through a local evidentiary hearing, requirements for state agency hearing after an adverse decision by local evidentiary hearing, state conduction of the hearing, matters that can be considered at the hearing, procedural rights of the applicant or recipient at the hearing (e.g., right to representation, access to documentation of person's case file, right to examine and cross-examine witnesses and present evidence),[46] parties involved in an eligibility determination, and mechanisms for rendering a hearing decision.[47] Regulations also stipulate that the individual has a right to receive written notice of the decision and any rights to judicial review to which he or she is entitled.[48] Note that participating providers in the Medicaid program may act as a beneficiary representative in these disputes in the hearing forum,[49] particularly because individual providers have only limited administrative relief and review available.[50] Hearings must be granted if requested in a timely manner unless the sole issue is one of federal or state law that requires an automatic change affecting all or some recipients.[51] In the latter circumstance, the agency may consolidate requests for hearings and hold a group hearing in lieu of individual hearings;[52] further, the state may terminate benefits in this situation if it informs the individuals affected in writing that services will be terminated or reduced pending the hearing.[53] In other cases, the state may continue benefits but may recoup any payments made during the pendency of the agency hearing if the state prevails; however, the state must make corrective payments if the agency does not prevail at the hearing level or if the decision ultimately is reversed and the individual has incurred expenses because of the adjudication.[54]

State judicial review is limited and generally can occur only after all administrative remedies have been exhausted.[55] Federal judicial review has been allowed in state actor suits under federal law[56] for violation of, for example, the laws regarding Social Security[57] and enforcement of a Medicaid waiver program.[58] Note that since federal administrative remedies generally are not accessible for review of state Medicaid policies, there is no issue of exhausting federal administrative remedies; in addition, state actor suits also generally do not require exhaustion of state administrative remedies.[59] In court adjudications, the plaintiff-beneficiary has the burden of proof;[60] and courts grant substantial deference to state administrative determinations,[61] granting relief only when

---

[42]42 U.S.C.A. §1396a(a)(3); 42 C.F.R. §§431.200–431.250 (1998).

[43]42 C.F.R. §431.210 (1998).

[44]42 C.F.R. §431.211 (1998).

[45]42 C.F.R. §431.240 (1998).

[46]42 C.F.R. §431.242 (1998).

[47]42 C.F.R. §§431.200 (1998) *et seq.*

[48]42 C.F.R. §431.245 (1998).

[49]42 U.S.C.A. §1396a(a)(32); 42 C.F.R. §447.10 (1998).

[50]42 C.F.R. §447.253 (1998).

[51]42 C.F.R. §§431.220 (1998), 431.221 (1998).

[52]42 C.F.R. §431.222 (1998).

[53]42 C.F.R. §431.230 (1998).

[54]42 C.F.R. §431.246 (1998).

[55]See, e.g., Provincial House, Inc. v. Department of Social Servs., 422 N.W.2d 241 (Mich. Ct. App. 1988) (issue review denied when exhaustion requirement was waived); Jordan Health Corp. v. Axelrod, 532 N.Y.S.2d 480 (1988) (when no factual issues need resolution, exhaustion is not required); Cowan v. Myers, 232 Cal.Rptr. 299 (Cal. Ct. App. 1986), *cert. denied* 484 U.S. 846 (1987) (direct challenge to state law does not require exhaustion of administrative remedies before judicial review).

[56]42 U.S.C.A. §1983.

[57]See, e.g., Maine v. Thiboutot, 448 U.S. 1 (1980); Wilder v. Virginia Hosp. Ass'n, 496 U.S. 498 (1990).

[58]See, e.g., Wood v. Wallace, 825 F.Supp. 177 (S.D. Ohio 1993); Case v. Weinberger, 523 F.2d 602 (2nd Cir. 1975).

[59]See, e.g., Wilder v. Virginia Hosp. Ass'n, 496 U.S. 498 (1990); Alacare, Inc.-North v. Baggiano, 785 F.2d 963 (11th Cir.), *cert. denied* 479 U.S. 829 (1986); but see New York City Health and Hosps. Corp. v. Heckler, 593 F.Supp. 226 (S.D. N.Y. 1984) (challenge in federal court of state law is not ripe until factual issues resolved in state administrative proceeding).

[60]See, e.g., Colorado Health Care Ass'n v. Colorado Dept. of Social Servs., 842 F.2d 1158 (10th Cir. 1988); Wisconsin Hops. Ass'n v. Reivitz, 733 F.2d 1226 (7th Cir. 1984).

[61]See, e.g., Unicare Health Facilities v. Miller, 481 F.Supp. 496 (N.D. Ill. 1979).

the state's actions were arbitrary, capricious, or violated federal law.[62]

Another limitation is relevant to challenges to state Medicaid determinations. The Eleventh Amendment of the U.S. Constitution provides that a suit may not be brought against a state unless that state consents to suit; states do not consent to suit merely by participating in the Medicaid program.[63] Although suits may be brought against the relevant officials that administer the program, relief is only prospective,[64] and state officials who are sued in their individual capacity usually are able to avoid liability under absolute or qualified immunity.[65] Retroactive relief that affects the state treasury is prohibited, and injunctive or declaratory relief may not be available if the state alters its regulations or procedures before relief is obtained through the court.[66] However, the state may be ordered to issue notices that inform Medicaid recipients of damages or other retroactive relief that may be available through state law in state courts or administrative actions, if the notice is ancillary to another form of permissible relief.[67]

Medicaid and Medicare

Beneficiaries of the Medicare program also may qualify for Medicaid. If the Medicare beneficiary falls within the general qualifications of a particular group in Medicaid, the Medicaid program will extend its service coverage to the Medicare beneficiary for all services not covered by Medicare. In addition, four other Medicare groups may receive partial state Medicaid coverage. First, qualified Medicare beneficiaries (QMBs) are Medicare beneficiaries who have resources at or below two times the standard allowed under the SSI program and income at or below 100% of the federal poverty level. The states' Medicaid programs pay Medicare Part A and B copayments and premiums for QMBs, subject to state limita-

tions on payment rates. Second, specified low-income Medicare beneficiaries (SLMBs) are Medicare beneficiaries with resources like QMBs but have incomes up to 120% of the federal poverty level. SLMBs are eligible for state Medicaid payment of Medicare Part B premiums. Third, qualified disabled and working individuals (QDWIs), according to the Medicare statute, are persons who previously qualified for Medicare due to disability but then lost eligibility due to a return to work. They are permitted to purchase Medicare Part A and B if they have incomes below 200% of the federal poverty level and do not meet any Medicaid category criteria. These QDWIs are eligible for state Medicaid program payment of their Part A premium if their incomes are between 150 and 200% of the federal poverty level; the state must pay their Part A premiums if their incomes are less than 150% of the federal poverty level. Fourth, qualifying individuals (QIs) also may be eligible for assistance. QIs must be eligible for Medicare Part A, have resources no greater than two times the standard allowed under the SSI program, and income no greater than 175% of the federal poverty limit. For those QIs with incomes at or up to 135% of the federal poverty limit, designated QI-1s, the state will pay the QI-1 beneficiaries' Medicare Part B premium. If the QI has an income between 135% and 175% of the federal poverty level, the state Medicaid program may pay part of the Medicare Part B premium.[68]

Waivers

Medicaid waivers allow states to experiment with service provision and financing in the state Medicaid program. States engage in these waiver efforts through two primary means: program waivers and research and demonstration waivers. These waiver authorities, particularly section 1115 research and demonstration waivers, have been used extensively by states in an effort to reduce program expenditures, generally by formation of some Medicaid managed care program.

Program Waivers

Two common program waivers are the home- and community-based service (HCBS) waivers and the free-

[62]See, e.g., Colorado Health Care Ass'n v. Colorado Dept. of Social Servs., 842 F.2d 1158 (10th Cir. 1988); Mississippi Hosp. Ass'n v. Heckler, 701 F.2d 511 (5th Cir. 1983); Temple Univ. v. White, 941 F.2d 201 (3d Cir. 1991), *cert. denied* 502 U.S. 1032 (1992).

[63]See, e.g., Florida Dep't of Health and Rehab. Servs. v. Florida Nursing Home Ass'n, 450 U.S. 147 (1981).

[64]See, e.g., Papasan v. Allain, 478 U.S. 265 (1986); Edelman v. Jordan, 415 U.S. 651 (1974); Amisub (PSL), Inc. v. Colorado Dept. of Social Servs., 879 F.2d 789 (10th Cir. 1989), *cert. denied* 496 U.S. 935 (1990); Hillhaven Corp. v. Wisconsin Dept. of Health and Social Servs., 733 F.2d 1224 (7th Cir. 1984).

[65]See, e.g., AGI-Bluff Manor, Inc. v. Reagen, 713 F.Supp. 1535 (W.D. Mo. 1989).

[66]See, e.g., Green v. Mansour, 474 U.S. 64 (1985).

[67]See, e.g., Quern v. Jordan, 440 U.S. 332 (1979).

[68]Health Care Financing Administration, *1998 Guide to Health Insurance for People with Medicare,* available at http://www.hcfa.gov/pubforms/98guide1.htm; Health Care Financing Administration, *Programs That Help Low-Income Beneficiaries,* available at *http://www.hcfa.gov/pubforms/*mhbkc04.htm; Health Care Financing Administration, "Program Memorandum: Medicaid State Agencies," transmittal no. 97-3 (December 1997), available at *http://www.hcfa.gov/transmit/97317.htm.*

dom of choice (FOC) waiver. HCBS program waivers focused on attempting to develop innovative methods to avoid placing Medicaid benficiaries into long-term care facilities such as nursing homes. Under Section 1915(c) of the Social Security Act,[69] states may apply to waive certain federal requirements under the Medicaid program, such as mandated statewide provision of the same levels of care, comparability of services, and community income and resource rules. HCBS program services specifically contemplated by the Social Security Act include case management, homemaker services, home health services, personal care services, adult day health, rehabilitation, and respite care. In addition, other services may be within the state waiver if they support the objective of avoiding placement into a medical facility, including transportation, in-home support services, meal services, special communications services, minor home modifications, adult day care, partial hospitalization services, psychosocial rehabilitation services, and clinical services for individuals with chronic mental illness. States may apply for HCBS program waivers that cover the entire state or that are limited in geographic scope and that cover many or specific eligible populations or disease states. Further, states may make HCBS available to persons who otherwise would qualify for Medicaid only if they were residents of a medical care facility.

States that wish to obtain an HCBS program waiver must apply to HCFA and indicate that the program will not exceed the cost associated with the care for the proposed covered population if institutionalized. Further, the state also must document that appropriate patient safeguards are in place to ensure the health and welfare of the individuals in the program. If the HCBS program waiver is granted, it initially is approved for three years and is renewable at five-year intervals. The HCBS program waivers are within the purview of HCFA's Office of Long-Term Care Services.

FOC program waivers are also authorized under Section 1915(b) of the Social Security Act.[70] Generally, Medicaid beneficiaries have the freedom of choice to obtain services from any provider that participates in the Medicaid program.[71] Under the FOC waivers, states may waive certain mandated provisions for Medicaid beneficiaries, including the beneficiaries' right to select their own providers, comparability of services, and the statewide service level requirement, if the appropriate criteria are met.[72] Usually, these waivers have been used to enroll certain Medicaid beneficiaries into managed care plans and primary case management programs (gatekeeper programs). FOC program waivers generally

are approved initially for two years and are renewable in two-year intervals. Note that not all state programs using managed care require FOC waivers; programs in which beneficiaries may choose between fee for service or managed care do not require FOC waivers. The FOC waiver programs are assessed and monitored by the Office of Managed Care, Medicaid Managed Care Team within the HCFA.

Research and Demonstration Waivers

Under section 1115 of the Social Security Act,[73] states may apply for much broader waivers for Medicaid services and financing projects. These projects, however, must be designed so that formal, rigorous evaluation can be performed for policy assessment. Research and demonstration waivers ordinarily are granted for up to five years to allow for greater experimentation in health policy. However, these programs must demonstrate that they will be budget neutral; that is, they cannot cost more during their proposed project time period than the Medicaid program would have spent without the demonstration. Typical projects include requiring beneficiaries to stay enrolled in a particular managed care plan for longer periods in mandatory Medicaid HMO enrollment programs, using a broader array of providers, covering new services, offering different service packages across the state, testing new reimbursement methodologies, and changing Medicaid eligibility to cover more persons in the program. However, research and demonstration waivers *cannot* be used to waive services for pregnant women and children, copayment and other cost-sharing requirements for current categorically needy beneficiaries, FMAP rates, quality assurance monitoring, HCFA approval authority, or the requirements of ERISA.

The Office of Research and Demonstrations within the HCFA is responsible for the section 1115 research and demonstration waivers. Further, the office implements and monitors research and demonstration waiver programs with the assistance of the Medicaid Bureau, the Office of Managed Care, and the HCFA's regional offices.

Spending Down for Nursing Home Care

Since Medicaid is a program for those with limited resources, it is available only to individuals with limited income and assets. However, because of its coverage of nursing home care and Medicare's lack of coverage in this area, many senior citizens utilize the strategy of reducing their financial resources to become eligible for the program to defray the extensive costs of nursing home

---

[69]42 U.S.C.A. §1396n.

[70]42 U.S.C.A. §1396n(b); 42 C.F.R. §430.25 (1998).

[71]42 U.S.C.A. §1396a(a)(23).

[72]42 C.F.R. §431.55 (1998).

[73]42 U.S.C.A. §1315.

coverage. Nursing home coverage in this context includes nursing home care, home health care, personal care, and various home- and community-based services as necessary.[74] Thus, Medicaid has become the largest third-party payer of nursing home coverage in the United States.

To become eligible for nursing home care, an individual must meet certain financial criteria.[75] Note, however, that each state may have different financial criteria as long as they meet baseline federal requirements.[76] Of general importance is that states also may provide eligibility for Medicaid to otherwise ineligible individuals who are institutionalized in nursing or other facilities or to persons who are receiving alternative services in their homes or in their communities.[77] In these situations, states may establish an income standard known as the *300% rule*:[78] Under the 300% rule, these individuals are eligible for Medicaid as long as their income does not exceed 300% of the SSI cash welfare payment, which is set by Department of Health and Human Services annually.[79]

If one spouse in a couple requires nursing home care and the other desires the state Medicaid program to pay for it, the spouse who lives at home (i.e., the "community spouse") may continue to maintain a certain level of financial resources on which to live[80] but not above a state-set ceiling amount. This amount is deemed the *community spouse income allowance*.[81] This spousal impoverishment protection prohibits use of the community spouse's income when determining the nursing home spouse's eligibility for the program unless the income actually is made available to the institutionalized spouse.[82] Resources in addition to this base amount are allowed if dependents will live with the community spouse, actual shelter costs are high, and in other circumstances.[83] Further, the community spouse also may keep some other assets such as a personal residence, automobile, personal effects, burial expenses, and other assets as deemed by the state; this is known as the *community spouse resource allowance*.[84] Note that states are required

to recover amounts paid on behalf of the institutionalized recipient from his or her estate after the death of both the institutionalized resident and the community spouse;[85] states are required to recover amounts paid by Medicaid for nursing facility services, home- and community-based care, and related hospital and prescription drug services from an individual beneficiary's estate if the beneficiary was at least 55 years of age.[86] States may broaden the number of services for which such a recovery is to be obtained.[87]

These resource allowances also are amenable to transfer by the institutionalized spouse to reduce the institutionalized spouse's assets for Medicaid purposes. From the combined set of available resources, the community spouse may generally keep up to one-half of the couple's resources based on state ceilings; this amount must be no greater than a maximum level and above a minimum level set by the federal government, which issues these figures annually.[88] If the one-half amount is less than the state-set standard, the institutionalized spouse may transfer to the community spouse his or her portion up to the state level. This makes spending down for the institutionalized spouse more accessible.

If there is no community spouse, the applicant for Medicaid nursing home coverage must "spend down" his or her assets to the levels at which he or she will qualify for the program.[89] Spending down assets requires that the applicant use up his or her assets in arm's length transactions (that is, genuine commercial transactions) and have a limited income under rules of the program.[90] Note that, in addition to traditional assets, annuities that still are accumulating income[91] and retirement plans that allow the retiree to retrieve lump-sum benefits are considered resources that must be spent down for Medicaid eligibility.[92] The applicant generally is allowed to keep between $30 and $100 per month for personal expenses, since Medicaid reimbursements will cover virtually all daily living expenses when the individual lives in the nursing facility.[93]

For the purposes of applying for Medicaid to fund nursing home coverage, the applicant will be asked by

[74]42 C.F.R. §447.253 (1998).

[75]42 U.S.C.A. §1396p.

[76]42 U.S.C.A. §1396p.

[77]Staff of House Committee on Ways and Means, 104th Cong., 2d Sess., Overview of Entitlement Programs: 1996 Green Book 884, 909 (Committee Print 1996).

[78]42 C.F.R. §435.1005 (1998).

[79]Staff of House Committee on Ways and Means, 104th Cong., 2d Sess., Overview of Entitlement Programs: 1996 Green Book 884 (Committee Print 1996).

[80]42 U.S.C.A. §1382b.

[81]42 U.S.C.A. §1396r-5(d)(3).

[82]42 U.S.C.A. §1382b.

[83]42 U.S.C.A. §1396r-5(d)(3).

[84]42 U.S.C.A. §§1396r-5(f)(2), 1396r-5(g).

[85]42 U.S.C.A. §1382b(a).

[86]42 U.S.C.A. §1396p(b)(1).

[87]42 U.S.C.A. §1396p(b)(4).

[88]Staff of House Committee on Ways and Means, 104th Cong., 2d Sess., Overview of Entitlement Programs: 1996 Green Book 884 (Committee Print 1996).

[89]Staff of House Committee on Ways and Means, 104th Cong., 2d Sess., Overview of Entitlement Programs: 1996 Green Book 906 (Committee Print 1996).

[90]42 C.F.R. §435.1005 (1998).

[91]42 U.S.C.A. §1396p.

[92]42 U.S.C.A. §1396p(e).

[93]45 C.F.R. §436.831 (1998).

the caseworker to provide 36 months' worth of detailed financial records of outright asset transfers[94] and five years' worth of information for transfers into trusts.[95] Analysis generally will extend to any substantial transfer by the applicant over $1000, usually determined through assessment of bank account records; however, other records such as bonds, stocks, real estate, mortgages, notes, life insurance policies, and business interests also are requested and used in assessing asset transfers. If the caseworker identifies a transfer without full consideration (i.e., for less than fair market value) within the 36-month "look-back" period, a "penalty period" is calculated, determined by taking the value of any such transaction (which is considered a gift) and dividing it by the average monthly nursing home cost in the area. This results in a number that represents the number of months of ineligibility (the penalty period) that will delay Medicaid coverage.[96]

Other exemptions from asset calculations for Medicaid applications by those wishing nursing home coverage are determined by the federal and state regulations. For example, a home can be transferred to a minor or a disabled adult child,[97] to a child who has resided in the home and cared for the applicant for two or more years or a brother or sister of the applicant with an equity interest in the house who has resided there for more than one year,[98] or to a trust established solely for the benefit of disabled persons under age 65.[99] Further, a taxpayer now may include long-term care expenses as qualified medical expenses that are deductible from federal income taxes if they exceed 7.5% of the taxpayer's adjusted gross income.[100] In addition, payments made under long-term care insurance are excluded from federal taxation;[101] employers are able to claim the cost of premiums paid for employees for long-term care as a business expense;[102] and individuals may deduct premiums paid for long-term care insurance as a medical expense.[103]

Concomitant with these benefits, federal law has established specific requirements for the long-term care industry. Long-term care policies must be guaranteed renewable and cannot be canceled on the basis of the beneficiary's age or health deterioration.[104] The policy may be canceled only on the basis of nonpayment of premiums, but in these cases, the policy may be reinstated up to five months later if nonpayment resulted from cognitive impairment.[105] Insurers must coordinate their benefits with Medicare to avoid coverage duplication;[106] insurers must follow prescribed administrative and marketing practices;[107] insurance carriers must provide the beneficiaries with a guide describing the policy benefits and limits and provide a comparison with the policies offered by other companies;[108] and insurance carriers must report the number of claims denied and provide information on policy replacement sales and policy terminations annually.[109]

If after all these asset assessment and allowable transfers, the applicant is deemed eligible for Medicaid support of nursing home expenses, he or she is limited to a double room.[110]

Further Reading

Appeals

Furrow BR et al. Medicaid Appeals and Judicial Review. In: *Health Law*. St. Paul, MN: West Publishing Co., 1995;§14–15.

Kinney ED. The Role of Judicial Review Regarding Medicare and Medicaid Program Policy: Past Experience and Future Expectations. *St Louis U L J* 1991;35:759–92.

Lever AB, Eastman HA. "Shake It Up in a Bag": Strategies for Representing Beneficiaries in Medicaid Litigation. *St Louis U L J* 1991;35:863–92.

See Also

Kinney ED. The Medicare Appeals System for Coverage and Payment Disputes: Achieving Fairness in a Time of Constraint. *Admin L J* 1987;1:1–106.

Covered Groups and Eligibility

Coughlin TA, Holahan JO et al. *Medicaid Since 1980: Costs, Coverage and the Shifting Alliance Between the Federal Government and the States*. Washington, DC: Urban Institute Press, 1994.

---

[94]42 U.S.C.A. §§1396p(c)(1)(A)–1396p(c)(1)(B)(ii).

[95]42 U.S.C.A. §1396p(c)(1)(B)(i).

[96]42 U.S.C.A. §§1396p(c)(1)(E), 1396p(c)(1)(D).

[97]42 U.S.C.A. §1396p(c)(2)(A).

[98]42 U.S.C.A. §1396p(c)(2)(A); see also N.Y. Comp. Codes R. & Regs, tit. 18, §360-4.4(c)(ii).

[99]42 U.S.C.A. §§1396p(c)(2)(A)(ii), 1396p(c)(2)(B)(IV).

[100]26 U.S.C.A. §§213(a), 213(d)(1)(C).

[101]26 U.S.C.A. §§7702B, 6050Q; Pub. L. No. 104-191, 110 Stat. 1936 (1996).

[102]26 U.S.C.A. §7702B(d)(4).

[103]26 U.S.C.A. §213(a).

[104]26 U.S.C.A. §§7702B(a)(5), 7702B(b)(C).

[105]Pub. L. No. 104-91, 110 Stat. 1936 (1996).

[106]42 U.S.C.A. §1395ss.

[107]Pub. L. No. 104-91, 110 Stat. 1936 (1996).

[108]Pub. L. No. 104-91, 110 Stat. 1936 (1996).

[109]42 U.S.C.A. §4980c.

[110]42 C.F.R. §483.70 (1998).

Furrow BR et al. Eligibility. In: *Health Law*. St. Paul, MN: West Publishing Co., 1995;§§14-2–14-4.

Henderson TM. *Outstanding Medicaid Eligibility Workers at Community and Migrant Health Centers*. Washington, DC: National Governors Association, 1992.

Kronebusch K. Medicaid and the Politics of Groups: Recipients, Providers, and Policy Making. *J Health Pol Pol'y & L* 1997;22:839–78.

Pellegrino C. Medicaid Eligibility. In: *Florida Jurisprudence*, 2d ed. New York: Lawyers Cooperative Publishing Co., 1996;§77.

Solomon LD, Asaro T. Community-Based Health Care: A Legal and Policy Analysis. *Fordham Urb L J* 1997;24:235–313.

Medicaid and Medicare

Coffin CL. Recent Decisions: The United States Court of Appeals for the 4th Circuit. *Md L Rev* 1998;57:1233–55.

Greenpield MA. *Medicare and Medicaid*. Westport, CT: Greenwood Publishing Group, 1983.

Lohr KN, Marquis MS. *Medicare and Medicaid: Past, Present and Future*. Santa Monica, CA: Rand Corporation, 1984.

Mehlman MJ, Visocan KA. Medicare and Medicaid: Are They Just Health Care Systems? *Hous L Rev* 1992;29:835–65.

Parnagian CP. New York City Health and Hospitals Corporation v. Perales: Unclear Congressional Intent, Permissible Agency Interpretation. *St John's L Rev* 1993;67:105–23.

Payment

Buck JA, Kamlet MS. Problems with Expanding Medicaid for the Uninsured. *J Health Pol Pol'y & L* 1993;18:1–24.

Coleman TS, Champbers SK. *Legal Aspects of Medicare and Medicaid Reimbursement: Payment for Hospital and Physician Services*. Kansas City, MO: National Health Lawyers Association, 1990.

Furrow BR et al. Medicaid Payment for Services. In: *Health Law*. St. Paul, MN: West Publishing Co., 1995;§§14-8–14-10.

Krauskopf JM et al. Payment for Services — in General. In: *Elder Law Advocacy for the Aging,* 2d ed. St. Paul, MN: West Publishing Co., 1997;§11.94.

Perkine J. Increasing Provider Participation in the Medicaid Program: Is There a Doctor in the House? *Soc Sec Rep Ser* 1989;26:846–76.

Services

Furrow BR et al. Covered Services. In: *Health Law*. St. Paul, MN: West Publishing Co., 1995;§§14-5–14-6.

Rosenberg JM, Zaring DT. Managing Medicaid Waivers: Section 1115 and State Health Care Reform. *Harv J on Legis* 1995;32:545–56.

Spending Down for Nursing Home Care

Bove AA. *The Medicaid Planning Handbook: A Guide to Protecting Your Family's Assets from Catastrophic Nursing Home Costs*, 2d. ed. Boston: Little Brown and Co., 1996.

Budish AD. *Avoiding the Medicaid Trap: How Every American Can Beat the Catastrophic Costs of Nursing Home Care*, 3d. ed. New York: Avon Books, 1996.

Dunlop BD et al. Medicaid Estate Planning Implementation of OBRA '93 Provisions in Florida: A Policy Context. *Nova L Rev* 1995;19:533–86.

Krauskopf JM et al. Persons Who Qualify — State Options for Long-Term Care. In: *Elder Law Advocacy for the Aging*, 2d ed. St. Paul, MN: West Publishing Co., 1993;§11.15.

Spence DA, Wiener JM. Estimating the Extent of Medicaid Spend-Down in Nursing Homes. *J Health Pol Pol'y & L* 1990;15:607–25.

Waivers—Program Waivers

Anderson E. Administering Health Care: Lessons from the Health Care Financing Administration's Waiver Policy-Making. *J L & Pol* 1994;10:215–62.

Krieger M. *Characteristics of Medicaid Home- and Community-Based Waiver Program Applications*. Washington, DC: Urban Institute Press, 1982.

Lindsey PA, Jacobson PD et. al. *AIDS Specific Home- and Community-Based Waivers for the Medicaid Population*. Santa Monica, CA: Rand Corporation, 1989.

Randall V et al. Section 1115 Medicaid Waivers: Critiquing the State Applications. *Seton Hall L Rev* 1996;26:1069–1142.

Waivers—Research and Demonstration Waivers

Anderson E. Administering Health Care: Lessons from the Health Care Financing Administration's Waiver Policy-Making. *J L & Pol* 1994;10:215–62.

Bulter PA, Tobler L. *Medicaid Research and Demonstration Programs*. Denver: National Conference of State Legislators, 1995.

Other Reading

Barrett CL. *Estate Planning in Depth: 1997 Elder Law Issues*. Pub. No. SB90 ALI-ABA 1365. Chicago: American Law Institute–American Bar Association, 1997.

Clark LW. The Demise of the Boren Amendment: What Comes Next in the Struggle over Hospital Payment Standards Under the Medicaid Act? *Health Law Digest* 1998;26(1):11–18.

Gallant MH. Medicaid Payment. In: National Health Lawyers Association, *Health Law Practice Guide.* Deerfield, IL: West Group, 1997.

Inglehart JK. The American Health Care System: Medicaid. *New Eng J Med* 1993;328:896–900.

Koss GK et al. ORYX: The Next Evolution in Accreditation. *Hosp Phys* 1998;34(8):36–43, 58.

Liang BA. *Continuing Mandatory Medicaid HMO Enrollment Programs: A Description of State, HMO, and Delivery Site Characteristics.* Chicago: University of Chicago, 1989. Thesis.

NCSL Health Program Staff. *Medicaid Survival Kit.* Denver: National Conference of State Legislators, 1996.

Perkins J. Living in a Land of Confusion: Health Care Litigation and the Eleventh Amendment. *Clearinghouse Rev* 1988;22:1114–17.

Web Sites

Health Care and Medicaid: *http://www.welfareinfo.org/healthcare.htm*

Joint Commission on Accreditation of Healthcare Organizations: *http://www.jcaho.org*

The Kaiser Commission on Medicaid and the Uninsured: *http://www.kff.org/state_health/*

The Medicaid Clearinghouse: *http://www.familiesusa.org/medicaid/*

Medicaid Consumer Network: *http://pw1.netcom.com/~rcauchi/mdg/intro.html*

Medicaid eligibility: *http://www.medicaidservices.com/*

Medicaid information: *http://www.hcfa.gov/medicaid/medicaid.htm*

The Medicaid Managed Care Program: *http://www.chcs.org/CHCS/mmcp.htm*

Medicaid services: *http://www.fdhc.state.fl.us/medicaid/index.html*

Medicaid — State-by-state descriptions and plans: *http://pw1.netcom.com/~rcauchi/mdg/states.html*

Medicaid waivers: *http://www.hcfa.gov/ob7.htm*

Medicare and Medicaid statistics and data: *http://www.hcfa.gov/stats/stats.htm*

Mining Co. guide to Medicaid and Medicare: *http://healthcare.miningco.com/msub6.htm*

Murphy's unofficial Medicaid page: *http://www.geocities.com/CapitolHill/5974/*

SeniorLaw — Medicare and Medicaid recent developments: *http://www.seniorlaw.com/recent.htm*

9

Managed Care

Managed care is a phrase that has different meanings to different parties. Generally, managed care can be seen as a method by which health care is arranged for patients under rules minimizing overutilization through the use of specific providers chosen by the managed care entity. This definition encompasses a very broad spectrum of organizational forms. Some general characteristics of managed care organizations (MCOs), such as health maintenance organizations (HMOs), include:

1. Selective criteria for and contracting with providers.
2. Review of medical necessity and appropriateness by parties other than the direct provider.
3. Constant quality assurance, utilization review, and outcomes measure assessments.
4. Financial or program coverage incentives and penalties for patients who do not use MCO-selected providers.
5. Provider risk sharing and other incentive arrangements to minimize costs.
6. Systems limitations on access to expensive care.
7. Management focus on cost-efficient providers and care.

Although these are common characteristics, the myriad of health delivery forms under the rubric of managed care makes its definition difficult to narrow further. However, critical in the concept of all managed care forms is the attempt to limit expenditures by limiting costs and maximizing the use of cost-effective resources. This focus has been one of the underlying reasons why the managed care revolution has swept the United States, with private and public entities embracing this health delivery method.

Managed Care Delivery Forms

With the caveat that standard managed care delivery forms are general models and many MCOs have only some of

these characteristics, several basic MCO delivery forms are recognized when describing managed care. Traditionally, managed care forms have been divided between HMOs and preferred provider organizations (PPOs).

HMOs

HMOs are organized delivery systems responsible for arranging for and financing health care for their enrolled populations, in contrast to traditional indemnity insurance, which is simply responsible for financing care. HMOs generally finance health delivery through prepaid, fixed fees and assume the risk for the costs of health delivery services. HMOs often utilize a gatekeeper system, which requires that the patient see his or her physician or other primary care provider (PCP) for all nonemergency care; care from specialists is available and paid for only if a referral is obtained from the PCP. The standard models of HMOs are the staff model, the group model, the network model, the independent or individual practice association (IPA) model, and the direct contract model.

Staff Model HMOs

In staff model HMOs the entity arranging for and financing the health care services employ physicians to provide these services. The physicians generally are paid a salary, possibly with productivity and performance bonuses. Due to the nature of providing services through an employed set of physicians, the staff model HMO must contract for a broad array of general and specialist physicians to take care of its enrollees' needs. If other services are needed, they are provided through outside contract physicians. Generally, staff model physicians practice at a centralized site, which contains all office and supporting capital and services for complete diagnosis and treatment of enrollees. These HMOs either own their own hospitals or contract with community hospitals for inpatient services.

Group Model HMOs

Group model HMOs are structured to provide medical care services to enrollees through contracting with a large, multispecialty medical group practice. It should be emphasized that the group contracts with the HMO; thus, the physicians are not employees of the HMO but of the group itself. There are two types of group model HMOs: the captive group model and the independent group model.

The captive group model HMO, reassuringly, is captive to the HMO and exists to serve the HMO's enrollees exclusively. In the majority of cases, the group was formed by the HMO to provide services to its members only.

In the independent group model HMO, the HMO contracts with the group practice, but the group generally continues to see other, non-HMO patients. Often, the independent group model HMO will have begun as a group practice, with the group practice then forming the HMO.

Both types of group model HMOs are considered "closed panel HMOs" because physicians must be members of the particular group practice to render services to the HMO's enrollees.

Network Model HMOs

Network model HMOs are structured to provide medical services to enrollees through contract with more than one group practice. The group practices can be similar to, on the one hand, the multispecialty group practices of group model HMOs or, on the other hand, to smaller groups of primary care and specialty providers. When the network model HMO contracts with predominantly primary care providers, the model often is referred to as a *primary care network model HMO*. If referrals to specialists are needed in this model, generally an outside physician is paid to see the patient and the group from which the referral is requested or emanates is responsible for the costs associated with the referral. Network model HMOs can be "closed panel" (like the group model) or "open panel" (i.e., any physician who meets the HMO's and specific group practice's requirements may join and serve the HMO's enrollees).

IPA Model HMOs

IPA model HMOs are structured to provide medical services to enrollees through contract with an IPA. An IPA, which is a separate and distinct legal entity, is an association of independent providers who maintain individual practices in their separate offices. Generally, the IPA is formed to obtain managed care contracts. IPA physicians, beyond their specific managed care contract, continue to see non-HMO patients and operate independently from other physicians by maintaining their own support staff,

records, and office activities. IPA model HMOs generally are of the open model form, since any community physician can join if he or she meets the IPA and HMO criteria. In addition to an IPA that seeks managed care contracts and usually has contracts with several HMOs on a nonexclusive basis, an HMO can be the impetus of creating an IPA for its exclusive use. In this latter circumstance, the HMO seeks out community physician leaders and assists them to create an IPA, which then participates and accepts the HMO's contract to provide services to its enrollees.

Other variations of IPAs, and thus IPA model HMOs, exist, for example, hospital-based provider IPAs. In these IPA model HMOs, the hospital and its staff provide all medical services to an HMO's enrollees. HMOs can contract with several of these IPAs to limit the number of providers that will be terminated from the HMO if their contracts are not renewed as compared to communitywide IPAs.

Direct Contract HMOs

Direct contract HMOs are structured to provide medical services to enrollees through contracts with individual physicians. These HMOs attempt to contract with a broad array of community physicians to provide services. These models are advantageous to HMOs because of the ease through which providers may be terminated from the HMO without adversely affecting other providers.

PPOs

PPOs are agglomerations of medical providers who usually contract directly with employers with self-funded employee benefit plans or with health insurance carriers to provide services to their particular population. What differentiates PPOs generally from traditional HMOs is that PPOs usually do not assume risk, usually charging on the basis of discounted fee for service, like an indemnity plan. Further, PPOs allow patients to go outside the PPO for services, albeit for a higher cost-sharing amount than when using PPO providers. Generally, PPOs have a selective provider panel, negotiated payment rates, rapid payment terms, strong utilization management of providers, and expanded access to non-PPO providers with higher copayments or deductibles.

Note that there are occasional references to "silent PPOs." Silent PPOs are not some form of medical care delivery but a methodology through which a provider's discounted fee schedule is used (or abused) by others and usually is unintended by the provider. This use generally occurs in two ways. In the first, a bona fide entity has arranged for a service contract with a PPO with a set discounted fee schedule. The entity with the contract then expands the discounted fee schedule to be used by others, including patients within or patients outside the entity. Thus, the discounted fee schedule is now used by a greater number of patients than originally contemplated. The second general way that the discounted fee schedule is utilized by a number of patients outside the contemplation of the PPO is through a "PPO broker." The PPO broker somehow obtains various discounted fee schedules from PPOs, sometimes through a kickback arrangement with the party who supplies the information. The broker then sells this information and the fee schedules to interested groups such as other employers, who then use the fee schedules to pay participating providers. In this way, additional patients and entities can pay less for care than they might have if they were not sold the information.

The legal status of silent PPOs is in question. On the one hand, because PPOs generally do not have provisions to limit the dissemination and use of their payment terms and schedules, entities and brokers who use them argue that such use is permitted. Providers, on the other hand, argue that these discounted fee schedules and payment methodologies are limited to the parties and patients in existence at the time the contract is drafted and signed. For providers, the major difficulty is that, to try to stem the use of silent PPOs, every payment submitted must be examined to determine whether the party appropriately or inappropriately used a PPO discount.

Other Managed Care Forms

Several other managed care forms are becoming part of the health delivery landscape.

Exclusive Provider Organizations

The exclusive provider organization (EPO) is an entity quite similar to PPOs, except that EPOs do not allow for expanded access and require that their patients obtain services only from preferred providers. EPOs generally are sponsored by employers who are concerned about cost escalations in health care.

Point-of-Service HMOs

The point-of-service (POS) HMO is a very popular form of managed care, combining aspects of traditional HMOs and PPOs. The POS HMO, also known as an *open access HMO*, operates like standard HMOs except it allows enrollees to decide at the point they need care, or at the "point of service," whether they wish to obtain services from the provider in the HMO or an outside physician or provider. If the enrollee obtains services from the outside provider, generally that provider's fees are paid using a traditional indemnity method with the enrollee responsible for significant cost sharing as well as more stringent utilization review.

Specialty HMOs

Specialty HMOs also have become more common on the U.S. health delivery landscape. As the name implies, specialty HMOs generally focus on a particular area of health care, such as dental HMOs, or disease state, such as mental health or cancer. In addition, disease-specific management also has resulted in some HMOs focusing on particular disease states such as diabetes, asthma, and other chronic disease states.

Integrated Delivery Systems

Integrated delivery system (IDS) is an umbrella term that encompasses any organization that provides the full spectrum of health care needs to patients, including physician and hospital services. Note that IDSs focus on the medical services side of the health care delivery system; they require no financial component. Thus, IDSs are not necessarily MCOs. Of course, some IDSs also have the financial component and thus are MCOs. IDSs can be controlled by hospitals or physicians and often are formed by providers to obtain managed care contracts. The advantage they represent to the MCO is that contracting with an IDS represents "one-stop shopping" for the MCO: The complete spectrum of physician and hospital care is available from this single entity.

Management Services Organizations

A management services organization (MSO) usually is an organization that provides services to physicians and physician groups as well as, less frequently, hospitals. MSOs often are hospital based and use the expertise gained there in billing, utilization review, quality assurance, negotiating medical supply discounts, and other areas to assist physicians in streamlining their operations and providing for a full package of physician and hospital services for managed care contracts. MSOs are particularly useful for hospitals that do not have established relationships with large, multispecialty physician groups. The difficulty with MSOs is allegiance; if issues arise that put the interests of physicians and the hospital in conflict, there may be no way to resolve whose interests should be superior. MSOs usually negotiate a percentage of practice income or a flat payment amount as their management fee.

Physician Practice Management Entities

Physician practice management entities (PPMs; also known as *physician management companies*, PMCs) are generally physician-owned and -operated companies that assist physicians in obtaining managed care contracts and streamlining operations. Their modus operandi usually is to acquire the assets of group practices and provide management services through a long-term (e.g., 40 years) contractual arrangement. PPMs also provide capital for needed expansion and computer systems for utilization review, quality assurance, and other monitoring and billing purposes. Note that the group's physicians are not employees of the PPM; if this were the case, such an arrangement might run afoul of some states' prohibitions regarding the corporate practice of medicine. The PPM can and does employ nurses and other ancillary staff. PPMs often exchange cash and stock in the PPM for the assets of the practice to align incentives of the provider with the PPM's success, thus inducing or maintaining high productivity. Generally, PPMs negotiate a percentage of practice income as their management fee.

Provider-Sponsored Organizations

Provider-sponsored organizations (PSOs; also known as *provider-sponsored networks*, PSNs) are agglomerations of providers that provide and finance health care directly, in whole or in part, rather than contracting with an HMO or other MCO. Since the *PSN* label is an umbrella term, many organizational structures fall within its purview, including provider joint ventures, provider affiliations by contract, and other risk-sharing arrangements between hospitals and physicians, generally known as *physician–hospital organizations* (PHOs; also *physician–hospital arrangements*, PHAs), *management services organizations* (MSOs), *nonprofit medical foundations,* and *physician networks*. These entities, because of their diversity, may be subject to some or all state laws that dictate requirements for more traditional managed care entities such as HMOs and PPOs. State regulation also will dictate to what extent PSOs can assume risk like HMOs and insurance companies. PSOs are granted somewhat favorable treatment for Medicare risk contracts under the BBA (see below).

Payment Methodologies

Compensation by MCOs to providers usually involves some risk-based methodology; this is especially true for payment to physicians. Contrary to the traditional fee-for-service days, when no controls were placed on utilization, current methods focus on giving the provider incentives to minimize costs.

For primary care physicians (PCPs), there are two predominant modes of payment: capitation and discounted fee for service. The classic method of risk sharing is capitation, the prepayment for services for an MCO enrollee on a per-member, per-month (PMPM) basis. Hence, each month, the PCP receives a standard amount for each

patient for whom he or she is responsible regardless of the extent of services required. If the costs for services that are required for a PCP's patients are less than the sum of all capitation payments, the PCP makes a profit; if the costs for services that are required is more than the aggregate PMPM amount, then the PCP loses money for that month. Thus, capitation provides a strong incentive for the provider to limit the expenditures used to treat patients. Capitation payments may vary on the basis of the scope of services for which the provider is responsible; the age, gender, and health status of the patients; and other factors. Capitation also may extend only to a certain set of delineated services; MCOs may require full capitation where the provider is responsible for all costs for patient care (although for physician capitation, this generally does not include hospital services unless capitation is provided to an integrated delivery system), or some financial arrangement in between.

In addition, a variation on straight capitation is capitation with a withhold arrangement. A *withhold arrangement* is a risk-based system that provides additional incentives for providers to hold down costs. In a withhold arrangement, a certain percentage of the physician's capitation or discounted fee-for-service payment (e.g., 20–30%) is withheld from the physician's remuneration. If utilization goals are met for the MCO, then part or all of the withheld amount is paid to the physician at the end of the year; if not, the physician forfeits some or all of the withheld amount. These arrangements are defined by contract.

MCOs also may pay physicians bonuses if they meet the utilization goals of the MCO. However, this is less common because bonus arrangements are not as successful in holding down utilization and costs as withhold arrangements.

An alternative method of paying physicians and other providers is the "percentage of premium" arrangement. This is similar to capitation in that a fixed amount is paid the provider regardless of the amount and scope of services rendered. However, this method differs from strict capitation by shifting some of the risk of collection of the premium to the physician and other providers; if the premium is not collected, for example, the payment is not provided. In addition, percentage of premium payment methods are more difficult to assess in terms of adequacy for services; for example, percentage of premium payments may be for a family, yet the providers do not know how many individuals in the family are covered under this arrangement. Percentage of premium methods, as might be expected, are also subject to withhold and bonus arrangements.

Providers may limit their risk by using reinsurance or stop-loss ("threshold") insurance. Although the terms of these policies vary, in general they limit the holder's limit for liability up to a certain point or threshold, above which the provider is responsible for only a percentage of care costs. These policies may cover aggregate expenses, stop a provider's loss for an individual patient, or both. Thus, for example, a stop-loss policy could cover all referral expenses for a PCP above 200% of capitation for purposes of determining the withhold amount to be returned at the end of the year. Or, a PCP's stop-loss could cover 80% of all costs above $3000 per patient. Individual patient stop-loss is more common than aggregate expense stop-loss. Further, there are many variations of these policies; for example, the stop-loss amount for each patient may vary on the basis of the number of patients for whom the PCP is responsible and is paid through capitation or stepwise stop-loss coverage could allow for 80% coverage between $3000 and $5000 referral expenses, 90% coverage if this amount is between $5,001 and $10,000, and 100% coverage of referral expenses above $10,000. For providers, stop-loss insurance may be obtained from the plan or a reinsurance company.

The shared risk between MCOs and providers can be either with the individual provider alone, the entire network of providers, or some level in between. This arrangement varies with the needs and structures of the MCO and its providers. For example, an HMO may capitate an IPA; the IPA uses this capitation amount to pay PCPs within it on a discounted fee-for-service rate with withhold, bonus, productivity, or other incentive schemes. Or, an HMO may capitate a group practice, which in turn capitates its providers with incentive structures for productivity. Of course, the difficulties with all these systems are that they give the provider a very strong incentive to avoid sick patients; providers with small numbers of patients may undergo adverse selection where by chance they simply have the more expensive patients; they present the scenario where the most valuable patient from a financial perspective is the one who is never seen; and even with stop-loss insurance, one very sick patient may use up all the stop-loss and withhold amounts.

Fee-for-service payment is utilized as indicated previously by MCOs. PPOs almost exclusively use discounted fee-for-service payment methods. Fee for service also is utilized by MCOs attempting to sign up providers in a particular market with low managed care penetration because of its acceptability to physicians. As managed care has become the predominant form of health delivery, alterations to the fee-for-service method have been created that vary from the straight fee for service in the indemnity world. Fee-for-service payments may be performance based (with the provider, plan, or some combination being measured), depend on relative work (e.g., using the work values from the Medicare resource-based relative value scale), represent global fees (fees that cover all services for a particular episode of care, e.g., surgical fees that cover preoperative, intraoperative, and postoperative care), or use other methods. Often, specialists and other non-PCPs are paid using some form of discounted fee for service.

Regulatory Structure

MCOs are regulated primarily by the states. Federal law, of course, has an impact on how MCOs operate, but states have specific requirements to which these organizations must adhere to provide services within the state.

First, note that, in 1973, Congress passed the HMO Act,[1] which provided a set of guidelines and incentives for HMO creation. Within this act, HMOs could become "federally qualified" if they hewed closely to the requirements of the act. Federally qualified status was completely voluntary; although this status provided several advantages with respect to contracting with the federal government and exemption from some state laws, the benefits package and financial requirements for qualification required a "Cadillac" level care.[2] Thus, these HMOs' costs are higher, and flexibility is rather limited in the current health delivery markets.

State laws applicable to HMOs generally are less restrictive but broader in their coverage. Generally, MCOs are regulated by state departments of insurance, departments of corporations, departments of health, or departments of commerce. Regulation encompasses licensing, MCO organization, mandated health services, provider contracting rules, insolvency requirements (including deposit, capital, reserve, net worth, and surplus levels), subscriber contract requirements, enrollee participation in MCO policy-making requirements, acceptable payment methods, disclosure requirements, enrollment and termination mechanisms, continuation requirements, grievance procedures, quality assurance requirements, utilization review requirements, rate regulation, information filing requirements, scope of financial examinations and site visits by states, permissible marketing and solicitation of enrollees, allowable MCO powers and investments, reporting requirements, inspections, and penalties for MCO noncompliance.[3] Note also that states may pass laws that affect MCOs such as any willing provider laws, patient protection laws, laws regarding direct access to particular providers, mandated benefits laws, and others.

---

[1]42 U.S.C.A. §§300e *et seq.*

[2]See, e.g., 42 U.S.C.A. §§300e(b)(1), 300e-1; 42 C.F.R. part 417 (1998).

[3]See, e.g., National Association of Insurance Commissioners, *Health Maintenance Organization Model Act* (Kansas City, MO: NAIC, 1990); U.S. Department of Health and Human Services, Health Care Financing Administration, Office of Managed Care, *A Report to the Governor on State Regulation of Health Maintenance Organizations* (Washington, DC: Department of Health and Human Services, 1996); National Association of Insurance Commissioners, *Preferred Provider Arrangements Model Act* (Kansas City, MO: NAIC, 1987); National Association of Insurance Commissioners, *HMO Examination Handbook* (Kansas City, MO: NAIC, 1990).

Liability

MCOs may face legal liability by a variety of methods. These liability forms follow similar issues that face hospitals and other organizational health delivery structures.

Negligent Selection of Providers

MCOs contract with providers to render services to their enrollees. However, MCOs are responsible for selecting those providers with due care, so as not to subject their enrollees to substandard medical care. Therefore, the MCO has a duty to the patient to select qualified providers using an adequate assessment system;[4] such a responsibility is one similar to that imposed on hospitals.[5] This duty is separate from the independent duty of the provider to render nonnegligent care. Overall, under a negligence rule,[6] the MCO has a preexisting duty to obtain competent health care providers to their enrollees; the MCO may breach that duty if it does not adequately assess the physicians and other providers selected for its enrollees. If that breach causes injury or damage to the enrollee, the MCO may be liable for negligent selection of the provider.

Note that although the MCO has a duty to nonnegligently select its providers, this does not make the MCO a guarantor of the services provided by the physician or other providers. As long as the process by which the MCO selects its providers is reasonable, the MCO will not face liability for the actions of its contracting providers.

Utilization Review

The MCO also has the responsibility to nonnegligently and in good faith perform utilization review (UR) for approval and denial of care requests and payments. Often, an MCO will contract with a UR company to perform these services for the MCO. If the UR company is negligent in its review process or performs it in bad faith, the MCO can also be held liable if the enrollee reasonably believed the UR company was an agent of the MCO when it made its decision and the MCO acted to reasonably lead the patient to that belief, even if the UR company is a separate and distinct legal entity. This attribution of agency to extend liability, known as *ostensible agency*, also may be applied to hospitals for some of their physicians (e.g., emergency room physicians, hospital-based physicians).[7] Of course, MCOs may also be liable for negligent selection of the UR company.

Early cases of utilization review generally held that the physician has an independent duty to advocate and appeal utilization review decisions that adversely affect patients and that the utilization review entity was not liable for patient injury due to its denial of services.[8] This stance has been eroded somewhat by subsequent cases that have held that if the utilization review entity was engaged in conduct that can be considered a substantial factor in the patient's suffered injury or harm (e.g., cost-containment concerns leading to denial of care), the utilization review entity can be held liable with the physician.[9] Note that MCO physicians who act as reviewers with the authority to deny authorization for care may be liable to the patient; at least one court has ruled that there is a physician–patient relationship established that subjects the physician reviewer to a malpractice liability.[10]

UR companies may also be held liable for negligence and bad faith relating to their process of review. The UR company has a duty to the enrollee to use an appropriate, nonnegligent, and good faith method to review the care proposed; it may breach that duty by not adequately investigating all clinical factors to assess medical appropriateness (e.g., making a decision on an incomplete chart, taking inadequate time to review clinical data, taking no action to obtain relevant information, using inappropriate personnel to review the claim); if that breach causes injury or damage to the enrollee, the UR company may be liable for negligent review and bad faith denial.[11] Of course, MCOs that engage in such utilization review in-house also will be subject to such analyses.[12] In addition, UR activities will be subject to state law with regard to appeals, clinical criteria, retrospective and prospective denial, registration, certification, licensure, grievance requirements, and penalties for noncompliance (but see below).

Note that ERISA[13] may have an impact on the ability of ERISA plan enrollees and physicians to challenge UR

---

[4]See, e.g., Harrell v. Total Health Care, Inc., 781 S.W.2d 58 (Mo. 1989); Moshe v. Anchor Org. for Health Maintenance, 557 N.E.2d 451 (Ill. App. Ct. 1990); McClellan v. Health Maintenance Organization of Pa., 604 A.2d 1053 (Pa. Super. Ct. 1992).

[5]See, e.g., Darling v. Charleston Comm. Mem. Hosp., 211 N.E.2d 253 (Ill. 1965), *cert. denied* 383 U.S. 946 (1966); Elam v. College Park Hosp., 183 Cal.Rptr. 156 (Cal. Ct. App. 1982); Mitchell County. Hosp. Auth. v. Joiner, 189 S.E.2d 412 (Ga. 1972); Johnson v. Misericordia Comm. Hosp., 301 N.W.2d 156 (Wis. 1981); Thompson v. Nason Hosp., 591 A.2d 703 (Pa. 1991); Blanton v. Moses H. Cone Mem. Hosp., Inc., 354 S.E.2d 455 (N.C. 1987); Rule v. Lutheran Hosp. & Homes Soc'y of America, 835 F.2d 1250 (8th Cir. 1987).

[6]See Chapter 1.

---

[7]See Chapter 2.

[8]See, e.g., Wickline v. State of Cal., 239 Cal.Rptr. 810 (Cal. Ct. App. 1986), *review dismissed and case remanded* 741 P.2d 613 (Cal. 1987); see also Corcoran v. United Healthcare Inc., 965 F.2d 1321 (5th Cir. 1992); Steineke v. Share Health Plan, 518 N.W.2d 904 (Neb. 1994).

[9]See, e.g., Wilson v. Blue Cross of Southern Cal., 271 Cal.Rptr. 876 (Cal. Ct. App. 1990); see also Long v. Great West Life & Annuity Ins. Co., 957 P.2d 823 (Wyo. 1998).

[10]Hand v. Tavera, 864 S.W.2d 678 (Tex. App. 1993).

decisions. For example, in *Corcoran v United Healthcare Inc.*,[14] a woman whose pregnancy was at high risk requested extended inpatient hospitalization as per her physician's recommendation. The UR company during the precertification process denied her request and provided authorization for only ten hours of home nursing. Unfortunately, at a time when no nurse was on duty, the fetus went into distress and died. The woman brought suit against the UR company. The federal appellate court held that the woman's claims were preempted by ERISA. It held that although the UR entity gives medical advice, it does so in the context of determining benefits; since the plaintiff's claims were based on possibly inappropriate levels of care and prayed for state tort-based compensatory damages, they "relate[d] to" the benefit determination and fell squarely with ERISA. Therefore, her state-based tort claims were preempted and her cause of action dismissed, even though this result left the plaintiffs no remedies for their injury.

Similarly, in *Varol v. Blue Cross and Blue Shield of Michigan*,[15] psychiatrists brought a claim against a health plan and its preauthorization and concurrent review methodology, claiming that the process provided inappropriate authority to utilization reviewers to the point of being illegal as an unauthorized practice of medicine. However, the federal court rejected these claims as preempted by ERISA. Because the UR mechanism "relate[d] to" the employee benefit plan that contracted with the MCO and was integral to the plan's purpose of reducing overutilization, it was preempted by the statute. Even though this left the psychiatrists with no forum to which they could bring their case, the court then dismissed the psychiatrists' suit.

Respondeat Superior or Vicarious Liability

MCOs and other organizational entities such as hospitals may be liable under a respondeat superior (or vicarious liability) theory for the actions of their employee providers. Respondeat superior (Latin for "let the master answer") is the legal rule that makes the employer liable for actions of the employee if the employee's actions are performed within the scope of the employment.

Note, however, that although employers who hire independent contractors are not generally liable for the actions of the independent contractors, employers *may* be liable under a theory of ostensible agency (also known as *apparent agency*) if the organization reasonably causes the patient to believe that the physician or other provider is the organization's employee or agent and the patient reasonably understands this to be the case and relies on this representation.[16] Further, the independent contractor may be considered an employee if an assessment of a variety of factors indicates the contractor is more like an employee. The primary focus is on control: Can the entity significantly control the actions of the independent contractor? Since physicians usually in fact are independent contractors,[17] are considered independent by most parties, use their own implements for treatment, maintain discretion over performance of their duties, and have the ability to contract with a variety of employers, they usually are not considered employees by the courts. The major implications of this status are that physicians will usually retain all liability for patient injury and the organizational entity will not be implicated, even when the MCO dictates significant practice limitations to providers.[18] However, courts have sometimes imposed liability on both hospitals[19] and MCOs.[20] MCO liability is significantly affected and intertwined with ERISA, a topic considered next.

---

[11]See, e.g., Hughes v. Blue Cross of Northern Cal., 245 Cal.Rptr. 273 (Cal. Ct. App. 1988); see also Salley v. E.I. Du Pont de Nemours & Co., 966 F.2d 1011 (5th Cir. 1992) (ERISA employer acting as plan administrator is liable for terminating beneficiary hospitalization using inadequate review); Aetna Life Ins. Co. v. Lavoie, 470 So.2d 1060 (Ala. 1984), *vacated on grounds* 475 U.S. 813 (1986), *on remand* 505 So.2d 1050 (Ala. 1987) (insurer is liable for compensatory and punitive damages due to its claims denial based on inadequate record review, use of inappropriate procedures in assessing claim, and communication to beneficiary that claim was reviewed by a physician when it was not); Linthicum v. Nationwide Life Ins. Co., 723 P.2d 675 (Ariz. 1986) (insurer is liable for inadequate review when claim denied without physician review); Davis v. Blue Cross of Northern Cal., 600 P.2d 1060 (Cal. 1979) (insurer must inform enrollees of right to challenge claim denial as part of its review process); Sarchett v. Blue Shield of Cal., 729 P.2d 267 (Cal. 1987) (insurer has the duty to inform a beneficiary of rights after claim denial); Kent v. Central Benefits Mut. Ins. Co., 573 N.E.2d 144 (Ohio. Ct. App. 1989), *appeal dismissed* 539 N.E.2d 166 (Ohio 1989); but see Nazay v. Miller, 949 F.2d 1323 (3d Cir. 1991) (health plan penalty due to subscriber not following utilization review precertification upheld); McGee v. Equicor-Equitable HCA Corp., 953 F.2d 1192 (10th Cir. 1992) (insurance company is not liable for institutional care provided after physician withdrew initial approval for care even though patient improved clinically).

[12]See, e.g., Rederscheid v. Comprecare, Inc., 667 P.2d 766 (Colo. Ct. App. 1983); Williams v. Health America, 535 N.E.2d 717 (Ohio Ct. App. 1987); see also McEvoy v. Group Health Co-op., 570 N.W.2d 397 (Wis. 1997).

[13]See Chapter 6.

[14]965 F.2d 1321 (5th Cir. 1992).

[15]708 F.Supp. 826 (E.D. Mich. 1989).

[16]See, e.g., Jones v. Chicago HMO, 703 N.E.2d 502 (Ill. App. 1998).

[17]See, e.g., Jones v. Philpott, 702 F.Supp. 1210 (W.D. Pa. 1988); Chase v. Independent Practice Association, Inc., 583 N.E.2d 251 (Mass. App. Ct. 1991); Huber v. Protestant Deaconess Hosp. Ass'n of Evansville, 133 N.E.2d 864 (Ind. Ct. App. 1956); Biddle v. Sartori Mem. Hosp., 518 N.W.2d 795 (Iowa 1994); James v. Ingalls Mem. Hosp., 701 N.E.2d 207 (Ill. App. 1998).

ERISA and Managed Care

Although MCOs can be subject to fiduciary requirements under ERISA,[21] ERISA also may play a role in direct and indirect liability claims against MCOs. Generally, direct claims against MCOs for patient injury due to a denial of benefits have been held to be preempted if these MCOs

deliver care through an ERISA EBP. State law–based causes of action that have been preempted by federal appeals courts include cases that have pled breach of contract and wrongful death;[22] wrongful death, improper refusal to authorize benefits, medical malpractice against the plan, insurance bad faith, breach of contract, negligent retention of health services by the MCO, loss of consortium;[23] wrongful death due to negligent administration;[24] medical malpractice against the plan, emotional distress, tortious interference with ERISA beneficiary's right to contract for medical care, breach of contract;[25] and wrongful revocation of EBP health plan insurance, breach of contract, tort of outrage, fraudulent denial of insurance coverage, wrongful death.[26] Further, other claims have been held preempted by federal trial courts.[27] As a result of ERISA, parties who have suffered these harms have no forum in which to seek a remedy.

Although it would appear that the ERISA shield is strong, other courts have allowed for causes of action

[18]See, e.g., W. Page Keeton et al., *Prossor and Keeton on the Law of Torts*, 5th ed. (St. Paul, MN: West., 1984); Lee v. Regal Cruises, 916 F.Supp. 300 (S.D. N.Y. 1996) (ship doctor considered independent contractor and thus ship owner not liable for purported malpractice of physician); Johnson v. Commodore Cruise Lines, 897 F.Supp. 740 (S.D. N.Y. 1995) (ship owner not liable for malpractice of physician except directly due to negligent selection of physician); Freedman v. Kaiser Foundation Health Plan of Colorado, 849 P.2d 811 (Colo. Ct. App. 1992) (patients cannot hold HMO responsible for medical malpractice of its independent contractor physicians due to statutory bar of HMOs from practicing medicine); Chase v. Independent Practice Association, Inc., 583 N.E.2d 251 (Mass. App. Ct. 1991) (independent practice association that arranged with HMO to provide services to HMO members is not vicariously liable for actions of physicians in treating HMO patients); Raglin v. HMO Illinois, Inc., 595 N.E.2d 153 (Ill. App. Ct. 1992) (health insurer and its HMO are not liable vicariously for negligence of physicians under contract with them to provide medical services to members of health plan); Jones v. Philpott, 702 F.Supp. 1210 (W.D. Pa. 1988) (physician is not an actual or ostensible agent of hospital for purposes of malpractice claims); Williams v. Good Health Plus, Inc., 743 S.W.2d 373 (Tex. Ct. App. 1987) (HMO is not liable for alleged negligence of physicians because it was incapable by statute of practicing medicine and physicians delivering services were independent contractors); G.L. v. Kaiser Foundation Hosps., Inc., 757 P.2d 1347 (Or. 1988) (no managed care organization liability for independent contractors); Mitts v. H.I.P. of Greater N.Y., 478 N.Y.S.2d 910 (N.Y. App. Div. 1984) (HMO is not liable for independent contractor physician actions); Hale v. Sheikholeslam, 724 F.2d 1205 (5th Cir. 1984) (plaintiff instituting suit against independent contractor physician who allegedly committed malpractice at county hospital cannot hold hospital liable for physician actions).

[19]See, e.g., Smith v. Baptist Mem. Hosp. Sys., 720 S.W.2d 618 (Tex. App. 1986); Brownsville Med. Ctr. v. Gracia, 704 S.W.2d 68 (Tex. App. 1985); Torrence v. Kusminsky, 408 S.E.2d 684 (W.Va. 1991); Latham v. Ohio State Univ. Hosp., 594 N.E.2d 1077 (Ohio Ct. App. 1991); Casucci v. Kenmore Mercy Hosp., 534 N.Y.S.2d 606 (N.Y. App. Div. 1988); Sword v. NKC Hosps., Inc., 661 N.E.2d 10 (Ind. Ct. App. 1996); Mitchell v. Shepperd Mem. Hosp., 797 S.W.2d 144 (Tex. App. 1990); Stratso v. Song, 477 N.E.2d 1176 (Ohio Ct. App. 1984); Pamperin v. Trinity Mem. Hosp., 423 N.W.2d 848 (Wis. 1988); Kashishian v. Port, 481 N.W.2d 277 (Wis. 1992).

[20]See, e.g., Boyd v. Albert Einstein Med. Ctr., 547 A.2d 1229 (Pa. Super. Ct. 1988); Sloan v. Metropolitan Health Council, 516 N.E.2d 1104 (Ind. Ct. App. 1987); Schleier v. Kaiser Foundation Health Plan, Inc., 876 F.2d 174 (D.C. Cir. 1989).

[21]See Chapter 6.

[22]See, e.g., Turner v. Fallon Comm. Health Plan, Inc., 127 F.3d 196 (1st Cir. 1997); Pilot Life Ins. Co. v. Dedeaux, 481 U.S. 41 (1987).

[23]See, e.g., Tolton v. American Biodyne, 48 F.3d 937 (6th Cir. 1995).

[24]See, e.g., Spain v. Aetna Life Ins. Co., 11 F.3d 129 (9th Cir. 1993).

[25]See, e.g., Kuhl v. Lincoln Nat'l Health Plan of Kansas City, Inc., 999 F.2d 298 (8th Cir. 1993).

[26]See, e.g., Settles v. Golden Rule Ins. Co., 927 F.2d 505 (10th Cir. 1991).

[27]See, e.g., Andrews-Clarke v. Travelers Ins. Co., 984 F.Supp. 49 (D. Mass. 1997) (holding state law claims for denial of mental health benefits by ERISA provider and utilization review company are preempted by ERISA); Schmid v. Kaiser Foundation Health Plan of the Northwest, 963 F.Supp. 942 (D. Or. 1997) (state law claims for breach of contract and negligence directly against MCO are preempted by ERISA); Lancaster v. Kaiser Foundation Health Plan of Mid-Atlantic States, 958 F.Supp. 1137 (E.D. Va. 1997) (ERISA preempts direct negligence and fraud claims against HMO); Kearney v. U.S. Healthcare, 859 F.Supp. 182 (E.D. Pa. 1994) (direct liability claims against MCO for wrongful death, misrepresentation, and breach of contract are preempted by ERISA); Elsesser v. Hospital of the Philadelphia College of Osteopathic Medicine, Parkview Div., 802 F.Supp. 1286 (E.D. Pa. 1992) (claims seeking to hold HMO directly liable for refusing to pay for Halter monitoring equipment under EBP, misrepresentation, and breach of contract are preempted by ERISA); Kohn v. Delaware Valley HMO, Inc., 1991 WL 275609 (E.D. Pa. Dec. 20, 1991) (state law claims against HMO in ERISA plan resulting from failure to provide promised benefits and discouraging referrals are preempted by ERISA); Altieri v. CIGNA Dental Health, Inc., 753 F.Supp. 61 (D. Conn. 1990) (ERISA preempts claims that MCO was negligent in determining provider's competence and claims that MCO misrepresented quality of benefits offered); see also In re Estate of Frappier, 678 So.2d 884 (Fla. Dist. Ct. App. 1996) (direct corporate liability and implied contract claims are preempted by ERISA).

against ERISA MCOs based on quality claims rather than a denial of benefits assessment. In *Dukes v U.S. Healthcare, Inc.*,[28] the plaintiff-patients brought suit against the ERISA MCO, claiming direct and indirect negligence on the part of the plan in providing for health care services that harmed them. The federal appeals court held that because the plaintiffs were merely attacking the quality of the benefits they received rather than challenging a denial of care (i.e., the quantity), the plaintiffs' claims could be heard in state court. However, the state court would have to assess whether the negligence claims "relate[d] to" the EBP. This holding has been the anchor on which many other courts have allowed claims against ERISA MCOs to go forward.

Beyond direct claims against ERISA MCOs, indirect or vicarious liability or ostensible agency claims against ERISA MCOs also are affected by ERISA. These claims are based on an actual or reasonably expected "control" by the MCO of the actions of the physician, whether a reasonable person would expect that the entity is responsible for the care, and whether the entity leads the patient to reasonably believe this, respectively. There appears to be a split in authority as to whether ERISA preempts indirect claims against MCOs for the actions of their independent contractor physicians. Some courts have concluded that there is no preemption and plaintiffs may pursue their claims against the MCO for actions of their contractor physicians;[29] others have concluded that ERISA preempts these indirect claims.[30]

Note, however, that although in many circumstances ERISA preempts claims against MCOs, it does not preempt claims against physicians and other providers who contract with these MCOs to provide care to their enrollees.[31] Because physicians generally contract with entities to provide services as independent contractors,[32]

[28]57 F.3d 350 (3d Cir. 1995).

[29]See, e.g., Pacificare of Oklahoma v. Burrage, 59 F.3d 151 (10th Cir. 1995); Newton v. Tavani, 962 F.Supp. 45 (D. N.J. 1997); Dykema v. King, 959 F.Supp. 736 (D. S.C. 1997); Prihoda v. Shpritz, 914 F.Supp. 113 (D. Md. 1996); Santitoro v. Evans, 935 F.Supp. 733 (E.D. N.C. 1996); Jackson v. Roseman, 878 F.Supp. 820 (D. Md. 1995); Kusznir v. Lutheran Gen. Hosp., 1995 WL 404860 (N.D. Ill. May 31, 1995), *motion for reconsideration denied* 1995 WL 408208 (N.D. Ill. July 7, 1995); Gibson v. Webb, 1995 WL 716640 (N.D. Ill. Nov. 30, 1995); Haas v. Group Health Plan, Inc., 875 F.Supp. 544 (S.D. Ill. 1994); Dearmas v. Av-Med., Inc., 865 F.Supp. 816 (S.D. Fla. 1994); Kearney v. U.S. Healthcare, Inc., 859 F.Supp. 182 (E.D. Pa. 1994); Burke v. Smithkline Bio-Science Labs., 858 F.Supp. 1181 (M.D. Fla. 1994); Paterno v. Albuerne, 855 F.Supp. 1263 (S.D. Fla. 1994); see also "Nascimento v. Harvard Community Health Plan," *Mass. Lawyers Weekly* (February 2, 1998), p. 2; Tufino v. New York Hotel and Motel Trades Council, 646 N.Y.S.2d 799 (N.Y. App. Div. 1996); In re Estate of Frappier, 678 So.2d 884 (Fla. Dist. Ct. App. 1996); Andujar v. Lenox Hill Hosp., 641 N.Y.S.2d 532 (N.Y. App. Div. 1996).

[30]See, e.g., Jass v. Prudential Health Care Plan, 88 F.3d 1482 (7th Cir. 1996); Clark v. Humana Kansas City, Inc., 975 F.Supp. 1283 (D. Kan. 1997); Bailey-Gates v. Aetna Life Ins. Co., 890 F.Supp. 73 (D. Conn. 1994); Pomeroy v. Johns Hopkins Medical Servs., Inc., 868 F.Supp. 110 (D. Md. 1994); Butler v. Wu, 853 F.Supp. 125 (D. N.J. 1994); Nealy v. U.S. Healthcare HMO, 844 F.Supp. 966 (S.D. N.Y. 1994); Ricci v. Gooberman, 840 F.Supp. 316 (D. N.J. 1993); Diaz v. Texas Health Enterprises, 822 F.Supp. 1258 (W.D. Tex. 1993); Craft v. Northbrook Life Ins. Co., 813 F.Supp. 464 (S.D. Miss. 1993); Altieri v. CIGNA Dental Health, Inc., 753 F.Supp. 61 (D. Conn. 1990).

[31]See, e.g., Lancaster v. Kaiser Foundation Health Plan, 958 F.Supp. 1137 (E.D. Va. 1997); Painters of Philadelphia Dist. Council No. 21 Welfare Fund v. Price Waterhouse, 879 F.2d 1146 (3d Cir. 1989); Vickers v. Nash Gen. Hosp. Inc., 78 F.3d 139 (4th Cir. 1996); Edelen v. Osterman, 943 F.Supp. 75 (D. D.C. 1996).

[32]See, e.g., Lee v. Regal Cruises, 916 F.Supp. 300 (S.D. N.Y. 1996) (ship doctor is considered independent contractor and so ship owner not liable for purported malpractice of physician); Johnson v. Commodore Cruise Lines, 897 F.Supp. 740 (S.D. N.Y. 1995) (ship owner is not liable for malpractice of physician except directly due to negligent selection of physician); Freedman v. Kaiser Foundation Health Plan of Colorado, 849 P.2d 811 (Colo. Ct. App. 1992) (patients cannot hold HMO responsible for medical malpractice of its independent contractor physicians due to statutory bar of HMOs from practicing medicine); Chase v. Independent Practice Association, Inc., 583 N.E.2d 251 (Mass. App. Ct. 1991) (independent practice association that arranged with HMO to provide services to HMO members is not vicariously liable for actions of physicians in treating HMO patients); Raglin v. HMO Illinois, Inc., 595 N.E.2d 153 (Ill. App. Ct. 1992) (health insurer and its HMO are not liable vicariously for negligence of physicians under contract with them to provide medical services to members of health plan); Jones v. Philpott, 702 F.Supp. 1210 (W.D. Pa. 1988) (physician is not an actual or ostensible agent of hospital for purposes of malpractice claims); Williams v. Good Health Plus, Inc., 743 S.W.2d 373 (Tex. Ct. App. 1987) (HMO is not liable for alleged negligence of physicians because it was incapable by statute of practicing medicine and physicians delivering services were independent contractors); Hale v. Sheikholeslam, 724 F.2d 1205 (5th Cir. 1984) (plaintiff instituting suit against independent contractor physician who allegedly committed malpractice at county hospital cannot hold hospital liable for physician actions); Propst v. Health Maintenance Plan, Inc., 582 N.E.2d 1142 (Ohio Ct. App.), *juris motion overruled* 562 N.E.2d 898 (Ohio 1990) (HMOs cannot be liable for physicians' alleged medical malpractice); Pickett v. CIGNA Health Plan of Texas, Inc., 1993 WL 209858 (Tex. App. 1993) (medical malpractice vicarious liability action against HMO dismissed because HMO cannot practice medicine under corporate practice of medicine doctrine); but see Boyd v. Albert Einstein Med. Ctr., 547 A.2d 1229 (Pa. Super. Ct. 1988) (remanding indirect liability claim against MCO due to statements in advertisements and brochures that HMO itself provides medical care and guarantees and assumes responsibility for the quality of care provided enrollees).

the MCOs will shoulder no liability for patient injury because standard tort law holds that, as independent contractors rather than employees (the latter generally are considered under the "control" of the MCO and so liability would reach the MCO), these physicians are solely responsible for their own actions and any resultant patient injury.[33] This result generally is true regardless of whether the MCO payment, utilization review, authorization requirements, and practice parameters are set up by the MCO.[34] However, one federal appellate court held that financial incentive disclosure is an ERISA fiduciary duty and remanded a case against an MCO for adjudication on this claim; but the court rejected plaintiff's state law claims for misrepresentation and fraudulent nondisclosure as preempted by ERISA.[35]

Medicaid and Managed Care

Due to the tremendous costs associated with medical care, virtually all states have turned to managed care in an effort to stem the rise in expenditures for their Medicaid populations and coordinate care for these beneficiaries. Although there have been some voluntary and mandatory state Medicaid MCO programs in the past through program and research and demonstration waivers, the Balanced Budget Act of 1997 (BBA)[36] dramatically changed the landscape of MCO use and made enrolling Medicaid beneficiaries into MCOs much easier for states. Under the BBA, states may mandate that their Medicaid beneficiaries enroll in an MCO without first obtaining waiver authority to do so if the state permits a choice between at least two such entities. Note, however, that the BBA also indicates that children with certain special needs, some Native Americans, dually eligible Medicare and Medicaid beneficiaries, and qualified Medicare beneficiaries are excluded from this provision.[37] The law requires that MCOs provide important information to Medicaid enrollees, including a list of items and services available to the beneficiary under the state–MCO contract. Each year, the state must provide Medicaid enrollees with a comparative list of the managed care entities, outlining the benefits, cost-sharing requirements, and quality performance reports of the MCOs.

Consistent with this liberalization, states with research and demonstration waivers are provided automatic renewals and extensions if the Secretary of the Department of Health and Human Services does not respond to the state's written request within six months.[38] Further, the BBA repeals the former requirement that MCOs with Medicaid risk contracts enroll at least 25% non-Medicaid–eligible subscribers (originally known as the *75–25 rule*); the BBA also allows states to guarantee contracting MCOs that enrolled Medicaid beneficiaries will be eligible for Medicaid for up to six months.[39] Because of this expansion in use of managed care, the BBA has added several requirements on MCOs enrolling Medicaid beneficiaries, including mandates for coverage of emergency services, prohibition on limitation of patient–provider communications (i.e., gag clauses), mandates for grievance procedures, prohibition of liability against enrollees for payment, mandates for quality assurance standards, provision of certain plan solvency standards, and mandates for protections against fraud and abuse.[40]

In addition, beyond the BBA, federal regulations also mandate other aspects of Medicaid managed care, including beneficiary access,[41] availability of specialists,[42] records

[33] Keeton et al., *Prossor and Keeton on the Law of Torts*, 5th ed. (St. Paul, MN: West, 1984), pp. 499–508; but see Mitts v. H.I.P. of Greater N.Y., 478 N.Y.S.2d 910 (N.Y. App. Div. 1984) (staff model HMO physician employee is solely liable for patient injury since HMO does not treat patients); Williams v. Good Health Plus, 743 S.W.2d 373 (Tex. App. 1987) (HMO is not liable for potential negligence of its employed physicians because HMO cannot practice medicine as a corporation); see also Sloan v. Metropolitan Health Council, 516 N.E.2d 1104 (Ind. Ct. App. 1987) (independent contractor is deemed an employee due to extensive control over physician actions); Dunn v. Praiss, 606 A.2d 862 (N.J. Super. Ct. App. Div. 1992) (HMO is liable for actions of independent contractor physician due to extensive HMO control of scheduling, policy, number of patients, medical records, practice parameters, billings); Schleier v. Kaiser Foundation Health Plan, 876 F.2d 174 (D.C. Cir. 1989) (outside consultant is deemed employee of HMO and HMO is vicariously liable for consultant actions due to consultant being answerable to HMO primary care physician); Decker v. Saini, 1991 WL 277590 (Mich. Cir. Ct. Sept. 17, 1991) (IPA model HMO is liable for negligence of independent contractor physician and outside consultant on ostensible agency theory for public policy reasons).

[34] See, e.g., Lancaster v. Kaiser Foundation Health Plan, 958 F.Supp. 1137 (E.D. Va. 1997); Pell v. Shmokler, 1997 WL 83743 (E.D. Pa. Feb. 20, 1997); Kearney v. U.S. Healthcare, Inc., 859 F.Supp. 182 (E.D. Pa. 1994); Kohn v. Delaware Valley HMO, Inc., 1991 WL 275609 (E.D. Pa. Dec. 20, 1991); see also Albain v. Flower Hosp., 553 N.E.2d 1038 (Ohio 1990) (even when hospital conducts quality assurance and peer review of physicians, this does not establish level of control that would allow vicarious liability to attach).

[35] Shea v. Esensten, 107 F.3d 625 (8th Cir. 1997); but see Ehlmann v. Kaiser Found. Health Plan, 20 F.Supp.2d 1008 (N.D. Tex. 1998) (MCO has no duty to disclose physician compensation terms under ERISA).

[36] Pub. L. No. 105-33, 111 Stat. 251 (1997).

[37] 42 U.S.C.A. §1396u-2(a)(2).

[38] 42 U.S.C.A. §1315(e)(3).

[39] 42 U.S.C.A. §1396r-6.

[40] 111 Stat. 251 §4704 (1997).

[41] 42 C.F.R. §434.20(c)(2) (1998).

[42] 42 C.F.R. §434.20(c)(2) (1998).

systems,[43] internal quality assurance systems and patient satisfaction surveys,[44] medical records audits by the states,[45] grievance procedures approved by the state,[46] and monitoring of enrollment and disenrollment practices.[47] Penalties against MCOs of up to $25,000 per violation also may be assessed, and exclusion from the program may occur if MCO activities result in: a failure to provide necessary care; imposition of excessive premiums; discrimination against possible enrollees with potentially high utilization requirements; failure to pay claims promptly; falsification of information submitted to HCFA, an individual, or other entity; and failure to comply with physician-incentive payment requirements.[48] However, these extensive requirements and generally low payment rates may be limiting managed care participation in Medicaid,[49] similar to the recent Medicare program experience.[50]

The physician-incentive payment requirements are applicable to both Medicaid and Medicare managed care arrangements. Physician incentives that act as an inducement to withhold or limit medically necessary services are prohibited; if the plan places the physician at "substantial financial risk" for services other than his or her own, stop-loss insurance must be obtained by the provider.[51] HCFA indicates that providers are under no substantial financial risk unless the providers' patient panel is at least 25,000 Medicaid or Medicare patients alone or with Medicaid or Medicare patients pooled with commercial enrollees when the pooled patients' services are under a similar risk arrangement.[52] Stop-loss insurance may be obtained from the MCO, an intermediate entity, or a physician group.[53] MCOs must disclose physician-incentive plans to the HCFA and state Medicaid agencies if they currently provide services or are at the end of the application process to provide services but they currently do not have contracts.[54] These disclosures must occur annually. In addition, MCOs must also make general disclosures regarding the physician-incentive plans to Medicaid and Medicare beneficiaries on request if the MCO uses such plans itself or if its subcon-

tracting contractor intermediaries also use such plans, regardless of whether the beneficiary actually is enrolled in the plan or not. However, provider-specific incentive plan disclosure is not required.

Medicare and Managed Care

As indicated already, Medicare has mandates and limitations on physician-incentive plans. However, like the Medicaid program, the Medicare program has undergone significant increases in costs and looked toward managed care to limit the rise of such costs. Although Medicare managed care enrollment as a percentage of all enrollment remains relatively small (e.g., approximately 15%[55]), significant increases are predicted due to changes in the opportunities for managed care.

The primary impetus for managed care in Medicare, like Medicaid, is the BBA. The BBA created a new Part C of Medicare, also known as *Medicare+Choice*.[56] Under this new law, previous rules regarding Medicare managed care were replaced with a new program that allows Medicare beneficiaries the choice of using Medicare in the traditional fee-for-service system or enrolling in a variety of other systems. If the beneficiary does not choose to stay in the traditional fee-for-service Medicare, the options under Medicare+Choice include:

1. A coordinated benefits managed care organization such as an HMO, PPO, or newly established PSO.
2. A high-deductible Medical Savings Account (MSA) plan,[57] which will sunset in 2002.
3. A Medicare+Choice private fee-for-service plan.

Coordinated benefits MCO plans will be paid using a PMPM methodology, taking into account national and local costs. To reduce the differences in patient mix between those in fee for service versus managed care, the BBA adjusts payments to providers by factoring into payment the provider's patient case mix (e.g., age, gender, health status).[58] In addition, Medicare beneficiaries will be restricted as to when they can opt out of a coordinated benefits MCO, with a six- to three-month disenrollment period being phased in.[59] Each Medicare+Choice plan is required to remit an annual fee to the Secretary of Health and Human Services for enrollment purposes and dis-

[43]42 C.F.R. §434.6(a)(7) (1998).

[44]42 C.F.R. §434.34 (1998).

[45]42 C.F.R. §434.53 (1998).

[46]42 C.F.R. §434.32 (1998).

[47]42 C.F.R. §434.63 (1998).

[48]See 42 C.F.R. §§417.500 (1998), 434.22 (1998), 434.42 (1998), 434.63 (1998), 434.67 (1998), 434.80 (1998); 42 C.F.R. §§1003.100–1003.106 (1998).

[49]See G. Aston, "Widespread HMO Defections Starting to Hit Medicaid, Too," *American Medical News* (December 14, 1998), pp. 5–6.

[50]See the next section, "Medicare and Managed Care."

[51]61 Fed. Reg. 69,034 (Dec. 31, 1996).

[52]42 C.F.R. §417.479(h)(1)(v) (1998).

[53]42 C.F.R. §417.479(g)(2)(ii) (1998).

[54]42 C.F.R. §§417.479(h)(2) (1998), 434.70(a)(3) (1998).

[55]K. Terry, "Managed Care 1998: Medicare Takes the Spotlight," *Medical Economics* 23 (March 1998), p. 60.

[56]See 42 U.S.C.A. §1395w-21; see also 64 Fed. Reg. 7968 (February 17, 1999).

[57]See 42 U.S.C.A. §1395w-28(3)(A).

[58]See 42 U.S.C.A. §§1395w-23(a)(1)(A), 1395w-23(a)(3), as added by 111 Stat. 251, 299 §4001 (1997).

[59]See 42 U.S.C.A. §1395w-21(e)(2), as added by 111 Stat. 251, 276 §4001 (1997).

semination of comparative plan information to Medicare beneficiaries.

Also notable about Medicare+Choice is the new use of PSOs. PSOs, under the Medicare+Choice program, are important because the BBA allows for PSOs to directly contract with the Medicare program without state licensure. The BBA indicates that providers such as physicians and hospitals may form a PSO[60] as a separate corporate entity and may operate for three years as a risk-based MCO without fulfilling state insurance regulations regarding solvency or other requirements if (1) they fulfill federal requirements and (2) the PSO has filed an application for licensure with the state in which it proposes to operate and the state has not acted on the application within 90 days, or the PSO has not met the state's requirements while meeting the federal standards. The PSO must directly provide a substantial portion of health care services and have at least a majority financial interest in the entity.[61] On the basis of the interim final rules,[62] PSOs must have a minimum net worth of $1.5 million, of which $750,000 must be in cash or cash equivalents at startup. All of the PSOs' assets may be counted toward the $1.5 million minimum. Providers may affiliate to be able to provide the substantial portion of Medicare-required benefits; *substantial portion* is defined as no less than 70% of services for nonrural PSOs and no less than 60% for rural PSOs.[63]

The other health plan available under Medicare+Choice is the private fee-for-service plan.[64] No limits are placed on the amounts that the fee-for-service Medicare+Choice plan can charge, and balance billing is available on a limited basis.[65] However, because this plan is most likely to be expensive relative to the managed care option, there may be only a limited market for it. In addition, difficulties may arise with inadvertent acceptance of a private fee schedule by physicians who treat Medicare patients without having knowledge of beneficiary enrollment in a specific private fee-for-service plan.

Providers under Medicare+Choice are subject to penalties for violations of the BBA; the statute allows the Secretary of Health and Human Services to impose large civil penalties on providers for violation of its provisions.[66] It remains to be seen how popular this new managed care mandate will be; preliminary results are not encouraging.[67]

---

[60]See 42 U.S.C.A. §1395w-25(d)(1).
[61]See 42 U.S.C.A. §1395w-25(d)(1)(B)–(C).
[62]See 63 Fed. Reg. 25,360 (1998).
[63]See 63 Fed. Reg. 18,124 (1998).
[64]See 42 U.S.C.A. §§1395w-21(a)(2)(C), 1395w-28(b)(2).
[65]See 42 U.S.C.A. §§1395w-22(k)(2)(A), 1395w-24(b)(2).
[66]See 42 U.S.C.A. §1395w-27(g).
[67]S. Teske, "Forty-Five HMOs Leave Program, 54 Reduce Service for 1999, HCFA Reports," *BNA Managed Care Report* 4 (1998), pp. 1219–20.

Other Federal Programs

Federal Employees Health Benefit Program

The Federal Employees Health Benefit Program (FEHBP) is the largest employer-sponsored health care plan, covering virtually all federal employees (other than the military) and their families.[68] The FEHBP is administered by the Office of Personnel Management (OPM), which enters into contracts with MCOs for provision of health care to its employees.[69] With regard to managed care, the FEHBP uses a formula to set payment levels, usually at approximately 60% of premiums. The amount is based on the average premium price of six plans that are considered typical of the overall system, including high options plans offered by Blue Cross/Blue Shield and Aetna, the two largest employee organization plans, and the two largest HMOs. OPM cannot pay more than 75% of any plan's premium, even if the premium is at or below the government's threshold for contribution.

Civilian Health and Medical Program of the Uniformed Services

The Civilian Health and Medical Program of the Uniformed Services (CHAMPUS) is the federal government health program for civilian members of the uniformed services under the authority of the Department of Defense (DOD). DOD has created a managed care program for its CHAMPUS members, known as the *TRICARE program*.[70] TRICARE works with MCOs in coordination with military medical treatment facilities (MMTF). Three types of TRICARE alternatives are available: an HMO-type program, TRICARE Prime; a civilian PPO program, TRICARE Extra; and an option to use nonnetwork providers with reimbursement for services under the standard CHAMPUS program, TRICARE Standard.

Accreditation

HMOs may be accredited by the JCAHO or the National Committee for Quality Assurance (NCQA). By far, the NCQA serves as the accreditor for most HMOs and other MCOs that choose to become accredited. NCQA accreditation requires that the MCO comply with federal and state laws and regulations; engage in appropriate quality management and improvement, utilization review, and credentialing; fulfill standards of member rights and

---

[68]5 U.S.C.A. §§8901 *et seq.*
[69]5 U.S.C.A. §8902.
[70]60 Fed. Reg. 52,078 (1995).

responsibilities; provide preventive health services; and adhere to specific medical records requirements. Although NCQA accreditation is voluntary, like JCAHO accreditation of hospitals, it may assist in licensing under state law, provide a quality measure for employers seeking health services for employees, and be evidence of meeting the standard of care in tort suits. NCQA may grant full accreditation, meaning the entity meets all of the NCQA's standards and is granted full accreditation status for three years; one-year accreditation, meaning the plan meets most of the NCQA standards and will be reviewed after one year for full accreditation; provisional accreditation, meaning the plan meets some of the NCQA standards but is required to show further progress before qualifying for higher accreditation status; and denial of accreditation, meaning the plan does not qualify for any level of accreditation. In addition, NCQA has developed the healthplan employer data and information set (HEDIS). HEDIS's purpose is to measure performance indicators and allow for comparison among managed care plans on the basis of data relating to the process and outcome of treatment derived from administrative data of the plan. HEDIS, in combination with accreditation status information, is used to generate quality compass reports from NCQA for a particular MCO, another mechanism that allows for cross-comparison of MCOs. Similarly, NCQA also allows for comparisons via its quality compass–HEDIS comparative results system. Finally, HCFA has mandated that Medicare managed care plans report quality performance data using HEDIS for assessment of Medicare MCO performance.

Further Reading

Accreditation

Dasco ST, Dasco CC. *Managed Care Answer Book,* 2d ed. Frederick, MD: Aspen Publishers, 1997;8-9–8-22.
O'Kane ME. External Accreditation of Managed Care Plans. In: Kongstvedt PR, *The Managed Health Care Handbook,* 3d ed. Gaithersburg, MD: Aspen Publishers, 1996;593–607.

ERISA and Managed Care

Ayling CJ. New Developments in ERISA Preemption and Judicial Oversight of Managed Care. *Creighton L Rev* 1998;31:403–34.
Dasco ST, Dasco CC. *Managed Care Answer Book,* 2d ed. Frederick, MD: Aspen Publishers, 1997;9-2–9-10, 5-41–5-47.
ERISA: The Law and the Code 1998. (Serial). Washington, DC: BNA Books, 1998.
Farrell MG. ERISA Preemption and Regulation of Managed Health Care: The Case for Managed Federalism. *Am J L & Med* 1997;23:251–89.

Grosso SM. Rethinking Malpractice Liability and ERISA Preemption in the Age of Managed Care. *Stan L & Pub Pol'y Rev* 1998;9:433–51.
Liang BA. Patient Injury Incentives in Law. *Yale L & Pol'y Rev* 1998;17:1–93.
Penhallegon JR. Emerging Physician and Organization Liabilities Under Managed Health Care. *Def Counsel J* 1997;64:347–56.
Richardson B. Health Care: ERISA Preemption and HMO Liability — A Fresh Look at Preemption in the Context of Subscriber Claims Against HMOs. *Okla L Rev* 1996;49:677–730.
Rooney CD. The States, Congress, or the Courts: Who Will Be the First to Reform ERISA Remedies? *Annals Health Law* 1998;7:73–106.
U.S. General Accounting Office. *Employer-Based Managed Care Plans: ERISA's Effect on Remedies for Benefit Denials and Medical Malpractice.* Pub. no. GAO/HEHS-98-154. Washington, DC: U.S. General Accounting Office, 1998.
Walsh AF. The Legal Attack on Cost Containment Mechanisms: The Expansion of Liability for Physicians and Managed Care Organizations. *J Mar L Rev* 1997;31:207–44.

HMOs

Brown VY, Hartung BR. Managed Care at the Crossroads: Can Managed Care Organizations Survive Government Regulation? *Annals Health Law* 1998;7:25–72.
Hillman AL. Health Maintenance Organizations, Financial Incentives, and Physicians' Judgments. *Ann Int Med* 1990;112:891–93.
Jones RW. *HMO 101: Introduction to HMOs,* 2d ed. Colorado Springs, CO: T.T.M. Publishing, 1997.
Kongstvedt PR. *Essentials of Managed Health Care.* Gaithersburg, MD: Aspen Publishers, 1995.
Moore P. *Evaluating Health Maintenance Organizations.* Westport, CT: Quorum Books, 1991.
Platt BD, Stream LD. Dispelling the Negative Myths of Managed Care: An Analysis of Anti-Managed Care Legislation and the Quality of Care Provided by Health Maintenance Organizations. *Fla St U L Rev* 1995;23:489–511.
Weiner EP. Managed Health Care: HMO Corporate Liability, Independent Contractors, and the Ostensible Agency Doctrine. *J Corp L* 1990;15:535–71.

HMOs—Direct Contract

Dasco ST, Dasco CC. *Managed Care Answer Book,* 2d ed. Frederick, MD: Aspen Publishers, 1997;3-22–3-25.
Kongstvedt PR. Health Maintenance Organization Models. In: *Essentials of Managed Health Care.* Gaithersburg, MD: Aspen Publishers, 1995;33.

HMOs—Group Model HMOs

Freeborn DK, Pope CR. *Promise and Performance in Managed Care: The Prepaid Group Practice Model.* Baltimore: Johns Hopkins University Press, 1994.

Hitchner CH et al. Integrated Delivery Systems: A Survey of Organizational Models. *Wake Forest L Rev* 1994; 29:273–304.

Kongstvedt PR. Health Maintenance Organization Models. In: *Essentials of Managed Health Care.* Gaithersburg, MD: Aspen Publishers, 1995;30.

HMOs—IPA Model HMOs

Dasco ST, Dasco CC. *Managed Care Answer Book,* 2d ed. Frederick. MD: Aspen Publishers, 1997;4-6–4-94-14-4-18.

Kongstvedt PR. Health Maintenance Organization Models. In: *Essentials of Managed Health Care.* Gaithersburg, MD: Aspen Publishers, 1995;31–33.

McGuire D: Industry Transition From Group/Staff to IPA May Adversely Affect Quality. *Managed Care Outlook* 1997;May 16:1.

Todd MK: *IPA, PHO, MSO Development Strategies: Building Successful Provider Alliances.* Westchester, IL: HFMA, 1997.

HMOs—Network Model HMOs

Kongstvedt PR. Health Maintenance Organization Models. In: *Essentials of Managed Health Care.* Gaithersburg, MD: Aspen Publishers, 1995;31.

HMOs—Staff Model HMOs

Hitchner CH et al. Integrated Delivery Systems: A Survey of Organizational Models. *Wake Forest L Rev* 1994;29:273–304.

Kongstvedt PR. Health Maintenance Organization Models. In: *Essentials of Managed Health Care.* Gaithersburg, MD: Aspen Publishers, 1995;29–30.

Liability

Allred AD, Tottenham TO. Liability and Indemnity Issues for Integrated Delivery Systems. *St Louis U L J* 1996;40:457–542.

Bearden DJ, Maedgen BJ. Emerging Theories of Liability in the Managed Health Care Industry. *Baylor L Rev* 1995;47:285–356.

Brewbaker WS. Medical Malpractice and Managed Care Organizations: The Implied Warranty of Quality. *Law & Contemp Probs* 1997;60:117–57.

Grosso SM. Rethinking Malpractice Liability and ERISA Preemption in the Age of Managed Care. *Stan L & Pol'y Rev* 1998;9:433–51.

Leitner DL. *Managed Care Liability: Examining Risks and Responsibilities in a Changing Health Care System.* Chicago: American Bar Association, 1997.

Liang BA. Patient Injury Incentives in Law. *Yale L & Pol'y Rev* 1998;17:1–93.

Liability—Negligent Selection of Providers

Benesch K. Emerging Theories of Liability for Negligent Credentialing in HMOs, Integrated Delivery and Managed Care Systems. *Health Law* 1996;Fall:14–19.

Dasco ST, Dasco CC. *Managed Care Answer Book,* 2d ed. Frederick, MD: Aspen Publishers, 1997;5-48–5-49.

Dasco ST, Dasco CC. *Managed Care Answer Book, 1998 Supplement.* Frederick, MD: Aspen Publishers, 1998;5-17–5-19.

Dorros TA, Stone TH. Implications of Negligent Selection and Retention of Physicians in the Age of ERISA. *Am J L & Med* 1995;21:383–418.

Liability—Respondeat Superior or Vicarious Liability

Keeton WP et al. Respondeat Superior. In: *Prosser and Keeton on the Law of Torts,* 5th ed. St. Paul, MN: West Publishing Co., 1984;499–522.

Kionka EJ. *Torts: In a Nutshell,* 2d ed. St. Paul, MN: West Publishing Co., 1992;§§8-10–8-12.

Liability—Utilization Review

Dasco ST, Dasco CC. *Managed Care Answer Book,* 2d ed. Frederick, MD: Aspen Publishers, 1997;5–49, 7-17–7-21.

Dasco ST, Dasco CC. *Managed Care Answer Book, 1998 Supplement.* Frederick, MD: Aspen Publishers, 1998;5-17–5-19.

Furrow BR et al. Utilization Review Liability. In: *Health Law.* St. Paul, MN: West Publishing Co., 1995;§8-7.

Liang BA. Patient Injury Incentives in Law. *Yale L & Pol'y Rev* 1998;17:1–93.

Medicaid and Managed Care

Dasco ST, Dasco CC. *Managed Care Answer Book*, 2d ed. Frederick, MD: Aspen Publishers, 1997;6-1–6-29.

Dasco ST, Dasco CC. *Managed Care Answer Book, 1998 Supplement.* Frederick, MD: Aspen Publishers, 1998;6-2–6-10.

Furrow BR et al. Medicaid Managed Care. In: *Health Law.* St. Paul, MN: West Publishing Co., 1995;§14-11.

Kongstvedt PR. Medicaid and Managed Care. In: *Essentials of Managed Health Care*. Gaithersburg, MD: Aspen Publishers, 1995;234–42.

Oberg CN, Polich CL. *Medicaid — Entering the Third Decade: Enrollment in HMOs and Alternative Health Systems*. Bloomington, MN: Interstudy, 1986.

Medicare and Managed Care

Baker J. Medicare Nuts and Bolts. *PLI/EST* 1998;263:65–82.

Brooks TA. Provider Sponsored Organizations Under the Medicare+Choice Program. *Health Law Digest* 1998; 26(6):3–16.

Dasco ST, Dasco CC. *Managed Care Answer Book,* 2d ed. Frederick, MD: Aspen Publishers, 1997;6-29–6-47.

Dasco ST, Dasco CC. *Managed Care Answer Book, 1998 Supplement*. Frederick, MD: Aspen Publishers, 1998;5-47–5-49.

Kongstvedt PR. Medicare and Managed Care. In: *Essentials of Managed Health Care*. Gaithersburg, MD: Aspen Publishers, 1995;209–33.

Kronick R, De Beyer J. *Medicare HMOs: Making Them Work for the Chronically Ill*. Chicago: Health Administration Press, 1998.

Visocan K. Recent Changes in Medicare Managed Care: A Step Backwards For Consumers? *Elder L J* 1998;6:31–48.

Other Federal Programs—CHAMPUS

Dasco ST, Dasco CC. *Managed Care Answer Book,* 2d ed. Frederick, MD: Aspen Publishers, 1997;6-48–6-49.

Sloss EM, Hosek SD. *Evaluation of the CHAMPUS Reform Initiative: Beneficiary Access and Satisfaction*. Santa Monica, CA: RAND Corporation, 1993.

Other Federal Programs—Federal Employees Health Benefit Program

Dasco ST, Dasco CC. *Managed Care Answer Book*, 2d ed. Frederick, MD: Aspen Publishers, 1997;6-47–6-48.

Dasco ST, Dasco CC. *Managed Care Answer Book, 1998 Supplement*. Frederick, MD: Aspen Publishers, 1998; 6-23–6-25.

Other Managed Care Forms—Exclusive Provider Organization

Dasco ST, Dasco CC. *Managed Care Answer Book*, 2d ed. Frederick, MD: Aspen Publishers, 1997;3–7.

Kongstvedt PR. Exclusive Provider Organizations. In: *Essentials of Managed Health Care*. Gaithersburg, MD: Aspen Publishers, 1995;27.

Other Managed Care Forms—Point-of-Service HMO

Dasco ST, Dasco CC. *Managed Care Answer Book*, 2d ed. Frederick, MD: Aspen Publishers, 1997;2-13–2-14, 3-7–3-8.

Kongstvedt PR. Point-of-Service Plan. In: *Essentials of Managed Health Care*. Gaithersburg, MD: Aspen Publishers, 1995;27.

Other Managed Care Forms—Specialty HMOs

Dasco ST, Dasco CC. *Managed Care Answer Book*, 2d ed. Frederick, MD: Aspen Publishers, 1997;3–9.

Kongstvedt PR. Specialty Health Maintenance Organizations. In: *Essentials of Managed Health Care*. Gaithersburg, MD: Aspen Publishers, 1995;28.

Other Managed Care Forms—Integrated Delivery Systems

Dasco ST, Dasco CC. *Managed Care Answer Book*, 2d ed. Frederick, MD: Aspen Publishers, 1997;5-12–5-17.

Integrated Delivery Systems: Creation, Management, and Governance. Chicago: Health Administration Press, 1997.

Johnson EA, Brown M et al. *The Economic Era of Health Care: A Revolution in Organized Delivery Systems*. San Francisco: Jossey-Bass, 1996.

Kongstvedt PR. Integrated Health Care Delivery Systems. In: *Essentials of Managed Health Care*. Gaithersburg, MD: Aspen Publishers, 1995;35–48.

Other Managed Care Forms—Management Services Organizations

Dasco ST, Dasco CC. *Managed Care Answer Book*, 2d ed. Frederick, MD: Aspen Publishers, 1997;4-21–4-24.

DeMuro PR. Management Services Organizations. *Topics in Health Care Finance* 1994;20(3):19–27.

Gorey TM. *Management Services Organizations: Cases and Analysis (Spotlight Series)*. Chicago: Health Administration Press, 1997.

Kongstvedt PR. Managed Service Organization. In: *Essentials of Managed Health Care*. Gaithersburg, MD: Aspen Publishers, 1995;42–43.

Other Managed Care Forms—Physician Practice Management Entities

Dasco ST, Dasco CC. *Managed Care Answer Book*, 2d ed. Frederick, MD: Aspen Publishers, 1997;4-22–4-24.

McCally JF. *Physician Practice Management Redefines: The Move to Integrate Practice Organizations*. New York: McGraw-Hill, 1998.

Physician Practice Management Companies: What You Need to Know. Chicago: American Medical Association, 1997.

Other Managed Care Forms—Provider-Sponsored Organizations

Dasco ST, Dasco CC. *Managed Care Answer Book*, 2d ed. Frederick, MD: Aspen Publishers, 1997;3-25–3-29.

Grant PN, Hirsch WR. *Medicare Provider-Sponsored Organizations: A Practical Guide to Development and Certification.* Chicago: American Hospital Pub., 1998.

Venable RS. *Capitation: Tools, Trends, Traps, and Techniques: A Textbook for Provider-Sponsored Organizations.* Los Angeles: Practice Management Information Corp., 1998.

PPOs

Dasco ST, Dasco CC. *Managed Care Answer Book*, 2d ed. Frederick, MD: Aspen Publishers, 1997;3-4–3-7.

Dechene JC. Preferred Provider Organization Structures and Agreements. *Annals Health L* 1995;4:35–70.

Furrow BR et al. Regulation of Preferred Provider Arrangements. In: *Health Law.* St. Paul, MN: West Publishing Co., 1995;§11–12.

Hubner M. Sounding Out Silent PPOs Could Save Practice Plenty. *Am Med News* 1997;27 Mar:14.

Payment Methodologies

Dasco ST, Dasco CC. *Managed Care Answer Book*, 2d ed. Frederick, MD: Aspen Publishers, 1997;2-28–2-32.

Dasco ST, Dasco CC. *Managed Care Answer Book, 1998 Supplement.* Frederick, MD: Aspen Publishers, 1998;8–15.

Kerr EA. Managed Care and Capitation in California: How Do Physicians at Financial Risk Control Their Own Utilization? *Ann Int Med* 1995;123:500–504.

Kongstvedt PR. Compensation of Primary Care Physicians in Open Panels. In: *Essentials of Managed Health Care.* Gaithersburg, MD: Aspen Publishers, 1995;76–89.

Ruskin A. Capitation: The Legal Implications of Using Capitation to Affect Physician Decision-Making Processes. *J Contemp Health L & Pol'y* 1997;13:391–421.

Regulatory Structure

Dasco ST, Dasco CC. *Managed Care Answer Book,* 2d ed. Frederick, MD: Aspen Publishers, 1997;5-82–5-85, 7-17, 7-43, 8-43, 12-62.

Kongstvedt PR. Regulating Managed Care at the State Level. In: *Essentials of Managed Health Care.* Gaithersburg, MD: Aspen Publishers, 1995;19–21.

Other Reading

Aston G. Widespread HMO Defections Starting to Hit Medicaid, Too. *Am Med News* 1998;Dec. 14:5–6.

Clancy CM, Hillner BE. Physicians as Gatekeepers—The Impact of Financial Incentives. *Arch Int Med* 1989;149:917–20.

Coile RC. *The Five Stages of Managed Care: Strategies for Providers, HMOs, and Suppliers.* Chicago: Health Administration Press, 1997.

Corcoran ME. *Managed Care Contracting: Advising the Managed Care Organization.* Washington, DC: Bureau of National Affairs, 1996.

Dasco ST, Dasco CC. *Managed Care Answer Book*, 2d ed. Frederick, MD: Aspen Publishers, 1997.

Dasco ST, Dasco CC. *Managed Care Answer Book, 1998 Supplement.* Frederick, MD: Aspen Publishers, 1998.

Davis GS. *Managed Care Contracting: Advising the Provider.* Washington, DC: Bureau of National Affairs, 1996.

Demetriou AJ, Dutton TE. *Health Care Integration: Structural and Legal Issues.* Washington, DC: Bureau of National Affairs, 1996.

Hillman AL et al. HMO Managers' Views on Financial Incentives and Quality. *Health Affairs* Winter 1991:207–19.

Hillman AL et al. How Do Financial Incentives Affect Physicians' Clinical Decisions and the Financial Performance of Health Maintenance Organizations? *N Engl J Med* 1989;321:86–92.

Kongstvedt PR, ed. *The Managed Health Care Handbook,* 3d ed. Gaithersburg, MD: Aspen Publishers, 1996.

Latham SR. Regulation of Managed Care Incentive Payments to Physicians. *Am J L & Med* 1996;22:399–432.

Liang BA. Deselection Under *Harper v. Healthsource:* A Blow for Maintaining Patient-Physician Relationships in the Era of Managed Care? *Notre Dame L Rev* 1997;72:799–861.

Liang BA. General Considerations for Managed Care Contracting. *Hosp Phys* 1995;31(5):41–51.

Liang BA. *Mandatory Medicaid HMO Enrollment Programs: A Description of State, HMO, and Delivery Site Characteristics.* Chicago: University of Chicago, 1989. Thesis.

Liang BA. The Practical Utility of Gag Clause Legislation. *J Gen Int Med* 1998;13:419–21.

McCormick B. Where Are Your Discounts? 'Silent PPOs' Broker Them to Insurers Costing Doctors and Hospitals Money. *Am Med News* 1995;6 Feb:1.

McWilliams MC, Russell HE. Hospital Liability for Torts of Independent Contractor Physicians. *S C L Rev* 1996;47:431–74.

Nash DB, ed. *The Physician's Guide to Managed Care.* Gaithersburg, MD: Aspen Publishers, 1994.

National Committee for Quality Assurance. *Draft Standards for the Accreditation of Managed Care Organizations.* Washington, DC: National Committee for Quality Assurance, 1997.

National Committee for Quality Assurance. *HEDIS 3.0,* vols. I–III. Washington, DC: National Committee for Quality Assurance, 1998.

Painter WS. *Provider Sponsored Managed Care Organizations: A Compendium of Key Legal Issues.* Pub. no. SB51 ALI-ABA 1065. Chicago: American Law Institute–American Bar Association, 1997.

Pauly MV. *Paying Physicians: Options for Controlling Cost, Volume, and Intensity of Services.* Ann Arbor, MI: Health Administration Press, 1992.

Peter GR. Organizational and Business Issues Affecting Integrated Delivery Systems. *Topics in Health Care Financing* 1994;20(3):1–12.

Reightner RC. State Regulation of Capitated Reimbursement for Physician-Hospital Organizations. *Health Matrix* 1997;7:301–31.

Robinson JC. Consolidation of Medical Groups into Physician Practice Management Organizations. *JAMA* 1998;279:144.

Rothschild IS et al. Recent Developments in Managed Care. *Tort & Ins L J* 1997;32:463–80.

Tokarski C. Running the Obstacle Course: PPMs. *Am Med News* 1998;13 Apr:13–15.

U.S. General Accounting Office. *Medicaid Managed Care: Challenge of Holding Plans Accountable Requires Greater State Effort.* Pub. No. GAO/HEHS-97-86. Washington, DC: General Accounting Office, 1997.

Web Sites

American Accreditation Healthcare Commission/URAC: *http://www.urac.org*

American Association of Health Plans: *http://www.aahp.org*

California Consumer Health Care Council: *http://www.cchcc.org*

Citizens Who Care: *http://www.visi.com/~crbowman/cchc/index.html*

CNN: The HMO debate: *http://cnn.com/HEALTH/specials/HMOs/*

Dr. David Trueman's site to fight HMOs: *http://www.truemanlaw.com*

Fight managed care: *http://www.his.com/~pico/usa.htm*

Fight your HMO: http://www.bright.net/~ewp/fight_your_hmo.html

Health Administration Responsibility Project: *http://www.harp.org*

Health care industry — Living in an HMO world: *http://healthcare.miningco.com/library/weekly/aa060998.htm*

Health care industry — Managed care: *http://healthcare.miningco.com/*

Health Care Liability Alliance: *http://www.wp.com/HCLA*

HMO Facts Inc.: *http://www.hmosearch.com/*

HMO house of horrors: *http://www.hmowatch.org/*

The HMO page: *http://www.hmopage.org/*

How I fought my HMO and won: *http://members.aol.com/jasonwolff/hmomain.htm*

HMO monitor — Tracking, reporting, and appealing HMO denials: *http://www.hmomonitor.com/*

Impact of managed care on clinical research: http://www.ncrr.nih.gov/newspub/mancare.htm

Impact of managed care on minorities: *http://www.udayton.edu/~health/manage02.htm*

Insurance industry — Managed care, HMOs and PPOs: *http://insurance.miningco.com/msubmco.htm*

Joint Commission on Accreditation of Healthcare Organizations: http://www.jcaho.org

Managed care links: http://home.sprintmail.com/~dmurray008/

Medicare and HMO program overview: http://www.panpha.org/Guide01.htm

Medicare+Choice contracting, quality assurance guidance: *http://www.hcfa.gov/medicare/opl077.htm* and *http://www.hcfa.gov/medicare/extnfinl.htm*

National Committee for Quality Assurance: *http://www.ncqa.org*

National Managed Health Care Congress: http://www.nmhcc.org/

Overview — Managed care: http://www.wnet.org/archive/mhc/Overview/essay.html

Physicians who care: *http://www.hmopage.org*

Policy.com issue of the week — Can managed care be managed?: *http://www.policy.com/issuewk/98/0608/index.html*

PART III
Modern Delivery Considerations

10

Physician Contracting and Employee Considerations

Physicians and other health care providers do not treat patients and render medical services in a vacuum. Generally, the relationship with patients and, indeed, access to patients are defined through contracts. Broadly viewed, contracts govern the rights and responsibilities of each party in providing care, paying or being paid for that care, and terminating the relationship. Therefore, it is important to have a firm grasp on a reasonable mode of assessment when considering entrance into these relationships. It should be emphasized that, in any contractual process, the assistance of legal counsel is imperative to provide guidance as to the legal effect of the terms and conditions of the contract.

The first part of this chapter uses contracts between providers and MCOs as a paradigm. The principles gleaned from this discussion are applicable to other health care contract situations. The second part of the chapter focuses on issues associated with employer–employee relationships.

Independent Contractors

Physicians generally contract with MCOs as independent contractors.[1] As such, all terms and conditions must be expressly indicated within the contract so that the rights and responsibilities of each party are as clear as possible. Three stages generally govern all contractual assessments before final signing: performing due diligence, preparing for negotiations, and reviewing the terms of the proposed contract.

Due Diligence

Before entering into contract negotiations, providers must pursue due diligence and ascertain the status of several

preliminary issues with regard to the entities with which they are contemplating a contract. For example, is the entity in compliance with all state and federal licensing and regulatory schemes? Has the entity been involved in any previous or current investigations? Is the entity financially sound? Is the entity appropriately accredited? This background legal information is essential to assess before engaging in the long-term and costly process of negotiating a contract.

In addition, operational issues to be determined include an assessment of other contractors with the entity and their relationships. For example, which party controls utilization and authorization for medical services? Who owns the entity? What other providers contract with the entity, and do they have legal authority to provide services or been subject to investigations? What is the malpractice history of the entity? How long does it take to be paid by the entity? What is the entity's patient-enrollee base? What is the public's perception of the entity? Does the entity have insurance? Does any third party that contracts with the entity, such as a utilization review company, also have insurance? If these and other relevant queries support continued assessment of the entity as a contracting partner, then the provider may wish to enter into negotiations with the entity. Note that it is important, even if a contract is signed, to continuously monitor this information throughout the life of the contract to allow for identification of problems at their early stages and so less costly (in terms of time and money) corrective action can be implemented if necessary.

Preparing for Negotiations

Once due diligence has been performed, the provider must prepare for negotiations with the entity. This requires an honest assessment of the provider's strengths

---

[1]See Chapter 9.

and weaknesses from an external point of view. These characteristics include factors such as number of physicians and specialties, support personnel and capital, geographic locations, outcomes measures, accreditations, computer systems, entity culture, and other factors as related to the proposed contracting partner. In addition, the provider must assess how contracting with the entity will allow the provider any opportunity to take advantage of its strengths. Finally, the provider must assess how its weaknesses can be seen as a threat to successful contracting and provision of services. This is known as SWOT (strengths, weaknesses, opportunities, threats) analysis.[2] In addition, the provider must also assess its BATNA (best alternative to a negotiated agreement). Critically, the BATNA will assist the provider in determining how far it wishes to negotiate and what minimum terms and conditions are necessary for the agreement to be acceptable. Finally, the provider, as best as possible, should do the same analysis for the proposed contracting partner to anticipate potential conflicts, potential joint benefits, and areas where compromise could be reached.

Terms to Be Considered

A large number of areas are covered by managed care contracts, and many will be provider, MCO, time, and geographically specific. However, some basic terms should be considered when entering into contract negotiations to understand the rights and responsibilities of the parties. Note that because the contract will define the rights and responsibilities of the parties, there should be no reliance on oral representations or promises between the parties, the memory of the parties, or a "gentleman's agreement." If there is a dispute regarding the terms and their interpretation, generally the naked terms of the agreement will govern, which will be interpreted by parties such as administrators, other physicians, and courts — parties not there at the time of negotiation.

That being said, one of the first aspects of the contract to which attention should be paid is the *definitions of important terms* within the agreement. A particular term used in lay language should not be assumed to have the same meaning within the contract as in casual conversation. Terms must be carefully assessed and evaluated as to how they have been defined; clarification may be necessary. It is important that no substantive legal obligations are implicated in these definitions. Value-laden terms such as *high-quality care, cost-effective care,* and so forth

should be avoided and the use of objective terms should be emphasized as much as possible.

Another aspect of the contract to assess is the *term of the agreement.* It is critical to determine for what total term the contract is to last (e.g., one year), whether there is an "evergreen clause" (i.e., an automatic renewal unless one of the parties exercises rights to terminate the agreement within the prescribed notice period, say, 60 days), and whether there are automatic updates for provider fee increases or whether these updates must be negotiated within some period of time before renewal. Note that a contract for one year but providing for allowable termination with 60 days' notice is simply a 60-day contract. In addition, any restrictive covenants after the contract is over, such as limitations in where the provider may practice, what kind of services can be performed, and the time during which this is in effect should be noted and reviewed.

Another termination clause should be reviewed as well. The *termination without cause clause* is a clause that allows either party to terminate the agreement for any or no reason at all as long as the prescribed notice is provided (e.g., 30 days). Thus, if the entity provides such notice as prescribed, the contract is legally terminated. Challenges to these termination without cause clauses almost always have been rejected by the courts.[3] Note that termination clauses may indicate that a termination can be only "for cause" or a "material breach." These clauses are not substantive and require further explanation in the agreement; specific instances and circumstances (e.g., late payment of capitation for six consecutive months or provider loss of privileges at a particular hospital) should be detailed so confusion is minimized in interpretation of terms. In addition, the rights of the provider on termination should be specified with regard to a hearing and other review in addition to that required by state and federal statutes.[4] In addition, it should be ascertained whether any bylaws of the organization are applicable to the parties of the contract, and the

[2]R. Fisher and W. Ury, *Getting to Yes,* 2d ed. (Boston: Houghton-Mifflin, 1991).

[3]See, e.g., Abrahamson v. NME Hosps., Inc., 241 Cal.Rptr. 396 (Cal. Ct. App. 1987) (wrongful discharge or breach of duty of good faith and fair dealing suit is untenable for independent contractors); B. A. Liang, "An Overview and Analysis of Challenges to Medical Exclusive Contracts," *Journal of Legal Medicine* 18 (1997), pp. 1–45; B. A. Liang, "Deselection Under Harper v. Healthsource: A Blow for Maintaining Patient-Physician Relationships in the Era of Managed Care?" *Notre Dame Law Review* 72 (1997), pp. 799–861, and the references therein.

[4]See, e.g., 42 U.S.C.A. §11111 *et seq.; Florida Statutes Annotated* (St. Paul, MN: West, 1997), section 395.0193; *Rhode Island General Laws* §23-17-23 (1997); *New York Public Health Law* (St. Paul, MN: West, 1997), section 2801-b; *Georgia Code Annotated,* §31-7-7 (1998).

specific terms of rights granted by them; bylaws have been held to constitute the terms of a contract.[5]

Another important issue to assess is *who is permitted to provide services?* Will physicians be mandated to see all patients, or may physician extenders such as physician assistants or nurse practitioners be permitted as well? What are the qualifications of providers that can provide services? Will they need to be accredited? Board certified? Board eligible? How will this information be ascertained and reviewed? Will malpractice history be taken into account and, if so, how? What are the obligations of providers with regard to entity accreditation if any? In addition, is the arrangement exclusive? Or, are other providers rendering care to the same patients? Related to this consideration is who owns the medical records, the provider or the proposed contracting entity? Who has access to these records and under what conditions?

The *scope of services to be provided* is still another important aspect of the contract that requires careful review. If the scope of services is more extensive than the provider can offer, there may be difficulty in avoiding a breach of contract. As well, if the scope is beyond the ken of the provider, is the provider permitted to subcontract for such service provision? The provider should assess how this set of services can be altered: can the provider unilaterally change the amount of services to be provided? Can the potential contracting partner do so? Further, the provider should determine if there is any overlap between services other providers will be responsible for and the scope of services in the contract at hand. In addition, a significant issue relates to experimental treatments: Who defines what treatment is experimental? Who determines

if it is covered and whether the provider is responsible for rendering it? Finally, it should be determined whether practice guidelines are to be used, whether they are mandatory or voluntary, and whether they are subject to review and revision. Are these guidelines used to evaluate performance? If so, are there outlier considerations? If not, by what processes is clinical performance assessed?

A related topic is the *utilization review process.* Often, utilization review requires providers to make available their medical records, fill out encounter forms, report clinical outcomes, obtain preauthorization for particular procedures, and take responsibility for all patient care outcomes, even though these utilization review requirements are set up by other parties. Because they often shoulder patient injury responsibility alone, even when utilization review might be a factor in attempting to render care,[6] physicians should be very circumspect about their obligations under this part of the contract and should perform due diligence of any third-party utilization reviewer. Further, ascertaining how the utilization review is accomplished is important: Who reviews the cases? What are their reputations? What are the appeals mechanisms? Is there any consultation with the provider before treatment or claims are denied? By what standards are treatment care or claims authorized or denied?

Of course, services are not provided to just anyone under the contract. The contract should specify *what parties are eligible for services under the agreement.* The contract should specify what party (parties) is (are) the payer(s) and which patients are to be treated. The specific patients generally are those enrolled with the particular payer (e.g., MCO); however, it is imperative that these be defined to avoid the problems encountered with silent PPOs.[7] If the contracting party is acting for others, those parties should be identified specifically and a reasonable opportunity given to verify their existence and ensure compliance with the terms of the agreement. As such, providers should be able to terminate the agreement with those parties not in compliance with the terms agreed to by its broker. In addition, providers should determine whether the potential contracting party is serving as a broker for an ERISA EBP. This will have implications as to potential obligations and liability.[8] Further, the contract should detail how conflicts with regard to eligibility are to be resolved.

If a relationship is in place, will the parties be able to *market the association between the parties?* Often, the question is not whether the parties can market their association, but to what extent and in what form. Will approval for marketing materials be performed by both parties, or

---

[5]See, e.g., American Med. Int'l, Inc. v. Scheller, 590 So.2d 947 (Fla. Dist. Ct. App. 1991); Lewisburg Comm. Hosp., Inc. v. Alfredson, 805 S.W.2d 756 (Tenn. 1991); Bartley v. Eastern Maine Med. Ctr., 617 A.2d 1020 (Me. 1992); Katz v. Children's Hosp., 602 N.E.2d 598 (Mass. App. Ct. 1992); see also Hospital Corp. of Lake Worth v. Romaguera, 511 So.2d 559 (Fla. Dist. Ct. App. 1986) (amendment to bylaws validly modified physician contract with hospital); but see Dutta v. St. Francis Regional Med. Ctr., 867 P.2d 1057 (Kan. 1994) (hospital bylaws regarding due process hearing are not applicable when physician's employment is terminated for administrative, and not quality, reasons); Saint Louis v. Baystate Med. Ctr., 568 N.E.2d 1181 (Mass. App. Ct. 1991) (same); Anne Arundel Gen. Hosp., Inc. v. O'Brien, 432 A.2d 483 (Md. Ct. Spec. App. 1981) (same); Kramer v. Kent Gen. Hosp., 1992 WL 91130 (Del. Super. Ct. Feb. 28, 1992) (same); but see St. Mary's Hosp. v. Radiology Professional Corp., 421 S.E.2d 731 (Ga. Ct. App. 1992) (bylaws do not create contractual rights); Keskin v. Munster Med. Research Foundation, 580 N.E.2d 354 (Ind. Ct. App. 1991) (bylaws do not necessarily constitute a contract); Gianetti v. Norwalk Hosp., 557 A.2d 1249 (Conn. 1989) (bylaws do not constitute contract due to legal duty to adopt them).

---

[6]See Chapter 9.
[7]See Chapter 9.
[8]See Chapters 6 and 9.

will the decision as to the extent and scope of marketing be allowed for each unilaterally? Will only one party be able to market freely while the other must obtain approval?

Another issue relates to communications. Will physicians and other providers be able to speak freely about patient care options even if not covered by the potential contracting party; that is, *does the contract contain gag clauses?* Many states have banned gag clauses, so even if one is in place, gag clauses may not be legally viable. However, the difficulty arises when a contract provision is not expressly a gag clause but deemed an "antidisparagement" provision (e.g., "Physician shall agree not to take an action or make any communication which undermines or could undermine the confidence of enrollees . . . in [the MCO] or the quality of [the MCO's] coverage").[9] Hence, it is important to ensure which communications are allowed, which are not, and how disputes regarding communications between the provider and patient and the provider and contracting partner are deemed and treated under the contract.

Once the services required under the contract, the persons to whom they are to be provided, and the scope of communications between the provider and patients are assessed, *the terms of payment* can be considered. How will the provider be paid? Discounted fee for service? Capitation?[10] Percentage of premium? Per diem? Are emergency room services included on the per diem rate? Per case? Is capitation fixed or adjusted by factors such as age, gender, or health status? Some contracts will vary payment terms by the number of patients treated or the number of patients for which the provider is responsible. Will the volume of services change these payment terms? In addition, other risk sharing such as using withhold arrangements[11] are common: Are there withhold arrangements in the proposed contract? If so, what percentage is withheld? What are the terms of obtaining payments from the withhold arrangement? Are there any productivity incentives? Is stop-loss insurance available? Are ceilings placed on the costs allocated toward the withhold arrangement? Are withhold assessments based on individual or group performance? Another important issue is experimental treatment. Are experimental treatments counted toward the withhold arrangement or to be provided under capitation? Are experimental treatments paid for through other payment schemes separate from nonexperimental care?

Obviously the form of payment and the relative aggregate amount as compared with costs are critical in assessing the acceptability of the contract. However, what happens if the enrollee population changes significantly, such as a much larger Medicare population is added? Can payment rates be renegotiated? Also, who pays for care provided to patients who are later determined to be ineligible for coverage? Further, who is responsible for care costs for services rendered out of the network? In addition, is there a hold-harmless clause, which requires that all payments made by the entity be payment in full to the provider, with no recourse to collect fees from the patient? This type of provision is mandated by law in some states and common in many HMO contracts. Further, how will payments be transferred to the provider? What grace period is allowed for such payments? What penalties incur for late payments? Note that some states have instituted a prompt payment requirement and penalty scheme for MCO payments to providers.[12]

Another area of contention is *indemnification for lawsuits.* Does either party indemnify the other against any, some, or all claims against the other? Note that if an indemnity clause is signed by the provider, often malpractice insurers will not pay for claims arising under the contractual provision. Related to this, who is responsible for malpractice insurance payments? What kind of malpractice insurance is required and at what levels?

Other considerations include *special enrollees* such as Medicare and Medicaid subscribers or ERISA beneficiaries. Should the provider be aware of any special requirements for serving these populations (e.g., utilization review, documentation, encounter forms)? Who is responsible for deductible and coinsurance amounts, if applicable? Do providers need specific physician identification numbers or other specific credentials to serve special enrollees? Are there fiduciary or other duties and compliance issues mandated for these populations?[13] Are there financial arrangements (e.g., physician incentive plans) that require approval or other review?

Of course, within the time period during which the contract is in force, changes may occur in the circumstances of the health delivery environment or the parties themselves. Therefore, *provisions for amending the contract* are very important. Generally, it is important to determine how the contract is to be amended, whether both parties need to assent to the amendment, and

---

[9]See B. A. Liang, "The Practical Utility of Gag Clause Legislation," *Journal of General Internal Medicine* 13 (1998), pp. 419–21; J. V. King and B. A. Liang, "The Silencing of the Physician: Gag Rules in a Managed Care Environment," *Hospital Physician* 34, no. 7 (1998), pp. 64–69.

[10]See *California Health and Safety Code* (St. Paul, MN: West, 1997), section 1345(f); Opinion Cal. Comm'r Dep't of Corps., No. 4600H (department of corporations' interpretation that capitation payments fall under HMO statutory licensing requirements for the state).

[11]See Chapter 9.

[12]*Florida Administrative Code Annotated* r. 4-191.066 (1997); *Maryland Code Annotated, Health—General I* §19-712.1 (1997); 28 *Texas Administrative Code* (St. Paul, MN: West, 1997), section 11.1604(1)(A); *Wisconsin Administrative Code* §106.04 (1997).

[13]See 29 U.S.C.A. §1133 (ERISA plans must notify and explain to participants any action that results in denied claims and must provide full and fair review of the decision).

whether acceptance of the amendment must be active or passive. The last is particularly important; if an active acceptance is required, then any amendment by either party must be affirmatively accepted through the procedures indicated in the contract. If only passive acceptance is required, then the amendment is deemed accepted if there is no objection within a certain period of time. Passive acceptance therefore can be done inadvertently. Another concern regarding changed circumstances is what happens if there is any sale of assets, mergers, changes of control, or the like to either party: Is there a notice requirement? Can either party assign the contract? Can either party terminate the contract on these events?

Finally, if conflict arises between the parties, *how will disputes be resolved?* Will there be alternative dispute resolution (ADR) processes? Arbitration? Mediation? Some combination? Is the process binding, or can the parties go to court? Which party will pay for the process if it is used? Which jurisdiction's law will govern? Note that although ADR processes are valuable, parties must be aware that sometimes they are inapplicable to resolve disputes.[14]

Employees

In addition to the more common independent contractor status of physicians, physicians may be employees. For example, staff model HMOs employ physicians to provide care to patients in their facilities; physicians also may be employees of medical groups. Similarly, health care professionals such as nurses, technicians, and others are employees. This section discusses important considerations regarding employee status and the general legal concepts describing the rights of employees.

At-Will Employment

Generally, individual employees are considered to be employees at will, absent other factors such as an employment contract. As employees at will, physicians and their employers may terminate the relationship at any time, with the caveat that such termination does not violate civil rights laws. While the allowable extent to which employment can be terminated by employers is quite broad,[15] three major exceptions to the unfettered termination of at-will employment by employers exist: the implied in-fact contract exception, the public policy

exception, and the breach of an implied covenant of good faith and fair dealing exception.

Implied In-Fact Contract Exception

Implied in-fact contracts as applied to at-will employment relationships allow the traditional at-will employee to maintain a breach of contract action when an act by the employer has induced the employee to reasonably believe that his or her employment tenure will continue or that the employer has promised some set of actions that will occur before the employment is terminated.[16] The classic circumstance where this arises is through modification of an employment at-will relationship. For example, procedural restraints on termination of employment added to an employee handbook have been held to have formed an implied in-fact contract between the at-will employee and the employer.[17]

[15]See, e.g., Payne v. Western & Atlantic Railroad, 81 Tenn. 507 (1884), *overruled on other grounds*, Hutton v. Watters, 179 S.W. 134 (Tenn. 1915) (termination of employment at-will contracts can be "for good cause, for no cause, or even for cause morally wrong"); NLRB v. McGahey, 233 F.2d 406 (5th Cir. 1956) (termination of an at-will agreement may be for "good cause, bad cause, or no cause at all"); Fawcett v. G.C. Murphy & Co., 348 N.E.2d 144 (Ohio 1976) (employer's right to discharge is absolute and not limited by considerations and principles that protect individuals from gross or reckless conduct, willful, wanton, or malicious acts, or acts done intentionally, with insult, or in bad faith); Wagenseller v. Scottsdale Mem. Hosp., 710 P.2d 1025 (Ariz. 1985) (termination can be "for no cause, or even for a cause morally wrong"); W. P. Keeton et al., *Prosser and Keeton on the Law of Torts,* 5th ed. (St. Paul, MN: West, 1984), section 1027 (termination can be "even for reasons of spite or malice").

[16]See Minihan v. American Pharmaceutical Association, 812 F.2d 726 (D.C. Cir. 1987) (indicating that the employment at-will doctrine is a rebuttable presumption).

[17]See, e.g., Pine River State Bank v. Mettille, 333 N.W.2d 622 (Minn. 1983); Duldulao v. St. Mary of Nazareth Hosp. Ctr., 505 N.E.2d 314 (Ill. 1987) (hospital must comply with employee manual when firing nurse); Sides v. Duke Univ. Hosp., 328 S.E.2d 818 (N.C. Ct. App. 1985) (implied contract under employee manual legally supported by nurse changing locations); but see Lee v. Sperry Corp., 678 F. Supp. 1415 (D. Minn. 1987) (granting summary judgment for an employer due to a postemployment amendment to the employee manual that transformed the employment relationship into one terminable at will is considered accepted by employee's continuation of work after receiving it); Hrehorovich v. Harbor Hosp. Ctr., 614 A.2d 1021 (Md. Ct. Spec. App. 1992) (employee manual can create an implied contract if employee reasonably relied on it, but disclaimer in manual can defeat reliance); Bearden v. Human Health Plan, 1992 WL 245604 (N.D. Ill. 1992) (employee manual with disclaimer and written employment agreement trumped information in manual).

[14]B. A. Liang, "Understanding and Applying Alternative Dispute Resolution Methods in Modern Medical Conflicts," *Journal of Legal Medicine* 19 (1998), pp. 397–430. See Chapter 14.

Generally, the requisite components for an implied in-fact modification of an at-will relationship are a promise by the employer related to employment,[18] legal consideration given by the employee and an employee acceptance, and a breach of that promise through inappropriate employment termination.[19] Note, however, that bylaws generally do *not* create an implied contract for employment that modifies the at-will nature of the employer–employee relationship.[20]

Public Policy Exception

Another major legal doctrine that has carved out an exception to the traditional terminable at-will employment doctrine is based on public policy: If the termination of the employment was against some clear manifestation of public policy and the employer has no requisite legitimate business interest or just cause that overrides the public policy interest, the termination can be held to be wrongful. However, note that the background rule under this public policy exception remains that the employment relationship is at will and only if the employee can manifest some evidence that there has been a violation of some articulable public policy will he or she have the potential to prevail.[21]

The public policies that have been implicated in this exception are quite broad but have the underlying feature of employer actions that simply violate some specific statutory or common law notion of legal morality;[22] that is, persons cannot be fired for actions that specifically are indicated acceptable by statutory mandate. Therefore, a litany of actions has been considered in concert with the public policy exception.

Several statutory frameworks are effective support for the public policy exception. For example, discriminatory dismissal in violation of Title VII of the Civil Rights Act of 1964, prohibiting discrimination on the basis of race, color, religion, sex, or national origin, is within the exception.[23] Discharge discrimination on the basis of age also is prohibited under the Age Discrimination in Employment Act of 1967[24] and on the basis of disability under the Rehabilitation Act of 1973.[25] Discharge for engaging in union activities also violates public policy under federal statutory law.[26]

Somewhat more variable are the common law public policy exceptions. Generally, these exceptions frame the concept that an employment cannot be terminated for an employee refusing to engage in activities that violate the law or prevent an employee from performing a civic duty. The cases cover an extensive subject matter. For example, the public policy exception has extended to circumstances where an employee refused to give false testimony,[27] refused to engage in a price-fixing scheme,[28] insisted that the employer comply with the Food, Drug and Cosmetics Act requirements,[29] reported

---

[18]See Thompson v. St. Regis Paper Co., 685 P.2d 1081 (Wash. 1984) (holding that employees who justifiably rely on expressed policies in employment manuals make these policies binding on the employer, and the employer cannot treat these policies as illusory promises).

[19]But see Broussard v. C.A.C.I., Inc., 780 F.2d 162 (1st Cir. 1986) (holding that express promises regarding employment security are distinguishable from implied promises from employee handbooks and negotiations, with implied promises insufficient to sustain a wrongful termination claim).

[20]See, e.g., Hrehorovich v. Harbor Hosp. Ctr., 614 A.2d 1021 (Md. Ct. Spec. App. 1992) (director of department could not rely on bylaws to support claim that there was an implied contract); Paul v. Lankenau Hosp., 543 A.2d 1148 (Pa. Super. Ct. 1988), *rev'd on other grounds* 569 A.2d 346 (Pa. 1990) (medical staff bylaws do not create an implied contract vitiating the at-will status of employee); see also St. Yves v. Mid State Bank, 748 P.2d 633 (Wash. Ct. App. 1987), *rev'd on other grounds* 757 P.2d 1384 (Wash. 1988); but see Hale v. Stoughton Hosp. Assoc., 376 N.W.2d 89 (Wis. Ct. App. 1985) (bylaw created more than an "at-will" employer–employee relationship, and hospital could not fire employee for any cause or even no cause).

[21]See, e.g., Cleary v. American Airlines, 168 Cal.Rptr. 722 (Ct. App. 1980) (indicating that plaintiff-employee has the burden of proof of unjust termination that the employer can refute).

[22]See, e.g., Haynes v. Zoological Society of Cincinnati, 567 N.E.2d 1048 (Ohio C.P. 1990), *rev'd on other grounds* 652 N.E.2d 948 (Ohio 1995) (violation of public policy is "deeply ingrained in community and moral values").

[23]42 U.S.C.A. §§2000(e)(2) *et seq.*

[24]29 U.S.C.A. §§623 *et seq.*; but see Yoho v. Triangle P.W.C. Inc., 336 S.E.2d 204 (W.Va. 1985) (clause of collective bargaining agreement mandating termination of seniority after employee's absence from work for one year for work-related injury was not contrary to public policy, even though loss of seniority also resulted in termination of employment).

[25]29 U.S.C.A. §794; see also Ambrosino v. Metropolitan Life Ins. Co., 899 F.Supp. 438 (N.D. Cal. 1995) (podiatrist's termination as a provider under contract violated state antidiscrimination statute and thus was discriminatory and in violation of his civil rights).

[26]29 U.S.C.A. §§158 *et seq.*

[27]See, e.g., Petermann v. International Brotherhood of Teamsters, 344 P.2d 25 (Cal. Ct. App. 1959).

[28]See, e.g., Tameny v. Atlantic Richfield Co., 610 P.2d 1330 (Cal. 1980).

[29]See, e.g., Boyle v. Vista Eyewear, 700 S.W.2d 859 (Mo. Ct. App. 1985); Sheets v. Teddy's Frosted Foods, 427 A.2d 385 (Conn. 1980); but see Smith v. Calgon Carbon Corp., 917 F.2d 1338 (3d Cir. 1990) (reversing employee verdict for $400,000 for an employee whose employment had been terminated after he reported water pollution activities for which he was not responsible).

violations of public health and safety statutes,[30] attempted to comply with jury duty,[31] filed a workers' compensation claim,[32] engaged in whistleblowing,[33] or refused to take a polygraph test that would violate a state's statute.[34] Other egregious behavior within the public policy exception beyond actions by employers in retaliation for an employee's refusal to violate the law include actions that, although potentially couchable in legal terms, simply offend the sensibilities of social and professional norms. For example, public policy exceptions to the at-will rule include situations where an employee was fired due to her rejection of a foreman's sexual advances[35] and where the employment of a radiology technician was terminated after not performing a procedure to which her license did not extend.[36] How-

ever, there are circumstances in which a violation of personal beliefs may not be enough to support a wrongful discharge claim under the public policy exception.[37]

Good Faith and Fair Dealing Exception

The covenant of good faith and fair dealing is a specific, legally implied promise that is imputed to an employer and imposes a legally enforceable obligation not to terminate employment in bad faith or in violation of public policy.[38] Therefore, it can be considered a subset of the public policy exception to at-will agreements.[39]

This duty generally has been recognized in two distinct circumstances: when employment is terminated without cause after long years of service by the employee, and when an employer terminates employment to avoid paying the employee bonuses or compensation.[40] Note, however, the implied covenant is one of the least recognized exceptions to the employer's ability to fire at will. The majority of states assessing this issue in fact have refused to recognize this cause of action.[41] Even those courts that have accepted the exception still severely limit its application:

> the implied obligation [of good faith and fair dealing] is in aid and furtherance of terms of the agreement of the parties. No obligation can be implied, however, which would be inconsistent with other terms of the contractual relationship. [Here], . . . plaintiff's employment was at-will, a relationship which the law accords the employer an unfettered right to terminate the employment at any time. In the context of such employment it would be incongruous to say that an inference may be drawn that

---

[30]See, e.g., Skillsky v. Lucky Stores, Inc., 893 F.2d 1088 (9th Cir. 1990) (reversing summary judgment for an employer who terminated the job of an employee for filing a complaint with the federal Occupational Safety and Health Administration); see also Occupational Health and Safety Act, 29 U.S.C.A. §660 (providing protection against employers who fire employees on the basis of reporting violations of the act); Clean Air Act, 42 U.S.C.A. §7622(a), and the Employee Retirement Income Security Act, 29 U.S.C.A. §1140 (providing statutory protection against termination of employment for reporting violations of its dictates).

[31]See, e.g., Reuther v. Fowler & Williams, Inc., 386 A.2d 119 (Pa. Super. Ct. 1978); see also Juror Protection Act, 28 U.S.C.A. §1875 (1988) (allowing for compensatory and punitive damages by an employee who is dismissed or threatened to be dismissed for jury service).

[32]See, e.g., Hartlein v. Illinois Power Co., 568 N.E.2d 520 (Ill. App. 1991); Smith v. Smithway Motor Xpress, 464 N.W.2d 682 (Iowa 1991); Sventko v. Kroger Co., 245 N.W.2d 151 (Mich. App. 1976); Hopkins v. Tip Top Plumbing & Heating Co., 805 S.W.2d 280 (Mo. App. 1991); but see Smith v. Gould, 918 F.2d 1361 (8th Cir. 1990); Kelly v. Mississippi Valley Gas Co., 397 So.2d 874 (Miss. 1981) (no cause of action for challenging termination after filing workers' compensation claim).

[33]See, e.g., Palmer v. Brown, 752 P.2d 685, 689 (Kan. 1988) ("Public policy requires that citizens in a democracy be protected from reprisals for performing their civil duty of reporting infractions of rules, regulations, or the law. . . ."); see also 10 U.S.C.A. §2409, *General Statutes of Connecticut Annotated* (St. Paul, MN: West, 1984), section 31-51m; *Michigan Compiled Laws Annotated* (St. Paul, MN: West, 1984), sections 15.361–15.369; *Maine Revised Statutes Anniotated* (St. Paul, MN: West, 1984), title 26, sections 831–33 (whistleblowers cannot be penalized for actions allowed by statute).

[34]See, e.g., Wilcox v. Hy-Vee Food Stores, 458 N.W.2d 870 (Iowa App. 1990); Perks v. Firestone Tire & Rubber Co., 611 F.2d 1363 (3d Cir. 1979); but see Larsen v. Motor Supply Co., 573 P.2d 907 (Ariz. Ct. App. 1977) (indicating that no cause of action is sustainable for employee's refusal to take polygraph test and subsequent termination of employment).

[35]Monge v. Beebe Rubber Co., 316 A.2d 549 (N.H. 1974).

[36]O'Sullivan v. Mallon, 390 A.2d 149 (N.J. Super. Ct. Law. Div. 1978).

[37]See, e.g., Farnam v. Crista Ministries, 807 P.2d 830 (Wash. 1991); Warthen v. Toms River Comm. Mem. Hosp., 488 A.2d 229 (N.J. Super. Ct. App. Div. 1985), *cert. denied* 501 A.2d 926 (N.J. 1985); see also Pierce v. Ortho Pharmaceutical Corp., 417 A.2d 505 (N.J. 1980).

[38]H. H. Perritt, *Employee Dismissal Law and Practice,* 4th ed. (New York: Aspen, 1997).

[39]See, e.g., Sheppard v. Morgan Keegan Co., 266 Cal.Rptr. 784 (Cal. Ct. App. 1990) (holding that the implied covenant of good faith and fair dealing may be violated by terminating an employee's job immediately after his move across country to take the job offered to him by the employer even though he clearly was employed at will); Luck v. Southern Pacific Transportation Co., 267 Cal.Rptr. 618 (Cal. Ct. App.), *cert. denied* 498 U.S. 939 (1990) (holding that termination of employment for an employee's refusal to take a drug test might violate the implied covenant of good faith and fair dealing).

[40]See, e.g., Cleary v. American Airlines, 168 Cal.Rptr. 722 (Cal. Ct. App. 1980); Fortune v. National Cash Register Co., 364 N.E.2d 1251 (Mass. 1977).

[41]C. J. Bakaly and J. M. Grossman, *The Modern Law of Employment Relationships* (New York: Aspen, 1989), section 10.1.

the employer impliedly agreed to a provision which would be destructive of his right of termination.[42]

Other cases have held that there is no implied covenant exception to the at-will rule.[43] Even in the jurisdictions that have accepted the implied covenant as applied to employment relationships, these courts have *not* extended the doctrine to require that at-will employment be terminated only for good cause.[44] Of course, the burden is on the employee to show that there was bad faith in termination of his or her employment.[45]

Finally, it has been specifically held that the implied covenant of good faith and fair dealing may *not* apply to health care contracts.[46] However, for employees, an employer such as a hospital has a duty to investigate allegations against an employee before firing him or her; lack of investigation may be considered a violation of good faith and fair dealing.[47]

Other Statutes

Other statutes that are applicable to employer–employee relationships are relevant to the health care context. Several of these statutes are reviewed next. Also see the Family and Medical Leave Act, which was discussed in Chapter 6.

National Labor Relations Act

The National Labor Relations Act (NLRA)[48] is a federal statute that governs the relationship between employers and employees, including unionizing activities and collective bargaining over terms and conditions of employment.

[42]Murphy v. American Home Products Corp., 461 N.Y.S.2d 232 (1983); see also Orthomet v. A.B. Medical, Inc., 990 F.2d 387, 392 (8th Cir. 1993) (independent claim of breach of implied covenant of good faith and fair dealing cannot stand independent of underlying breach of contract claim); Alan's of Atlanta, Inc. v. Minolta Corp., 903 F.2d 1414, 1429 (11th Cir. 1990) (implied duty of good faith and fair dealing is not an independent contract term subject to breach apart from other contract terms but only modifies meaning of express terms); Tollefson v. Roman Catholic Bishop of San Diego, 268 Cal.Rptr. 550 (1990) (implied covenant of good faith and fair dealing cannot contradict an express contract term); Foley v. Interactive Data Corp., 254 Cal.Rptr. 211 (1988) (implied covenant of good faith and fair dealing cannot be invoked to contradict an express term and prevent employer from terminating an at-will contract); and Brehany v. Nordstrom, Inc., 812 P.2d 49 (Utah 1991) (implied covenant of good faith and fair dealing assists in interpreting contract rights but cannot add rights or override express provisions).

[43]See, e.g., Grant v. Butler, 590 So.2d 254 (Ala. 1991); Burk v. K-Mart Corp., 770 P.2d 24 (Okla. 1989); Elliott v. Tektronix, Inc., 796 P.2d 361 (Or. Ct. App. 1990); Hillesland v. Federal Land Bank Association, 407 N.W.2d 206 (N.D. 1987); Breen v. Dakota Gear & Joint Co., 433 N.W.2d 221 (S.D. 1988); Minihan v. American Pharmaceutical Association, 812 F.2d 726 (D.C. Cir. 1987); Morriss v. Coleman Co., 738 P.2d 841 (Kan. 1987); Thompson v. St. Regis Paper Co., 685 P.2d 1081 (Wash. 1984); Sadler v. Basin Electric Power Co-op, 409 N.W.2d 87 (N.D. 1987); Brandenburger v. Hilti, Inc., 556 N.E.2d 212 (Ohio Ct. App. 1989); Harrison v. Sears, Roebuck & Co., 546 N.E.2d 248 (Ill. App. Ct.), *appeal denied* 548 N.E.2d 1068 (Ill. 1989); Cockels v. International Business Expositions, Inc., 406 N.W.2d 465 (Mich. Ct. App. 1987); Keystone Carbon Co. v. Black, 599 N.E.2d 213 (Ind. Ct. App. 1992); Hostettler v. Pioneer Hi-Bred Int'l Inc., 624 F.Supp. 169 (S.D. Ind. 1985); Melnick v. State Farm Mutual Auto. Ins. Co., 749 P.2d 1105 (N.M.), *cert. denied* 488 U.S. 822 (1988); Hunt v. IBM Mid-America Employees Federal Credit Union, 384 N.W.2d 853 (Minn. 1986); Horne v. Gibson Well Serv. Co., 894 F.2d 1194 (10th Cir. 1990); Mobil Coal Producing Inc. v. Parks, 704 P.2d 702 (Wyo. 1985); Neighbors v. Kirksville College, 694 S.W.2d 822 (Mo. Ct. App. 1985); English v. General Electric Co., 765 F.Supp. 293 (E.D. N.C. 1991), *aff'd*, 977 F.2d 572 (4th Cir. 1992); Satterfield v. Lockheed Missiles & Space Co., 617 F.Supp. 1359 (D. S.C. 1985); Wyant v. SCM Corp., 692 S.W.2d 814 (Ky. Ct. App. 1985); Armstrong v. Richland Clinic, Inc., 709 P.2d 1237 (Wash. Ct. App. 1985); Magnan v. Anaconda Indus. Inc., 479 A.2d 781 (Conn. 1984); Larrabee v. Penobscot Frozen Foods, 486 A.2d 97 (Me. 1984); White v. Ardan, Inc., 430 N.W.2d 27 (Neb. 1988); Kelly v. Gill, 544 So.2d 1162 (Fla. Dist. Ct. App. 1989); Perry v. Sears, Roebuck & Co., 508 So.2d 1086 (Miss. 1987); Winograd v. WIllis, 789 S.W.2d 307 (Tex. Ct. App. 1990); Hew-Len v. F.W. Woolworth, 737 F.Supp. 1104 (D. Haw. 1990); Parnar v. Americana Hotels, Inc., 652 P.2d 625 (Haw. 1982); Shell v. Metropolitan Life Ins. Co., 396 S.E.2d 174 (W.Va. 1990).

[44]See, e.g., Crossen v. Foremost-McKesson, Inc., 537 F.Supp. 1076 (N.D. Cal. 1982) (holding that an employment agreement that expressly provides for termination at will of either party will not have an implied term not to terminate except for good cause); Magnan v. Anaconda Indus., 479 A.2d 781 (Conn. 1984) (accepting the implied covenant of good faith and fair dealing but indicating that a claim for breach cannot be based simply on the absence of good faith in the termination); Cort v. Bristol-Meyers Co., 431 N.E.2d 908 (Mass. 1982) (holding that there is no breach of good faith or fair dealing implied covenant on the basis of lack of good cause in termination, and even if employer provides a pretext or false reason for the discharge, the employer is not liable unless the actual reason is contrary to public policy); Wagenseller v. Scottsdale Mem. Hospital, 710 P.2d 1025 (Ariz. 1985) (holding that a no-cause termination of employment does not breach the implied covenant of good faith and fair dealing in an at-will employment relationship).

[45]See, e.g., Kravetz v. Merchants Distributors, Inc., 440 N.E.2d 1278, 1281 (Mass. 1982) (burden of proving breach of good faith and fair dealing implied covenant on the plaintiff-employee).

[46]See, e.g., Hrehorovich v. Harbor Hospital Center, 614 A.2d 1021 (Md. Ct. Spec. App. 1992) (holding that there is no implied covenant of good faith and fair dealing for at-will employees such as physicians on a hospital staff); Aung v. Fontenot, 1992 WL 57471 (Tex. App. Mar. 24, 1992) (no implied covenant of good faith if bargaining power between parties is not unequal).

[47]See, e.g., Crenshaw v. Bozeman Deaconess Hosp., 693 P.2d 487 (Mont. 1984).

[48]29 U.S.C.A. §§151 *et seq.*

Supervisory personnel[49] are not within the purview of the NLRA's dictates and protections.[50] Further, only employees may create unions for collective bargaining purposes; independent contractors, such as physicians, cannot, even though they have attempted to do so.[51] Note also that interns and residents are not covered by the NLRA due to their status as "students."[52] The NLRA also serves to delineate what activities are considered unfair labor practices; firing employees acting in a concerted fashion to improve the terms and conditions of employment clearly is an example of an unfair labor practice[53] and is applicable to the health care industry.[54] The National Labor Relations Board (NLRB) is the federal agency that enforces the NLRA.

The NLRA did not apply to private hospitals or other health care organizations until the 1974 Health Care Amendments were passed.[55] Health care organizations have specific treatment under the NLRA. Typically, notice for termination or modification of collective bargaining agreements in non–health care contexts requires that one party provide 60 days' notice to the other before expiration of the contract.[56] However, for health care institutions, the notice is at least 90 days; in addition, the parties must provide notice to the Federal Mediation and Conciliation Service as well as any similar state agency within 30 days of any proposed action.[57]

In addition, the NLRA prohibits a health care labor organization from striking or picketing a health care institution unless it provides a ten-day written notice, indicating the day and time of the strike; deviation from this notice requirement can occur only if the proposed action is still within 72 hours of the originally scheduled time and the health care institution is provided at least 12 hours' notice as to the actual time picketing is to begin.[58] Noncompliance with this rule constitutes an unfair labor practice. Note that, under these parameters of the NLRA, the labor organization need not be organized as a union; however, this section does not apply to strikes or picketing performed by nonunion employees.

Bargaining units in hospitals have been established by the NLRB after much litigation.[59] Generally, eight bargaining units are appropriate for acute care hospitals: physicians, registered nurses, other professional employees, technical employees, business office clerical employees, skilled maintenance employees, other nonprofessional employees, and security guards. These union units may be combined for collective bargaining but only under limited circumstances.[60]

Remedies for violations of the NLRA generally are equitable orders to cease and desist the unfair labor practice and back pay and reinstatement, if applicable, of the employees adversely affected.[61]

Title VII of the Civil Rights Act

Title VII of the Civil Rights Act of 1964 (Title VII)[62] prohibits discrimination against employees on the basis of race, color, religion (including moral and ethical beliefs and persons with atheist beliefs[63]), gender (including pregnancy), and national origin, by employers, employment agencies, and labor organizations (employment entities) that have 15 or more employees for at least 20 weeks in either the current or previous calendar year.[64] The issue in health care with regard to who is an employee and who is not is considerably complex, and courts have assessed health care employees differently.[65]

---

[49]29 U.S.C.A. §152(11).

[50]29 U.S.C.A. §152(3).

[51]29 U.S.C.A. §§157, 152(3).

[52]29 U.S.C.A. §§152(3), 158.

[53]29 U.S.C.A. §158.

[54]See, e.g., Misericordia Hosp. Med. Ctr. v. NLRB, 623 F.2d 808 (2d Cir. 1980) (hospital that fired a nurse for assisting in preparing critical report to JCAHO was ordered to reinstate the nurse); NLRB v. Mount Desert Island Hosp., 695 F.2d 634 (1st Cir. 1982) (unfair labor practice to fire employees for airing patient care concerns to newspapers); Community Hosp. of Roanoke Valley, Inc. v. NLRB, 538 F.2d 607 (4th Cir. 1976); Montefiore Hosp. and Med. Ctr. v. NLRB, 621 F.2d 510 (2d Cir. 1980).

[55]29 U.S.C.A. §152.

[56]29 U.S.C.A. §158(d)(1).

[57]29 U.S.C.A. §158(d)(3); 29 C.F.R. pt. 1420 (1998).

[58]29 U.S.C.A. §159.

[59]See American Hosp. Ass'n v. NLRB, 499 U.S. 606 (1991); 54 Fed. Reg. 16,336 (1989).

[60]See 29 U.S.C.A. §159, 29 C.F.R. §159 (1998).

[61]29 U.S.C.A. 160(c).

[62]42 U.S.C.A. §§2000e et seq.

[63]29 C.F.R. §1605.1 (1998).

[64]29 U.S.C.A. §2000e(b).

[65]See, e.g., Sibley Mem. Hosp. v. Wilson, 488 F.2d 1338 (D.C. Cir. 1973) (private duty nurse from employment registry is considered an employee of hospital under Title VII); Shrock v. Altru Nurses Registry, 810 F.2d 658 (7th Cir. 1987) (nurse from referral agency is not an employee under Title VII); Mitchell v. Frank R. Howard Mem. Hosp., 853 F.2d 762 (9th Cir. 1988), cert. denied 489 U.S. 1013 (1989) (physician with staff privileges is not an employee); Diggs v. Harris Hosp.–Methodist, Inc., 847 F.2d 270 (5th Cir.), cert. denied 488 U.S. 956 (1988) (same); Ikpoh v. Central DuPage Hosp., 1992 WL 211074 (N.D. Ill. Aug. 21, 1992) (physician is an employee not due to staff privileges but due to opportunities available controlled by hospital); Vakharia v. Swedish Covenant Hosp., 765 F.Supp. 461 (N.D. Ill. 1991) (anesthesiologist was an employee of the hospital due to the hospital's control over practice); Ross v. Beaumont Hosp., 678 F.Supp. 680 (E.D. Mich. 1988) (physician is an employee of the hospital due to the physician's committee activity and derivation of complete livelihood from the hospital); Mousavi v. Beebe Hosp. for Sussex County, 674 F.Supp. 145 (D. Del. 1987), aff'd 853 F.2d 919 (3d Cir. 1988) (physician's exclusive contract and recruitment agreement supported a Title VII employment claim); Pao v. Holy Redeemer Hosp., 547 F.Supp. 484 (E.D. Pa. 1982) (preference of patients for the hospital where provider located supports an employment relationship under Title VII).

The Equal Employment Opportunity Commission (EEOC) is the agency that enforces Title VII and has the power to file judicial actions of discrimination.[66]

Title VII claims can be tried using jury trials, and claims for monetary damages are allowed if discrimination is intentional.[67] The discrimination itself may be established through direct or circumstantial evidence. In disparate impact cases (i.e., claims of discrimination when an employer's facially neutral criteria have a disparate impact on one of the protected Title VII groups), the burden of proof can be shifted to the employer entity.[68] To bring this type of claim, the aggrieved employee must first show he or she is a member of a Title VII protected class; then, the employee must show that he or she was treated differently from an individual of another class in a similar situation. If these two criteria are shown, then the burden shifts to the employer entity to show a legitimate, nondiscriminatory reason for the treatment. If the employer entity makes such a showing, the burden then shifts back to the employee to show that the employer entity's reason is mere pretext or that the discriminatory reason was the primary basis for the employer entity's decision.

Title VII also is applicable in suits by employees claiming the employer entity engaged in a pattern or practice of discrimination against a protected class. In these cases, the employee or potential employee must show that he or she applied for a job or was deterred from applying for a job and the employer entity did not hire the applicant because of discriminatory practices. Discriminatory practices may be shown using statistical analysis.[69] If this method is used, the employer entity must then establish that the statistical analysis is faulty or inaccurate; further, the employer entity may defend a particular pattern or practice by showing the potential employee was not hired due to legitimate reasons.

More specifically, employer entities are mandated to reasonably accommodate religious beliefs and practices unless they pose an undue hardship on the business and this hardship can be demonstrated.[70] Interestingly, religious organizations and corporations are for the most part exempt from Title VII's religious discrimination mandates,[71] although employer entities that wish to "inject"

religious beliefs and practices into the workplace are subject to the prohibitions of Title VII.[72]

With regard to gender discrimination, Title VII mandates that employer entities apply similar performance and evaluation standards for both genders. In addition, Title VII prohibits sexual harassment and discrimination on the basis of gender stereotypes.[73] What is important to note, however, is that Title VII gender discrimination mandates do not extend to sexual orientation[74] nor to sexual attractiveness, sexual activity, or sexual morality.[75]

Sexual harassment cases are generally divided into two classes, generally referred to as *quid pro quo* cases and *hostile environment* cases. Using the totality of circumstances to assess the claims, quid pro quo harassment is present when employer entities require sexual favors from a subordinate to obtain economic or job benefits or if employer entities punish a subordinate employee for refusing these advances.[76] Note that an employer entity may be liable for the actions of its agents and supervisors for such harassment if the employer entity knew or should have known of its occurrence.[77] Hostile environment cases occur when unwelcome sexual advances, requests for sexual favors, or other verbal or physical conduct of a sexual nature exists in the workplace.[78] Employer entities have significant potential liability in these circumstances, since they may be liable for constructive discharge due to the harassment if the harassment made the working situation too onerous to stay, for conduct of other employees if the employer entity knew or should have known of the harassment (unless the employer entity took immediate and appropriate action), or even for the conduct of nonemployees if the employer knew or should have known of the conduct and failed to take appro-

---

[66]42 U.S.C.A. §2000e-4.

[67]42 U.S.C.A. §§1981a(a)(1), 1981a(b), 1981a(c).

[68]See, e.g., McDonnell Douglas Corp. v. Green Corp., 411 U.S. 792 (1973).

[69]International Brotherhood of Teamsters v. United States, 431 U.S. 324 (1977).

[70]42 U.S.C.A. §2000e(j); see also Trans World Airlines, Inc. v. Hardison, 432 U.S. 63 (1977) (religious need to not work Saturday unreasonable because employer would be required to pay a premium to other workers to cover Saturday shifts).

[71]42 U.S.C.A. §2000e-1.

[72]See, e.g., EEOC v. Townlety Engineering & Mfg. Co., 859 F.2d 610 (9th Cir. 1988), *cert. denied* 489 U.S. 1077 (1989); EEOC v. Kamehameha Schools, 990 F.2d 458 (9th Cir. 1993).

[73]See, e.g., Price Waterhouse v. Hopkins, 490 U.S. 228 (1989) (employer engaged in gender discrimination when evaluating an employee on basis of female stereotypes).

[74]See, e.g., DeSantis v. Pacific Telephone & Telegraph Co., 608 F.2d 327 (9th Cir. 1979); Williamson v. A.G. Edwards and Sons, Inc., 876 F.2d 69 (8th Cir.), *cert. denied* 493 U.S. 1089 (1989); see also Wrightson v. Pizza Hut of America, Inc., 99 F.3d 138 (4th Cir. 1996); DeCintio v. Westchester County Med. Ctr., 807 F.2d 304 (2d Cir. 1986); Fox v. Sierra Development Co., 876 F.Supp. 1169 (D. Nev. 1995).

[75]See, e.g., Thomas v. Metroflight, Inc., 814 F.2d 1506 (10th Cir. 1987).

[76]See, e.g., Chamberlin v. 101 Realty, Inc., 915 F.2d 777 (1st Cir. 1990); Henson v. City of Dundee, 682 F.2d 897 (11th Cir. 1982); Dees v. Johnson Controls World Servs., Inc., 938 F.Supp. 861 (S.D. Ga. 1996); see also Sparks v. Pilot Freight Carriers, Inc., 830 F.2d 1554 (11th Cir. 1987); Does 1,2,3, and 4 v. Covington County School Bd., 969 F.Supp. 1264 (M.D. Ala. 1997).

[77]29 C.F.R. §1604.11(c) (1998).

[78]29 C.F.R. §1604.11(a) (1998).

priate action.[79] To show such harassment, the employee must establish that the complained-of conduct unreasonably interfered with the employee's work or created an intimidating, hostile, or offensive work environment[80] and that the conduct was unwelcome.[81]

However, note that Title VII does allow employer entities to make employment decisions on the basis of religion, gender, and national origin if there is a bona fide occupational qualification that is reasonably necessary for business operations (e.g., gender-specific lavatory attendants).[82] Class stereotypes cannot be used in determining bona fide occupational qualifications.[83]

Title VII remedies generally are focused on the EEOC. The employee first must make his or her charges against the employer within 180 days of occurrence of the discrimination.[84] The EEOC then investigates the claim and, if a violation has been found, uses informal methods by which to try to resolve the dispute.[85] If informal methods are not successful within 30 days, the EEOC may then bring a civil action against the employer (although it is prohibited from suing a government or government agency; the U.S. Attorney General has jurisdiction over these claims).[86] Individuals may intervene if the EEOC (or Attorney General) files suit. In addition, if the EEOC (or Attorney General) does not file a suit, individuals may file their own suit within 90 days of such EEOC (or Attorney General) notice of nonsuit.[87] It is important to note that administrative remedies with the EEOC must be exhausted before an employee may sue.[88] Employee suits must be filed in federal court, and remedies available to aggrieved employees include equitable orders against unlawful practices, back pay, reinstatement, rehiring, and possibly attorneys' fees.[89]

Americans with Disabilities Act

The Americans with Disabilities Act (ADA)[90] prohibits discrimination on the basis of disabilities in the areas of employment, public transportation, public accommodation, and telecommunications. These mandates apply to employer entities,[91] including the employer entities' agents, with 15 or more employees, working or having worked 20 or more weeks in the current or previous calendar year. Part-time workers are counted in this assessment.

With regard to employment, generally the ADA protects individuals who are qualified with a disability; further, the ADA's protections extend to discrimination by employer entities against individuals associated with an individual with a known disability.[92] Note that employer entities must make applications and application sites accessible to individuals with disabilities, employer entities must provide assistance if needed for applicants to provide the information, and employer entities must limit their application inquiries to performance of essential job functions. However, an employer entity may require that applicants successfully complete a physical examination after a conditional job offer is given, as long as all individuals are required to do so.[93] This examination may be the basis for rescinding the offer if the individuals pose a direct threat to health or safety.

A qualified employee is one who has "the skill, experience, education, and other job-related requirements of a position held or desired, and who, with or without reasonable accommodation, can perform the essential functions of a job."[94] An individual with a disability is one who has "a physical or mental impairment that substantially limits one or more of his or her major life activities,"[95] or an individual regarded as having such an impairment, or an individual who has a record of such impairment.[96] A *major life activity* is defined in the regulations as functions including (but not limited to) caring for one's self, walking, seeing, speak-

---

[79] 29 C.F.R. §§1604.11(d) (1998), 1604.11(e) (1998); see also Splunge v. Shoney's Inc., 97 F.3d 488 (11th Cir. 1996) (constructive knowledge adequate for liability against employer in sexual harassment case); Varner v. National Super Markets, Inc., 94 F.3d 1209 (8th Cir. 1996), *cert. denied* 117 S.Ct. 946 (1997) (employer liable for sexual harassment despite policy of reporting such actions and employee not following such policy due to failure of employer to take appropriate corrective action).

[80] See, e.g., Ellison v. Brady, 924 F.2d 872 (9th Cir. 1991); Fuller v. City of Oakland, 47 F.3d 1522 (9th Cir. 1995); Fox v. Sierra Development Co., 876 F.Supp. 1169 (D. Nev. 1995); see also Ransom v. Secretary of Navy, 977 F.2d 590 (9th Cir. 1992); Henson v. City of Dundee, 682 F.2d 897 (11th Cir. 1982).

[81] See, e.g., Meritor Savings Bank, FSB v. Vinson, 477 U.S. 57 (1986); see also T.L. v. Toys 'R' Us, Inc., 605 A.2d 1125 (N.J. Super. Ct. App. Div. 1992); Lipsett v. University of Puerto Rico, 864 F.2d 881 (1st Cir. 1988).

[82] 29 U.S.C.A. §623(f)(1).

[83] See, e.g., Weeks v. Southern Bell Telephone & Telegraph Co., 408 F.2d 228 (5th Cir. 1969) (heavy lifting not a bona fide occupational qualification justifying exclusion of women).

[84] 42 U.S.C.A. §2000e-5(e)(1).

[85] 42 U.S.C.A. §2000e-5(b).

[86] 42 U.S.C.A. §2000e-5(f)(1).

[87] 42 U.S.C.A. §2000e-5(f)(1).

[88] See, e.g., Shannon v. Ford Motor Co., 72 F.3d 678 (8th Cir. 1996) (compliance with administrative process is a prerequisite to filing suit).

[89] 42 U.S.C.A. §§2000e-5(g)(1)–2000e-5(k).

[90] 42 U.S.C.A. §§12101 *et seq.*

[91] 29 C.F.R. §1630.2(b) (1998).

[92] 29 C.F.R. §1630.8 (1998).

[93] 29 C.F.R. §1630.14(a) (1998).

[94] 29 C.F.R. §1630.2(m) (1998).

[95] 29 C.F.R. §1630.2(g)(1) (1998).

[96] 29 C.F.R. §§1630.2(g)(2) (1998), 1630.2(g)(3) (1998), 1630.2(h)(1) (1998), 1630.2(h)(2) (1998).

ing, and working.[97] The substantial limitation requirement is quite broad[98] but does not include inability to perform a *single* job; rather, it must be a *class* of jobs.[99] The essential functions of a particular job are assessed on the basis of whether the position exists to perform the function, a limited number of employees are available to perform the function, the position with the function requires an individual with special expertise, and removing the function from the position would fundamentally change the job.[100] To determine whether the function is essential, assessment of the following factors is important: the employer's judgment, the written job description, the amount of time spent performing the function, the result of not requiring an individual in the job to perform the function, the terms of a collective bargaining agreement, and the work experience of people who have performed the job in the past and who currently perform similar jobs.[101] What constitutes reasonable accommodation is extremely varied and intentionally broad.[102] However, accommodations that impose an undue hardship on employers (i.e., that would be unduly costly, extensive, substantial, or destructive or that would fundamentally alter business operations) are not required.[103] Note that employer entities must have knowledge of the need for reasonable accommodation for liability to attach.[104]

Several conditions do not qualify for protection under the ADA. The ADA does not protect: individuals *currently* using illegal drugs, transvestitism, transsexualism, pedophilia, exhibitionism, voyeurism, gender identity disorders, sexual behavior disorders, compulsive gambling, kleptomania, pyromania, homosexuality, and bisexuality.[105] Other claims of disability that are in conflict with employee statements, that are temporary or emotionally based with minimal residual effects, or that are self-imposed are not within the purview of ADA.[106] There is a significant amount of disagreement within the courts with respect to pregnancy and fertility as the basis of ADA claims.[107] In addition, an employer entity may refuse to hire an individual if he or she poses a direct threat to the health or safety of the individual or others.[108]

---

[97] 29 C.F.R. §1630.2(i) (1998); see also Bragdon v. Abbott, 524 U.S. 624 (1998) (holding that *major life activity* includes reproduction and is implicated in an asymptomatic HIV patient's ADA claim against a provider).

[98] 29 C.F.R. §1630.2(j) (1998).

[99] 29 C.F.R. §1630.2(j)(3) (1998); see also Bridges v. City of Bossier, 92 F.3d 329 (5th Cir. 1996), *cert. denied* 117 S.Ct. 770 (1997) (inability to perform a single, particular job does not constitute substantial limitation in the major life activity of working).

[100] 29 C.F.R. §§1630.2(n)(1) (1998), 1630.2(n)(2) (1998).

[101] 29 C.F.R. §1630.2(n)(3) (1998).

[102] 29 C.F.R. §1630.2(o) (1998).

[103] 29 C.F.R. §1630.2(p) (1998); see also Monette v. Electronic Data Systems Corp., 90 F.3d 1173 (6th Cir. 1996) (employer holding a job open for an employee without knowledge of if or when employee will return an undue hardship); Eckles v. Consolidated Rail Corp., 94 F.3d 1041 (7th Cir. 1996), *cert. denied* 117 S.Ct. 1318 (1997) (accommodation that would have conflicted with collective bargaining agreement is not an appropriate reasonable accommodation); Garza v. Abbott Labs., 940 F.Supp. 1227 (N.D. Ill. 1996) (employee who proposes an accommodation must show that the accommodation would allow performance of the job and the costs do not substantially outweigh the benefits).

[104] See, e.g., Beck v. University of Wis. Bd. of Regents, 75 F.3d 1130 (7th Cir. 1996); Simpkins v. Specialty Envelope Inc., 94 F.3d 645 (6th Cir. 1996); Taylor v. Principal Financial Group, Inc., 93 F.3d 155 (5th Cir.), *cert. denied* 117 S.Ct. 586 (1996); Tan v. Runyon, 91 F.3d 133 (4th Cir. 1996); Hedberg v. Indiana Bell Telephone Co., 47 F.3d 928 (7th Cir. 1995).

[105] 29 C.F.R. §§1630.3(a) (1998), 1630.3(d) (1998), 1630.3(e) (1998).

[106] See, e.g., McNemar v. Disney Store, Inc., 91 F.3d 610 (3d Cir. 1996), *cert. denied* 117 S.Ct. 958 (1997) (HIV-positive person cannot support ADA claim if, on the one hand, he claims he is disabled, and on the other, he can work); Kennedy v. Applause Inc., 90 F.3d 1477 (9th Cir. 1996) (ADA claim not supported by an employee's statement on a disability benefits application that employee was totally disabled but that reasonable accommodation would have allowed her to perform her job); Sanders v. Arneson Products, Inc., 91 F.3d 1351 (9th Cir. 1996), *cert. denied* 117 S.Ct. 1247 (1997) (emotional leaves that are temporary with little residual effects do not qualify as disabilities under ADA); Johnson v. New York Hosp., 96 F.3d 33 (2d Cir. 1996) (vacationing nurse who came to workplace drunk and engaged in violent actions could be discharged even though alcoholism may be a disability under ADA); Dauen v. Board of Fire and Police Comm'rs, 656 N.E.2d 427 (Ill. App. Ct. 1995) (employee firing due to commission of a crime does not violate ADA); Siefken v. Village of Arlington Heights, 65 F.3d 664 (7th Cir. 1995) (firing of diabetic after blackout behind wheel of police car not in violation of ADA due to employee not making effort to control disease).

[107] See, e.g., Banks v. Hit or Miss, Inc., 946 F.Supp. 569 (N.D. Ill. 1996) (heel and bone spurs from pregnancy resulting in inability to walk a disability under the ADA); Cerrato v. Durham, 941 F.Supp. 388 (S.D. N.Y. 1996) (pregnancy-related conditions a disability under ADA due to an impairment of reproductive system); Patterson v. Xerox Corp., 901 F.Supp. 274 (N.D. Ill. 1995) (pregnancy not a disability but resulting conditions may be considered disabilities for purpose of ADA); Pacourek v. Inland Steel Co., 916 F.Supp. 797 (N.D. Ill 1996) (infertility a disability under ADA on basis of reproduction as a major life activity); but see Zatarain v. WDSU-Television, Inc., 881 F.Supp. 240 (E.D. La. 1995), *aff'd* 79 F.3d 1143 (5th Cir. 1996) (infertility may not be basis for ADA claim); Krauel v. Iowa Methodist Med. Ctr., 915 F.Supp. 102 (S.D. Iowa 1995), *aff'd* 95 F.3d 674 (8th Cir. 1996) (same).

[108] See, e.g., EEOC v. Kinney Shoe Corp., 917 F.Supp. 419 (W.D. Va. 1996), *aff'd* Martinson v. Kinney Shoe Corp, 104 F.3d 683 (4th Cir. 1997) (firing of an employee with epileptic seizures that disrupted store is permissible); Moses v. American Nonwovens, Inc., 97 F.3d 446 (11th Cir. 1996), *cert. denied* 117 S.Ct. 964 (1997) (an employee with epileptic seizures working near fast moving press machines and rollers could be fired without violating ADA because there was no way to accommodate his disability).

Remedies for ADA violations include equitable relief such as is available under Title VII, provision of employee back pay, hiring the applicant, reinstatement of the employee, promotion of the employee, reasonable accommodation for the employee, and provision of "front pay" (i.e., financial compensation instead of reinstatement if reinstatement is not appropriate or possible[109]); attorneys' fees and other legal costs may also be available.[110] As well, compensatory and punitive damages may be available in cases of intentional discrimination.[111]

Age Discrimination in Employment Act

The Age Discrimination in Employment Act of 1967 (ADEA)[112] prohibits discrimination against individuals who are 40 years of age or older. The ADEA is applicable to employers with 20 or more employees who work at least 20 weeks per year. The statute is derived mostly from Title VII and its general interpretation follows it. Overall, the ADEA mandates that employer entities may not discriminate on the basis of age in the hiring, firing, or denying employment of an employee.[113]

Further Reading

Employees—At-Will Employment

Calamari JD, Perillo JM. *Contracts,* 3d ed. St. Paul, MN: West Publishing Co., 1987;61–63.
Fick BJ. *The American Bar Association Guide to Workplace Law: Everything You Need to Know About Your Rights as an Employee or Employer.* Chicago: American Bar Association, 1997.
Liang BA. Deselection Under *Harper v. Healthsource:* A Blow for Maintaining Patient-Physician Relationships in the Era of Managed Care? *Notre Dame L Rev* 1997;72:799–861.

Employees—Good Faith and Fair Dealing Exception

Calamari JD, Perillo JM. *Contracts,* 3d ed. St. Paul, MN: West Publishing Co., 1987;508–12.
Liang BA. Deselection Under *Harper v. Healthsource:* A Blow for Maintaining Patient-Physician Relationships in the Era of Managed Care? *Notre Dame L Rev* 1997;72:799–861.

Schaber GD, Rohwer CD. *Contracts: In a Nutshell,* 3d ed. St. Paul, MN: West Publishing Co., 1987;§§95–96.

Employees—Implied In-Fact Contract Exception

Calamari JD, Perillo JM. *Contracts,* 3d ed. St. Paul, MN: West Publishing Co., 1987;61–63.
Liang BA. Deselection Under *Harper v. Healthsource:* A Blow for Maintaining Patient-Physician Relationships in the Era of Managed Care? *Notre Dame L Rev* 1997;72:799–861.
Schaber GD, Rohwer CD. *Contracts: In a Nutshell,* 3d ed. St. Paul, MN: West Publishing Co., 1987;§142.

Employees—Public Policy Exception

Kuhlmann-Macro VF. Blowing the Whistle on the Employment At-Will Doctrine. *Drake L Rev* 1992;41:339–50.
Liang BA. Deselection Under *Harper v. Healthsource:* A Blow for Maintaining Patient-Physician Relationships in the Era of Managed Care? *Notre Dame L Rev* 1997;72:799–861.
Timmernan TR. Legislative Attempts to Modify the Employment At-Will Doctrine: Will the Public Policy Exception Be the Next Step? *J Corp L* 1988;14:241–64.
Westman DP. Implied Limitations on Employer's Exercise of Discretion in At-Will Setting. *PLI/LIT* 1997;558:605–61.

Independent Contractors

Fishman S. *Hiring Independent Contractors: The Employers' Legal Guide.* Berkeley, CA: Nolo Press, 1997.
Keeton WP et al. *Prosser and Keeton on Torts,* 5th ed. St. Paul, MN: West Publishing Co., 1984;509–16.
Kionka EJ. *Torts: In a Nutshell,* 2d ed. St. Paul, MN: West Publishing Co., 1992;§8–12.
Shenson HL. *The Contract and Fee-Setting Guide for Consultants and Professionals.* New York: John Wiley & Sons, 1989.

Other Statutes—Age Discrimination in Employment Act

Lake MB. *Age Discrmination in Employment Act: A Compliance and Litigation Manual for Lawyers and Personnel Practitioners.* Washington, DC: Equal Employment Advisory Council, 1982.
Moberly MD. Reconsidering the Discriminatory Motive Requirement in ADEA Disparate Treatment Cases. *N M L Rev* 1994;24:89–124.
Rutherglen G. From Race to Age: The Expanding Scope of Employment Discrimination Law. *J Legal Stud* 1995;24:491–521.
Ziegler M. Disparate Impact Analysis and the Age Discrimination in Employment Act. *Minn L Rev* 1984;68:1038–76.

---

[109]See, e.g., Fitzgerald v. Sirloin Stockade Inc., 624 F.2d 945 (10th Cir. 1980).
[110]42 U.S.C.A. §12117(a).
[111]42 U.S.C.A. §1983.
[112]29 U.S.C.A. §§621 *et seq.*
[113]29 U.S.C.A. §623(a)(1)

Other Statutes—Americans with Disabilities Act

Anderson WL, Roth ML. Deciphering the Americans with Disabilities Act. *Mo B J* 1995;51:142–47.

Breen PM. The Americans with Disabilities Act: Planning for Compliance. *Practising Law Institute* 1991;412:233–47.

Court PG, O'Conner LK. A Selected Bibliography on Employment and the Americans with Disabilities Act. *Cornell J L & Pub Pol'y* 1992;2:63–87.

Dickson M, Keppler K. *The Americans with Disabilities Act: Hiring, Accommodating and Supervising Employees with Disabilities.* Menlo Park, CA: Crisp Publications, 1995.

Pfeiffer D, Finn J. Survey Shows State, Territorial, Local Public Officials Implementing ADA. *Mental & Physical Disability L Rep* 1995;19:537–39.

Terry E. *Americans with Disabilities Act Facilities Compliance: A Practical Guide.* New York: John Wiley & Sons, 1992.

Other Statutes—National Labor Relations Act

Heilman MJ. The National Labor Relations Act at Fifty: Roots Revisited, Heart Rediscovered. *Duq L Rev* 1985;23:1059–82.

Lipsky AA. Participatory Management Schemes, the Law, and Workers' Rights: A Proposed Framework Analysis. *Am U L Rev* 1990;39:667–720.

Other Statutes—Title VII of the Civil Rights Act

Bourdeau JA. Individual Liability of Supervisors, Managers, or Officers for Discriminatory Actions. In: *American Law Reports, Federal.* New York: Lawyers Cooperative Publishing Co., 1997;131:221–91.

Buckley JF. Discrimination in Employment: Title VII of the Civil Rights Act of 1964. In: *Texas Jurisprudence,* 3d ed. New York: Lawyers Cooperative Publishing Co., 1993;12:§19.

Jovanovic TB. Title VII of Civil Rights Act of 1964. In: *New York Jurisprudence,* 2d ed. New York: Lawyers Cooperative Publishing Co., 1998;18:§6.

Other Reading

Behinfar DJ. Exclusive Contracting Between Hospitals and Physicians and the Use of Economic Credentialing. *DePaul J Health Care Law* 1996;1:71–91.

Borkon PE. Commentary: Exclusive Contracts: Are Constructively Terminated Incumbent Physicians Entitled to a Fair Hearing? *J Legal Med* 1996;17:143–68.

Cooper A. Restrictive Covenants. *JAMA* 1982;248:3091–92.

Fisher R, Ury W. *Getting to YES,* 2d ed. Boston: Houghton-Mifflin, 1991.

Jurgeleit PB. Note: Physician Employment Under Managed Care: Toward a Retaliatory Discharge Cause of Action for HMO-Affiliated Physicians. *Ind L J* 1997;73:255–96.

King JV, Liang BA. The Silencing of the Physician: Gag Rules in a Managed Care Environment. *Hosp. Phys* 1998;34(7):64–69.

Liang BA. Deselection Under *Harper v. Healthsource:* A Blow for Maintaining Patient-Physician Relationships in the Era of Managed Care? *Notre Dame L Rev* 1997;72:799–861.

Liang BA. General Considerations for Managed Care Contracting. *Hosp Phys* 1995;31(5):41–51.

Liang BA. An Overview and Analysis of Challenges to Medical Exclusive Contracts. *J Legal Med* 1997;18:1–45.

Liang BA. The Practical Utility of Gag Clause Legislation. *J Gen Int Med* 1998;13:419–21.

Liang BA. Understanding and Applying Alternative Dispute Resolution Methods in Modern Medical Conflicts. *J Legal Med* 1998;19:397–430.

Lowe MR. Stirring Muddled Waters: Are Physicians with Hospital Medical Staff Privileges Considered to Be Employees Under Title VII or the Disabilities Act When Alleging an Employment Discrimination Claim? *Labor Lawyer* 1997;13:225–62.

Web Sites

Americans with Disabilities Act home page: *http://www.usdoj.gov/crt/ada/adahom1.htm*

Americans with Disabilities Act document center: *http://janweb.icdi.wvu.edu/kinder/*

The Family and Medical Leave Act pro—Department of Labor FMLA hotline: *http://www.fmla.com/fmlalink.html*

A guide to basic law and procedures under the National Labor Relations Act: *http://www.ibewfifthdistrict.org/legal.htm*

Human resources policy: *http://www.ppspublishers.com/home.htm*

The independent contractor report: *http://workerstatus.com/*

Independent contractor resources: *http://www.altstaffing.com/index.html*

Independent contractor vs. employee—Do you know which you are?: *http://www.bizcoach.org/independ.htm*

Labor law resources: *http://www.dsmo.com/laborres.htm*

Nolo's Legal Encyclopedia—Independent contractors: *http://www.nolo.com/ic/*

Title VII, Civil Rights Act of 1964: *http://www.dol.gov/dol/oasam/public/regs/statutes/2000e-16.htm*

11
Licensure and Practice Regulation

To practice medicine,[1] an individual generally must be licensed by the state in which he or she wishes to practice. The state has the power to regulate health care professionals under the state's police power to protect the health, safety, and general welfare of the community.[2] Once an individual is granted a license by the state, he or she can practice medicine; therefore, a state license is an extremely valuable property right.[3] Since a medical license represents a property right, specific procedures must be fulfilled before a license can be suspended or revoked. A quasi-public entity, usually called a *Board of Medical Examiners* or *Medical Licensing Board,* composed of medical professionals as well as others, is given jurisdiction by a state medical practice act or similar statute to grant medical licensure, monitor the actions of physicians within the state, and discipline errant practitioners within its purview.[4] In addition, these boards have the authority to review and discipline those who attempt to practice medicine but are not authorized to do so.

Other agreements also may limit the scope and ability to practice. Individual hospital grants of staff and clinical privileges as well as private covenants not to compete provide the basis on which an individual practitioner, although licensed, may be limited in what services he or she can provide and to whom those services may be provided.

State Licensure and Revocation

Individual state medical examining boards typically set the qualification standards and rules by which licenses to practice medicine are granted. Licensing by these boards is based on overlapping concerns that unqualified practice could pose a serious risk to an individual patient's health, safety, or economic well-being; this risk would be likely to occur without a licensing system; the public could not adequately assess a practitioner's qualifications without guidance; and the benefits of licensure would be greater than the potential harmful effects of licensing. Those with a license to practice may perform the services that are indicated by state law; those without cannot. Note that certification or registration is separate and distinct from licensure. Even though certification and registration may prescribe certain qualifications and rules for an individual to be certified or registered, generally persons not so certified or registered still may perform services that certified or registered practitioners perform. In contrast, only licensed practitioners may perform the activities covered by licensure.

Physicians in the United States generally must sit for examinations as well as show proof of postgraduate training to obtain a medical license within a state. Other requirements also may need to be fulfilled, such as a personal interview.[5] Note that licensure assessments may

---

[1]This chapter uses the physician and physician licensure as a model for state licensing considerations. These considerations will be similar for other medical personnel, including nurses, chiropractors, and psychologists, and their respective boards.

[2]See, e.g., Barsky v. Board of Regents, 347 U.S. 442 (1954); Graves v. Minnesota, 272 U.S. 425 (1926); Reetz v. Michigan, 188 U.S. 505 (1903); Hawker v. New York, 170 U.S. 189 (1898); Lambert v. Yellowley, 272 U.S. 581 (1926); Dent v. West Virginia, 129 U.S. 114 (1889).

[3]See, e.g., Damino v. O'Neil, 702 F.Supp 949 (E.D.N.Y. 1987); Balian v. Board of Licensure in Medicine, 722 A.2d 362 (ME 1999); Telong v. Commonwealth of Pa., 714 A.2d 1109 (Comm. Ct. Pa. 1998).

[4]See, e.g., Graves v. Minn., 272 U.S. 425 (1926); State v. Rosenkrans, 75 A. 491 (R.I. 1925), *aff'd* 225 U.S. 698 (1912); Douglas v. Noble, 261 U.S. 165 (1923).

[5]See, e.g., *Colorado Revised Statutes Annotated* (St. Paul, MN: West, 1998), section 12-36-107; *Florida Statutes Annotated* (St. Paul, MN: West, 1998), section 458.311; *Official Compilation Rules and Regulations of the State of Georgia* r. 360-2-.01 (1998); *Hawaii Revised Statutes Annotated* (Charlottesville, VA: Michie, 1997), section 453-2; *Iowa Code Annotated* (St. Paul, MN: West, 1997), section 148.3; *New Jersey Administrative Code* tit. 13, §35-3.2 (1998); *New Mexico Statutes Annotated* (Charlottesville, VA: Michie, 1998), section 61-6-11; 49 *Pennsylvania Code* §§17.1–17.8; 22 *Texas Administrative Code* (St. Paul, MN: West, 1998), section 166.2 (West 1998); *Wisconsin Administrative Code* §1.02 (1998).

include evidence of good moral character and ethics.[6] In the past, most physicians fulfilled the examination portion of licensure through passing the National Board of Medical Examiners examination or the Federal Licensing Examination.[7] However, since December 1993, these examinations have been replaced by the United States Medical Licensing Examination (USMLE), which is composed of three parts or steps. Step 1 tests information related to biomedical sciences and concepts describing underlying disease and therapy. Step 1 generally is taken at the end of the second year of medical school. Step 2 tests concepts of clinical sciences in a supervised setting and generally is taken at the end of the third year of medical school. Finally, Step 3 tests concepts of clinical sciences in a nonsupervised setting and generally is taken after the first year of postgraduate training. The USMLE may be taken for licensing purposes by students and physicians who attend medical school or train both in the United States and abroad.

Once examination, training, and other state-specific requirements are met, physicians and other health care workers are granted a time-limited license to practice. However, state medical boards also have the power, after an administrative hearing by the board, to revoke or suspend medical licenses if a practitioner violates the state-prescribed statutory or administrative standards and rules. Note that injury to patients or proof of such injury is not a prerequisite for these actions.[8] This is the area most replete with legal challenge in medical licensing.

The practitioner must be provided with adequate prior notice of the hearing by the board or a hearing officer and the opportunity to present his or her case before

any suspension or revocation of his or her medical license can occur; that is, he or she must be provided with due process before the board, representing the state, takes away the valuable property right of licensure.[9] The board may suspend a practitioner's license summarily without a hearing if allowing the practitioner to continue practice would endanger the public. However, this action must be followed by a prompt due process hearing.[10]

The notice encompasses specification of both the time of the hearing and the charges to be brought against the provider. Generally, notice difficulties are challenged on the latter basis,[11] although notice of the time of the hearing has been challenged because the notice did not provide adequate time for preparation of the practitioner's

---

[6]See, e.g., Hawker v. New York, 170 U.S. 189 (1898); Barnes v. State, 151 So.2d 619 (Ala. 1963); Hughes v. State Bd. of Medical Examiners, 134 S.E. 42 (Ga. 1926); Gilpin v. Bd. of Nursing, Dept. of Commerce, 837 P.2d 1342 (Mont. 1992); Horoshko v. Ambach, 504 N.Y.S.2d 838 (N.Y. App. Div. 1986); Bevacqua v. Sobol, 579 N.Y.S.2d 243 (N.Y. App. Div. 1992).

[7]American Medical Association, *Medical Licensure Statistics and Current Licensure Requirements* (Chicago: American Medical Association, 1991).

[8]See, e.g., Colorado v. Hoffner, 832 P.2d 1062 (Colo. Ct. App. 1992); Kearl v. Board of Med. Quality Assurance, 236 Cal.Rptr. 526 (Cal. Ct. App. 1986); In re Guess, 393 S.E.2d 833 (N.C. 1990); Medical Licensing Bd. of Indiana v. Ward, 449 N.E.2d 1129 (Ind. Ct. App. 1983); see also Wassermann v. Board of Regents, 182 N.E.2d 264 (N.Y. 1962); Colorado St. Bd. of Med. Examiners v. Boyle, 924 P.2d 1113 (Colo. Ct. App. 1996).

[9]See, e.g., Dent v. State of West Virginia, 129 U.S. 114 (1889); Semler v. Oregon State Bd. of Dental Examiners, 294 U.S. 608 (1935); Greenfield v. Hamrick, 341 So.2d 136 (Ala. 1976); Aylward v. State Bd. of Chiropractic Examiners, 192 P.2d 929 (Cal. 1948); Wills v. Composite Bd., 384 S.E.2d 636 (Ga. 1989); Fleury v. Clayton, 847 F.2d 1229 (7th Cir. 1988); Lowe v. Scott, 959 F.2d 323 (1st Cir. 1992).

[10]See, e.g., Barry v. Barchi, 443 U.S. 55 (1979).

[11]See, e.g., Jutkowitz v. Department of Health Serv., 596 A.2d 374 (Conn. 1991) (notice of legal basis on which chiropractor licensed was challenged, although somewhat unclear, still served as adequate notice for the charge against the licensee); Re Van Hyning, 241 N.W. 207 (Mich. 1932) (in an administrative proceeding, charges in practitioner notice not required to be stated as clearly as they would be if stated by an attorney for adequate notice); Melone v. State Educ. Dept., 495 N.Y.S.2d 808 (N.Y. App. Div. 1985) (dentist accused of sexual contacts with patients ranging in age from 7 to 15 at different times between 1981 and 1983 was found to have adequate notice and was not required to be presented with specific dates for each action); Amarnick v. Sobol, 569 N.Y.S.2d 780 (N.Y. App. Div. 1991) (statute for disciplinary action does not require administrative body to identify each element for each misconduct charge for notice purposes); Med. Licensing Bd. v. Ward, 449 N.E.2d 1129 (Ind. Ct. App. 1983) (in state board proceedings revoking chiropractor's license for massaging genitalia of female patients was not in violation of due process when term used in charge was *vagina*); cf. State Licensing Bd. for Healing Arts v. Alabama Bd. of Podiatry, 249 So.2d 611 (Ala. 1971) (letter from state board merely stating podiatrist should appear before state board on a given date and listing a general state code section failed in notice specificity and thus due process notice requirement); Schaffer v. State Bd. of Vet. Med., 237 S.E.2d 510 (Ga. Ct. App. 1977) (notice of hearing failing to specify statement of facts on which board was relying for revocation of license was inadequate for due process purposes); Celaya v. Dept. of Prof. Reg., Bd. of Med., 560 So.2d 383 (Fla. Dist. Ct. App. 1990) (board did not provide adequate notice or due process when it questioned physician and reached the conclusion to revoke his license on the basis of matters not alleged in the administrative complaint against him); Burdge v. State Bd. of Med. Examiners, 403 S.E.2d 114 (S.C. 1991) (board decision to revoke a physician's license, where the complaint was based on incompetent care and violation of protocol but the decision was based on falsifying documents, is overturned since the administrative complaint did not give the physician notice of the allegations on which the board decision was based).

case[12] and in circumstances when a rescheduled hearing time is not provided to the practitioner and actions are taken against him or her at the rescheduled hearing.[13] The policy of requiring a notice is to allow the practitioner a full and fair opportunity to challenge the charges against him or her. However, it is important to note that failure to object to an inadequate notice and demand a remedy generally waives the defects in the notice by the practitioner.[14]

Although notice and an opportunity to be heard are necessary for a valid hearing, practitioners usually are not entitled to a level of proceeding that mirrors a judicial proceeding; that is, a practitioner need not be told that he or she has a right to legal counsel,[15] the charges by the board need not meet the level of specificity as in a criminal trial,[16] nor does the board need to provide notice as to the witnesses who will be at the hearing or the materials to be

used in it.[17] However, the practitioner may call and cross-examine witnesses. Challenges in this area generally focus on whether the practitioner was given an adequate opportunity to cross-examine witnesses, with the results, as in the notice area, a general function of state law.[18]

Finally, note that there is no requirement that the practitioner be in attendance for the hearing to be valid, as long as the practitioner had adequate notice.[19] In addition, courts have held that the administrative powers of the board allow it to make its decision on the record of the proceedings alone;[20] full hearings often are not required when disciplinary sanctions are based on criminal convictions,[21] find-

---

[12]See, e.g., State *ex rel.* Tullidge v. Hollingsworth, 146 So. 660 (Fla.), *later proceeding* 158 So. 277 (Fla. 1933) (action of the board revoking the license is invalid because physician was not served with charges against him); Rhodes v. Oregon State Vet. Med. Examining Bd., 223 P.2d 804 (Or. 1950) (board action revoking the license is invalid because no evidence showed practitioner ever was served with notice); State *ex rel.* Frenzel v. Wyoming State Bd. of Examiners, 74 P.2d 343 (Wyo. 1937) (state board actions are invalid because board is under duty to give notice that never was received); Colorado St. Bd. of Med. Examiners v. Palmer, 400 P.2d 914 (Colo. 1965) (board that received returned notice and provided actual notice only two days before hearing was inadequate due to statutory requirement of 30 days); Grether v. Indiana St. Bd. of Dental Examiners, 159 N.E.2d 131 (Ind. 1959) (when statute conflicted between requirement of 5 or 15 days' notice for license hearing, statutory construction required that 15-day notice be applied), cf. Cooper v. Board of Med. Examiners, 123 Cal.Rptr. 563 (Cal. Ct. App. 1975) (adequate notice on basis of statutory definition); Davis v. Arizona State Dental Bd., 112 P.2d 877 (Ariz. 1941) (dentist given notice of charges on which license to practice hearing was based received the notice after the hearing had begun but before it finished was deemed to have adequate notice); Stern v. Ambach, 516 N.Y.S.2d 319 (N.Y. App. Div.), *appeal dismissed without opinion* 522 N.Y.S.2d 114 (N.Y.), *appeal dismissed without opinion* 543 N.Y.S.2d 399 (N.Y. 1987) (dentist who failed to notify board of current address could not invalidate board decision on the basis of inadequate notice).

[13]See, e.g., Wright v. Roller, 111 So.2d 485 (Fla. Dist. Ct. App. 1959); Bruce v. Dept. of Reg. & Educ., 187 N.E.2d 711 (Ill. 1963).

[14]See, e.g., Jaffe v. State Dept. of Health, 64 A.2d 330 (Conn. 1949); Sheppard v. Board of Dentistry, 385 So.2d 143 (Fla. Dist. Ct. App.), *petition denied* 392 So.2d 1379 (Fla. 1980); Levinson v. Connecticut Bd. of Chiropractic Examiners, 560 A.2d 403 (Conn. 1989).

[15]See, e.g., Bills v. Weaver, 544 P.2d 690 (Ariz. Ct. App. 1976); Adams v. Texas St. Bd. of Chiropractic Examiners, 744 S.W.2d 648 (Tex. Ct. App. 1988).

[16]See, e.g., Maun v. Dept. of Prof. Reg., 701 N.E.2d 791 (Ill. App. 1998).

[17]See, .e.g., Norton v. Colorado Bd. of Med. Examiners, 821 P.2d 897 (Colo. Ct. App. 1991), *cert. denied* Norton v. Colorado St. Bd. of Med. Examiners, 1992 Colo. LEXIS 22 (Colo. 1992); Langlitz v. Board of Registration of Chiropractors, 486 N.E.2d 48 (Mass. 1985) (due process does not require an administrative entity to provide a detailed description of the evidence it will use in disciplinary hearing); Davidson v. District of Columbia Bd. of Med., 562 A.2d 109 (D.C. Cir. 1989); Erwin v. State Dept. of Prof. & Occupational Reg., etc., 320 So.2d 2 (Fla. Dist. Ct. App.), *cert. denied* 334 So.2d 605 (Fla. 1975); Angerman v. Ohio State Med. Bd., 591 N.E.2d 3 (Ohio Ct. App. 1990); Serian v. State, 297 S.E.2d 889 (W.Va. 1982).

[18]See, e.g., State Bd. of Reg. for the Health Arts v. Masters, 512 S.W.2d 150 (Mo. Ct. App. 1974) (a physician who did not appear to offer any additional evidence when requested, even though he stated that, "I have other witnesses here who will repudiate this man's testimony" in response to earlier adverse testimony was held not to have been deprived of his right to present witnesses); Ohio State Med. Bd. v. Zwick, 392 N.E.2d 1276 (Ohio Ct. App. 1978) (denial of the right to cross-examine witnesses is harmless error when board decision to suspend physician's license is supported in absence of witnesses' testimony); Zaman v. Board of Med. Examiners, 408 S.E.2d 213 (S.C. 1991) (failure of physician to appear at board proceeding waived the right to cross-examination); cf. Dragan v. Connecticut Med. Examining Bd., 591 A.2d 150 (Conn. App. Ct.), *appeal granted* 593 A.2d 967 (Conn.), *aff'd.* 223 Conn. 618 (1991) (denial of practitioner's right to cross-examine crucial witness is reversible error); Bruce v. Dept. of Reg. & Educ., 187 N.E.2d 711 (Ill. 1963) (a dentist's denial of the right to cross-examine witnesses against him is a denial of due process).

[19]See, e.g., Appeal of Beyer, 453 A.2d 834 (N.H. 1982); Dorsey v. Board of Regents, 449 N.Y.S.2d 337 (N.Y. App. Div. 1982); Lazachek v. Board of Regents, 475 N.Y.S.2d 160 (N.Y. App. Div. 1984); Marcus v. Ambach, 523 N.Y.S.2d 241 (N.Y. App. Div. 1988); Revici v. Commissioner of Educ., 546 N.Y.S.2d 240 (N.Y. App. Div. 1989); Reed v. State Med. Bd., 532 N.E.2d 189 (Ohio Ct. App. 1988).

[20]See, e.g., Cooper v. State Bd. of Med. Examiners, 217 P.2d 630 (Cal. 1950); Lieberman v. Dept. of Prof. Reg., Bd. of Med., 573 So.2d 349 (Fla. Dist. Ct. App. 1990); Bruns v. Dept. of Reg. & Educ., 376 N.E.2d 82 (Ill. App. Ct. 1978); Pundy v. Dept. of Prof. Reg., 570 N.E.2d 458 (Ill. App. Ct. 1991).

[21]See, e.g., Galang v. State, 484 N.W.2d 375 (Wis. Ct. App. 1992); Paiano v. Sobol, 572 N.Y.S.2d 440 (N.Y. App. Div. 1991).

ings of other state agencies,[22] or other state action against a practitioner's license.[23] Indeed, to be valid, this information can be simply from a summary of the hearing officer to the medical board or some other reasonable source from which the board can base its assessment.[24] However, in certain circumstances, proceedings and conclusions based on these kinds of records have been invalidated.[25]

---

[22]See, e.g., Choi v. State, 550 N.Y.S.2d 267 (N.Y. App. Div. 1989); Camperlengo v. Barell, 578 N.Y.S.2d 504 (N.Y. App. Div. 1991); Pacific Coast Med. Enterprises v. Department of Benefit Payments, 189 Cal.Rptr. 558 (Cal. Ct. App. 1983); see also Hughes v. Board of Arch. Examiners, 80 Cal.Rptr.2d 317 (Cal. Ct. App. 1998).

[23]See, e.g., McKay v. Board of Med. Examiners, 788 P.2d 476 (Or. Ct. App. 1990); In the Matter of Cole, 476 A.2d 836 (N.J. Super. App. Div. 1984); Marek v. Board of Podiatric Med., 20 Cal.Rptr.2d 474 (Cal. Ct. App. 1993); Yellen v. Board of Med. Quality Assurance, 220 Cal.Rptr. 426 (Cal. Ct. App. 1985); Shea v. Board of Med. Examiners, 81 Cal.App.3d 564 (Cal. Ct. App. 1978).

[24]See, e.g., Bernstein v. Board of Med. Examiners, 22 Cal.Rptr. 419 (Cal. Ct. App. 1962); Davis v. State Bd. of Psychologist Examiners, 791 P.2d 1198 (Colo. Ct. App. 1989), *cert. denied* 1990 Colo LEXIS 410 (Colo 1992); You v. Minami, 652 P.2d 632 (Haw. 1982); Chock v. Bitterman, 678 P.2d 576 (Haw. Ct. App.), *cert. denied* 744 P.2d 781 (Haw. 1984); McCabe v. Dept. of Reg. & Educ., 413 N.E.2d 1353 (Ill. App. Ct.), *cert. denied* 454 U.S. 838 (1980); Chapman v. Ohio State Dental Bd., 515 N.E.2d 992 (Ohio Ct. App. 1986).

[25]See, e.g., Dossick v. Florida State Bd. of Osteopathic Med. Examiners, 359 So.2d 12 (Fla. Dist. Ct. App.), *cert. denied* 366 So.2d 881 (Fla. 1978) (board action to increase the penalty beyond recommendation of hearing officer is in violation of due process when only an incomplete record was before board); State *ex. rel* Wolfe v. Missouri Dental Bd., 221 S.W. 70 (Mo. 1920) (state dental board order revoking a dentist's license is invalid when no transcript of proceedings made up to the decision and the dentist was not provided an opportunity to argue the case); State v. Carroll, 376 N.E.2d 596 (Ohio Ct. App. 1977) (state medical board proceeding with only one member of the board to administer hearing and no other member of board considering evidence presented in hearing rendered the decision in violation of due process); In re Zar, 434 N.W.2d 598 (S.D. 1989) (state board adoption of hearing officer's recommendation in a psychologist's license proceeding without, at a minimum, reviewing hearing officer's findings rendered the board decision invalid).

[26]Statutory provisions also may require that the specific law that has been violated by the practitioner be identified in the administrative complaint. See, e.g., Stalder v. Board of Med. Examiners, 588 P.2d 659 (Or. Ct. App. 1978) (state board hearing notice must include particular rule or law on which license revocation based as required by state law). See also Bills v. Weaver, 544 P.2d 690 (Ariz. Ct. App. 1976) (notice of board proceeding is valid even though notice referred to wrong statute); Mannan v. District of Columbia Bd. of Med., 558 A.2d 329 (D.C. Cir. 1989) (notice of board proceeding is valid even though notice referred to a repealed statute).

The specific requirements for adequate due process often, but not always, are indicated by state statutory or administrative law.[26] Substantive fulfillment of these due process requirements is subject to judicial review, with a standard simply of whether the decision is supported by the evidence on the record. Invalidation and remand are the general remedies for inadequate due process;[27] but outside these challenges, the decision of the board, like other administrative proceedings, is given great deference by the courts. It is important to note that a license provides the individual with a right to practice within the confines of the laws of the state; it does not guarantee the right to practice nor does it guarantee the right to practice in a particular manner or provide particular services.[28]

Concept.

State medical board actions against a practitioner's license must be preceded by adequate notice of the proceeding and a hearing where the practitioner may present his or her case and cross-examine witnesses brought forward against him or her. Judicial review is limited to a determination of whether the decision was supported by the evidence on the record.

Case. Dr. C, a psychologist, was investigated by the Psychology Examining Committee (the committee) of the State Board of Medical Examiners (the board) after complaints were lodged against him for inappropriate drug prescriptions and sexual activities with his patients. On investigation of these complaints, the committee charged Dr. C with four causes for disciplinary action. Notice of the hearing indicated that the charges "included, but were not limited to" illegal prescribing of drugs and inappropriate sexual relations with patients. Notice of the hearing that was to be scheduled for August 7, 8, and 9 was sent on July 28; these dates represented a rescheduling from an earlier May set of dates. At the hearing, the hearing officer offered to take Dr. C's witnesses in any order convenient for him, to consider holding evening sessions, or to reschedule the hearing for the last three days of the week (rather than the scheduled first three days). Dr. C, through his attorney, refused. On these dates, the board submitted the testimony of Dr. F, who testified that Dr.

---

[27]See, e.g., Lopez v. New Mexico Bd. of Medical Examiners, 754 P.2d 522 (N.M. 1988); Moranu v. Board of Med. Examiners, 32 Cal.2d 301 (Cal. 1948); Murphy v. Board of Med. Examiners, 75 Cal.App.2d 161 (Cal. 1946); Hohreiter v. Garrisa, 81 Cal.App.2d 384 (Cal. 1947).

[28]See, e.g., In re Guess, 393 S.E.2d 833 (N.C. 1990); Majebe v. North Carolina Bd., 416 S.E.2d 404 (N.C. Ct. App.), *rev. denied* 421 S.E.2d 355 (N.C. 1992); Williams v. Medical Licensure Comm., 453 So.2d 1051 (Ala. Ct. App. 1984); Idaho Assn. of Naturopathic Physicians v. U.S. Food and Drug Adm., 582 F.2d 849 (4th Cir. 1978), *cert. denied* 440 U.S. 976 (1979).

C's actions constituted an "extreme departure from the standard of practice of psychology." After these three days, the hearing was continued until October 18, 19, and 20. At that time, Dr. C did not indicate he would have any difficulty with the October dates. On October 18, neither Dr. C nor his attorney attended the scheduled hearing. Instead, on that morning, the hearing officer received a letter from Dr. C's attorney indicating that Dr. C and the attorney would not attend and objected to the hearing being continued to October 18. The hearing officer telephoned Dr. C's counsel to clarify the attorney's position and offered to continue the matter. Dr. C's counsel did not indicate his position or make any request as to the future hearing. The hearing therefore was held in their absence, and the committee concluded that three of the four charges against Dr. C were true and recommended the penalty be revocation of Dr. C's license. The board adopted this recommendation. Dr. C sought judicial review of the board decision on the basis that the evidence was insufficient, that the charges against him were too vague for him to prepare a defense because of the "included but not limited to" language, that he was not provided with statutorily adequate notice, that he was not provided with a full and fair opportunity to present his case due to changes in hearing dates, and therefore he was not provided with adequate due process.

Legal Discussion.   Dr. C's license revocation was affirmed in the case on which this illustration is based.[29] First, in administrative decisions, review is limited to whether the trial court found that the evidence supported the board's decision. The trial court concluded it did; Dr. F's expert testimony, patient testimony of Dr. C's actions, and the action of prescribing drugs by Dr. C, a psychologist with no authority to do so, all were adequate to support the actions of the board. Second, the charges against Dr. C were not too vague for him to prepare a defense. Liberal rules of administrative pleading require that Dr. C simply be informed of the substance of the charges against him so that he could prepare a defense. The mere use of "included but not limited to" was not so vague as to limit Dr. C from preparing a defense because the substance of the accusations, illegal prescribing of drugs and inappropriate sexual relations with patients, was clearly indicated on the notice. Third, Dr. C's claim of inadequate notice also failed; his claim that he should have been provided with ten days' notice by statute was fulfilled: The statute specifically indicated that the time of notice was to be calculated by excluding the first day and including the last. On that basis, he was provided the ten-day notice required. Fourth, Dr. C was provided with a full and fair opportunity to have his case heard. Administrative agencies are given great flexibility to proceed with their charge; this includes the days on which to sit to hear cases. Although there was a change of dates, the hearing officer offered to accommodate Dr. C's presentation of witnesses or move the dates to the end of the week or both; he also telephoned Dr. C's attorney and offered to continue the hearing. Having refused every offer of accommodation by the hearing officer, Dr. C could not claim that he was precluded from presenting an adequate defense. Because the board decision was based on the trial court's review of the evidence on the record; Dr. C was provided with adequate notice; and Dr. C was provided with an adequate opportunity to present his case, he was afforded due process, and the decision to revoke his license was affirmed.

Notes on State Licensure and Revocation

Expert Witness Testimony

There is a significant debate as to whether physician expert testimony should be subject to medical board review as the practice of medicine and possible suits for negligence. Groups such as the AMA support extending board authority to testimony provided by physicians. And at the present time, most courts do not accept malpractice or other suits based on the physician's expert testimony since witness testimony in court or some other forum generally is immune from lawsuit,[30] although courts have indicated that such testimony is not absolutely immune from board review because such professional regulation is not a judicial proceeding.[31]

Additional Reading.   D. S. Agliano, "Focus: Peer Review of Expert Witnesses," *Medical Malpractice Law and Strategy* 15, no. 11 (1998), pp. 1–4; R. A. Clifford, "Are Physician Expert Witnesses Practicing Medicine?" *Medical Malpractice Law and Strategy* 15, no. 11 (1994),

---

[29]Cooper v. Board of Medical Examiners of the State of Cal., 123 Cal.Rptr. 563 (Cal. Ct. App. 1975).

[30]See, e.g., Restatement (Second) of Torts, §588; see also Briscoe v. LaHue, 460 U.S. 325 (1983); Frazier v. Bailey, 957 F.2d 920 (1st. Cir. 1992); Griffin v. Summerlin, 78 F.3d 1227 (7th Cir. 1996); Hamed v. Pfeifer, 647 N.E.2d 669 (Ind. App. 1995); Kahn v. Burman, 673 F.Supp. 210 (E.D. Mich. 1987), *aff'd without opinion* 878 F.2d 1436 (6th Cir. 1989); Moore v. Conliffe, 871 P.2d 204 (Cal. 1994).

[31]See, e.g., Deatherage v. Washington Examining Bd. of Psychology, 948 P.2d 828 (Wash. 1997); Moses v. Parwatikar, 813 F.2d 891 (8th Cir. 1987) (psychiatrist's absolute immunity from lawsuit for damages does not extend to other corrective actions); Moses v. McWilliams, 549 A.2d 950 (Pa. Super. Ct. 1988) (physician's immunity from lawsuit does not bar professional discipline); see also Imbler v. Pachtman, 424 U.S. 409 (1976) (prosecutor is immune from lawsuit but not from professional discipline); Silberg v. Anderson, 266 Cal.Rptr. 638 (Cal. 1990) (immunity from lawsuit for lawyer does not preclude professional discipline).

p. 4; C. T. Drechsler, "Expert Testimony," in *American Jurisprudence,* 2d ed., vol. 61 (Rochester, NY: Lawyers Cooperative Publishing Co., 1998), §345–56; D. R. Eitel et al., "Physicians' Attitudes About Expert Medical Witnesses," *Journal of Legal Medicine* 18 (1997), pp. 345–60; J. Erikson, "Arizona Review Board Sides with HMO," *American Medical News* (January 4, 1999), p. 7; D. M. Gianelli, "Nonexpert Witnesses Raise Delgates' Ire," *American Medical News* (January 4, 1999), p. 7; D. L. Keith, "Medical Expert Testimony in Texas Medical Malpractice Cases," *Baylor Law Review* 43 (1991), pp. 1–138; L. R. Masterson, "Witness Immunity or Malpractice Liability for Professionals Hired as Experts?" *Review of Litigation* 17 (1998), pp. 393–418; G. N. McAbee, "Improper Expert Medical Testimony: Existing and Proposed Mechanisms of Oversight," *Journal of Legal Medicine* 19 (1998), pp. 257–72; A. B. McNaughton and S. McNaughton, "Divided Loyalty: The Dilemma of the Treating Physician Advocate," *Oklahoma City University Law Review* 22 (1997), pp. 1051–66; D. L. Merideth, "The Medical Expert Witness in Mississippi: Outgunning the Opposition," *Mississippi Law Journal* 64 (1994), pp. 85–115.

Medical Directors

An increasingly important issue for medical boards is the extent to which physicians who act as medical directors of managed care and other organizations are within the board's jurisdictional purview under the board's authority as the regulator of the practice of medicine within the state. Although cases are scant, it appears that the courts are split on this issue, with some courts concluding that the board may reach medical directors while others indicating that such activities do not constitute the practice of medicine.[32] This area most likely will sustain burgeoning growth as managed care becomes the standard for health delivery.

Additional Reading. V. Y. Brown et al., "Managed Care at the Crossroads: Can Managed Care Organizations Survive Government Regulations?" *Annals of Health* 7 (1998), pp. 25–59; "Chamber of Commerce Targets Health Care Legislation," *California Health Law Monitor* 5, no. 10 (1997), pp. 5–10; M. W. Sage, "Enterprise Liability and the Emerging Managed Healthcare System," *Law and Contemporary Problems* 60 (1997), pp. 159–210.

National Practitioner Data Bank

In addition to governing malpractice payment reports,[33] the National Practitioner Data Bank (NPDB), created by the Health Care Quality Improvement Act of 1986,[34] requires that state medical and dental licensing boards report adverse actions against a practitioner's license relating to care.[35] An important corollary is that if medical or dental professional societies, which are mandated to report adverse actions against practitioner membership to state medical or dental boards, report such actions to the appropriate board, the board must forward a copy of this report to the NPDB.[36]

Additional Reading. R. N. Ankney et al., "Physician Understanding of the National Practitioner Data Bank," *Southern Medical Journal* 88 (1995), pp. 200–203; H. M. Barton, "National Practitioner Data Bank: To Report or Not?" *Texas Medicine* 89 (1993), pp. 35–37; B. A. Liang, "Beyond the Malpractice Suit: The National Practitioner Data Bank," *Hospital Physician* 31, no. 7 (1995), pp. 11–14; E. W. Martz, "National Practitioner Data Bank," *Delaware Medical Journal* 67 (1995), pp. 492–93; W. E. Neighbor et al., "Rural Hospitals' Experience with the National Practitioner Data Bank," *American Journal of Public Health* 87 (1997), pp. 663–66.

Requirement for Expert Witness Support for Board Action

Authorities are split as to whether license suspension or revocation actions require the board to substantiate its action using expert testimony. First, there appears to be no question that expert testimony *may* be introduced if relevant; however, the major issue is *must* it be used. On the one hand, courts have held that expert testimony is not necessary, primarily on the basis that the board itself, with its professional members, can determine the appropriate standard of care and what a breach of that standard would be without a need for expert witnesses.[37] On the other hand, some

---

[32]See, e.g., Murphy v. Board of Medical Examiners of the State of Ariz., 949 P.2d 530 (Ariz. Ct. App.), *rev. denied* (Ariz. Jan. 21, 1998) (medical director decision making is the practice of medicine and subject to regulation by the medical board); cf. Morris v. District of Columbia Bd. of Med., 701 A.2d 364 (D.C. Cir. 1997) (medical director of an insurance company is not practicing medicine and not subject to board discipline).

[33]See Chapter 2.

[34]42 U.S.C.A. §§11101 *et seq.*

[35]42 U.S.C.A. §11132.

[36]42 U.S.C.A. §11132.

[37]See, e.g., Weiss v. New Mexico Bd. of Dentistry, 798 P.2d 175 (N.M. 1990); Croft v. Arizona St. Bd. of Dental Examiners, 755 P.2d 1191 (Ariz. Ct. App. 1988); Sillery v. Bd. of Med., 378 N.W.2d 570 (Mich. Ct. App.), *appeal denied* 425 Mich. 858 (Mich. 1985); State Bd. of Chiropractic Examiners v. Clark, 713 S.W.2d 621 (Mo. Ct. App. 1986); Appeal of Beyer, 453 A.2d 834 (N.H. 1982); Kundrat v. Commonwealth State Dental Council & Examining Bd., 447 A.2d 355 (Pa. Cmmw. Ct. 1982); Washington St. Med. Disciplinary Bd. v. Johnston, 663 P.2d 457 (Wash. 1983); Davidson v. State, 657 P.2d 810 (Wash. Ct. App.), *rev. denied* 99 Wash.2d 1011 (1983); Jaffe v. State Dept. of Health, 64 A.2d 330 (Conn. 1949).

courts indicate that expert testimony is required to substantiate license suspension or revocation, primarily on the basis of providing a record for judicial review.[38] However, even in the latter circumstances, courts have found exceptions to the need for expert testimony, including where the board has the power to take official notice of scientific facts within the expertise of the board or administrative body hearing the case,[39] where the practitioner admits or stipulates to the charges of misconduct,[40] or when the circumstances are within the understanding of laypersons.[41]

Unauthorized Practice

Generally, persons who hold themselves out as medical professionals who are not entitled to do so are practicing medicine without a license, including using the title of *doctor* in their representations.[42] Representation of a person indicating he or she is authorized to practice medicine to the public need not actually mean that a person must advertise or show in some other public manner that he or she is providing medical services for liability to attach.[43] Consent of or demand by the patient also generally is no defense of unauthorized practice of medicine.[44] Note also that the actions by licensed practitioners to assist another to practice unlawfully also is an unauthorized practice of medicine and may result in license revocation.[45]

Additional Reading.   G. F. Indest and B. Egolf, "Is Medicine Headed for an Assembly Line? Exploring the Doctrine of the Unauthorized Corporate Practice of Medicine," *Augusta Business Law Today* 6 (1997), pp. 32–36; L. M. Rosenberg, "Notice of Revocation of License Not Required to Prosecute for Unauthorized Practice of Medicine," *New York Health Law Update* 4, no. 10 (1997), pp. 3–6.

Staff and Clinical Privileges

Once a practitioner has obtained a license to practice medicine, he or she generally will desire hospital privileges for the inpatient requirements of his or her patients. Therefore, the practitioner will seek to obtain staff privileges at a particular hospital. This process of applying

---

[38]See, e.g., State Bd. of Medical Examiners v. McCroskey, 880 P.2d 1188 (Colo. 1994); Jutkowitz v. Department of Health Services, 596 A.2d 374 (Conn. 1991); Obasi v. Department of Prof. Regulation, 639 N.E.2d 1318 (Ill. App. Ct. 1994); Franz v. Board of Medical Quality Assurance, 642 P.2d 792 (Cal. 1982) (administrative record in license action must contain expert testimony to allow for a lay judge to provide an adequate judicial review); Medical Licensing Bd. v. Ward, 449 N.E.2d 1129 (Ind. Ct. App. 1983) (expert testimony is necessary to support license action, particularly in a case where not all members of the board are educated in specific professional area and for purposes of judicial review); Arthurs v. Bd. of Reg. in Med., 418 N.E.2d 1236 (Mass. 1981) (material facts, including expert testimony, must appear on the administrative record for purposes of judicial review); Dotson v. Texas State Bd. of Medical Examiners, 612 S.W.2d 921 (Tex. 1981) (expert testimony on the record is required to support suspension of medical licenses).

[39]See, e.g., Perez v. Missouri State Bd. of Registration for the Healing Arts, 803 S.W.2d 160 (Mo. Ct. App. 1991); Franz v. Board of Medical Quality Assurance, 642 P.2d 792 (Cal. 1982); Arthurs v. Bd. of Registration in Med., 418 N.E.2d 1236 (Mass. 1981); Re Appeal of Schramm, 414 N.W.2d 31 (S.D. 1987); Dotson v. Texas State Bd. of Medical Examiners, 612 S.W.2d 921 (Tex. 1981); Wood v. Texas State Bd. of Medical Examiners, 615 S.W.2d 942 (Tex. Ct. App. 1981).

[40]See, e.g., Board of Dental Examiners v. Brown, 448 A.2d 881 (Me. 1982); Arlen v. Ohio St. Med. Bd., 399 N.E.2d 1251 (Ohio 1980); Re Appeal of Schramm, 414 N.W.2d 31 (S.D. 1987); Martinez v. Texas State Bd. of Med. Examiners, 476 S.W.2d 400 (Tex. Ct. App.), *writ ref n r e, appeal dismissed* 409 U.S. 1020 (1972).

[41]See, e.g., Franz v. Board of Med. Quality Assurance, 642 P.2d 792 (Cal. 1982); Medical Licensing Bd. v. Ward, 449 N.E.2d 1129 (Ind. Ct. App. 1983); Arthurs v. Bd. of Registration in Med., 418 N.E.2d 1236 (Mass. 1981); Sillery v. Bd. of Med., 378 N.W.2d 570 (Mich. Ct. App.), *appeal denied* 425 Mich. 858 (1985); Re Appeal of Schramm, 414 N.W.2d 31 (S.D. 1987).

[42]See, e.g., Williams v. State, 453 So.2d 1051 (Ala. Ct. App. 1984) (naturopath use of title *doctor* violated medical practice act as unauthorized practice of medicine); Cooper v. State Bd. of Public Health, 229 P.2d 27 (Cal. Ct. App. 1951) (laboratory technologist using title of *M.D.* appropriately deprived of his license); Dare v. Bd. of Med. Examiners, 136 P.2d 304 (Cal. 1943) (psychologist using title *doctor* with no indication of type of doctor degree cited for unprofessional conduct).

[43]See, e.g., Medical Lic. Bd. v. Stetina, 477 N.E.2d 322 (Ind. Ct. App. 1985) (unauthorized person merely preparing to offer services to public in violation of medical practice act); Forrest v. Eason, 123 Utah 610 (Utah 1953); Hall v. Warren, 632 P.2d 848 (Utah 1981); Orr v. BYU, 960 F.Supp. 1522 (Utah 1994).

[44]See, e.g., Board of Med. Quality Assurance v. Andrews, 260 Cal.Rptr. 113 (Cal. Ct. App. 1989); State v. Howard, 337 S.E.2d 598 (N.C. Ct. App. 1985), *rev. denied, appeal dismissed* 341 S.E.2d 581 (N.C. 1986); Bowland v. Municipal Court, 134 Cal.Rptr. 630 (Cal. 1976); State v. Southworth, 704 S.W.2d 219 (Mo. 1986); Majebe v. North Carolina Bd., 416 S.E.2d 404 (N.C. Ct. App.), *rev. denied* 421 S.E.2d 355 (N.C. 1992); Mitchell v. Clayton, 995 F.2d 772 (7th Cir. 1993).

[45]See, e.g., Magit v. Bd. of Med. Examiners, 17 Cal.Rptr. 488 (Cal. 1961); State Bd. of Medical Educ. & Licensure v. Ferry, 94 A.2d 121 (Pa. Super. Ct. 1953); Blazic v. Ohio State Dental Bd., 611 N.E.2d 802 (Ohio 1993); State Bd. of Dental Examiners v. Savelle, 8 P.2d 693 (Colo.), *appeal dismissed* 287 U.S. 562 (Colo. 1932); Chalmers-Francis v. Nelson, 6 Cal.2d 402 (Cal. 1936); Hausen v. Bd. of Med. Examiners, 128 Cal.App. 35 (Cal. Ct. App. 1933); Rilcoff v. State Bd. of Med. Examiners, 90 Cal.App.2d 603 (Cal. Ct. App. 1949).

for and obtaining hospital privileges is often known as *credentialing* practitioners. Note that obtaining a license to practice medicine in a particular state does not guarantee that individual the right for staff privileges at a particular hospital.

Typically a physician first must apply to the hospital for staff privileges; that is, he or she must apply to become a member of the medical staff.[46] Membership of the medical staff is important because JCAHO mandates that the medical staff have responsibility for the quality of professional services provided by individuals with clinical privileges.[47] Medical staff membership also provides the physician with the rights and subjects him or her to responsibilities defined by the hospital bylaws. Once granted membership, the physician may apply for specific clinical privileges for the particular services he or she desires to provide at the hospital.[48] These two functions may be incorporated into the same application instrument. Generally, the application for staff and clinical privileges is reviewed for accuracy, sent to the appropriate division director or department chair for review (which may include a personal interview with the practitioner), and then sent to the credentials committee for evaluation of the applicant's documentation of clinical competence. The credentials committee then makes a recommendation to the executive committee of the medical staff; if the executive committee of the medical staff concurs in the credentials committee's evaluation, the application usually is sent to the hospital board of directors for final action. Generally, privileges and reappointments to the medical staff must be reviewed every two years.[49]

Decisions challenging denial or termination of staff and clinical privileges typically are unsuccessful, although providers have used a variety of theories, including antitrust,[50] breach of contract,[51] and constitutional due

process[52] in their efforts. Denial of staff and clinical privileges, like licensure, generally is considered denial of a property interest.[53] However, aggrieved physicians must exhaust internal procedures first before accessing the courts.[54] Only when practitioners claim that staff and clinical privilege decisions violate federal antidiscrimination statutes is the internal administrative exhaustion requirement waived.[55] Once these administrative procedures are fulfilled, the practitioner may obtain judicial review of the hospital decision; but like other administrative actions, such as licensure, courts grant great deference to these administrative assessments.[56]

The requisite type of judicial review for practitioner application for denial or termination of staff and clinical privileges ostensibly is affected by the private or public nature of the hospital. Private hospitals generally are not subject to constitutional claims, such as violation of due process, whereas publicly owned or operated institutions, as state (i.e., government) actors, generally are.[57] Note that the mere receipt of public funding does not render the institution a state actor subject to constitu-

[46]Joint Commission on Accreditation of Healthcare Organizations, *1995 Accreditation Manual for Hospitals* (Oakbrook Terrace, IL: JCAHO, 1995), M.S. 1.1.1.

[47]Ibid., M.S.1.

[48]Ibid., M.S. 1.1.2.

[49]Ibid., M.S. 2.13.

[50]See, e.g., Jefferson Parish Hosp. Dist. No. 2 v. Hyde, 466 U.S. 2 (1984); Beard v. Parkview Hosp., 912 F.2d 138 (6th Cir. 1990); Coffey v. Healthtrust, Inc., 955 F.2d 1388 (10th Cir. 1992); Patel v. Scotland Mem. Hosp., 1995 WL 319213 (M.D. N.C. March 31, 1995); Tomlinson v. Humana, Inc., 495 So.2d 630 (Ala. 1986); Collins v. Associated Pathologists, Ltd., 844 F.2d 473 (7th Cir. 1988); see also Capital Imaging Assocs., P.C. v. Mohawk Valley Medical Assn., 791 F.Supp. 956 (N.D. N.Y. 1992) (no antitrust injury when a managed care organization chose to exclusively contract with one radiology group rather than another); cf. Oltz v. St. Peter's Comm. Hosp., 861 F.2d 1440 (9th Cir. 1988) (nurse anesthetist showed an antitrust injury when department anesthesiologists acted to exclude him and increased their income from anesthesia services).

[51]See, e.g., Saint Louis v. Baystate Medical Ctr., 568 N.E.2d 1181 (Mass. Ct. App. 1991); Bartley v. Eastern Maine Medical Ctr., 617 A.2d 1020 (Me. 1992); Jefferson Parrish Hosp. Dist. No. 2 v. Hyde, 466 U.S. 2 (1984); Balaklau v. Lovell, 14 F.3d 793 (2d Cir. 1994); Konik v. Champlain Valley Physicians Hosp. Med. Ctr., 733 F.2d 1007 (2d Cir. 1984).

[52]See, e.g., Keskin v. Munster Medical Research Found., 580 N.E.2d 354 (Ind. Ct. App. 1991); Ezpeleta v. Sisters of Mercy Health Corp., 800 F.2d 119 (7th Cir. 1986); Anne Arundel Gen. Hosp., Inc. v. O'Brien, 432 A.2d 483 (Md. Ct. App. 1981); Holt v. Good Samaritan Hosp. and Health Ctr., 590 N.E.2d 1318 (Ohio Ct. App. 1990); Hutton v. Memorial Hosp., 824 P.2d 61 (Colo. Ct. App. 1991).

[53]See, e.g., Northeast Georgia Radiological Assoc. v. Tidwell, 670 F.2d 507 (5th Cir. 1982); Daly v. Sprague, 675 F.2d 716 (5th Cir. 1982); Shahawy v. Harrison, 875 F.2d 1529 (11th Cir. 1989); Bloom v. Hennepin County, 783 F.Supp. 418 (D. Minn. 1992).

[54]See, e.g., Seontgen v. Quain & Ramstad Clinic, 467 N.W.2d 73 (N.D. 1991); Eufemio v. Kodiak Island Hosp., 837 P.2d 95 (Alaska 1992); Garrow v. Elizabeth Gen. Hosp., 401 A.2d 533 (N.J. 1979); Voight v. Snowden, 923 P.2d 171 (Alaska 1982); Eidelson v. Archer, 645 P.2d 171 (Alaska 1982).

[55]See, e.g., Chowdhury v. Reading Hosp. and Medical Center, 677 F.2d 317 (3d Cir. 1982), *cert. denied* 463 U.S. 1229 (1983); Doe v. St. Joseph's Hosp. of Fort Wayne, 788 F.2d 411 (7th Cir. 1986); Chester Residents Concerned for Quality Living v. Seif, 132 F.3d 925 (3d Cir. 1997); Fynes v. Weinberger, 677 F.Supp. 315 (E.D. Pa. 1985); Spence v. Straw, 54 F.3d 196 (3d Cir. 1995); Wood v. Rendell, 1995 WL 120648 (E.D. Pa. 1995).

[56]See, e.g., Keskin v. Munster Med. Research Found., 580 N.E.2d 354 (Ind. Ct. App. 1991); Redding v. St. Francis Medical Ctr., 255 Cal.Rptr. 806 (Cal. Ct. App. 1989); Lewin v. St. Joseph's Hosp., 146 Cal.Rptr. 892 (Cal. Ct. App. 1978).

tional claims.[58] Although this private versus public distinction is useful, ultimately courts look to the actual governmental influence or control and its relationship with institutional decisions to assess state actor status.[59] If the hospital is deemed a state actor, it must conform with constitutional due process procedures, similar to licensure revocation and suspension reviews, such as providing the practitioner with adequate notice, the opportunity to present his or her case, the opportunity to cross-examine witnesses, and so forth.[60]

Although due process claims based on state action are not available on constitutional grounds for nongovernment-owned or -operated facilities, some due process protections are available for practitioners who have staff and clinical privileges denied or terminated by private hospitals and hospitals not considered state actors. These protections usually are enumerated in the bylaws of the hospital; further, these protections exist within the context

of a common law requirement that the process is "fundamentally fair"[61] as well as state and federal statutes that mandate all hospitals to provide hearing and appeals procedures.[62] Indeed, many of the requirements for bylaw due process are indicated by state statute. On judicial review, courts generally limit their assessment to whether the bylaw provisions for due process were followed and once again grant great deference to the administrative body.[63]

Medical staff and clinical privilege decisions usually focus on quality-of-care issues and other competency criteria,[64] including the ability to work with others.[65] Further, in the current highly competitive health delivery climate, hospitals have used economic methods such as exclusive contracts and other arrangements to minimize costs. These methodologies generally have been accepted by the courts as a valid mode by which the hospital may structure its medical departments.[66] Assuredly, as costs

[57]See, e.g., Blum v. Yaretsky, 457 U.S. 991 (1982); Ezekwo v. NYC Health and Hosps. Corp., 940 F.2d 775 (2d Cir.), *cert. denied* 502 U.S. 1013 (1991); Northeast Georgia Radiological Assocs., P.C. v. Tidwell, 670 F.2d 507 (5th Cir. 1982); Engelstad v. Virginia Municipal Hosp., 718 F.2d 262 (8th Cir. 1983); Ezpeleta v. Sisters of Mercy Health Corp., 800 F.2d 119 (7th Cir. 1986); St. Mary's Hosp. v. Radiology Prof. Corp., 421 S.E.2d 731 (Ga. Ct. App. 1992); Long v. Houston Northwest Medical Center, 1991 WL 19837 (Tex. Ct. App. 1991); Mahmoodian v. United Hosp. Center, 404 S.E.2d 750 (W.Va.), *cert denied* 502 U.S. 863 (1991); Stiller v. La Porte Hosp., 570 N.E.2d 99 (Ind. Ct. App. 1991); Albert v. Carovano, 851 F.2d 561 (2d Cir. 1988); Carter v. Norfolk Comm. Hosp. Ass'n, Inc., 761 F.2d 970 (4th Cir. 1985); see also Mathis v. Pacific Gas and Electric Co., 891 F.2d 1429 (9th Cir. 1989).

[58]See, e.g., Keskin v. Munster Medical Research Found., 580 N.E.2d 354 (Ind. Ct. App. 1991); Mendez v. Belton, 739 F.2d 15 (1st Cir. 1984); Richardson v. St. John's Mercy Hosp., 674 S.W.2d 200 (Mo. Ct. App. 1984); Loh-Seng Yo v. Cibola Gen. Hosp., 706 F.2d 306 (10th Cir. 1983); Hodge v. Padi Mem. Hosp., 576 F.2d 563 (3d Cir. 1978).

[59]See, e.g., Kiracofe v. Reid Mem. Hosp., 461 N.E.2d 1134 (Ind. Ct. App. 1984); Weston v. Carolina Medicorp Inc., 402 S.E.2d 653 (N.C. Ct. App.), *rev. denied* 409 S.E.2d 611 (N.C. 1991); Jatoi v. Hurst-Euless-Bedford Hosp. Authority, 807 F.2d 1214 (5th Cir. 1987), *cert. denied* 484 U.S. 1010 (1988); Milo v. Cushing Municipal Hosp., 861 F.2d 1194 (10th Cir. 1988); Silver v. Castle Mem. Hosp., 497 P.2d 564 (Haw. 1972); Kelly v. St. Vincent Hosp., 692 P.2d 1350 (N.M. Ct. App. 1984); Pepple v. Parkview Mem. Hosp., Inc., 511 N.E.2d 467 (Ind. Ct. App. 1991); Keskin v. Munster Medical Research Found., 580 N.E.2d 354 (Ind. Ct. App. 1991).

[60]See, e.g., Huellmantel v. Greenville Hosp. System, 402 S.E.2d 489 (S.C. Ct. App. 1991); South Carolina Dept. of Labor v. Girgis, 503 S.E.2d 490 (S.C. Ct. App. 1998); Lew v. Kona Hosp., 754 F.2d 1420 (9th Cir. 1985); Goss v. Lopez, 419 U.S. 565 (1975); Armstrong v. Mazo, 380 U.S. 545 (1975); Wolff v. McDonnell, 418 U.S. 539 (1974).

[61]See, e.g., Rosenblit v. Fountain Valley Regional Hosp., 282 Cal.Rptr. 819 (Cal. Ct. App. 1991); Christenson v. Mount Carmel Health, 112 Ohio App.3d (Ohio 1996); Goodstein v. Cedars-Sinai Med. Ctr., 78 Cal. Rptr. 2d 577 (Cal. 1998); Ende v. Cohen, 686 A.2d 1239 (N.J. Super. Ct. 1997).

[62]See Health Care Quality Improvement Act of 1986, 42 U.S.C.A. §§11101 *et seq.*

[63]See, e.g., Stiller v. La Porte Hosp., 750 N.E.2d 99 (Ind. Ct. App. 1991); Mahmoodian v. United Hosp. Ctr., 404 S.E.2d 570 (W.Va.), *cert. denied* 502 U.S. 863 (1991); Huellmantel v. Greenville Hosp. Sys., 402 S.E.2d 489 (S.C. Ct. App. 1991).

[64]See, e.g., Weston v. Carolina Medicorp, Inc., 402 S.E.2d 653 (N.C. Ct. App.), *rev. denied* 409 S.E.2d 611 (N.C. 1991); Paskon v. Salem Mem. Hosp. Dist., 806 S.W.2d 417 (Mo. Ct. App.), *cert. denied* 502 U.S. 908 (1991); Blum v. Yaretsky, 457 U.S. 991 (1982); Albright v. Longview Police Dept., 884 F.2d 835 (5th Cir. 1989); Lubin v. Crittenden Hosp. Assn., 713 F.2d 414 (8th Cir. 1983).

[65]See, e.g., Everhart v. Jefferson Parish Hosp. Dist. No. 2, 757 F.2d 1567 (5th Cir. 1985); Mahmoodian v. United Hosp. Center, 404 S.E.2d 750 (W.Va.), *cert. denied* 112 S.Ct. 185 (1991); Rooney v. Medical Ctr. Hosp., 1994 WL 854372 (S.D. Ohio 1994); Hyde v. Jefferson Parish Hosp. Dist. No. 2, 764 F.2d 1139 (5th Cir. 1985); Shaw v. The Hosp. Authority of Cobb County, 614 F.2d 946 (5th Cir. 1980); Ezekwo v. American Bd. of Internal Med., 18 F.Supp.2d 271 (S.D. N.Y. 1998).

[66]See, e.g., Keskin v. Munster Med. Research Found., 580 N.E.2d 354 (Ind. Ct. App. 1991); Kramer v. Kent Gen. Hosp., 1992 WL 91130 (Del. Super. Ct. 1992); Hutton v. Mem. Hosp., 824 P.2d 61 (Colo. Ct. App. 1991); Bartley v. Eastern Maine Med. Ctr., 617 A.2d 1020 (Me. 1992); Lewin v. St. Joseph's Hosp., 146 Cal.Rptr. 892 (Cal. Ct. App. 1978); Alonso v. Hosp. Authority of Henry Cty., 332 S.E.2d 884 (Ga. Ct. App. 1985); Radiology Professional Corp. v. Trinidad Area Health Assn., 195 Colo. 253 (Colo. 1978); Jefferson Parish Hosp. Dist. No. 2 v. Hyde, 466 U.S. 2 (1984); Redding v. St. Francis Med. Ctr., 208 Cal.App.3d 98 (Cal. Ct. App. 1989); Belmar v. Cipolla, 96 N.J. 199 (N.J. 1984); Brandon v. Combs, 666 S.W.2d 755 (Ky. Ct. App. 1984); Williams v. Hobbs, 9 OhioApp.3d 331 (Ohio 1983).

continue to be the focus in the health delivery environment in the United States, hospitals will continue to use economic criteria to assess physician applications for privileges.

Note that although practitioners generally have a right to some form of due process if privileges are not extended, are reduced, or are terminated for quality-of-care reasons, usually no such protections are mandated when the hospital acts on the basis of economic reasons, such as when one exclusive contractor is replaced by another or one exclusive contractor already provides all services in a particular area and the hospital needs no additional providers.[67] Therefore, physicians may have adverse effects on their ability to practice at the hospital due to a change in contractor. This effect on the ability to practice usually does not invoke any right to due process hearings; generally, only poor-quality care leading to potential privilege reduction or termination invokes such rights.

Concept.

Staff and clinical privilege reduction or termination by the hospital without a hearing is permitted if the reduction or termination is due to a valid, nonquality basis. When physician privileges are to be reduced or terminated due to quality concerns, the physician is entitled to due process notice and hearing rights.

Case.   Dr. H was an emergency room physician with an exclusive contract with the Hospital to provide all emergency room services. Dr. H had staff and clinical privileges at the Hospital. Dr. H's contract included a 90-day termination without cause clause, which allowed either party to terminate the contract with such notice. The Hospital gave Dr. H 90 days' notice, indicating that it had entered into a new exclusive contract with another physician to supply all emergency room services. The Hospital was exercising appropriate action in entering into an exclusive contract. The Hospital indicated that Dr. H would retain medical staff privileges; however, he could not provide, nor bill for, any emergency room services once the new emergency room physician contractor began providing services. Dr. H was then replaced with the new

contracting physician. Dr. H was not provided any bylaw termination hearing. Dr. H sued the Hospital, claiming that he was entitled to a due process termination hearing before the Hospital entered into a new exclusive contract because his ability to practice (i.e., clinical privileges) was terminated.

Legal Discussion.   Dr. H was not entitled to a termination hearing according to the case on which this illustration is based.[68] Here, the Hospital was within its rights to enter into an exclusive contract. Dr. H's ability to practice was not terminated for quality reasons; therefore, at least on this basis, he was not entitled to a termination hearing. In addition, a simple exchange of contractors, regardless of the adverse effect on one of them, also does not provide a basis for a due process hearing. Finally, there was no change in Dr. H's status; Dr. H's privileges were not revoked or reduced. Dr. H was still a member of the medical staff; he still had the same privileges as to his permitted scope of practice. Although he was prevented from providing services in the emergency room, Dr. H's reputation or ability to practice medicine was not placed in jeopardy by the Hospital; although Dr. H has a right to practice medicine, he does not have the right to do so at any particular hospital. Hence, Dr. H's ability to practice in the emergency room was reduced or terminated by a valid, nonquality action on the Hospital's part, and as such, Dr. H was not entitled to any termination hearing. Indeed, Dr. H retained his staff privileges and permissible scope of practice at the Hospital; therefore, his privileges in fact were never reduced. He merely was unable to exercise them and bill for them at the Hospital.

Notes on Staff and Clinical Privileges

Contracting Out of Hearing Rights

Generally, physicians are entitled to due process hearings indicated in the medical staff bylaws. However, physician contracts may contain a provision that contracts away those rights as part of an agreement between the hospital and its contracting physician. These contract provisions generally are upheld.[69] In addition, hospitals may insert into contracts "clean sweep" provisions that automatically provide hospital management with the power to unilaterally terminate the physician's privileges on termination of the provider's contract. Therefore, it behooves physicians who enter into these agreements to closely scrutinize the contracts for such provisions, as

[67]See, e.g., Anne Arundel Gen. Hosp., Inc. v. O'Brien, 432 A.2d 483 (Md. Ct. App. 1981); Holt v. Good Samaritan Hosp. and Health Ctr., 590 N.E.2d 1318 (Ohio Ct. App. 1990); Hutton v. Memorial Hosp., 824 P.2d 61 (Colo. Ct. App. 1991); Dutta v. St. Francis Regional Medical Ctr., 867 P.2d 1057 (Kan. 1994); Dramer v. Kent Gen. Hosp., 1992 Del. Super. LEXIS 160 (Del. Super. Ct.); Bryant v. Glen Oaks Medical Ctr., 650 N.E.2d 622 (Ill. App. Ct. 1995); Redding v. St. Francis Medical Ctr., 255 Cal.Rptr. 806 (Cal. Ct. App. 1989); but see Garibaldi v. Applebaum, 653 N.E.2d 42 (Ill. App. Ct.), *cert. denied* 660 N.E.2d 1268 (Ill. 1995) (physician is entitled to bylaw termination proceeding after being replaced by another exclusive contractor).

[68]Holt v. Good Samaritan Hosp. and Health Center, 590 N.E.2d 1318 (Ohio Ct. App. 1990).

[69]See, e.g., Abrams v. St. John's Hosp., 30 Cal.Rptr.2d 603 (Cal. Ct. App. 1994).

they may adversely affect the practitioner's due process rights in the event of termination of the contract.

Additional Reading. P. M. Rosen, "Medical Staff Peer Review: Qualifying the Qualified Privilege Provision," *Loyola of Los Angeles Law Review* 27 (1993), pp. 357–90; M. D. Roth, "Peer Review Pitfalls: The Data Bank and Beyond," *Whittier Law Review* 13 (1992), 387–89.

Criteria for Review in Staff and
Clinical Privilege Assessments

A wide variety of criteria may be used in granting and renewing staff and clinical privileges. Diverse characteristics such as ability to work with others relating to quality of care,[70] board certification,[71] ability to obtain and retain a medical school faculty appointment,[72] and geographic proximity to the hospital[73] have been found to be acceptable criteria for assessing privilege applications and renewals. However, requiring the physician to have an office and practice within the same county in which the hospital is located,[74] to join a medical group that includes physicians already on the medical staff,[75] to be a member of a particular medical society,[76] or to be an allopathic rather than osteopathic physician with similar qualifications[77] have been held to be impermissible by courts.

Additional Reading. P. E. Borken, "Exclusive Contracts: Are Constructively Terminated Incumbent Physicians Entitled to a Fair Hearing?" *Journal of Legal Medicine* 17

(1996), pp. 143–68; M. A. Kadzielski, "Provider Deselection and Decapitation in a Changing Healthcare Environment," *St. Louis University Law Journal* (1997), pp. 891–914; B. A. Liang, "An Overview and Analysis of Challenges to Medical Exclusive Contracts," *Journal of Legal Medicine* 18 (1997), pp. 1–45; C. Scott, "Medical Peer Review, Antitrust, and the Effect of Statutory Reform," *Maryland Law Review* 50 (1991), pp. 316–407.

Peer Review and Quality Assurance—States

Hospitals generally assess the overall quality of their practitioners at the credentialing stage, as well as monitor their physicians after a grant of privileges through quality assurance activities such as peer review. Generally, these peer review activities are mandated or strongly encouraged by state law as well as JCAHO accreditation requirements.[78] Peer review discussions, oral and written peer review assessments, and quality assurance material generated by peer review and quality assurance committees are intended to be protected from legal discovery by state peer review privilege statutes[79] as well as the common law.[80] Note, however, that generally only the discussions and assessments of and conclusions based on the materials are privileged; the materials on which these are based (e.g., medical records, incident reports) are *not* within the peer review privilege[81] or even the attorney–client

[70]See, e.g., Robinson v. Magovern, 521 F.Supp. 842 (W.D. Pa. 1981), *aff'd mem.* 688 F.2d 824 (3d Cir.), *cert. denied* 459 U.S. 971 (1982); Truly v. Madison Gen. Hosp., 673 F.2d 763 (5th Cir.), *cert. denied* 459 U.S. 909 (1982); Weiss v. York Hosp., 745 F.2d 786 (3d Cir. 1984), *cert. denied* 470 U.S. 1060 (1985); cf. Mahmoodian v. United Hosp. Ctr., Inc., 404 S.E.2d 750 (W.Va.), *cert. denied* 502 U.S. 863 (1991); Yellen v. Bd. of Med. Quality Assurance, 220 Cal.Rptr. 426 (Cal. Ct. App. 1985).

[71]See, e.g., Khan v. Suburban Comm. Hosp., 340 N.E.2d 398 (Ohio 1976); Sarasota County Pub. Hosp. Bd. v. Shahawy, 408 So.2d 644 (Fla. Dist. Ct. App. 1981).

[72]See, e.g., Adamsons v. Wharton, 771 F.2d 41 (2d Cir. 1985); Dillard v. Rowland, 520 S.W.2d 81 (Mo. Ct. App. 1974).

[73]See, e.g., Kennedy v. St. Joseph Mem. Hosp., 482 N.E.2d 268 (Ind. Ct. App. 1985); Robinson v. Magovern, 521 F.Supp. 842 (W.D. Pa. 1981), *aff'd mem.* 688 F.2d 824 (3d Cir.), *cert. denied* 459 U.S. 971 (1982).

[74]See, e.g., Sams v. Ohio Valley Gen. Hosp. Ass'n, 413 F.2d 826 (4th Cir. 1969).

[75]See, e.g., Desai v. St. Barnabas Medical Ctr., 510 A.2d 662 (N.J. 1986).

[76]See, e.g., Foster v. Mobile Cty. Hosp., 398 F.2d 227 (5th Cir. 1968).

[77]See, e.g., Weiss v. York Hosp., 745 F.2d 786 (3d Cir. 1984), *cert. denied* 470 U.S. 1060 (1985).

[78]Joint Commission for Accreditation of Healthcare Organizations, *1994 Accreditation Manual for Hospitals* (Oakbrook Terrace, IL: JCAHO, 1994), standard PI.1.

[79]See, e.g., Samuelson v. Susen, 576 F.2d 546 (3d Cir. 1978); Harding v. Dana Transport, Inc., 914 F.Supp. 1084 (D.N.J. 1996); Bredice v. Doctors Hosp., Inc., 50 F.R.D. 249 (D.D.C. 1970); Utterback v. Yoon, 121 F.R.D. 297 (W.D. Ky. 1987); Balk v. Dunlap, 163 F.R.D. 360 (D. Kan. 1995); Brem v. DeCarlo, 162 F.R.D. 94 (D. Md. 1995); Spinks v. Childrens Hosp. National Med. Ctr., 124 F.R.D. 9 (D.D.C. 1989); Gillman v. U.S., 53 F.R.D. 316 (S.D. N.Y. 1971).

[80]See, e.g., Bredice v. Doctors Hosp., Inc., 50 F.R.D. 249 (D.D.C. 1970), *aff'd* 479 F.2d 920 (D.C. Cir. 1973); Segal v. Roberts, 380 So.2d 1049 (Fla. App. 1979); Oviatt v. Archbishop Bergan Mercy Hosp., 214 N.W.2d 490 (Neb. 1974); Armstrong v. Dwyer, 155 F.3d 211 (3d Cir. 1998); Meistrell v. McPhail, 788 P.2d 1387 (Okla. Ct. App. 1989); Faroog v. Coffey, 206 A.D.2d 879 (N.Y. App. Div. 1994); Jaffee v. Redmand, 518 U.S. 1 (1996); Brunt v. Hunterden Cty., 183 F.R.D. 181 (D.N.J. 1998).

[81]See, e.g., State of Missouri *ex rel.* Dixon v. Darnold, 939 S.W.2d 66 (Mo. Ct. App. 1997); Columbia/HCA Health Care Corp. v. Eighth Judicial Dist. Ct., 936 P.2d 844 (Nev. 1997); Harper v. Cadenhead, 926 S.W.2d 588 (Tex. Ct. App. 1995); Hollard v. Muscatine Gen. Hosp., 971 F.Supp. 385 (S.D. Iowa 1997); Century Med. Ctrs. v. Marin, 686 So.2d 606 (Fla. Dist. Ct. App. 1996); Monroe Regional Med. Ctr. v. Roundtree, 721 So.2d 1220 (Mo. 1998).

privilege.[82] In addition, utilization review of medical necessity decisions is not protected from discovery.[83] Therefore, simply presenting information to a peer review or quality assurance committee does not make it privileged from discovery in a legal suit. Note that because the peer review or quality assurance privilege is a function of state statute, the protections and the allowable disclosure necessarily require an assessment of each individual state's law. Finally, physicians who participate in these activities in good faith usually are immune from state lawsuits, again based on the specific state jurisdiction.[84] This is particularly important when these physicians impose sanctions on practitioners they have reviewed, and the sanctioned practitioners bring suit against them in retaliation.

Additional Reading. M. G. Sagsueen and J. L. Thompson, "The Evolution of Medical Peer Review in North Dakota," *North Dakota Law Review* 73 (1997), pp. 477–504; S. Scheutzow and S. Gillis, "Confidentiality and Privilege of Peer Review Information: More Imagined Than Real," *Journal of Law and Health* 7 (1992), pp. 169–97; P. L. Scibetta, "Restructuring Hospital-Physician Relations: Patient Care Quality Depends on the Health of Hospital Peer Review," *University of Pittsburgh Law Review* 51 (1990), pp. 1025–59.

Peer Review and Quality Assurance—Federal

State peer review statutes protect participants from state law–based suits for actions stemming from service on peer review committees; however, these statutes do not extend to suits claiming violations of federal law.[85] Consequently, Congress passed the Health Care Quality Improvement Act of 1986 (HCQIA)[86] to provide federal immunity from civil liability for peer review participants in and outside the hospital.[87] Participants are protected so long as pro-

fessional peer review is taken in the reasonable belief that the review is in furtherance of high-quality care, a reasonable attempt is made to obtain the facts of the matter, adequate hearing and notice are given to the practitioner being reviewed and that the procedure provided the practitioner is fair, and the actions of the participants are warranted on the basis of the facts obtained.[88] Persons who provide information to the review body also are protected unless the information given is false and the person providing it had actual knowledge it was false.[89] HCQIA does not preempt the effect of state law that is supplementary to it or provides greater protections.[90] HCQIA immunity does not apply to peer review of nonphysicians not covered within it[91] nor for prosecution brought by the federal government or state attorney general.[92]

Additional Reading.   J. D. Blum, "Medical Peer Review," *Journal of Legal Education* 38 (1998), pp. 525–33; T. S. Jost, "The Necessary and Proper Role of Regulation to Assure the Quality of Health Care," *Houston Law Review* 25 (1998), pp. 525–98; C. S. Morter, "The Healthcare Quality Improvement Act of 1986," *Virginia Law Review* 74 (1998), pp. 1115–40; T. J. Nodzenski, "Where Is the Quality in the Healthcare Improvement Act of 1986?" *Loyola of Los Angeles Law Journal* 22 (1991), pp. 361–408.

Peer Review and Medicare

The Medicare program also engages in peer review through its Medicare Utilization and Quality Control Peer Review Organization (PRO) program.[93] Generally, this program provides a mechanism by which the federal government can assess whether Medicare beneficiaries are obtaining medically appropriate as well as cost-effective care. The Department of Health and Human Services (DHHS) contracts with private PROs to perform this peer review; most of these organizations are physician sponsored,[94] although each PRO must have at least one consumer representative on its board.[95] PROs may contract to perform reviews for the Medicaid program[96] as well as private insurers.[97] Generally, PROs are provided data from the HCFA; PROs then

---

[82]See, e.g., State of West Virginia *ex rel.* United Hosp. Ctr., Inc. v. Bedell, 484 S.E.2d 199 (W. Va. 1997); State of West Virginia *ex rel.* United States Fidelity v. Canady, 194 W. Va. 431 (W. Va. 1995); McDougal v. McCommon, 193 W. Va. 229 (W. Va. 1995); State *ex rel.* Chaparro v. Wilkes, 190 W. Va. 395 (W. Va 1993).

[83]See, e.g., Missouri *ex rel.* Tennill v. Roper, 965 S.W.2d 945 (Mo. Ct. App. 1998).

[84]See, e.g., Spencer v. Community Hosp., 408 N.E.2d 981 (Ill. App. Ct. 1980); Bainhauer v. Manoukian, 520 A.2d 1154 (N.J. Super. Ct. App. Div. 1987); Garrow v. Elizabeth Gen. Hosp. & Dispensary, 401 A.2d 533 (N.J. 1979); Gill v. Hughes, 278 Cal.Rptr. 306 (Cal. Ct. App. 1991); Zoneraich v. Overlook Hosp. (N.J. 1986); Petrocco v. Dover Gen. Hosp. and Med. Ctr., 273 N.J.Super. 501 (N.J. Super. Ct. App. Div. 1994).

[85]See, e.g., Patrick v. Burget, 486 U.S. 94 (1988), *reh'g denied* 487 U.S. 1243 (1988).

[86]42 U.S.C.A. §§11101–11152.

[87]42 U.S.C.A. §§11151(8), 11151(9).

[88]42 U.S.C.A. §11112(a).

[89]42 U.S.C.A. §11111(a)(2).

[90]42 U.S.C.A. §11115(a).

[91]42 U.S.C.A. §11111.

[92]42 U.S.C.A. §11111(a)(1).

[93]42 U.S.C.A. §1320c-3(a)(1).

[94]42 C.F.R. §§462.102 (1998), 462.103 (1998); 42 U.S.C.A. §1320c-2(b)(1).

[95]42 U.S.C.A. §1320c-1(3).

[96]42 U.S.C.A. §1320c-7.

[97]42 U.S.C.A. §1320c-3(a)(11).

attempt to assess patterns of practice for identification of such patterns, education efforts regarding practice, and assessment of proposed changes such as corrective action plans.[98] PROs also have authority to recommend sanctions to the OIG (Office of Inspector General) of the DHHS.[99] Due process requirements must be fulfilled if the OIG accepts the PRO's recommendation and attempts to sanction the provider.[100] Sanctions are subject to review by an ALJ as well as judicial review, generally only after the sanctions are levied,[101] with the exception of physicians in rural areas.[102] Challenges to the postsanction nature of judicial review have survived constitutional challenge.[103] PROs also are mandated to review cases where hospitals indicate care is not covered by Medicare,[104] investigate Medicare beneficiary complaints regarding poor quality of care,[105] educate Medicare beneficiaries on the role and function of the PRO program,[106] and assess whether a provider has fulfilled prescribed duties under the Emergency Medical Treatment and Active Labor Act.[107]

Additional Reading.   T. S. Jost, "Administrative Law Issues Involving the Medicare Utilization and Quality Control Peer Review Organization (PRO) Program: Analysis and Recommendations," *Ohio State Law Journal* 50 (1989), pp. 1–71; P. M. Mellette, "The Changing Focus of Peer Review Under Medicare," *University of Richmond Law Review* 20 (1986), pp. 315–56; H. E. Morreim, "Cost Containment and the Standard of Medicare," *California Law Review* 75 (1987), pp. 1719–63.

Retaining Staff Privilege Membership But Termination of Ability to Practice

As seen previously, for economic reasons, practitioners effectively will have their clinical privileges terminated

when the hospital enters into an exclusive contract with other providers, who replace the original practitioners, although technically the original practitioners retain medical staff membership. In these situations, courts generally have indicated that no due process hearing requirement is attendant on the hospital because the old practitioners retain medical staff membership, even if they cannot actually practice within the hospital.[108] Note, however, that courts generally have held that bylaws may be considered part of the practitioner's contract with the hospital;[109] practitioners who retain staff privileges but have their clinical privileges reduced or terminated occasionally have been able to challenge hospitals that have not afforded them a pretermination hearing based on the requirements of the bylaws.[110] Similarly, if a practitioner's contract indicates that termination may be only "for cause," generally he or she must be provided a pretermination hearing.[111]

Additional Reading.   A. D. Allred and T. O. Tottenham, "Liability and Indemnity Issues for Integrated Delivery Systems," *St. Louis University Law Journal* 40 (1996), pp. 457–542; D. J. Behinfar, "Exclusive Contracting Between Hospitals and Physicians and the Use of Economic Credentialing," *DePaul Journal of Healthcare Law* 1 (1996), pp. 71–91; B. A. Liang, "An Overview and Analysis of Challenges to Medical Exclusive Contracts," *Journal of Legal Medicine* 18 (1997), pp. 1–45; J. D. Zellers and M. R. Paulin, "Termination of Hospital Medical Staff Privileges for Economic Reasons: An Appeal for Consistency," *Maine Law Review* 46 (1994), pp. 67–86.

---

[98]42 U.S.C.A. §1320c-5(b)(1)(A).

[99]42 U..S.C.A. §§1320c-5(b)(1), 1320c-5(b)(3).

[100]42 U.S.C.A. §§1320c-5(b)(5); 42 C.F.R. Part 1004; see also 42 U.S.C.A. §1320c-9(b)(1)(D) (a PRO that recommends sanction against a physician must notify the state medical license board of this).

[101]42 C.F.R. §1004.130 (1998).

[102]42 U.S.C.A. §1320c-5(b)(5).

[103]See, e.g., Thorbus v. Bowen, 848 F.2d 901 (8th Cir. 1988); Doyle v. Bowen, 848 F.2d 296 (1st Cir. 1988); Varandani v. Bowen, 824 F.2d 307 (4th Cir. 1987), *cert. denied* 484 U.S. 1052 (1988); Papendick v. Bowen, 658 F.Supp. 1425 (W.D. Wis. 1987).

[104]42 U.S.C.A. §1320c-3(e).

[105]42 U.S.C.A. §1320c-3(a)(14).

[106]42 U.S.C.A. §1320c-3(a)(4)(B).

[107]42 U.S.C.A. §1395dd(d)(3); see Chapter 12.

[108]See, e.g., Holt v. Good Samaritan Hosp. and Health Ctr., 590 N.E.2d 1318 (Ohio Ct. App. 1990); Bouquett v. St. Elizabeth Corp., 43 OhioSt.3d 50 (Ohio 1989); Williams v. Hobbs, 9 OhioApp.3d 331 (Ohio Ct. App. 1983); Redding v. St. Francis Med. Ctr., 208 Cal.App.3d 98 (Cal. Ct. App. 1989); Tomlinson v. Humana, Inc., 495 So.2d 630 (Ala. 1986); Brendon v. Combs, 666 S.W.2d 755 (Ky. 1983); Radiology Prof. Corp. v. Trinidad Area Health Ass'n, 195 Colo. 253 (Colo. 1978)

[109]See, e.g., Bartley v. Eastern Maine Medical Ctr., 617 A.2d 1020 (Me. 1992); Katz v. Children's Hosp., 602 N.E.2d 598 (Mass. Ct. App. 1992); Rees v. Intermountain Health Care, 808 P.2d 1069 (Utah 1991); St. Louis v. Baystate Medical Ctr., 568 N.E.2d 1181 (Mass. Ct. App. 1991); but see Gianetti v. Norwalk Hosp., 557 A.2d 1249 (Conn. 1989) (bylaws are not a contract between the hospital and physicians on staff); Murdoch v. Knollwood Park Hosp., 585 So.2d 873 (Ala. 1991) (same); St. Mary's Hosp. v. Radiology Prof. Corp., 421 S.E.2d 731 (Ga. Ct. App. 1992) (same).

[110]See, e.g., American Medical Int'l, Inc. v. Scheller, 590 So.2d 947 (Fla. Dist. Ct. App. 1991); Lewisburg Comm. Hosp., Inc. v. Alfredson, 805 S.W.2d 756 (Tenn. 1991).

[111]See, e.g., Northeast Georgia Radiological Assocs. v. Tidwell, 670 F.2d 507 (5th Cir. 1982); Bilek v. Tallahassee Mem. Regional Medical Ctr., No. 91-973, slip. op. (Fla. Dist. Ct. App. Apr. 29, 1991).

Public Safety Rationale Obviating Pretermination Hearings

Although both public and private hospitals generally are subject to due process requirements on constitutional or hospital bylaw grounds for quality-of-care reductions or for privilege termination, formal pretermination hearings may be dispensed with if the hospital's action is to protect the public or the provider represents an imminent danger to patients.[112] If summary termination occurs with no pretermination hearing, posttermination hearings must be held as soon as practicable to determine if the summary disposition was warranted.

Additional Reading. B. A. Liang, "An Overview and Analysis of Challenges to Medical Exclusive Contracts," *Journal of Legal Medicine* 18 (1997), pp. 1–45.

Staff Versus Clinical Privileges

Although in most cases, staff and clinical privileges are distinct, courts have not always considered them so, deeming a reduction or termination of clinical privileges a "constructive" revocation of all privileges necessitating a due process hearing.[113] However, most courts have indicated that retaining staff privileges while losing clinical privileges for nonquality (i.e., economic) reasons does not entitle the physician to a due process hearing.[114]

Additional Reading. D. J. Behinfar, "Exclusive Contracting Between Hospitals and Physicians and the Use of Economic Credentialing," *DePaul Journal of Healthcare Law* 1 (1996), pp. 71–91; D. H. Cowan, "Medical Staff Legal Issues," *University of Toledo Law Review* 17 (1986), pp. 851–65; L. A. Hagan, "Physician Credentialing: Economic Criteria Compete with the Hippocratic Oath," *Gonzaga Law Review* 31 (1995), pp. 427–74; B. A. Liang, "An Overview and Analysis of Challenges to Medical Exclusive Contracts," *Journal of Legal Medicine* 18 (1997), pp. 1–45; J. S. Schroder and M. A. Wiliams, "Critical Revisions in Medical Staff Bylaws—Part II,"

Health Law 7 (1994), pp. 1–5; S. Summers, "Medical Staff Credentialing: Physician Challenges to Board Certification Criteria," *American Journal of Trial Advocacy* 18 (1995), pp. 673–700.

Covenants Not to Compete

In addition to broader provisions on both the public and private levels that may regulate how, what, and where a practitioner may practice, private employment agreements between practitioners and employers such as group practices or managed care organizations also may limit the extent to which practitioners render medical services, particularly after the physician no longer works for the employer. These covenants are important for entities because of the desire of the contracting entity to keep patients within its practice or plan after the physician leaves. Because of the fact-specific nature of these contracts and state statutes, specific contractual limitations that are enforceable in one jurisdiction may not be in another.

Generally, these limitations on practice, known as *covenants not to compete* or *restrictive covenants*, are enforceable if they are ancillary to the employment contract,[115] supported by legal consideration,[116] and reason-

---

[112]See, e.g., Caine v. Hardy, 943 F.2d 1406 (5th Cir. 1991), *cert. denied* 503 U.S. 936 (1992); Charbonnet v. Board of Trustees, 782 F. Supp. 1507 (Kan. Ct. App. 1992); Copsey v. Swearingen, 36 F.3d 1336 (5th Cir. 1994); Mudge v. Macomb Cty., 580 N.W.2d 845 (Mich. 1998).

[113]See, e.g., Lewisburg Comm. Hosp. v. Alfredson, 805 S.W.2d 756 (Tenn. 1991).

[114]See, e.g., Dutta v. St. Francis Regional Med. Ctr., 867 P.2d 1057 (Kan. 1994); Bartley v. Eastern Maine Medical Ctr., 617 A.2d 1020 (Me. 1992); Engelstad v. Virginia Mun. Hosp., 718 F.2d 262 (8th Cir. 1983); Keskin v. Munster Medical Research Found., 580 N.E.2d 354 (Ind. Ct. App. 1991).

[115]See, e.g., Brecher v. Brown, 17 N.W.2d 377 (Iowa 1945), *overruled on other grounds* Ehlers v. Iowa Warehouse Co., 188 N.W.2d 368 (Iowa), *modified on other grounds* 190 N.W.2d 413 (Iowa 1971); Reeves v. Decorah Farmers Coop. Soc., 160 Iowa 194 (Iowa 1913); Swigert & Havard v. Tilden, 97 N.W. 82 (Iowa 1913); Trionic Assn., Inc. v. Harris Corp., 27 F.Supp.2d 175 (E.D. N.Y. 1998)

[116]See, e.g., Canfield v. Spear, 254 N.E.2d 433 (Ill. 1969) (a promise to limit practice in community is a valid legal consideration on which employer hired him); Taylor v. Lovelace Clinic, 432 P.2d 816 (N.M. 1967) (a restrictive covenant was enforceable on basis of promises in contract that constituted legal consideration); Loescher v. Policky, 173 N.W.2d 50 (S.D. 1969) (compliance with an employment contract through first year and from the end of this year to its termination and employer's desire to continue contract for indefinite period are a valid legal consideration making the restrictive covenant enforceable); Zellner v. Stephen D. Conrad, M.D., P.C., 589 N.Y.S.2d 903 (N.Y. App. Div. 1992) (a corporation's continued employment of an ophthalmologist constituted valid legal consideration for the noncompetition clause); *cf.* Parker v. Slayter, 238 S.W.2d 814 (Tex. Ct. App. 1951) (an employment agreement that was to last two years did not support the restrictive covenant when the employee chiropractor was fired after less than one year); Freeman v. Duluth Clinic, Ltd., 334 N.W.2d 626 (Minn. 1983) (a covenant not to compete was unenforceable for lack of consideration, where covenant not bargained for and executed after employment began).

able. State statutes also may place additional requirements or limitations on these contractual terms.

The major determinant, and the focus of legal challenge to these provisions, is the relative reasonableness of the covenant not to compete.[117] Reasonableness is assessed by courts balancing how the restrictive covenant affects the parties and the public, the geographic scope of the restriction on practice, the time duration of the restriction, and the services covered.[118] In this assessment, courts usually construe the covenants very narrowly, as they all represent restraints on trade; therefore, courts attempt to apply the restrictive effects on former employees only to the extent necessary to protect the legitimate interests of the employer.

Reasonableness is assessed from the employer's perspective by determining how to protect the interests of the employer after the employee physician has obtained access to patients during employment and has been provided with professional benefits by the employer. If the courts deem that the contact with the employer's patient and the professional benefits provided by the employer, such as the experience gained from the practice, are substantial, then they will enforce the covenants to protect the interest of the employer.[119] In addition, if courts find that the former employee has opportunities available to him or her elsewhere, courts may weigh this factor positively in the interests of the employer in enforcing the covenant.[120] Likewise, when a sufficient number of practitioners are in the area, courts have enforced practice

covenants, since they represent no harm to the public interest.[121] However, courts will not enforce limitations against practice when the former employee's activities are not deemed to damage the employer.[122] Also, if the public interest would suffer due to a shortage of competent

---

[117]See, e.g., Lessner Dental Labs., Inc. v. Kidney, 492 P.2d 39 (Ariz. Ct. App. 1971); Marshall v. Covington, 339 P.2d 504 (Idaho 1959); Cogley Clinic v. Martini, 112 N.W.2d 678 (Iowa 1962); Lovelace Clinic v. Murphy, 417 P.2d 450 (N.M. 1966); Reddy v. Comm. Health Found. of Man, 298 S.E.2d 906 (W.Va. 1982).

[118]See, e.g., Phoenix Orthopedic Surgeons, Ltd. v. Peairs, 790 P.2d 752 (Ariz. Ct. App. 1989), *rev. denied* (Ariz.) 1990 Ariz. LEXIS 96; Williams v. Hobbs, 460 N.E.2d 287 (Ohio Ct. App. 1983); Hosp. Consultants Inc. v. Potyka, 531 S.W.2d 657 (Tex. Ct. Civ. App. 1975).

[119]See, e.g., Freudenthal v. Espey, 102 P. 280 (Colo. 1909) (covenant not to compete in practice of medicine, surgery, or obstetrics for five years in the city of the employer is deemed reasonable); Mabray v. Williams, 291 P.2d 677 (Colo. 1955) (covenant prohibiting practice of medicine within a 50-mile radius of the city of the employer for five years is deemed reasonable); Reddy v. Comm. Health Found. of Man, 298 S.E.2d 906 (W.Va. 1982) (a restrictive covenant contained in the contract between the physician and a nonprofit health center limiting practice to areas beyond a 30-mile radius of clinic for three years is deemed reasonable and enforceable); Torbett v. Wheeling Dollar Sav., 314 S.E.2d 166 (W. Va. 1983); Ferrofluidics Corp. v. Advanced Vacuum Comp. Inc., 968 F.2d 1463 (1st. Cir. 1992) (finding a nondisclosure agreement is enforceable).

[120]See, e.g., Lareau v. O'Nan, 355 S.W.2d 679 (Ky. 1962) (a restrictive covenant was enforceable against a physician because the nationwide demand for physicians and geographic limitation did not cause enough harm to invalidate the covenant); Phoenix Orthopedic Surgeons, Ltd. v. Peairs, 790 P.2d 752 (Ariz. Ct. App. 1989) (a restrictive covenant was enforceable against an orthopedic surgeon when at least eight other hospitals and surgical facilities provided opportunity for him to practice); Vascular & Gen. Surgical Assoc., Ltd. v. Loiterman, 599 N.E.2d 1246 (Ill. App. Ct. 1992) (a restrictive covenant was enforceable because physician could practice elsewhere, outside geographic limitation).

[121]See, e.g., Cogley Clinic v. Martini, 112 N.W.2d 678 (Iowa 1962) (enforcing a restrictive covenant is not against the public welfare because a significant supply of physicians are in the geographic area); Lareau v. O'Nan, 355 S.W.2d 679 (Ky. 1962) (enforcing a restrictive covenant is not against public interest even when the county needed additional physicians because the community was not deprived of any services it had before contract was made); Horne v. Radiological Health Services, P.C., 371 N.Y.S.2d 948 (Misc. 1975) (a restrictive covenant is enforceable against former employee radiologist when the community appeared to have an adequate supply).

[122]See, e.g., Wilson v. Clarke, 470 F.2d 1218 (1st Cir. 1972) (new managerial duties directing the activities of subordinates in clinical practice did not damage the former employer and did not violate a restrictive covenant not to compete by providing clinical services); Lessner Dental Labs. Inc. v. Kidney, 492 P.2d 39 (Ariz. Ct. App. 1971) (a restrictive covenant that, for two years after terminating employment, employee would not directly engage in the repair, adjustment, creation, manufacture, or sale of dental prostheses and related devices and would not divulge any knowledge disclosed by employer regarding techniques or formulas, not disclose the names of customers or client lists was too broad to cover the legitimate interests of the employer because the employee would be prevented from using her skill and general knowledge for two years); PHP HealthCare Corp. v. EMSA Ltd. Partnership, 14 F.3d 941 (4th Cir. 1993) (a noncompetition agreement was unenforceable when the former employer did not compete in same market as former employees); Broome v. Ginsberg, 283 S.E.2d 1 (Ga. Ct. App. 1980) (a restrictive covenant was unenforceable because the terms would not benefit the other party, which was a corporation that was dissolved); Ellis v. McDaniel, 596 P.2d 222 (Nev. 1979) (a restrictive covenant was partially unenforceable as to orthopedic services when the orthopedic surgeon left a group that did not provide orthopedic services and patients with a need for those services would be significantly burdened if the covenant were applied to the services).

practitioners in an area, courts have held that the restrictive covenants are unenforceable.[123]

Note that covenants not to compete will not be invalidated simply because they are unlimited in time as long as they are reasonably limited as to geographic location.[124] Courts will imply a reasonable time for the purposes of protecting the employer's interests.[125] If stated in the contract, it appears that up to three to five years as a duration for the restrictive covenants are deemed enforceable under each situation's unique facts and circumstances.[126]

Geographic scope of the restrictive covenant generally is limited to the area where the employer practices or the locale from which the employer draws its patients. The focus of the inquiry is to what extent the geographic limitations on practice are necessary to protect the legitimate interests of the employer; this represents a highly fact-specific assessment.[127] Courts may enforce the covenants after they reduce the extent of the original geographic scope.[128]

The scope of the services that are limited by the covenant must also be limited to the level of restriction that would protect the employer's interests. These limitations cannot harm the public health if they are to be enforceable.[129]

Note that courts may enforce all, some, or none of the restrictive covenant. Remedies for breach may include damages against the breaching party (usually the physician), injunctive relief against the physician if monetary damages are not adequate, or an invalidation of some or all of the restrictive covenant if unenforceable.

Concept.

Covenants not to compete are enforceable if they are ancillary to the employment contract, supported by legal consideration, and reasonable in time and scope and if they do not adversely affect the public welfare.

---

[123]See, e.g., Odess v. Taylor, 211 So.2d 805 (Ala. 1968) (an anti-competition covenant is unenforceable when enforcing such a covenant would limit availability of otolaryngologists, already in short supply, in the community); Dick v. Geist, 693 P.2d 1133 (Idaho Ct. App. 1985) (a restrictive covenant prohibiting critical-care neonatologist pediatricians from practicing within 25 miles of Twin Falls, Idaho, was unenforceable because it would deprive the community of the only available specialists and have detrimental public health consequences); Iredell Digestive Disease Clinic, P.A. v. Petrozza, 373 S.E.2d 449 (N.C. Ct. App.), *aff'd* 377 S.E.2d 750 (N.C. 1988) (a restrictive covenant was unenforceable because it would lead to only one gastroenterologist in the community, with monopoly power, and have adverse consequences on the public health); cf. Medical Specialists v. Sleweon, 652 N.E.2d 517 (Ind. Ct. App. 1995) (a restrictive covenant was enforceable against an infectious disease physician who could not establish that other physicians in the area could not provide adequate medical care to patients with infectious diseases).

[124]See, e.g., Karpinski v. Ingrasci, 320 N.Y.S.2d 1 (N.Y. 1971) (restrictive covenant silent as to duration did not render agreement unenforceable); Keen v. Schneider, 114 N.Y.S.2d 126 (Misc.), *aff'd* 116 N.Y.S.2d 494 (N.Y. App. Div. 1952) (same).

[125]See, e.g., Hansen v. Edwards, 426 P.2d 792 (Nev. 1967) (time interval of one year is deemed reasonable in absence of time duration of restrictive covenant); Lewis v. Krueger, Hutchinson & Overton Clinic, 269 S.W.2d 798 (Tex. 1954) (restrictive covenants without time duration enforceable if limited in geographic scope, but court could limit time period to reasonable time to protect employer's interests); but see Mandeville v. Harman, 7 A. 37 (N.J. Eq. 1886) (restrictive covenant covering all of former employee's life deemed unreasonable time duration); Schneller v. Hayes, 28 P.2d 273 (Wash. 1934) (restrictive covenant that would forever prohibit employee from carrying on optometry business is deemed unenforceable).

[126]See, e.g., Long v. Huffman, 557 S.W.2d 911 (Mo. Ct. App. 1977) (five years); McMurray v. Bateman, 144 S.E.2d 345 (Ga. 1965) (three years); Marshall v. Covington, 339 P.2d 504 (Idaho 1959) (three years); Canfield v. Spear, 254 N.E.2d 433 (Ill. 1969) (three years).

[127]See, e.g., Hall v. Willard & Woolsey, P.S.C., 471 S.W.2d 316 (Ky. 1971) (50-mile radius from city where practice is located is deemed enforceable); Raiford v. Kramer, 204 S.E.2d 171 (Ga. 1974) (five-county area is deemed enforceable); Canfield v. Spear, 254 N.E.2d 433 (Ill. 1969) (25-mile radius from city and city is deemed enforceable); Gomez v. Chua Med. Corp., 510 N.E.2d 191 (Ind. Ct. App. 1987) (30-mile radius from practice is deemed enforceable); Isuani v. Manske-Sheffield Radiology Group, P.A., 805 S.W.2d 602 (Tex. Ct. App. 1991) (15-mile radius from hospital is deemed enforceable); cf. Brecher v. Brown, 17 N.W.2d 377 (Iowa 1945) (25-mile radius of city is deemed unenforceable); Parker v. Slayter, 238 S.W.2d 814 (Tex. Ct. App. 1951) (county restriction is deemed unenforceable); Rudolph Bros., Inc. v. Greulick, 21 N.Y.S.2d 971 (N.Y. 1940) (10-mile radius from any municipality where employer operates is deemed unenforceable); Cukjati v. Burkett, 772 S.W.2d 215 (Tex. Ct. App. 1989) (12-mile radius of employer is deemed unenforceable).

[128]See, e.g., Foltz v. Struxness, 215 P.2d 133 (Kan. 1950) (reduction from 100-mile radius to 5-mile radius); Hansen v. Edwards, 426 P.2d 792 (Nev. 1967) (reduction from 100-mile radius to boundary of the city); Total Health Physicians, S.C. v. Barrientos, 502 N.E.2d 1240 (Ill. App. Ct. 1986) (unreasonable geographic limitation may be limited to reasonable area to make restrictive covenant enforceable).

[129]See, e.g., Lloyd Damsey, M.D., P.A. v. Mankowitz, 339 So.2d 282 (Fla. Dist. Ct. App.), *cert. denied* 345 So.2d 421 (Fla. 1977) (covenant is unenforceable when it would require physician to leave the community where he made significant investments and where the community needed the physician's services); Geocaris v. Surgical Consultants, Ltd., 302 N.W.2d 76 (Wis. Ct. App. 1981) (covenant not to compete is valid only for services that the former employer supplied); Valley Med. Spec. v. Farber, 950 P.2d 1184 (Ariz. Ct. App. 1997) (found protectable interests in its current patients and referral sources); Gant v. Hygeia Fac. Foun., Inc., 384 S.E. 2d 842 (Ga. 1989) (found restrictive covenant enforceable based on clinic's patients' close proximity).

Case.   Neurosurgeon Dr. F hired neurologist Dr. C to be able to compete with several other neurological practices in the area. The contract between them stipulated that Dr. C was to associate with the practice of Dr. F to provide neurological services for one year in the area of the city of Malden. Within the contract, there was the following covenant not to compete:

> For a period of two (2) years after termination of the Agreement, the Employee [Dr. C] agrees not to solicit business from, nor engage in the practice of medicine, in the specialty of neurology, directly or indirectly, nor read EEG findings [at area hospitals]. The Employee [Dr. C] further agrees that for a period of two (2) years from the date of termination of this Agreement he will not open an office for the practice of medicine in the specialty of neurology, directly or indirectly, nor associate with any physician or professional medical corporation for the purpose of practicing said specialty of neurology, directly or indirectly, in or within a radius of five (5) statute miles from the borders of the City of Malden.

During the initial period of association, Dr. F assisted Dr. C in treating Dr. F's patients; Dr. F also assisted Dr. C in obtaining staff privileges in the area's hospitals where Dr. F practiced. However, five months later, significant disagreements erupted between the two in clinical and nonclinical care aspects of their relationship. The association was terminated by both parties. Dr. C immediately set up practice within the area. Dr. F sued, requesting the court to enjoin Dr. C from practicing in violation of the covenant.

Legal Discussion.   The restrictive covenant was a valid, enforceable part of the employment agreement and so Dr. C was enjoined from practicing in violation of it according to the case on which this illustration is based.[130] First, it appears that the restrictive covenant was ancillary to the contract. The contract was primarily to delineate the employment agreement between Dr. F and Dr. C; the restrictive covenant was not the primary portion of the contract. Second, the contract was supported by legal consideration. Each party promised to bind itself to a particular set of obligations that were not extant before the agreement. There was no evidence of fraud, duress, or unconscionability in the entry into the contract. Third, the geographic coverage was reasonable to protect Dr. F's interests and was not unreasonably broad. Dr. F actively practiced in each of the geographic areas that Dr. C claimed was too broad to reasonably protect his former employer's interests. Therefore, the geographic scope of the restrictive covenant was appropriate to protect Dr. F's legitimate interests. Fourth, the duration of two years was

reasonable. The goodwill that was to be protected by the covenant was a long-term benefit, which applies to both Dr. F's patients as well as potential referrals he may receive. Two years allowed these interests to be protected. Finally, this covenant was not against the public interest. A significant number of neurologists and neurosurgeons were in Malden and the surrounding areas; hence, no patients have suffered or will suffer due to the unavailability of Dr. C's neurological services. Therefore, the restrictive covenant was valid and Dr. C must terminate his practice, which was in violation of its terms.

Further Reading

Contracting Out of Hearing Rights

Rosen PM. Medical Staff Peer Review: Qualifying the Qualified Privilege Provision. *Loy LA L Rev* 1993;27:357–90.
Roth MD. Peer Review Pitfalls: The Data Bank and Beyond. *Whittier L Rev* 1992;13:387–89.

Covenants Not to Compete

Berg P. Judicial Enforcement of Covenants Not to Compete Between Physicians: Protecting Doctors' Interests at Patients' Expense. *Rutgers L Rev* 1992;45:1–48.
Sullivan MR. Covenants Not to Compete and Liquidated Damages Clauses: Diagnosis and Treatment for Physicians. *SC L Rev* 1995;46:505–23.

Criteria for Review in Staff and Clinical Privilege Assessments

Borken PE. Exclusive Contracts: Are Constructively Terminated Incumbent Physicians Entitled to a Fair Hearing? *J Legal Med* 1996;17:143–68.
Kadzielski MA. Provider Deselection and Decapitation in a Changing Healthcare Environment. *St Louis U L J* 1997;891–914.
Liang BA. An Overview and Analysis of Challenges to Medical Exclusive Contracts. *J Legal Med* 1997;18:1–45.
Scott C. Medical Peer Review, Antitrust, and the Effect of Statutory Reform. *Md L Rev* 1991;50:316–407.

Expert Witness Testimony

Drechsler CT. Expert Testimony. In: *American Jurisprudence,* 2d ed., vol. 61. Rochester, NY: Lawyers Cooperative Publishing Co., 1998 (update supplement); §§345–56.
Eitel DR et al. Physicians' Attitudes About Expert Medical Witnesses. *J Legal Med* 1997;18:345–60.
Keith DL. Medical Expert Testimony in Texas Medical Malpractice Cases. *Baylor L Rev* 1991;43:1–138.

---

[130]Middlesex Neurological Assocs., Inc. v. Cohen, 324 N.E.2d 911 (Mass. Ct. App. 1975).

McNaughton AB, McNaughton S. Divided Loyalty: The Dilemma of the Treating Physician Advocate. *Okla City U L Rev* 1997;22:1051–66.

Merideth DL. The Medical Expert Witness in Mississippi: Outgunning the Opposition. *Miss L J* 1994;64:85–115.

Medical Directors

Brown VY et al. Managed Care at the Crossroads: Can Managed Care Organizations Survive Government Regulations? *Annals Health Law* 1998;7:25–59.

Chamber of Commerce Targets Health Care Legislation. *Cal Health L Monitor* 1997;5(10):5–10.

Sage MW. Enterprise Liability and the Emerging Managed Healthcare System. *Law & Contemp Probs* 1997;60:159–210.

National Practitioner Data Bank

Ankney RN et al. Physician Understanding of the National Practitioner Data Bank. *South Med J* 1995;88:200–203.

Barton HM. National Practitioner Data Bank: To Report or Not? *Tex Med* 1993;89:35–37.

Liang BA. Beyond the Malpractice Suit: The National Practitioner Data Bank. *Hosp Phys* 1995;31(7):11–14.

Martz EW. National Practitioner Data Bank. *Del Med J* 1995;67:492–93.

Neighbor WE et al. Rural Hospitals' Experience with the National Practitioner Data Bank. *Am J Public Health* 1997;87:663–66.

Peer Review and Medicare

Jost TS. Administrative Law Issues Involving the Medicare Utilization and Quality Control Peer Review Organization (PRO) Program: Analysis and Recommendations. *Ohio St L J* 1989;50:1–71.

Mellette PM. The Changing Focus of Peer Review Under Medicare. *U Rich L Rev* 1986;20:315–56.

Morreim HE. Cost Containment and the Standard of Medicare. *Cal L Rev* 1987;75:1719–63.

Peer Review and Quality Assurance—Federal

Blum JD. Medical Peer Review. *J Legal Educ* 1998;38:525–33.

Jost TS. The Necessary and Proper Role of Regulation to Assure the Quality of Health Care. *Hous L Rev* 1998;25:525–98.

Morter CS. The Healthcare Quality Improvement Act of 1986. *Va L Rev* 1998;74:1115–40.

Nodzenski TJ. Where Is the Quality in the Healthcare Improvement Act of 1986? *Loy LA L J* 1991;22:361–408.

Peer Review and Quality Assurance—States

Sagsueen MG, Thompson JL. The Evolution of Medical Peer Review in North Dakota. *ND L Rev* 1997;73:477–504.

Scheutzow S, Gillis S. Confidentiality and Privilege of Peer Review Information: More Imagined Than Real. *JL & Health* 1992;7:169–97.

Scibetta PL. Restructuring Hospital-Physician Relations: Patient Care Quality Depends on the Health of Hospital Peer Review. *U Pitt L Rev* 1990;51:1025–59.

Retaining Staff Privilege Membership

Allred AD, Tottenham TO. Liability and Indemnity Issues for Integrated Delivery Systems. *St Louis U L J* 1996;40:457–542.

Behinfar DJ. Exclusive Contracting Between Hospitals and Physicians and the Use of Economic Credentialing. *DePaul J Healthcare L* 1996;1:71–91.

Liang BA. An Overview and Analysis of Challenges to Medical Exclusive Contracts. *J Legal Med* 1997;18:1–45.

Zellers JD, Paulin MR. Termination of Hospital Medical Staff Privileges for Economic Reasons: An Appeal for Consistency. *Me L Rev* 1994;46:67–86.

Staff and Clinical Privileges

Behinfar DJ. Exclusive Contracting Between Hospitals and Physicians and the Use of Economic Credentialing. *DePaul J Healthcare L* 1996;1:71–91.

Cowan DH. Medical Staff Legal Issues. *U Tol L Rev* 1986;17:851–65.

Hagan LA. Physician Credentialing: Economic Criteria Compete with the Hippocratic Oath. *Gonz L Rev* 1995;31:427–74.

Schroder JS, Wiliams MA. Critical Revisions in Medical Staff Bylaws — Part II. *Health Law* 1994;7:1–5.

Summers S. Medical Staff Credentialing: Physician Challenges to Board Certification Criteria. *Am J Trial Advoc* 1995;18:673–700.

State Licensure

Coleman P, Shellow RA. Restricting Medical Licenses Based on Illness Is Wrong — Reporting Makes It Worse. *J L & Health* 1997;9:273–302.

Darricades J. Medical Peer Review: How Is It Protected by the Health Care Quality Improvement Act of 1986? *J Contemp L* 1992;18:263–83.

Kadzielski MA. Provider Deselection and Decapitation in a Changing Healthcare Environment. *St Louis U L J* 1997;41:891–914.

Mars S. The Corporate Practice of Medicine: A Call for Action. *Health Matrix* 1997;7:241–81.

Zeve OL. Physician Discipline: Considerations for a National Policy. *In Pub Interest* 1993;13:1–32.

Unauthorized Practice

Indest GF, Egolf B. Is Medicine Headed for an Assembly Line? Exploring the Doctrine of the Unauthorized Corporate Practice of Medicine. *Aug Bus L Today* 1997;6:32–36.

Rosenberg LM. Notice of Revocation of License Not Required to Prosecute for Unauthorized Practice of Medicine. *NY Health L Update* 1997;4(10):3–6.

Other Reading

American Medical Association. *U.S. Medical Licensure Statistics and Current Licensure Requirements.* Chicago: American Medical Association, 1998.

Berg P. Judicial Enforcement of Covenants Not to Compete Between Physicians: Protecting Doctors' Interests at Patients' Expense. *Rutgers L Rev* 1992;45:1–48.

Blum JD. Economic Credentialing: A New Twist on Hospital Appraisal Process. *J Legal Med* 1991;12:427–75.

Drechsler CT. Physicians, Surgeons, and Other Healers. In: *American Jurisprudence,* 2d ed., vol. 61. Rochester, NY: Lawyers Cooperative Publishing Co., 1997;139–278.

Liang BA. Error in Medicine: Legal Impediments to U.S. Reform. *J Health Politics Pol'y Law* 1999;24:27–58.

Liang BA. An Overview and Analysis of Challenges to Medical Exclusive Contracts. *J Legal Medicine* 1997;18:1–45.

Smith SM. Construction and Application of Health Care Quality Improvement Act of 1986 (42 U.S.C.A. §§11101–11152). In: *American Law Reports, Federal,* vol. 121 (supp.). Rochester, NY: Lawyers Cooperative Publishing Co., 1997.

Springer EW, Casale HM. Hospitals and the Disruptive Health Care Practitioner: Is the Ability to Work with Others Enough to Warrant Exclusion? *Duquesne L Rev* 1986;24:377–423.

Web Sites

American Association of Medical Review Officers: *http://www.aamro.com*

Doc-Guard: *http://www.doc-guard.com*

The Health Care News server: *http://www.healthcare newsserver.com*

Healthcare Quality Improvement Resources, Inc.: *http://www.hqir.com*

Joint Commission on Accreditation of Healthcare Organizations: *http://www.jcaho.org*

Managed care information center: *http://www.themic.com*

Medical Society of the County of Erie: *http://www.eriemds.org*

Online continuing medical education CME at the Virtual Lecture Hall: *http://www.vlh.com*

Physician licensing service: *http://www.physicianlicensing.com*

Risk management consulting: *http://www.riskmanco.com*

USMLE news: *http://www.usmle.org*

12

Fraud and Abuse

Fraud and abuse in health care generally involves the fraudulent provision and billing for health care services. As the health care dollar becomes increasingly stretched, federal and state governments have become more aggressive in their attempts to limit the provision of unnecessary services and business relationships that may increase health care costs. Hence, this area has become one of the most important and expansive in health care law and policy and shows no sign of abating.

This chapter on health care fraud and abuse focuses on three basic areas: false claims and other fraudulent billing, bribes or kickbacks in exchange for referrals, and referrals to entities in which the referring providers have some financial interest. Each area is covered by specified areas of the law, although there is overlap between them. The major statutes that define these prohibitions, respectively, are the False Claims Act[1] (FCA), the Medicare/Medicaid Antikickback Statute[2] (Antikickback Statute), and Medicare/Medicaid self-referral provisions[3] (Stark laws; the laws are named after Fortney "Pete" Stark, the congressional representative who proposed these rules). Generally, the Office of the Inspector General (OIG) of the Department of Health and Human Services (DHHS), the Health Care Financing Administration (HCFA), and the Department of Justice (DOJ) are the primary enforcers of the fraud and abuse rules.

False Claims Act

The FCA is a broad statute that applies to any activities that involve billing the government for goods or services. With regard to health care, the FCA prohibits submission of false claims and fraudulent billing:

1. under any federal health care program;
2. for any item or services;
3. provided by a person who:
   a. knowingly and willfully has made or caused to be made any false statement or representation of a material fact in application for payment; or
   b. has furnished services or supplies that are determined to be substantially in excess of those needed or are so lacking as to be worthless.[4]

The FCA thus implicates as illegal much more than simple billing for services or products not provided. Indeed, the FCA may be invoked if the provider has actual knowledge, acts in deliberate ignorance of the truth or falsity of the information, or acts in reckless disregard of the truth or falsity of information.[5] Further, merely billing a federal program for products or services more expensive than the actual product or service provided, making claims for products or services not within coverage of the program as well as fraudulently misrepresenting the condition of the patient to obtain higher billing levels are also within the FCA's contemplation of an illegal and false claim. Penalties for violation of the FCA include treble damages for all false claims, a $5,000–$10,000 fine per false claim, potential exclusion from federal health programs, criminal penalties, and loss of tax-exempt status.[6]

Some Established Categories of Fraud Under the FCA

Claims for Services Not Provided or Medically Unnecessary Services

Claims for services not provided include both false claims for services that were not provided to the patient and

---

[1] 31 U.S.C.A. §§3729–3733; 18 U.S.C.A. §287; see also 42 U.S.C.A. §1320a-7a.

[2] 42 U.S.C.A. §1320a-7b(b).

[3] 42 U.S.C.A. §1395nn.

[4] 42 U.S.C.A. §1320a-7a.

[5] 31 U.S.C.A. §3729(b).

[6] 31 U.S.C.A. §3729(a).

claims for services with higher reimbursement in lieu of those actually rendered (also known as *upcoding*). Examples of the former are pharmacists who bill for durable medical equipment that is not provided[7] and physicians who bill for invasive procedures never rendered.[8] Upcoding examples include billing for an office visit when only telephone contact was made with a patient,[9] treatments such as an injection billed by the physician when the nurse performed the procedure,[10] and dental claims for oral cancer consultation when only a normal dental screening was performed.[11] In addition, claims for payment for medically unnecessary services are considered false claims. Therefore, any claims that cannot be substantiated as medically indicated and necessary for the patient's health may be considered medically unnecessary and subject the claimant to liability.

In an important qui tam action (discussed later in this chapter), *United States ex rel. Grossenbacher v Smith-Kline Beecham Clinical Laboratories, Inc.*,[12] SmithKline Beecham Clinical Laboratories (SKBL) designed laboratory testing profiles that could not be billed under a single code and were unbundled (i.e., billed for as if the tests were done separately) even though all the tests were performed simultaneously on automated equipment. Beyond these actions, SKBL also used a marketing tool that would allow physicians to bill private insurance companies using these profiles so as to make their own substantial profits. Using this strategy, as well as other questionable methods, SKBL increased its reimbursements for laboratory testing significantly. The federal government sued SKBL under the FCA, indicating that these activities were not related to medical necessity and by marketing the profiles in this manner, it encouraged physicians to order them from SKBL, which in turn billed Medicare and Medicaid at substantial profit. The federal government obtained a $325 million settlement from SKBL as well as an admission of guilt for violating the FCA.

Coinsurance and Deductible Waivers

Federal programs such as Medicare contain provisions that require cost sharing by the patient.[13] Providers are prohibited from waiving such coinsurance and deductible

cost sharing (except in the instance of indigence or nonpayment by patients after a good faith effort to collect by the provider). The basis of this insistence on collecting patient cost-sharing amounts is that the federal government is to pay only a part of the cost of the patient's care; by waiving cost sharing, providers thus make the government pay for 100% of the patient's care.[14] Thus, inappropriate waiver of cost sharing can constitute a false claim under the FCA. Liability also may result under the Health Insurance Portability and Accountability Act of 1996 for such waivers, if the provider knows or should know that the waivers (considered "remuneration") would induce a patient to obtain services from that provider. Note that no actual intent to induce a referral is necessary for liability, only that the entity providing the remuneration should have known that it would induce the patient to go to the specific provider who waived the patient's cost sharing.[15]

DRG Creep and DRG Payment Window Claims

The term *DRG creep* describes upcoding in hospitals that results in higher reimbursed DRGs (diagnosis-related groups) for their Medicare patients.[16] Because DRG payments are affected by a broad array of factors, such as principal and secondary diagnoses, procedures performed during hospitalization, and complications, misrepresentation can occur (intentionally or unintentionally), resulting in a DRG that has "crept" from a lower reimbursement category to a higher one. This form of maximizing the hospital's reimbursement is considered fraudulent. DRG payment window violations represent billing separately for outpatient services that should be covered by the DRG payment. Federal law indicates that all services provided by a hospital or any entity wholly owned or operated by the hospital 72 hours before admission are covered by the inpatient reimbursement rate.[17] Therefore, any separate claim for normal services rendered within that 72-hour DRG window, such as for preoperative laboratory services the day before surgery, may be considered a false claim.

False Cost Reporting

Annual cost reports reflecting the actual costs of delivering care to patients must be submitted by Medicare and Medicaid participating institutions, such as home health agencies, hospitals, and nursing homes. These cost

[7]United States v. Hershenow, 680 F.2d 847 (1st Cir. 1982).

[8]People v. American Med. Ctrs., 324 N.W.2d 782 (Mich. Ct. App. 1982), *cert. denied* 464 U.S. 1009 (1983).

[9]See, e.g., State v. Romero, 574 So.2d 330 (La. 1990); see also United States v. Krizek, 859 F.Supp. 5 (D.D.C. 1994).

[10]See, e.g., United States v. Larm, 824 F.2d 780 (9th Cir. 1987).

[11]See, e.g., United States v. Lorenzo, 768 F.Supp. 1127 (E.D. Pa. 1991).

[12]United States *ex rel.* Grossenbacher v. SmithKline Beecham Clinical Laboratories, Inc., 1998 WL 166256 (E.D. Pa. April 8, 1998).

[13]42 U.S.C.A. §§1395e, 1395l.

[14]Department of Health and Human Services, Office of Inspector General, *Special Fraud Alert: OIG Announcement 91023* (1991).

[15]Joint Explanatory Statement H.R. Doc. No. 104-736 3103, Health Insurance Portability and Accountability Act of 1996, 104 Cong., 2d Sess. (1996).

[16]See Chapter 7.

[17]42 U.S.C.A. §1395ww(a)(4); 42 C.F.R. §412.2(c)(5) (1998).

reports serve as one basis for calculating the specific reimbursement levels for the particular health care institution. False claims liability may arise if these cost reports contain cost amounts unrelated to patient care or that misrepresent a higher cost of patient care than actually expended. Examples of such activities considered false claims include incorrect cost apportionment, noncovered service or equipment inclusion in the allowable costs, bad debt cost claims with no genuine effort to collect, asset depreciation on assets already depreciated or sold, and statistical manipulation of cost report data to obtain additional, unwarranted payments.[18]

Managed Care False Claims

If an MCO desires to provide services under the auspices of a federal program, it is subject to potential false claims liability, although to a different extent in relation to other providers. For example, when an MCO desires to serve in the Medicare program, it must indicate to HCFA in its application that it can provide all necessary services in a cost-effective manner to the Medicare population. If information in this application is misrepresented, the MCO is subject to false claims liability. In addition, MCO false claims liability may attach if the MCO exceeds permitted premiums, falsifies information provided to the Medicare program, prevents or discourages potentially high-cost Medicare beneficiaries from enrolling in the MCO, or wrongfully disenrolls a beneficiary from the MCO.[19] In addition, MCOs may be subject to liability if they do not fulfill the requirements for physician incentive plans[20] or operate the plan in a way that is inconsistent with the rules and regulations of the Medicare and Medicaid programs.[21]

Physicians at Teaching Hospitals (PATH)

PATH audits are reviews by the OIG investigating past physician billing practices at academic medical centers. The OIG has indicated that false claims have been submitted by these physicians and institutions because the level of care billed was not supported by documentation and thus constituted upcoding; in particular, there is no documentation of attending physician presence during treatment by resident physicians. On the basis of Intermediary Letter 372 (IL 372),[22] which was issued in 1969,

the OIG indicated that an attending physician may bill for services only if the services were actually provided by the attending physician or if the attending physician directly and personally supervised the resident physician, such supervision was necessary, the attending physician was physically present, and documentation justified such supervision. Hence, supervision by an attending physician of a resident that is not necessary because the resident is capable of performing the procedure alone, supervision by an attending physician that is necessary but the physical presence and justification are not documented, and cosigning a resident's note and billing for the procedure all are considered false claims. Although academic physicians had supervised and billed for procedures without such documentation or supervision as indicated in IL 372 for years after IL 372 was issued, these billing methods were not questioned in the past even under past government audits,[23] and regulations were issued in December 1995 clarifying the language of IL 372.[24] The OIG has still targeted all 125 of the academic medical centers in the United States for audits for past false claims and has collected millions of dollars in settlement of false claims against the centers at which investigations have occurred.[25] However, the OIG has dropped audits for those facilities it deems did not have clear communication with their Medicare carriers before December 30, 1992, regarding the attending physician physical presence requirement, which has amounted to 16 dropped audits.[26] Under the PATH initiative, the OIG may perform the audit or the institution may voluntarily perform the audit under OIG supervision (with the institution assuming the cost). However, the perception in the health care community is that voluntary self-audits are necessary to avoid high legal costs and high punitive sanctions.[27] This is further supported by the OIG and DOJ's insistence that teaching hospitals waive statute of limitations defenses and any attorney–client and work product privileges that relate to PATH audit information.[28] Health care organizations have attempted to block these audits through the

[18]Health Care Financing Administration, *Medicare Intermediary Manual* (Washington, DC: Health Care Financing Administration, 1998), section 3951.

[19]42 U.S.C.A. §1395mm(i)(6); 42 C.F.R. §1003.103(f) (1998).

[20]42 C.F.R. Part 1003 (1998).

[21]42 U.S.C.A. §§1320a-7a, 1395mm(i)(8).

[22]Intermediary Letter No. 372 from Department of Health, Education, and Welfare, Bureau of Health Insurance to Intermediaries (April 1969).

[23]J. J. Cohen and R. M. Dickler, "Auditing the Medicare-Billing Practices of Teaching Physicians — Welcome Accountability, Unfair Approach," *New England Journal of Medicine* 336 (1997), pp. 1317–20.

[24]Ibid.

[25]"IG to Audit All Hospital Academic Institutions Under PATH, IG's Morris Says," *BNA Health Care Daily* (July 18, 1996), p. D2.

[26]"HHS Backs Off Anti-Fraud Initiative, Dropping Audits of 16 Teaching Hospitals," *BNA Health Care Fraud Report* 1 (1997), p. 442.

[27]Cohen and Dickler, "Auditing the Medicare-Billing Practices of Teaching Physicians."

[28]L. Aussprung, "Fraud and Abuse: Federal Civil Health Care Litigation and Settlement," *Journal of Legal Medicine* 19 (1998), pp. 1–62.

courts; however, these challenges have been rejected[29] and FCA PATH liability settlements continue.

Physician-Incentive Programs That Attempt to Limit Necessary Services

Physicians may be provided with financial incentives to limit the costs associated with health care. These incentive programs, however, may not be used as an inducement by hospitals to limit medically necessary care for patients with Medicare or Medicaid insurance.[30] Hospitals that knowingly make these payments and physicians who accept these payments are subject to civil penalties for each patient on whom payment is made.[31] Note that physician-incentive plans may be allowed if they base payments on the cost performance of a group of physicians rather than a single physician, evaluate performance over a longer (e.g., annual) period rather than a shorter (e.g., quarterly) period, and do not base payments on a single patient's costs.[32]

Poor Quality of Care

As a condition of participation in public health care programs such as Medicare and Medicaid, the providers must meet certain quality standards as to the care rendered. If it can be shown that the requisite level of quality is not reached, any claim for such services could constitute a false claim. For example, a nursing home and its contractees that did not provide adequate nutritional and wound care and billed for its care have paid large settlements under the FCA.[33] Similarly, a psychiatric facility was found to have submitted false claims when some of the facility's patients, former sexual offenders and physically aggressive patients, sexually abused and physically injured other residents in the facility.[34] Therefore, any circumstance where the quality of care at the facility is deemed to have dropped below the quality standard set by the government that is billed as a claim for service payment may be considered a false claim.

Unbundling and Fragmenting

A very important area of focus for false claims is unbundling of services. Unbundling constitutes the practice of billing for several separate services that in fact should be billed as one. For example, hospitals that unbundle certain clinical laboratory tests that generally are run together and then bill for each separately are considered to have submitted false claims. Similarly, fragmenting claims is the practice of separately claiming for services that should be billed under a global reimbursement rate. Examples of this practice are billing Medicare separately for surgical services and pre- and postoperative care when a global fee is supposed to cover all these services[35] and separate billing for a biopsy that was part of a surgical procedure. It is important to note that consultants who offer to "maximize" hospital revenue may engage in this activity as well as upcoding;[36] however, this consultant activity does not absolve the provider of liability, although the consultant also may face FCA suit.[37]

Qui Tam Suits

In addition to public enforcement activities, the FCA allows private plaintiffs, also known as *whistleblowers*, to sue on behalf of the United States for monetary damages.[38] The term *qui tam* results from the legal phrase *qui tam pro domino rege quam pro se ipso in hace parte sequitur* (he who brings the action for the king as well as for himself).[39] This provision of the FCA often is referred to as the *whistleblower's statute*, with this private cause of action known as a *qui tam action*.[40] The private individual who brings the cause of action, known as the *relator*, usually wishes to ferret out fraud or is a former employee or competitor of the entity being sued. Relators may not base their suits on previously disclosed public information unless the qui tam relator is the original source of the information.[41]

Generally, relator suits are filed with the government under seal for at least 60 days (which may extend to years as the government investigates the action) to allow the

---

[29]Ass'n of American Medical Colleges v. United States, No. SA-CV—97862 (D.C. Cal., filed Oct. 10, 1997).

[30]42 U.S.C.A. §1320a-7a(b).

[31]42 U.S.C.A. §1320a-7a(b).

[32]42 C.F.R. Part 1003 (1998).

[33]United States v. Tucker House Inc., No. 96-1271 (E.D. Pa. Feb. 21, 1996) (consent order with nursing home paying $25,000 and contractee paying $575,000 in settlement); see also United States v. Northern Health Facilities, Inc., 25 F.Supp.2d 690 (D. Md. 1998) (federal U.S. attorney files civil FCA action seeking injunctive relief and damages against nursing home for substandard care).

[34]United States *ex rel.* Aranda v. Community Psychiatric Ctrs. of Oklahoma, Inc., 945 F.Supp. 1485 (W.D. Okla. 1996).

[35]See, e.g., United States v. Erickson, 75 F.3d 470 (9th Cir. 1996); see also Texas St. Bd. of Med. Examiners v. Scheffey, 949 S.W.2d 431 (Tex. Ct. App. 1997).

[36]Department of Health and Human Services, Office of Inspector General, *Medicare Fraud Alert: Fraud Alert OIG-97-01* (1997).

[37]See, e.g., United States v. Metzinger Assocs., 1996 WL 412811 (E.D. Pa. July 18, 1996) (settlement agreement).

[38]31 U.S.C.A. §§3730(a), 3730(b).

[39]W. Blackstone, *Commentaries on the Laws of England,* 4th ed., book III (Chicago: Callaghan Publishing, 1899).

[40]31 U.S.C.A. §3730.

government to determine whether it will intervene in the suit.[42] An action may not be brought more than 6 years after the date on which the violation occurred or more than 3 years after the date when facts material to the right of action are known or reasonably should have been known by the government official charged with responsibility to act in the circumstances, but in no event more than 10 years after the date on which the violation occurred, whichever occurs last.[43] If the government decides to intervene and the qui tam action is successful (i.e., results in a settlement with the accused entity or a court decision with a monetary verdict), the relator generally will be entitled to between 10% and 30% of the recovery (as well as reasonable costs and attorneys' fees), depending on his or her contribution to the action and other factors.[44] If the government declines to intervene, the relator may bring the action him- or herself.[45] The violation must be proven by a preponderance of the evidence.[46] Note that the government may dismiss the action, regardless of objections by the relator, as long as the relator has had the opportunity to be heard; also, the government may settle the action, regardless of objections by the relator, as long as a court determines after a hearing that the settlement is fair, adequate, and reasonable.[47] Further, if the relator actually was involved and is convicted of criminal conduct arising from his or her role in the false claim, the relator must be dismissed from the action and cannot receive any share of the proceeds.[48] And, if the government does not proceed with the action but the relator does proceed and loses, the defendant may be awarded its reasonable attorneys' fees and expenses if the court finds that the relator's action was clearly frivolous, clearly vexatious, or brought primarily for the purposes of harassment.[49] However, the potential for high awards, in the millions of dollars, has provided an extremely powerful incentive for individuals to ferret out and report fraud.

It is important to note that because of the risks attendant with whistleblowing (e.g., potential termination of employment), the whistleblower's statute also has protections for relators. Relators and those who assist them have explicit statutory protections against employment demotion, discharge, discrimination, harassment, and suspension threats.[50] Remedies for violation of these provisions include double back pay, reinstatement, special damages, and an award of attorneys' and other fees.[51]

Antikickback Statute

The Antikickback Statute's primary focus is payment for referrals. The Antikickback Statute prohibits

1. any knowing and willful conduct involving:
   a. the solicitation, receipt, offer, or payment of any kind of remuneration;
   b. in return for referring an individual for services or recommending or arranging the purchase, lease, or ordering of an item;
   c. that may be wholly or partly paid by a federal health care program.

This statute is quite broad in its application. For example, a completed, actual referral is not necessary; mere recommendation is enough for liability. Further, actual payment by a federal health care program also is not necessary; the statute requires only that the services or products *may* be wholly or partly paid by such a program. Violations of the Antikickback Statute are subject to fines of up to $25,000 per violation or actual imprisonment for up to five years or both as well as potential exclusion from federal health care programs.[52]

What is extremely important to note is that the term *remuneration* is very broad and may include any kind of payment "in cash or in kind" made directly, indirectly, overtly, or covertly.[53] Clearly, payment for referrals disguised as payments for consulting, marketing, research, or

[41]1 U.S.C.A. §§3730(e)(4)(A), 3730(e)(4)(B); see also United States *ex rel.* Susan Remseyer v. Century Healthcare Corp. and Century Healthcare Development Corp., 3 *Medicare and Medicaid Guide* (Chicago: Commerce Clearing House, 1995), ¶42,978 (W.D. Okla. 1994) (qui tam action based on government audit that is part of public record is barred because plaintiff is not original source of information); U.S. *ex rel.* Jones v. Horizon Healthcare, 160 F.3d 326 (6th Cir. 1998) (individual who filed an action in state court for whistleblower protection could not sustain False Claim Act qui tam suit due to previous state suit disclosure); cf. United States *ex rel.* Stinson, Lyons, Gerlin & Bustamante v. Prudential Ins. Co., 944 F.2d 1149 (3d Cir. 1991) (law firm original source of information when obtained through representation of party in unrelated lawsuit); Cooper v. Blue Cross and Blue Shield, 19 F.3d 562 (11th Cir. 1994) (federal employee who gained knowledge of fraud through his own claims processing, research, and correspondence with federal officials is held to be original source even though information had been publicly disclosed earlier); but see United States *ex rel.* Foust v. Group Hospitalization and Med. Servs., Inc., 26 F.Supp.2d 60 (D.D.C. 1998) (federal auditors cannot be original sources under FCA due to their obligation to report fraud to government).
[42]31 U.S.C.A. §3730(b)(2).
[43]31 U.S.C.A. §3731(b).
[44]31 U.S.C.A. §§3730(d)(1), 3730(d)(2).
[45]31 U.S.C.A. §3730(b).
[46]31 U.S.C.A. §3731(c).
[47]31 U.S.C.A. §§3730(c)(2)(A), 3730(c)(2)(B).
[48]31 U.S.C.A. §3730(d)(3).
[49]31 U.S.C.A. §3730(d)(4).
[50]31 U.S.C.A. §3730(h).
[51]31 U.S.C.A. §3730(h).
[52]42 U.S.C.A. §1320a-7b.
[53]42 U.S.C.A. §1320a-7b(b).

other activities[54] and payments in the form of loan guarantees, hospital leasing of physician office space at above market rates, practice enhancement payments, and the like[55] are payments for referrals under the Antikickback Statute. It should be emphasized, however, that remuneration includes *any* economic benefit, including reduced or discounted rent; guarantees of a specific level of compensation, loans, administrative, billing, or other services; and business activities that would give a provider an opportunity to generate fees. Note also that if one purpose of the payment is to induce referrals, even though the remuneration also reimbursed the providers for actual services rendered, the payment still may violate the Antikickback Statute.[56] In addition, common business arrangements may violate the Antikickback Statute, such as commercial rental based in whole or in part on percentage of gross revenues if there is a potential referral arrangement between the landlord and tenant (e.g., landlord is a physician group and tenant is a pharmacy or clinical laboratory). Note, however, that remuneration does not include discounts or price reductions *that are disclosed and reflected in claims for reimbursement*[57] or for employee pay from an employer for normal services.[58]

Finally, there is significant debate as to whether a violation of the Antikickback Statute constitutes a false claim under the FCA. Because the FCA merely requires a reckless disregard of the law to impose liability whereas the Antikickback Statute appears to require specific intent to violate the law, the government has tried to extend the FCA to kickback situations. Courts are split on the issue as to whether the FCA applies[59] or does not[60] in antikickback circumstances.

OIG Special Fraud Alerts

Several arrangements have been the focus of attention by the OIG under the Antikickback Statute. When these arrangements come to light, OIG Special Fraud Alerts often are issued to warn providers of their concern with these arrangements and provide information and guidance on specific trends in health care fraud, which generally are focused on violations of the Antikickback Statute.[61] Other fraudulent activities are also reported in the Special Fraud Alerts. Some suspect arrangements that are the subject of OIG Special Fraud Alerts are reviewed here.

Home Health Fraud

The OIG has identified certain practices in the home health area that are suspect under the Antikickback Statute and FCA. For example, claims for home health visits not made to the beneficiary, to beneficiaries not homebound, to beneficiaries not requiring a qualifying service, and to beneficiaries without physician authorization are considered false claims. Further, home health agencies have been deemed by the OIG as submitting false claims in their Medicare annual cost reports (that report overhead and other general patient care costs) by claiming costs for entertainment, travel, lobbying, gifts, and other expenses unrelated to patient care. Finally, the OIG has identified home health service arrangements that are considered payment or receipt of kickbacks in exchange for Medicaid and Medicare referrals, a violation of the Antikickback Statute. These kickbacks include payment to physicians for each plan of care certified by the physician for the home health agency, disguising referral fees as salaries by paying referring physicians for care not provided or paying physicians at greater than fair market value for their services, offering free services to beneficiaries if they agree to switch home health providers, providing hospitals with discharge planners or other "liaisons" to induce referrals to the home health agency, and providing free services to retirement homes or adult living facilities for referrals to the home health agency. Finally, some home health agencies have engaged in aggressive marketing tactics that target health beneficiaries and offer noncovered services in exchange for beneficiary Medicare identification numbers; also, some

[54]See, e.g., United States v. Caremark, 1995 WL 422157 (D. Minn. 1995); In re Caremark Int'l Inc. Derivative Litigation, 698 A.2d 959 (Del. Ch. 1996).

[55]See, e.g., United States v. Horizon Group Enter. Inc., No. 3:97CR0022 (N.D. Ind. Apr. 28, 1997).

[56]See, e.g., United States v. Greber, 760 F.2d 68, 69 (3d Cir.), *cert. denied* 474 U.S. 988 (1985) ("if one purpose of the payment was to induce referrals, the [Antikickback] statute has been violated"); United States v. Kats, 871 F.2d 105 (9th Cir. 1989) (Antikickback Statute is violated unless payments are "wholly and not incidentally attributable to the delivery of goods and services"); see also United States v. Bay State Ambulance & Hosp. Rental Serv., 874 F.2d 20 (1st Cir. 1989); United States v. Lipkis, 770 F.2d 1447 (9th Cir. 1985).

[57]See, e.g., Polk County v. Peters, 800 F.Supp. 1415 (E.D. Tex. 1992); see also Homecare Leasing Corp. v. Harrisburg Med. Management, 1998 WL 36358 (E.D. Pa. 1988).

[58]See, e.g., Central Il. Public Service Co. v. United States, 540 F.2d 300 (7th Cir. 1976).

[59]See, e.g., United States *ex rel.* Pogue v. American Healthcorp, 914 F.Supp. 1507 (M.D. Tenn. 1996); United States v. Metzinger, 1995 WL 398714 (E.D. Pa. 1995); see also United States v. Columbia/HCA Healthcare Corp., 938 F.Supp. 399 (S.D. Tex. 1996).

[60]See, e.g., United States *ex rel.* Thompson v. Columbia Health Care, 938 F.Supp. 399 (S.D. Tex. 1996), *reh'g granted* 1997 U.S.App. LEXIS 29090 (5th Cir.), *aff'd in part and vacated in part* 125 F.3d 899 (5th Cir. 1997), *on remand* 20 F.Supp.2d 1017 (S.D. Tex. 1998); see also United States *ex rel.* Hopper v. Anton, 91 F.3d 1261 (9th Cir. 1996) (simple violation of the law does not give rise to FCA liability).

[61]Department of Health and Human Services, Office of the Secretary, Office of Inspector General, *Special Fraud Alerts,* No. HHS-OS-00401 (August 4, 1995), available at www.hhs.gov.

of these agencies have attempted to pressure physicians to order unnecessary personal care services by indicating to these physicians that their patients are requesting these services and will change to another physician unless their demands are met. These marketing activities may run afoul of both the FCA and the Antikickback Statute.

Hospital–Physician and Other Joint Ventures

Joint ventures between physicians and hospitals or other entities can result in increased service provision to the benefit of the patient. For example, a hospital may assist a surgical group to create an outpatient surgery center in a community without such access by investing funds with the surgical group. Such a new venture could increase access to services best provided in these facilities while decreasing costs associated with typical inpatient stays. However, joint ventures also may be created to increase referrals from one party to the other. Hence, the OIG has indicated that certain joint ventures will be considered suspect.[62] These suspect joint ventures include those in which investors are potential referral sources, if physicians likely to be referral sources are given the opportunity to purchase larger shares of the joint venture than smaller or nonreferral sources, if physicians who are likely investors are encouraged to refer to the joint venture, if physicians are encouraged to divest from the joint venture if their referral levels fall below some "acceptable" level, if physicians are mandated to divest if they retire or otherwise cannot refer patients to the joint venture entity, if the joint venture entity tracks and distributes information regarding referral sources, or if an investment interest is nontransferable. The OIG also looks to the actual business structure of the joint venture; for example, a party in a joint venture that already provides the services that the joint venture will need and to which the joint venture will refer patients is considered party to a suspect "shell arrangement" in violation of the Antikickback Statute. Finally, the OIG will examine financing and profit distribution methodologies. Suspect arrangements would include those in which the capital invested by the physician is disproportionately small and the returns disproportionately large in comparison to a typical investment in a new business, physicians have to invest only a nominal amount, physician investors are allowed to "borrow" the "investment" amount from the joint venture and pay it back through profit distribution deductions, or investors are paid extremely high returns for the investment risk involved.

Note that although the reach of the Antikickback Statute is broad in these joint venture situations, according to the leading case on the subject, *Hanlester Network v Shalala*,[63] to be in violation of the statute, an individual or entity must *knowingly and willfully* offer to or actually pay remuneration to induce referrals with the specific intent to violate the law (although knowledge of the specific law violated is not necessary[64]). Simply because a large number of referrals could benefit physician-investors or a low number of referrals could result in a failure of the venture is not sufficient proof that an offer or payment of remuneration was made to induce referrals.[65] However, even with this case on the books, joint venture arrangements should be closely scrutinized to avoid potential fraud and abuse liability.

Hospital Purchase of Physician Practices

Hospitals that purchase physician practices, continue to allow those physicians to practice at the hospitals, and refer patients there are subject to scrutiny under the Antikickback Statute. These hospital purchases can be deemed illegal remuneration to induce referrals because the purchase may interfere with the physicians' subsequent decision as to where to refer their patients.[66] If the practice purchase includes any amount paid for assets that relate to the continuing treatment of the practice's patients by the selling physicians, this would be considered a payment for referrals and a violation of the Antikickback Statute. This concern includes payment for goodwill, noncompetition covenants, exclusive dealing arrangements, patient lists, and patient records. In addition, another suspect situation would be paying any amount to the selling physicians after the sale, even if they are hospital employees; these payments would be considered payments, at least in part, for referrals and so would not be considered to be within the employee exemption.

Hospital Retention and Recruitment Incentives for Physicians

Antikickback risks exist if hospitals require that hospital-based physicians pay for hospital-provided services at greater than fair market rates.[67] These kinds of arrangements can be seen as hospital-based physicians paying

---

[62]Department of Health & Human Services, Office of Inspector General, *Special Fraud Alert: Joint Venture Arrangements*, OIG-89-04 (April 1989).

[63]Hanlester Network v. Shalala, 51 F.3d 1390 (9th Cir. 1995).

[64]United States v. Starks, 157 F.3d 833 (11th Cir. 1998).

[65]Hanlester Network v. Shalala, 51 F.3d 1390, 1400 (9th Cir. 1995).

[66]Letter from D. McCarthy Thronton, associate general counsel of the Department of Health and Human Services, Office of Inspector General, to the Internal Revenue Service, Office of Associate Chief Counsel (December 22, 1992).

[67]Department of Health and Human Services, *Memorandum: Office of Inspector General, Management Advisory Report: Financial Arrangements Between Hospitals and Hospital-Based Physicians* OEI-09-89-0030 (January 31, 1991).

the hospital remuneration for referrals from the hospital. Hence, agreements that would be considered suspect include those that require these physicians to pay more than fair market value for hospital services provided or that pay the physicians less than fair market value for services or goods they provide the hospital. Suspect arrangements would include any situations where physicians are required to split their income with hospitals; for example, emergency department physicians required to pay half of their fees over a floor amount to the hospital, hospitals that provide no or nominal payment to clinical pathologists for Medicare Part A services in return for the opportunity to perform Medicare Part B services, radiologists who are required to pay half of their gross receipts to an entity's endowment fund, radiologists required to pay one-third of all profits above a floor amount to the hospital (for capital improvements, equipment, and other department expenditures), radiologists required to purchase radiology equipment and then to donate them to the hospital at the termination of the radiologist–hospital contract, radiologists required to pay half their collections over a floor amount to the hospital with the hospital reserving the right to unilaterally adjust these amounts, radiologists required to pay one-quarter of their profits over a floor amount to the hospital for capital improvements, and radiologists required to pay for facilities, services, supplies, personnel, utilities, maintenance, and billing services of the hospital on a fee schedule if the radiologist's gross revenue does not exceed $1 million.

In addition, recruitment and retention of physicians using any method intended in whole or in part to influence referral decisions also constitutes a risk of violating the Antikickback Statute.[68] Suspect arrangements include incentive payments for each patient referred; no cost or significantly reduced cost office space, equipment, or staff services; compensation guarantees; interest-free or low-interest loans subject to forgiveness if certain referral patterns are met; certain hospital payments for physician travel expenses or continuing education courses; inappropriately low-cost insurance coverage on the hospital's insurance plan; and payments for physician services that are higher than fair market value.[69] Therefore, physicians being recruited or retained must closely assess all offers to assure themselves that all the components are based on fair market value to avoid fraud and abuse sanctions.

Medical Supplies to Nursing Facilities

Antikickback Statute and FCA liability may attend fraudulent activities in providing medical supplies to nursing facilities.[70] False claims include false or fraudulent billing for medical supplies that were not provided, not provided as claimed, claimed twice or more, and claimed for medically unnecessary services. Of particular note are claims for medical supplies and equipment not medically necessary that are paid for under the general Medicare cost report to the facility but also billed for by the medical supplier directly to Medicare Part B. In addition, billing for items not covered under the Medicare program by fraudulently misrepresenting the item (e.g., adult diapers are not covered; claim made instead for "female external urinary collection device") also is a violation of the FCA. Suppliers providing medical supplies for free to nursing facilities in exchange for ordering Medicare-reimbursable and nonreimbursable products, sending products to nursing facilities without the facilities ordering them in exchange for access to patient medical records and other information needed to bill Medicare, and related activities are violations of the Antikickback Statute (as well as other regulations that prohibit unauthorized release of patient records under the Medicare program[71]).

Nursing Home Arrangements with Hospices

Terminally ill patients often are best served by the specialized care provided in hospices. However, payment by hospices to nursing homes for referrals of terminally ill patients are illegal kickbacks under the Antikickback Statute.[72] The OIG specifically has indicated that certain arrangements are suspect, including those where the hospice offers free goods or goods for prices below market value to induce a nursing home to refer patients to the hospice, the hospice paying "room and board" payments to the nursing home in excess of what the nursing home would have received directly from Medicaid had the patient not been enrolled in the hospice, the hospice paying amounts to the nursing home for "additional" services that Medicaid considers to be included in its room and board payment to the hospice, the hospice paying greater than fair market value for "additional" services that Medicaid does not consider to be included in the nursing home's room and board payment, the hospice referring its patients to a nursing home to induce the nursing home to refer patients to the

[68]Department of Health and Human Services, *Special Fraud Alert: Hospital Incentives to Physicians* (May 7, 1992).

[69]See, e.g., Polk County Mem. Hosp. v. Peters, 800 F.Supp. 1451 (E.D. Tex. 1992) (interest-free loan, free office space, subsidies, and reimbursement for medical malpractice insurance subject to referrals to the hospital are in violation of the Antikickback Statute); Vana v. Vista Hosp. Sys. Inc., 1993 WL 597402 (Cal. App. Ct. Oct. 25, 1993) (low-rent lease entered into by physicians and hospital is void under the Antikickback Statute).

[70]Department of Health and Human Services, Office of Inspector General, *Special Fraud Alert: Medical Supplies to Nursing Facilities*, 60 Fed. Reg. 40849-40851 (August 10, 1995).

[71]42 C.F.R. §483.10(e) (1998).

[72]Department of Health and Human Services, Office of Inspector General, *Special Fraud Alert: Fraud and Abuse in Nursing Home Arrangements with Hospices* (March 1998).

hospice, the hospice providing free care or charging below market value for care to nursing home patients with the expectation that the patient (after exhausting the skilled nursing facility benefit under Medicare) will receive hospice services from the hospice, and the hospice providing staff to the nursing home to perform duties that otherwise would be performed by the nursing home.

Physician Liability for Certifications in the Provision of Medical Equipment and Supplies and Home Health Services

The Medicare program only pays for services that are medically necessary. Physicians generally determine, through certification of medical necessity, particular goods and services that are medically necessary for particular Medicare beneficiaries. Antikickback Statute violations can occur when physicians improperly sign certifications of medical necessity, particularly when the physician receives compensation in exchange for such a signature. The OIG has identified instances where physicians have inappropriately certified medical necessity in violation of the statute in areas of DME and home health services,[73] including: where a physician knowingly signs forms provided by a home health agency falsely representing that skilled nursing services are medically necessary so that the patient can qualify for home health services; a physician certifies that a patient is confined to the home and thus qualifies for home health services even though the patient informs the physician that her only restrictions are based on arthritis in her hands and she has no restrictions on routine activities; at the prompting of a DME supplier a physician signs a stack of blank certification forms for transcutaneous electrical nerve stimulator units and the certifications are used to support false claims for the equipment; a physician signs certification forms for respiratory medical equipment falsely representing that the equipment was medically necessary; a physician signs certification forms for wheelchairs and hospital beds without seeing the patients and then falsifies medical charts to indicate that he treated the patients; and a physician accepts cash payments from a DME supplier for each prescription he signs for oxygen concentrators and nebulizers.

Prescription Drug Marketing Schemes

The market for pharmaceuticals is highly competitive, and many manufacturers are becoming more aggressive in attempting to gain market share. Antikickback Statute violations may occur if these activities induce use of certain pharmaceuticals through some form of remuneration.[74] For example, prohibited arrangements include manufacturer cash payments to pharmacies when a drug prescription is changed from a competitor's brand to the company making the payment, "frequent flier" programs sponsored by a drug manufacturer where physicians are provided credit toward frequent flier programs each time they complete a questionnaire for a new patient placed on the company's drug, and "research grant" programs where the physician is paid high amounts for nominal record keeping for patients on the company's drug. The OIG indicates that suspect arrangements will be investigated if they have one or more of the following characteristics: company provision of prizes, cash, gifts, coupons, or bonuses in exchange for prescribing or supplying specific pharmaceuticals, particularly if based on volume; company provision of cash or other benefits to pharmacists or others who recommend prescription drug products in exchange for marketing activities; company provision of grants to physicians and other clinicians for studies of prescription drugs when these studies are of questionable value; and company provision of any benefit given to a patient, provider, or supplier for changing or requesting a change of a prescription to the company's product outside of normal federal rules allowing such change.

Provision of Clinical Laboratory Services

Since physicians generally choose the laboratory at which patient samples are analyzed, significant Antikickback Statute risks are associated with arrangements that can be seen as remuneration for referrals.[75] For example, if a clinical laboratory makes available the services of a phlebotomist to a physician office for sample collection but then allows this phlebotomist to perform other functions, such as nursing activities (e.g., taking vital signs), testing for the physician's office laboratory, or clerical services, there is a "strong inference" that a benefit is being provided for the purpose of inducing referrals to the laboratory. In addition, actions such as discounting one area of laboratory service to a facility below fair market value in exchange for having the facility refer all its other tests to the laboratory also runs the risk of an Antikickback Statute violation. In the managed care context, if a physician (who by contract with the MCO must refer all labo-

---

[73]Department of Health and Human Services, Office of Inspector General, *Special Fraud Alert: Physician Liability for Certifications in the Provision of Medical Equipment and Supplies and Home Health Services* (January 1999), available at http://www.hhs.gov/progorg/frdalert/index.htm.

[74]Department of Health and Human Services, Office of Inspector General, *Special Fraud Alert: Prescription Drug Marketing Schemes*, OIG-94-18 (August 1994).

[75]Department of Health and Human Services, Office of Inspector General, *Special Fraud Alert: Arrangements for the Provision of Clinical Lab Services*, OIG-95-03 (October 1994).

ratory work for that MCO to one laboratory) prefers another laboratory and sends all other, non-MCO laboratory work there, and if the preferred laboratory offers to do the physician's MCO work for free to maintain its non-MCO business with the physician, it would appear to the MCO that the physician has a reduced utilization rate for MCO patient laboratory costs. If this false appearance of lower utilization to the MCO results in a physician bonus, the arrangement may invoke the Antikickback Statute as a payment for referrals. Finally, other activities may run afoul of the Antikickback Statute, including free pickup and disposal of biohazardous waste materials not related to the collection of specimens for the clinical laboratory, provision of computers or fax machines unless such equipment is integral to and exclusively used for performance of the laboratory work, and provision of free laboratory testing for health care providers, their families, or their employees.

Provision of Services in Nursing Facilities

OIG has indicated that significant risks are associated with care provided to nursing home patients that falls within the ambit of the Antikickback Statute.[76] Major difficulties include falsifying bills and medical records to misrepresent the services, or extent of services, provided at the nursing facilities. In addition, claims falsified to circumvent program coverage limitations for certain medical specialty services have been the subject of OIG scrutiny. The OIG has indicated that certain activities may suggest fraud in terms of providing medically unnecessary services or false billing, including "gang visits" by one or more medical professionals where a large number of patients in the nursing facility are seen in a single day, frequent and recurring "routine visits" by the same medical professional, unusually active presence at the nursing facility of health care practitioners who are given or request unlimited access to resident medical records, and questionable documentation for medical necessity for professional services.

Routine Waiver of Deductibles Under Medicare Part B

Similar to FCA concerns, the Antikickback Statute deems illegal the routine waiver of deductibles for physician services or medical supplies.[77] From the government's perspective, providers effectively are paying remuneration (providing an economic benefit) to patients when the providers waive Medicare deductibles and thus are illegally inducing patients to purchase ser-

vices or products from them. Waiver of cost sharing is permitted only in hardship cases; however, this "hardship waiver" is not to be used routinely and is relevant only in the occasional circumstance to take into account a particular patient's specific needs. Outside these circumstances, a good faith effort to collect cost-sharing amounts from patients is required to avoid liability under the Antikickback Statute. The OIG has specifically indicated that certain activities of providers are suspect: advertisements that indicate that Medicare will be considered payment in full or that there is no out-of-pocket expense for the patient; advertisements that promise that "discounts" will be given Medicare beneficiaries; routine use of "financial hardship" forms; collection of cost-sharing amounts only when the beneficiary has Medigap insurance; higher charges to Medicare beneficiaries to offset the cost-sharing waiver; failure to collect cost-sharing amounts for a specific group of Medicare beneficiaries for reasons unrelated to indigence; and "insurance programs" that cover cost-sharing amounts only for goods or services provided by the entity offering the insurance.

Safe Harbors[78]

The DHHS is authorized by statute to promulgate regulations that specify payment methodologies that do not invoke the provisions of the Antikickback Statute.[79] Further, under the Health Insurance Portability and Accountability Act, the Secretary of Health and Human Services, through the OIG, is mandated to solicit proposals to amend existing safe harbors or create new ones.[80] The criteria for such amendment and creation require an assessment of eight factors: access to health care services, quality of health care services, competition among health care providers, patients' freedom of choice of providers, ability of health care facilities to provide services in medically underserved areas or populations, cost to federal health care programs, potential for overutilization of health care services, and financial benefits to health care professionals or providers that may affect referrals. To take advantage of these safe harbors, providers must comply fully and completely with the requirements of the safe harbor regulation; however, good faith efforts to comply will be assessed to determine if prosecution under the Antikickback Statute is warranted.[81]

[76]Department of Health and Human Services, Office of Inspector General, *Special Fraud Alert: Fraud and Abuse in the Provision of Services in Nursing Facilities*, 61 Fed. Reg. 30,623-30,625 (June 17, 1996).

[77]Department of Health and Human Services, Office of Inspector General, *Special Fraud Alert: Routine Waiver of Copayments or Deductibles Under Medicaid Part B*, OIG-91-23 (May 1991).

[78]42 C.F.R. Part 1001 (1998).

[79]42 U.S.C.A. §1320a-7b.

[80]42 U.S.C.A. §1320a-7d.

[81]42 C.F.R. §1001.952 (1998).

Discounts

Discounts for products or services can run the risk of Antikickback Statute violation if they are seen to be given in exchange for referrals. However, discounts are acceptable if buyers and sellers fulfill the safe harbor requirements. Discounts, in contemplation of the discount safe harbor:

1. Are defined as a reduction in the amount a seller charges a buyer (buying either directly or via a wholesaler or group purchasing organization) for a good or service based on an arm's length transaction.
2. Include rebate checks, credits, or coupons directly redeemable from the seller only to the extent that such reductions in price are attributable to the original good or service purchased or furnished.
3. Do not include any cash payment or furnishing one good or service without charge or at a reduced charge in exchange for any agreement to buy a different good or service.

Under the standards for entities such as hospitals that report costs on a cost report required by the DHHS or state agency, the following requirements must be met by the buyers:

1. The discount must be based on purchases of the same good or service bought within a single fiscal year.
2. The entity must claim the benefit of the discount in the fiscal year in which the discount is earned or in the following year.
3. The entity must fully and accurately report the discount in the applicable cost report.
4. The entity must provide the information sellers are obligated to provide under the regulation on request by the Secretary of Health and Human Services or a state agency.

The person or entity that sells discounted goods or services is required to meet one of the following two standards:

1. The seller must fully and accurately report the discount on the statement or invoice given to the buyer and inform the buyer of its obligations to report the discount.
2. Where the value of the discount is not known at the time of sale, the seller must fully and accurately report the existence of a discount program on the invoice or statement given to the buyer, inform the buyer of its reporting obligations, and, when the value of the discount becomes known, provide the buyer with documentation of the discount calculation identifying the goods or services to which the discount will be supplied.

Note that the discount safe harbor excludes bundled goods arrangements (e.g., free surgical pack with purchase of intraocular lens, credits toward free items that may be useful to the purchaser) due to the high abuse potential. Free items are of particular risk; the OIG will assess purchasing practices by determining the amount of the benefit reported and passed on to the program, whether the good itself is separately reimbursable, and the intent behind the arrangement. This safe harbor expressly exempts from the definition of *discount* a reduction in price applicable to one payer but not to Medicare or a state health care program, a reduction in price offered to a beneficiary (e.g., routine waiver of cost sharing), warranties, services provided through a personal or management services contract, and other remuneration in cash or in kind not explicitly described in the discount safe harbor rules.

Employees

Taken literally, the Antikickback Statute would find normal payments by employers to employees a potential kickback arrangement. The employee safe harbor allows an employer to pay an employee for normal rendering of services or providing goods.[82] The DHHS uses the IRS definition of *employee*[83] for this safe harbor. In addition, part-time employment is covered by this safe harbor, but independent contractors are not. Independent contractors should follow the personal services and management safe harbor to avoid Antikickback Statute risks.

Group Purchasing Organizations

Purchasing by groups at reduced prices may be considered an illegal kickback. The group purchasing organization (GPO) safe harbor allows for such purchasing.[84] Payments by vendors to GPOs as part of an agreement to furnish goods and/or services is allowed if:

1. The GPO has a written agreement with each individual or entity to which items or services are furnished and
   a. That agreement states that participating vendors from which the individual or entity will purchase goods or services will pay a fee to the GPO of 3% or less of the purchase price of the goods or services provided by the vendor.
   b. Or, if the fee paid to the GPO is not fixed at 3% or less, the agreement specifies the amount (or, if unknown, the maximum amount) the GPO will be paid by each vendor; the fee may be a fixed sum or a fixed percentage of the value of the purchases made from the vendor by the members of the group under the contract between the vendor and the GPO.
2. When the entity that receives the good or service from the vendor is a health care provider of services, the GPO must disclose in writing to the entity at least

---

[82]42 C.F.R. §1001.952(i) (1998).

[83]26 U.S.C.A. 3121(d)(2).

[84]42 C.F.R. §1001.952(j) (1998).

annually and to the Secretary of the DHHS on request the amount received from each vendor with respect to purchases made by or on behalf of the entity.

Note that this safe harbor mandates that written contracts indicate the specific amount the vendor pays to the GPO and the GPO must disclose to a health care provider the fees received from only those vendors that provide goods and services to that provider. In addition, it is important to recognize that the GPO safe harbor applies to payments made by a vendor of goods or services to an entity authorized to act as a GPO; therefore a vendor's discount payments to a health care provider must qualify under the discount safe harbor to receive protection.

Investment Interest

The investment interest safe harbor is designed to permit health care providers to invest in health care facilities in circumstances where the financial incentives to refer to these entities are limited. Providers may be investors and have an investment interest in health care entities if certain conditions are met. It should be noted that "investors" include an individual or entity that holds a direct investment interest in an entity or an indirect interest through family members or holds an investment interest through a legal or beneficial interest in another entity (e.g., holding company or trust) that owns the investment interest. The "investment interest" includes shares in a corporation, interest or units of a partnership, and bonds, debentures, notes, or other debt instruments.

The requirements of the investment interest safe harbor differ on the basis of whether the investment is in a large, publicly traded entity or in a smaller venture. For the large, publicly traded entity, there is no antikickback violation when the entity pays the provider a return on investment if:

1. The entity possesses more than $50 million in undepreciated, net tangible assets.
2. If the ownership interest is an equity security, the equity security is registered with the Securities and Exchange Commission as described by federal law.[85]
3. The investment interest of an investor in the position to make referrals is obtained on terms available to the public through trading on a registered national securities exchange.
4. The investor or the entity is not marketing or furnishing the entity's goods or services to passive investors differently than to noninvestors.
5. The entity is not loaning funds or guaranteeing loans for an investor in the position of making or influencing referrals or furnishing goods or services to or otherwise generating business for the entity if the investor

would use any part of the loan to acquire the investment interest.
6. Return-on-investment payment to the investor is directly proportional to the investor's capital investment.[86]

Smaller investment ventures require all the following to be met to avoid Antikickback Statute risks:

1. No greater than 40% of the value of the investment interests for each class of investment may be held in the previous fiscal year or 12-month period by investors in a position to refer or influence referrals, furnish goods or services to, or generate business for the entity.
2. Investment interest terms for passive investors in the position to make or influence referrals to, furnish goods or services to, or otherwise generate business for the entity must be the same as all other passive investors.
3. Investment interest terms for passive investors in the position to make or influence referrals to, furnish goods or services to, or otherwise generate business for the entity must not be related to previous or expected referrals, goods or services furnished, or amount of business otherwise generated from that investor to the entity.
4. The entity must have no requirement that a passive investor make or influence referrals to, furnish goods or services to, or otherwise generate business for the entity to remain an investor.
5. The entity and the investor cannot market or furnish the entity's goods or services to passive investors differently than to noninvestors.
6. No greater than 40% of the gross revenue of the entity in the previous fiscal year or 12-month period may come from referrals, goods or services furnished, or business otherwise generated from investors.
7. The entity may not loan funds to or guarantee a loan for an investor in the position to make or influence referrals to, furnish goods or services to, or otherwise generate business for the entity if the investor would use any portion of the loan to obtain the investment interest.
8. Return-on-investment payments to the investor must be directly proportional to the investor's capital investment.[87]

Note that physicians who are retired and no longer make or influence referrals, who reside and practice in a separate service area from the entity, or who sign a written agreement indicating that, for the life of the investment, the investor will not make referrals to, furnish items or services for, or otherwise generate business for the entity will not be considered one who is in a position to make referrals.[88]

[85]15 U.S.C.A. §§781(b), 781(g).

[86]42 C.F.R. §1001.952(a)(1) (1998).
[87]42 C.F.R. §1001.952(a)(2) (1998).
[88]See 56 Fed. Reg. 35,952, 35,963 (July 29, 1991).

Lease of Space and Equipment Rental

The safe harbors for renting space and equipment are designed to allow legitimate arrangements while deterring agreements that actually are kickbacks. Rental payments made by lessees to lessors for use of space[89] and equipment[90] must fulfill all the following requirements:

1. The lease agreement is in writing and signed by the parties.
2. The lease agreement specifies the premises, equipment, or services that will be provided.
3. If the lease agreement is only for the use of premises or equipment on a periodic, sporadic, or part-time basis, the agreement must specify the exact schedule of the intervals, their precise length, and exact charge for such intervals.
4. The term of the agreement must be no less than one year.
5. The total compensation paid over the term of the agreement is set in advance, consistent with fair market value, and not determined on the basis of volume or value of referrals or business otherwise generated between the parties of which Medicare or a state health program will provide payment in whole or in part.

A critical component of this safe harbor is the need for rental to reflect "fair market value." *Fair market value* is defined as "[t]he value of the equipment when obtained from a manufacturer or professional distributor, or rental property for general commercial purposes, but not adjusted to reflect the additional value that either the prospective lessee or the lessor would attribute to the equipment or property as a result of its proximity or convenience to sources of referrals or business otherwise generated for which payment may be made in whole or in part under Medicare or a state health program."[91] Therefore, it is essential that, to fall within the rental safe harbors, the actual pricing of the rent or lease be completely untainted by any potential to refer or generate business between lessor and lessee.

Managed Care Safe Harbors

Several safe harbors have been promulgated specifically for arrangements under managed care. These safe harbors are relevant to managed care enrollees, contract health care providers, and health plans. *Enrollees* are defined as persons who have entered into a contractual relationship with a health plan (or on whose behalf an employer or government or private entity has entered into such a relationship) where the person is entitled to receive health

care items and services or insurance coverage for these items or services in return for a premium payment. *Contract health providers* are individuals or entities under contract with the health plan to provide goods or services to enrollees covered by the health plan, Medicare, or state health program. *Health plan* means an entity that either provides or arranges under agreement with health care providers for the provision of items or services to enrollees or provides insurance coverage for the provision of such items and services in exchange for a premium. A health plan within the managed care safe harbor regulations must either operate according to a contract, agreement, or statutory demonstration project authority approved by HCFA or state health care program or have its premium structure regulated by a state insurance statute or state-enabling statute governing HMOs or PPOs. Note that employer self-insured plans do not appear to be included within this definition.

In the *increased coverage, reduced cost-sharing amounts, or reduced premium amounts offered by health plans to enrollees* managed care safe harbor,[92] health plans are permitted to offer additional coverage to an enrollee, reduce some or all of the enrollee's payment obligation to the health plan or contract health care provider for beneficiary cost-sharing amounts, or reduce premium amounts attributable to goods or services covered by the health plan, Medicare, or state health plan. To be within this safe harbor:

1. If the health plan is under contract with HCFA or state health care plan as a risk-based plan, it must offer the same increased coverage or reduced cost-sharing or premium amounts to all enrollees unless otherwise approved by HCFA or by a state health care plan.
2. If the health plan is under contract with HCFA or state health care plan as a non–risk-based plan, it must
   a. Offer the same increased coverage or reduced cost-sharing or premium amounts to all enrollees unless otherwise approved by HCFA or by a state health plan; and
   b. Not claim the costs of the increased coverage or reduced cost-sharing or premium amounts as a bad debt for payment purposes under Medicare or state health care program or otherwise shift the costs of increased coverage or reduced cost-sharing or premium amounts to Medicare, a state health care program, other payers, or individuals.

In the *price reductions offered to health plans by providers* managed care safe harbor, contract health care workers are permitted to offer a reduction in price to a health plan without running the risk of Antikickback Statute violation.[93] Health plans and contract health care providers must fulfill the following requirements:

[89]42 C.F.R. §1001.952(b) (1998).
[90]42 C.F.R. §1001.952(c) (1998).
[91]42 C.F.R. §1001.952(c)(5) (1998).
[92]42 C.F.R. §1001.952(l) (1998).
[93]42 C.F.R. §1001.952(m) (1998).

1. If the health plan is a prepaid health care plan organization under contract with the HCFA or a state agency, the contract health care provider must not claim payment in any form from the DHHS or a state agency for items or services provided in accordance with the agreement except as approved by the HCFA or state health care program or otherwise shift the cost of such an agreement to Medicare, a state health care program, other payers, or individuals.

2. If the health plan is a non–risk-based plan that has executed a contract or agreement with the HCFA or state health care program, the health plan and contract health care provider must fulfill the following requirements:
   a. The term of the agreement between the health plan and contract health care provider must be for no less than one year.
   b. The agreement between the health plan and the contract health care provider must specify in advance the covered items and services to be furnished to enrollees and the method for computing the plan's payment to the contract health care provider.
   c. The health plan must fully and accurately report on the relevant cost report or other claim form filed with the DHHS or state health care program the amount it has paid the contract health care provider under the agreement.
   d. The contract health care provider must not claim payment in any form from the DHHS or state health care program for items or services furnished through the agreement except as approved by the HCFA or state health care program nor may it shift the costs of the agreement to Medicare, the state health care program, other payers, or individuals.

3. If the health plan does not fit within preceding categories 1 or 2, both the health plan and contract health care provider must fulfill the following requirements:
   a. The term of the agreement must be for no less than one year.
   b. The agreement must specify in advance the covered items and services to be furnished to enrollees, which party is to file payment claims requests with Medicare or the state health care program, and the schedule of fees the contract health care provider will charge for providing items and services to enrollees.
   c. The fee schedule in the agreement between the health plan and contract health care provider must remain in effect throughout the term of the agreement unless a fee increase results directly from a payment update authorized by Medicare or state health care program.
   d. The party submitting payment claims or requests from Medicare or state health care programs for

items and services provided according to the agreement must not claim or request payments in excess of the fee schedule.
   e. The contract health care provider and health plan must fully and accurately report the fee schedule amounts charged according to the agreement on any cost report filed with Medicare or a state health care program.
   f. The party that does not have the responsibility to file payment claims or requests must not claim or request payment in any form from the DHHS or state health care program for the services provided under the agreement nor shift the costs of the agreement to Medicare, a state health care program, other payers, or individuals.

In the *risk-sharing arrangements* managed care safe harbor, created by the Health Insurance Portability and Accountability Act,[94] written risk-sharing arrangements providing for payments between MCOs and service providers as well as between service providers are permissible if the organization is a Medicare-certified HMO or the written agreement places the individual or entity at substantial financial risk for the cost or utilization of the items or services that the individual or entity is obligated to provide. This safe harbor significantly expands the potential agreements between MCOs and providers that allow for providers to assume risk and be paid for doing so while avoiding potential Antikickback Statute risks.

Personal Services and Management Contracts

Under certain circumstances, one provider requires the services of another for appropriate clinical care to be provided. However, there is the potential for financial situations where payments for services exceed fair market value and actually are payments for referrals. The personal services and management contracts safe harbor specifies requirements that provide the basis for legitimate arrangements that do not violate the Antikickback Statute.[95]

The safe harbor is applicable to payments made by a principal (such as a hospital) to an agent (such as a physician) as the agent's compensation and requires the following requirements to be met:

1. The agreement between the parties (the agency agreement) is in writing and signed by the parties.
2. The agency agreement specifies the services to be provided by the agent.
3. If the agency agreement is intended to provide for the services of the agent on a periodic, sporadic, or part-

---

[94]42 U.S.C.A. §1320a-7b(B)(3)
[95]42 C.F.R. §1001.952(d) (1998).

time basis, the agreement specifies the schedule of these intervals, their length, and the exact charge for such intervals.

4. The term of the agreement is for no less than one year.
5. The total compensation paid to the agent is set in advance, consistent with fair market value, and not determined by taking into account the volume or value of any referrals or business otherwise generated between the parties for which payment may be made in part or entirely by the Medicare program or a state health care program.
6. The services performed under the agreement do not involve counseling or promotion of a business arrangement or other activity that violates any state or federal law.

Note that the "agent of the principal" for the purposes of this safe harbor is "any person other than a bona fide employee of the principal who has an agreement to perform services for, or on behalf of, the principal." Note also that salespersons paid on commission are within the scope of the Antikickback Statute and so must fall within this safe harbor to avoid risk of prosecution under the statute. However, marketing and advertising activities contracted for by the principal generally are considered within this safe harbor because these agents have no direct contact with beneficiaries and are not involved in health care delivery.

Referral Services

The referral services safe harbor allows for payments to referral services organizations (e.g., a hospital) by a practitioner (e.g., a physician) that provide services to the referred patients if the payments do not depend on the number of referrals made to the practitioner.[96] This arrangement is allowed under the following circumstances:

1. The referral service does not exclude participants in the referral service that meet its qualifications for participation.
2. In addition to the preceding, any payment made by the participant to the referral service is assessed equally against and collected equally from all participants and is based on only the operating costs of the referral service and not on the volume or value of referrals to or business generated by the participants for the referral service for which some or all payment is made by the Medicare program or state health program.
3. The referral service has no requirements on the method by which the participant provides services to a referred person (other than when the referral service requires that the participant provide services at the same rate it charges other persons not so referred or

that the services be provided free or at a reduced charge).
4. The referral service makes the following disclosures to those seeking a referral and maintains a written record certifying this disclosure with a signature by those seeking a referral or by the individual making the disclosure:
   a. The manner in which the referral service selects participants.
   b. Whether the participant has paid a fee to the referral service.
   c. The manner by which the referral service selects a particular participant for those seeking referrals.
   d. The nature of the relationship between the referral service and the participants.
   e. Any restrictions that would exclude an individual or entity from continuing as a participant.

Note that *any* remuneration for the referral may constitute a kickback. Hence, if hospitals provide referral services to participating physicians without a specific fee but the participating physicians provide services to the hospital (such as serving on committees), this may constitute an illegal kickback. In addition, full disclosure must be made before the referral and provision of services; the information must be provided to those seeking the referrals so that the information can be used to make the decision as to whether to use the referral service.

Sale of Practice

One provider selling a practice to another raises the possibility of Antikickback Statute violation if part of the price includes payment for referrals. The sale of practice safe harbor allows for such a sale if the following requirements are met:[97] The period from the date of the first agreement with regard to the sale of the practice to the actual completion of the sale does not exceed one year; and the selling practitioner is not in a professional position to make referrals to or otherwise generate business for the purchasing practitioner for which some or all payment is made by the Medicare program or state health care programs after one year from the date of the first agreement relating to the sale. Also note that the requirements for option agreements on sales of physician practices must fulfill this safe harbor to avoid risk of prosecution under the Antikickback Statute.

Warranties

Warranties for products, as an inducement for a provider to purchase them, can be considered illegal kickbacks if they provide for more than simple replacement of a defective product. The warranties safe harbor prescribes

[96]42 C.F.R. §1001.952(f) (1998).

[97]42 C.F.R. §1001.952(e) (1998).

actions that must be taken for these warranties to avoid the risk of Antikickback Statute violation.[98] Warranties under this safe harbor are those defined under federal law[99] as well as agreements by a manufacturer or supplier to replace another manufacturer's or supplier's defective item. Separate requirements must be fulfilled by buyers and manufacturers or suppliers. For buyers, any payment or exchange of anything of value under a warranty provided by the manufacturer or supplier to the buyer is within the safe harbor if the buyer fully and accurately reports any price reduction of the item (including a free item) obtained as a part of the warranty through the relevant cost-reporting mechanism or claim for payment filed with the DHHS or a state agency and provides the information that manufacturers or suppliers must report to the buyer on request by the Secretary of Health and Human Services or the relevant state agency. The manufacturer or supplier is required to:

1. Fully and accurately report the item's price reduction (including a free item) on the invoice or statement submitted to the buyer that was obtained as part of the warranty and inform the buyer of its obligations.
2. Where the price reduction is not known at the time of sale,
   a. Fully and accurately report the existence of a warranty on the product invoice or statement.
   b. Inform the buyer of its obligations.
   c. Provide the buyer with documentation of the calculation of the price reduction resulting from the warranty when the price reduction becomes known.
3. Not pay any remuneration to any individual (other than the beneficiary) or entity for any medical, surgical, or hospital expense incurred by the beneficiary other than the cost of the item itself.

Note that this safe harbor is somewhat flexible since the OIG recognizes that warranties are beneficial to the Medicare and Medicaid programs as well as their beneficiaries.

Waiver of Beneficiary Cost Sharing

Waivers of beneficiary cost sharing can be seen to be a violation of the Antikickback Statute. However, under this safe harbor, hospitals may waive beneficiary cost sharing for inpatient services if the following requirements are met:[100]

1. The hospital must offer the benefit without regard to the Medicare beneficiary's reasons for admission, the length of stay, or diagnosis.

2. The hospital must not later claim the amount waived as a bad debt for payment purposes under Medicare or otherwise shift the burden of the waiver to the Medicare program, state health program, or other payers or individuals.
3. The hospital must not make the waiver a part of a price reduction agreement between itself and a third-party payer.

Note that this safe harbor does not apply to outpatient services, inpatient services in non-PPS units, and physician services. Waivers of beneficiary cost sharing in circumstances of true indigence by public hospitals outside the safe harbor (e.g., county hospital outpatient departments) do not invoke the statute as long as "the partial forgiveness of the copayment obligation was strictly a pragmatic financial decision and not an inducement to patients to purchase medical services."[101] The safe harbor also applies only to beneficiary cost sharing and does not apply to price reduction agreements between health care providers and third-party payers.

Advisory Opinions[103]

Under the HIPAA,[103] the Secretary of Health and Human Services is mandated to issue advisory opinions on issues relating to the Antikickback Statute, including what constitutes a prohibited remuneration, whether a business arrangement falls within a statutory exception or safe harbor, and if an action or activity is sufficient grounds for sanctions under the statute.[104] Note, however, that advisory opinions will not assess what constitutes fair market value in a particular transaction or whether a particular person is considered an employee for purposes of federal tax law.[105] Advisory opinions will not be provided if a request presents only a general question of interpretation or a hypothetical situation, if it does not relate to a named person or entity, if the same or similar actions or activities already are under government investigation, or if an informed opinion cannot be made without an extensive investigation or clinical study.[106] Advisory opinions generally are limited in applicability to the entity that requested it.

Advisory Opinion 97-1

This advisory opinion relates to whether donations by renal dialysis providers to an independent, 501(c)(3) charitable

---

[98]42 C.F.R. §1001.952(g) (1998).

[99]Magnuson-Moss Warranty — Federal Trade Commission Improvement Act, 15 U.S.C.A. §2301(6).

[100]42 C.F.R. §1001.952(k) (1998).

[101]42 U.S.C.A. §422.64.

[102]These are available at http://www.hhs.gov; 42 C.F.R. §1008.5 (1998); see 63 Fed. Reg. 38,311 (July 16, 1998) (outlining the final rule on advisory opinions under the Antikickback Statute).

[103]42 U.S.C.A. §1397ii.

[104]42 U.S.C.A. §1320a-7b; 42 C.F.R. §1008.41 (1998).

[105]I.R.C. §3121(D)(2).

[106]42 C.F.R. Part 1008 (1998).

organization to fund a program to pay for Medicare Part B or Medigap premiums for financially needy Medicare beneficiaries with end-stage renal disease who obtain services from the donor dialysis providers would be a violation of the Antikickback Statute, subjecting the providers to sanctions. The OIG concluded that this arrangement would not violate the statute because donations by the providers to the charitable organization do not constitute remuneration to an eligible beneficiary and the charitable organization's purchase of the premiums for the beneficiary is not likely to influence the beneficiary's choice of a particular provider.

Advisory Opinion 97-2

This advisory opinion relates to whether a state-funded program that pays for insurance premiums for financially needy Medicare beneficiaries with end-stage renal disease would be in violation of the Antikickback Statute, subjecting the requester to sanctions. The OIG concluded that this arrangement would not violate the statute because all funds for the state program premium payments are provided by the state and available to all chronic dialysis facilities in the state and to all eligible beneficiaries in the state. Such a state-financed arrangement would not likely influence the individual patients in their selection of a particular provider.

Advisory Opinion 97-3

This advisory opinion relates to whether a transfer of assets by Mrs. P to her nephew Mr. S and subsequent application for Medicaid benefits after the period of ineligibility for such benefits has run[107] subjects Mrs. P to sanctions in a violation of the Antikickback Statute. The OIG concluded that this arrangement would not violate the statute because Mrs. P will wait until after the period of ineligibility has run before applying for Medicaid; therefore, no period of ineligibility will be imposed because of her transfer of assets.

Advisory Opinion 97-4

This advisory opinion relates to whether declining to pursue copayments from certain patients who have employer-sponsored Medicare complementary coverage constitutes a violation of the Antikickback Statute, subjecting the requestor to sanctions. The OIG concluded that such an arrangement may be in violation of the statute because prohibited remuneration specifically includes waiver of beneficiary cost sharing and would influence a beneficiary's choice of a particular provider, does not provide for individual determinations of hardship, and does not include any bona fide collection efforts.

---

[107]See Chapter 8.

Advisory Opinion 97-5

This advisory opinion relates to whether an outpatient radiology imaging center joint venture owned by the radiology medical group and a hospital generates prohibited remuneration, is subject to sanctions, or satisfies a safe harbor. The hospital radiologists would make no referrals to the imaging joint venture; the imaging joint venture would not accept any such referrals; the hospital would take no action to induce its medical staff to use the imaging joint venture; the hospital would inform the medical staff of these facts and agreements; the hospital, radiology group, and joint venture would not track referrals; and the hospital would continue to use its own radiology units. The OIG indicated that the arrangement does not meet any safe harbor but does not generate any prohibited remuneration. According to the OIG, the arrangement does not satisfy the safe harbor for investment interests in small entities, the only safe harbor of relevance. However, there is no violation of the Antikickback Statute because there is no prohibited remuneration for referrals to the imaging joint venture by the radiology group or hospital, it is unlikely that the radiology group would generate a significant amount of referrals to the imaging joint venture since most tests are ordered by a patient's attending physician, and there is no prohibited remuneration for referrals outside the joint venture.

Advisory Opinion 97-6

This advisory opinion relates to whether a proposed arrangement for free restocking of municipal ambulance supplies and medications by hospital emergency rooms would constitute a violation of the Antikickback Statute. The OIG concluded that this arrangement would be in violation of the statute because at least one purpose of the arrangement may be to induce the ambulance services to bring patients to the restocking hospitals.

Advisory Opinion 98-1

This advisory opinion relates to whether a contractual arrangement for distribution and billing services between company A, the supplier, and company B, the distributor and billing contractor, where company B obtains remuneration for its services based on a percentage of collections, constitutes a violation of the Antikickback Statute, subjecting the parties to sanctions. The OIG concluded that such an arrangement violates the Antikickback Statute because the percentage of collections includes significant financial incentives that increase the risk of abusive marketing and billing practices that result in higher prices than when company A would sell the supplies alone, company B will have opportunities to unduly influence referral sources including physicians and patients, and the arrangement between the parties does not contain safeguards against fraud and abuse. In addition, the OIG noted the arrangement does not fall within safe harbor protections of the personal services and management contracts because the majority of the compensation to be paid by company A to company B is calculated on a percentage of reimbursements collected by company B for sales of company A products; therefore, compensation levels are not fixed in advance and take into account value or volume of business generated between the parties.

Advisory Opinion 98-2

This advisory opinion relates to whether pharmaceutical discount pricing arrangements (i.e., a fixed percentage price reduction for multisource generics with further reductions if certain limited marketing activities are performed by the wholesaler, which are limited to arrangements between a manufacturer and wholesaler and would fulfill the requirements of the Medicaid drug rebate program[108]) constitute a violation of the Antikickback Statute, subjecting the parties to sanctions. The OIG concluded that such an arrangement would not be a violation of the statute because this arrangement furthers legislative intent to encourage price competition; although wholesalers do not submit claims to Medicare or Medicaid for their purchases, the manufacturer disclosures will ensure that discounts are reported and reflected in the Medicaid rebate; the discount is not a commission; and there is little reason for disparate treatment between the bioequivalent products subject to the arrangement and a simple price reduction regardless of the marketing arrangement. The OIG also concluded that the arrangement would not qualify for the discount or personal services safe harbors.

Advisory Opinion 98-3

This advisory opinion relates to whether a hospital system's free provision of an ambulance to a municipal fire department constitutes a violation of the Antikickback Statute, subjecting the parties to sanctions. The OIG concluded that such a provision may not be in violation of the statute because, although potentially prohibited remuneration, the arrangement presents minimal risks of abuse to federal health care programs, allows for greater patient freedom of choice as to hospital providers, allows for greater competition between hospitals in the geographic area to be served, the ambulance use protocol limits the ability of the fire department to steer patients to the hospital's facilities, and does not include any financial incentive or reward to the fire department for referrals to the hospital.

---

[108]42 U.S.C.A. §1396r-8.

Advisory Opinion 98-4

This advisory opinion relates to whether a proposed management services contract between a medical practice management company and a physician practice, which provides that the management company will be reimbursed for its costs and paid a percentage of net practice revenues, would constitute a violation of the Antikickback Statute, subjecting the parties to sanctions. The OIG concluded that this arrangement could violate the Antikickback Statute because the arrangement may include financial incentives to increase patient referrals through the marketing arrangements and setup of provider networks to which the physician practice might refer, the arrangement does not contain safeguards against overutilization, and the arrangement may include financial incentives that increase the risk of abusive billing practices by the management company. The OIG also noted that this arrangement does not fall within the personal services and management contracts safe harbor because its compensation to the management company is not set in advance and is not an aggregate amount.

Advisory Opinion 98-5

This advisory opinion relates to whether a nursing home that provides subacute and rehabilitative services to an MCO under a coordination of benefits plan constitutes a violation of the Antikickback Statute, subjecting the parties to sanctions. The coordination of benefits agreement would release the MCO from any obligation to pay benefits when the nursing home already received payment from the patient's primary insurer, including Medicare, in an amount equal to or exceeding the MCO fee schedule amount and requires that the nursing home hold the MCO enrollees harmless from any charges, including copayments and deductibles. The OIG concluded that this arrangement may be in violation of the Antikickback Statute because the arrangement may involve prohibited remuneration as Medicare cost sharing may be waived in full or in part, thus resulting in a financial benefit to the MCO from the nursing home that could induce referrals from the MCO; the nursing home may have an incentive to increase lengths of stay or skimp on services to recoup such payments; and the MCO has no incentive to control costs associated with Medicare fee-for-service beneficiaries, since it pays little or nothing. In addition, the OIG concluded that the arrangement did not fit within the price reductions safe harbor, waiver of coinsurance safe harbor, or the discount safe harbor.

Advisory Opinion 98-6

This advisory opinion relates to whether waiving deductibles and coinsurance obligations for participants in the National Emphysema Treatment Trial (NETT) clinical study sponsored by HCFA and the National Heart, Lung, and Blood Institute would constitute a violation of the Antikickback Statute, subjecting the parties to sanctions. The OIG concluded that the proposed arrangement would not constitute a violation of the Antikickback Statute because it is unlikely to influence beneficiaries to obtain Medicare-covered services from NETT providers, it will not increase the risk of utilization of Medicare covered services, and it is a reasonable means of enhancing the likelihood of success of the NETT study.

Advisory Opinion 98-7

This advisory opinion relates to whether a free ambulance restocking and continuing education arrangement for ambulances and emergency medical services (EMS) personnel, in which all area hospitals participate, constitutes a violation of the Antikickback Statute. The OIG concluded that the arrangement could constitute prohibited remuneration if the underlying rationale was to induce referrals, but that OIG would not subject the arrangement to sanctions. The OIG indicated that the arrangement is viable because it is limited to emergency medical services and thus does not increase the risk of overutilization and costs to federal health care programs; there is no financial reason arising from the arrangement for ambulance personnel to steer patients to specific hospitals, since all area hospitals participate; the arrangement is not unilateral and is based on an ongoing effort to maintain and improve a regional emergency medical system; restocking is not a freestanding arrangement and is an integral part of a comprehensive and coordinated regional effort to improve emergency medical care in the area; regional and local programs have actively been encouraged by the federal government over the past 25 years to improve and coordinate quality emergency services; and the arrangement is likely to have a positive impact on the quality of patient care.

Advisory Opinion 98-8

This advisory opinion relates to whether a company that charges Medicare 21–32% higher prices for durable medical equipment (DME) than cash-and-carry retail customers would be subject to sanctions. Medicare charges would be higher due to the additional administrative costs associated with participating in the Medicare program. The OIG noted that charges substantially in excess of a supplier's usual charges are permissible only when they are "due to unusual circumstances or medical complications requiring additional time, effort, expense, or other good cause."[109] The OIG indicated that additional costs for dealing with the Medicare program could constitute a "good cause," but the higher Medicare charge should bear a direct

and reasonable relationship to the additional costs incurred. The OIG indicated that a possible benchmark to consider is profit margin; if the profit margin for the Medicare sale is less than or equal to the cash-and-carry retail sale, the good cause exception would be satisfied. However, on the basis of the information provided the OIG, it could not determine whether the company's proposed fee structure would be within the good cause exception.

Advisory Opinion 98-9

This advisory opinion relates to whether a compensation arrangement with a baseline that rises on the basis of the number of admissions for registered nurses and certain other employees pursuant to a collective bargaining agreement with the nurses' union constitutes prohibited remuneration under the Antikickback Statute, subjecting the parties to sanctions. The OIG concluded that, assuming the nurses are bona fide employees, the proposed arrangement requires the union employees to perform nursing and other health care–related services to be eligible for the compensation arrangement and thus falls within the plain language of the bona fide employee safe harbor.

Advisory Opinion 98-10

This advisory opinion relates to whether the payment of a sales commission, representing fair market value for such services, by the manufacturer of disposable medical supplies to an independent contractor sales agent who sells the supplies to large purchasers constitutes prohibited remuneration in violation of the Antikickback Statute. The OIG concluded that although the arrangement could constitute prohibited remuneration under the Antikickback Statute, it would not subject the arrangement to sanctions. The OIG first noted that the arrangement did not fall within the personal services and management contracts safe harbor because remuneration for services was not set out in advance. The OIG indicated that the arrangement would not be subject to sanctions because the manufacturer did not bill any payer for the items being sold; there was no contact between the sales agent and patients or physicians; the sales agent was not in a position to exert undue influence on medical decision making; the sales agent's contacts were with sophisticated purchasers (group purchasing organizations, purchasing units for multihospital systems), none of which were in a position to order specific products for individual patients; and the disposable medical supplies were not separately reimbursed by the federal health care programs and their costs were reimbursed through the fixed DRG payment.

Advisory Opinion 98-11

This advisory opinion relates to whether a purchasing arrangement involving a trade association, its nursing home

---

[109]42 C.F.R. §1007.701(c)(1) (1998).

members, and an electrical utility consultant, the latter of which would obtain payment by charging a fee of 17% of the cost savings achieved by the consultant, would constitute prohibited remuneration under the Antikickback Statute, subjecting its participants to penalties. The OIG indicated that this arrangement falls squarely within the GPO safe harbor. There is minimal risk of fraud or abuse between the nursing homes and the utility consultant, since neither party is likely to be a referral source for the other, the consultant's fee is based solely on electricity cost savings, the net cost savings will be accurately reflected in the nursing homes' cost reports, and the cost savings will be to the benefit of federal health care programs.

Advisory Opinion 98-12

This advisory opinion relates to whether the formation of a joint venture between several orthopedic surgeons and anesthesiologists specializing in pain management to establish an ambulatory surgical center would be in violation of the Antikickback Statute and subject the arrangement to sanctions. Each physician investor would be a shareholder of the corporation that forms the ambulatory surgical center, and each would contribute at least a certain amount of cash to the venture that is not dependent on expected volume of referrals with voting and profit distribution rights proportional to investment. At least 40% of each physician investor's medical practice income will be generated through performance of the joint venture's procedures. Further, the providers would disclose their ownership interest in the ambulatory surgical center. Although the proposed venture could violate the Antikickback Statute, the OIG concluded that it would not impose sanctions on the arrangement. Since HCFA promotes ambulatory surgical centers as a cost-effective alternative to higher-cost treatment settings, there are legitimate business and professional reasons for surgeons to want to own an ambulatory surgical center, including patient benefit and quality control; the physician investors are making substantial financial investments in the joint venture; a high percentage (at least 40%) of each physician's service income derives from the venture; the remuneration is based on capital investments and not referrals; and ownership interests are disclosed to patients. Therefore, the OIG concluded that there would be limited opportunity for Antikickback Statute concerns.

Advisory Opinion 98-13

This advisory opinion relates to whether an ambulance restocking program, coordinated through a local emergency medical services council composed of eight fire departments and a county ambulance district that provide emergency medical services, hospitals, ambulance providers, local educational facilities, and medical directors, would constitute prohibited remuneration under the Antikickback Statute, subjecting the arrangement to sanctions. The program would provide free exchange of drugs and medical supplies used by hospitals to EMS providers when they bring a patient to a hospital for emergency treatment. All hospitals and EMS providers in the county participate. The ambulance providers are not charged for nor do they pay for the restocked items, and the cost of the supplies is charged to the patient by the receiving hospital. The OIG concluded that the program could constitute prohibited remuneration under the statute if the intent is to induce referrals, but the OIG will not subject the program to sanctions. Because the program is not a unilateral arrangement and is an ongoing effort by the council throughout the county, the restocking aspects of the program are not freestanding but an integral part of a coordinated regional effort to integrate and improve the emergency medical care system, regional and local programs to improve and coordinate delivery and quality of EMS care have been encouraged and promoted by the federal government over the past 25 years, and the program is likely to have a positive impact on patient care, it is of benefit to beneficiaries and will not lead to program abuse.

Advisory Opinion 98-14

This advisory opinion relates to whether a pharmaceutical restocking program and medical supplies restocking program by several hospitals in the provision of emergency medical services constitute prohibited remuneration under the Antikickback Statute, subjecting the arrangement to sanctions. Ambulances will be stocked with pharmaceutical and medical supplies by receiving hospitals when these ambulances bring patients to the emergency rooms of the hospital. The pharmaceutical program would be arranged and run by a local emergency medical council, including EMS providers, hospitals, physicians, paramedics, education providers, and consumer representatives; the supply program would be implemented by a committee formed exclusively of hospital representatives. The OIG concluded that since the pharmaceutical restocking program is substantially similar to circumstances addressed by OIG Advisory Opinions 98–7 and 98–13, it would not subject the arrangement to sanctions. However, the supply program, although of potential community benefit, is implemented by only hospital representatives; therefore, the OIG concluded that the arrangement might violate the statute if one purpose was to induce federal health care program business. Without additional information, the OIG indicated it could not provide any additional conclusions on the acceptability of the arrangement.

Advisory Opinion 98-15

This advisory opinion relates to whether a contract arrangement between a university and pharmacy company to facilitate an outpatient pharmacy program for the university's hemophilia center under provisions of federal law would be in violation of the Antikickback Statute and subject the arrangement to sanctions. The company would provide and dispense hemophilia-related drugs through the university's hemophilia center and provide outpatient pharmacy services for those patients, including inventory management, billings, collections, and educational support. Because of restrictions in federal law, the arrangement would not have the university serve Medicaid patients, although they may obtain services from the company elsewhere. The company was selected on the basis of competitive bidding, and the compensation paid to the company will be based on a fee schedule that pays the company a fixed amount per unit of drug dispensed, with the payments being reduced per unit if the volume exceeds some threshold amount. Compensation will be renegotiated annually. The OIG first noted that the proposed arrangement does not fall within the personal services and management contract safe harbor because the nature of the services in the agreement precludes an exact specification of the schedule for their performance and the aggregate amount of compensation is not set in advance. However, the OIG concluded that the arrangement would not be subject to sanctions because it poses a minimal risk of fraud or abuse, since the proposed arrangement is consistent with congressional intent by fulfilling the requirements for such programs under federal law; the company will be paid fair market value for services rendered; the company is not paying for referrals of Medicaid fee-for-service patients; and the proposed arrangement preserves patient freedom of choice for Medicaid patients.

Advisory Opinion 98-16

This advisory opinion relates to whether a proposed arrangement, under which a mail-order pharmacy would assign an employee pharmacist to work in designated hospital transplant centers to provide pharmacy-related products and services, would constitute a violation of the Antikickback Statute and subject the arrangement to sanctions. The mail-order pharmacy would be responsible for all employee costs, including wages, benefits, and taxes; and the pharmacist's duties would include working with transplant teams to facilitate the patient's posttransplant care, preparing pharmaceutical care plans, overseeing patient compliance with such plans after discharge, securing the patient's insurance coverage for pharmaceuticals and services provided by the mail-order pharmacy, and processing prescriptions through the mail-order pharmacy's distribution center. These items and services, in whole or in part, may be paid for by a federal health care program. The transplant centers would incur no cost but would be responsible for providing the pharmacist a work area and patient access. The OIG concluded that the pro-

posed arrangement most likely would violate the statute because the mail-order pharmacy would be providing the transplant centers something of value in order to induce referrals; one purpose of the arrangement in fact is to induce referrals; and the arrangement contains no safeguards, conditions, or controls that mitigate against the risk of improper steering by transplant centers to the mail-order pharmacy due to the provision of free services by the pharmacist.

Advisory Opinion 98-17

This advisory opinion relates to whether donations by a company to a nonprofit, 501(c)(3) charitable organization for the purpose of funding a program to pay for Medicare Part B or Medigap premiums for financially needy Medicare beneficiaries with end-stage renal disease, where some or all of the beneficiaries may be receiving treatment from the company, would constitute a violation of the Antikickback Statute and subject the arrangement to sanctions. No restrictions would be placed on the donations from the company to the organization. The OIG concluded that the arrangement would not constitute prohibited remuneration for referrals because donations by the company are not made to or on behalf of an individual eligible for Medicare or a state health care program's benefits and the organization that receives the funds purchase of premiums for beneficiaries is not likely to induce a beneficiary's choice of a particular provider.

Advisory Opinion 98-18

This advisory opinion relates to whether an ophthalmologist's proposed sublease to an optometrist of certain imaging equipment would meet the criteria of the equipment rental safe harbor. The imaging equipment may be used by the ophthalmologist to conduct telemedicine consultations relating to the optometrist's patients. The telemedicine relationship would allow for the optometrist to have access to telemedicine consultations with the ophthalmologist; however, the optometrist will not advertise or market this access and will not charge a fee in connection with such consultations. The telemedicine arrangement permits the optometrist's patients to choose any ophthalmologist they wish, and there is no collateral arrangement regarding the referral of patients from either party to the other. The sublease would be in writing for a 12-month term, with a fixed rental per month and an annual aggregate amount fixed in advance based on fair market value. The OIG concluded that, first, the sublease would not constitute prohibited remuneration because it is not determined in a manner that takes into account the volume or value of any referrals or business generated between the parties. The sublease thus fulfills the requirements of the equipment rental safe harbor. The OIG also concluded that the telemedicine arrangement would also not constitute prohibited remuneration because the optometrist will obtain no fees for access to telemedicine consultations nor will the optometrist advertise such access and because the proposed arrangement allows the optometrist's patients to choose any ophthalmologist desired by them in the absence of any understanding that there will be referrals between the optometrist and the ophthalmologist.

Advisory Opinion 98-19

This advisory opinion relates to whether an arrangement through which an IPA would acquire an equity interest in an MCO would constitute a violation of the Antikickback Statute, subjecting the arrangement to sanctions. The IPA would acquire a less than 15% equity interest in the MCO and the consequent return on the equity investment. The IPA would assign the MCO the IPA's contract rights under several long-term provider service agreements. The IPA then would become the exclusive physician provider panel for all managed care agreements in which the MCO participated and would not serve as a provider panel for any other health care entity. Individual physicians in the IPA, however, would be permitted to serve on panels for other health plans under certain conditions. The IPA would be responsible for developing and maintaining the provider network for the MCO for ten years and the IPA and the MCO would enter into a ten-year agreement where the IPA shareholder physicians would develop and implement various programs for the MCO including credentialing, utilization management, quality improvement, and case management functions and the MCO would provide the IPA with administrative services including credentialing, accounting and auditing, utilization and quality management, and office administration services. Finally, the IPA will offer additional shares of stock to those of its shareholder physicians who agree to assume certain levels of financial risk. It is estimated that 90% of the IPA physicians will be eligible to participate. The OIG first noted that the proposed arrangement does not fall within the safe harbor for investment interests in small entities, particularly because the investment opportunities are limited to IPA physician shareholders. Although the proposed arrangement potentially violates the Antikickback Statute, the proposed arrangement does not appear to implicate sanctions because of the absence of any specific marketing efforts by the IPA physician shareholders to promote enrollment in the MCO's plans; the IPA was not formed for the purpose of entering into the proposed agreement; the ownership in the IPA is based on per capita share distribution and future shareholdings will be based in part on physician assumption of risk and performance on a number of preset quality of performance standards rather than referrals; the MCO provides at least some services on a capitated basis, discouraging unnecessary services; and all investor returns on investment will be commensurate with

their financial risk undertakings. The OIG next noted that the ten-year network services agreement and the ten-year administrative services agreement did not fall within the personal services and management contracts safe harbor, since the aggregate compensation to be paid over the term of the agreements are not set out in advance. However, because the IPA's compensation will represent fair market value and does not take into account volume or value of business generated between the parties, it does not appear to represent prohibited payment for referrals. However, the agreement with regard to the IPA providing credentialing, utilization review, quality improvement, and case management programs lacked specificity for the OIG to render judgment on its legality. Finally, the OIG concluded that the stock plan did not implicate the Antikickback Statute since the physicians receiving the stock would not be in a position to refer business to the IPA and eligibility for IPA stock is tied to the assumption of risk by the physician.

Advisory Opinion 99-1

This advisory opinion relates to whether an arrangement for provision of backup emergency ambulance services that would involve copayment and deductible waivers is in violation of the Antikickback Statute and would subject the arrangement to sanctions. Emergency services involve paramedic services, which do not have independent transport, and separate transport or basic ambulance services. Company X, a 501(c)(3) charitable organization, is the sole provider of paramedic services; it is generally prohibited by law from transporting patients in conjunction with its paramedic services. Volunteer first aid squads generally provide emergency transport services. Company X would provide emergency backup transport services when it responds to a paramedic service request and a volunteer transport squad fails to arrive at the scene; and when 911 public safety answering points request a volunteer first aid squad but one is unavailable to respond. Volunteer squads do not bill state, federal, or private insurance programs, whereas Company X bills insurers for paramedic services, including Medicare. Because patients in Company X's area typically do not pay for basic ambulance services and because collection of such fees would cast volunteer ambulance systems in a poor light, Company X desires to waive patient copayments and deductibles for backup emergency ambulance services. The OIG concluded that such a waiver, although it may constitute prohibited remuneration in violation of the statute, is of limited risk in this situation because there is no expectation on the part of an emergency patient that there will be a charge, much less a copayment, for emergency ambulance services. Therefore, Company X's failure to collect a copayment for isolated instances in which it provides backup emergency ambulance transport is not an inducement to use the service.

Advisory Opinion 99-2

This advisory opinion relates to whether an arrangement under which discounted ambulance services are provided residents of Medicare skilled nursing facilities would constitute prohibited remuneration, subjecting the arrangement to sanctions under the Antikickback Statute. Under consolidated billing, the Medicare program for the most part will pay skilled nursing facilities a per diem rate under Medicare Part A in the prospective payment system, which would include ambulance services. Skilled nursing facilities have Medicare patients who have such services covered under Part A, some who are covered under Part B, and some who have private insurance. The ambulance company proposes to provide discounts to these facilities for its ambulance services rendered to Medicare Part A patients. The OIG concluded that this arrangement may constitute illegal remuneration under the Antikickback Statute. The OIG first concluded that the arrangement did not fit within the discount safe harbor because federal health programs may not truly receive the benefit from the discount and may result in inappropriate increases in utilization or abusive billing practices to recoup losses on the discounted business. Second, the circumstances surrounding the arrangement suggest a possible nexus between the discount to the skilled nursing facilities' Medicare prospective payment system ambulance transports and referrals of other federal health care program business. Since the skilled nursing facilities are in a position to direct a significant amount of business to the ambulance company that is not covered by prospective payment system payment, both parties have obvious motives for agreeing to discounts on this business for referrals of nonprospective payment system business; and the ambulance company's request for an advisory opinion has come at a time when many informal inquiries indicate that such discount arrangements are being used to generate more lucrative Medicare Part B charges, the OIG concluded that these discounts may be improper "swapping" arrangements, where one form of business is swapped for other more lucrative forms. Therefore, the OIG indicated that the arrangement may run afoul of the Antikickback Statute.

Stark Laws

The Stark laws focus on provider self-referral of Medicare and Medicaid patients (i.e., referrals to entities in which the provider has a financial interest). The Stark laws prohibit a physician investor or a physician having a financial relationship (including through family members) with an entity to make a referral to that entity for any designated health care service reimbursable by Medicare or Medicaid. Both the physician and the entity

are subject to sanctions for violating the Stark laws. Note that the Stark laws are not criminal statutes, in contrast to the FCA, which has both criminal and civil components.

Stark I and Stark II

Two self-referral laws have been passed by Congress. In 1989, under the Ethics in Patient Referrals Act, known as *Stark I*, physicians are prohibited from referring Medicare patients to clinical laboratories in which they or a direct family member have a financial interest.[110] In 1993, under *Stark II*, self-referral prohibitions were extended from clinical laboratories and Medicare patients to physical therapy services, occupational therapy services, radiological services (including computerized axial tomography, CT, scans; magnetic resonance imaging, MRI, scans; and ultrasonography), radiation therapy treatment, durable medical equipment, parenteral and enteral nutrition and equipment, prosthetics, home health services, outpatient prescription drugs, and inpatient and outpatient hospital services as well as Medicaid patients.[111] The services included within the Stark laws are referred to as *designated services*. Formally, if the physician or immediate family member has a financial relationship with an entity, then

1. the physician may not make a referral to the entity to furnish designated health services for which payment otherwise may be made by a federal health program; and
2. the entity may not present or cause to be presented a claim to a federal health program, or bill any individual, third-party payor, or other entity for designated health services furnished pursuant to a referral prohibited by the law.[112]

A *referral*, in the context of the Stark laws, encompasses a broad set of actions and includes a request by a physician for any Medicare Part B reimbursable good or service. Further, beyond a simple referral by one physician to another, any test or procedure ordered, performed, or supervised by the referred-to physician is deemed a referral by the referring physician.[113] In addition, any request or establishment of a care plan by a physician that includes provision of any of the services included within the Stark laws is considered a referral by the physician for those services, even when those services are provided by that physician's practice. Note, however, that a pathologist requesting clinical laboratory

[110]42 U.S.C.A. §1395nn; 42 C.F.R. §§411.350–411.361 (1998).

[111]42 U.S.C.A. §1395nn(h)(6).

[112]42 U.S.C.A. §1395nn(a)(1).

[113]42 U.S.C.A. §1395nn(h)(5)(A).

services, a radiologist requesting diagnostic radiology services, and a radiation oncologist requesting radiation therapy services are not deemed referrals if the services are furnished or supervised by the pathologist, radiologist, and radiation oncologist, respectively, on the basis of a request by another physician for these services.[114]

A *financial relationship*, within the Stark laws, encompasses an ownership or investment interest in the entity as well as a compensation arrangement between the physician or an immediate family member and the referred-to entity.[115] Financial relationships encompass equity, debt, or other forms of entity interests. Note also that the ownership or investment interest extends to the entity's related corporate relationships; for example, a physician who has a financial relationship with a particular company has a financial relationship with all entities owned by that company.

Compensation agreement, under the Stark laws, also is a broadly applicable concept and includes any remuneration, direct or indirect, overt or covert, in cash or in kind, between a physician or immediate family member and an entity providing the designated services.[116] Note that, like the Antikickback Statute, the concept of remuneration generally includes any economic benefit.[117]

The definition of *immediate family member* is concomitantly broad. Such a family member includes the physician's spouse, natural or adoptive parent, child, sibling, stepparent, stepchild, stepbrother, stepsister, father-in-law, mother-in-law, son-in-law, daughter-in-law, grandparent, grandchild, and spouse of the grandparent or grandchild.[118]

It is essential to note that because the Stark self-referral prohibitions impose liability for simple self-referral, there is no requirement of any knowledge on the part of the provider that the acts were illegal or that the provider should have known that such referrals are illegal. Hence, even innocent violation of the Stark laws would subject the provider to their penalties, effectively making the Stark laws one of strict liability.

Exceptions

There are exceptions to the Stark laws' prohibitions on self-referrals. These exceptions modify the ownership or investment financial relationships and the compensation arrangement component aspect of the laws. In addition, some general exceptions are applicable to all financial relationships.

Exceptions to Ownership or Investment Financial Relationships

Hospitals in Puerto Rico. Stark II prohibitions on self-referral are not applicable for designated health services provided by hospitals in Puerto Rico.[119]

Ownership Interest in Hospitals. The Stark laws do not apply to designated health services provided by hospitals if "the referring physician is authorized to perform services at the hospital; and the physician's ownership or investment interest is in the hospital itself, not simply one of the hospital's subdivisions or departments."[120]

Ownership in Publicly Traded Securities and Mutual Funds. Certain forms of ownership are permissible under the Stark laws and allow physicians to refer to these entities.[121] Ownership of investment securities such as stock, bonds, debentures, notes, or other debt instruments is permissible if the securities:

1. May be purchased on terms generally available to the public.
2. Are listed on the New York Stock Exchange, the American Stock Exchange, or any regional exchange in which quotations are published daily; or are foreign securities listed on a recognized foreign, national, or regional exchange in which quotations are published daily; or are traded under an automated interdealer quotation system operated by the National Association of Securities Dealers.
3. Are in a corporation that has total assets exceeding $75 million at the end of its most recent fiscal year or on average during the previous three fiscal years (or, for securities purchased before January 1, 1995, assets exceeding $100 million).

Note that ownership of shares in a regulated investment company as defined by the Internal Revenue Code[122] also is permissible if the company has total assets exceeding $75 million at the end of its most recent fiscal year or on average during the previous three fiscal years.

Rural Providers. Stark laws do not apply to designated health services furnished in a rural area by an entity[123] if substantially all services provided by the entity are furnished to individuals who reside in the rural area and the entity is located in a rural area and primarily serves patients residing in that same area. Note that a provider

---

[114]42 U.S.C.A. §1395nn(h)(5)(c).

[115]42 U.S.C.A. §1395nn(h)(6).

[116]42 U.S.C.A. §1395nn(h)(1).

[117]42 U.S.C.A. §1395nn(h)(1)(C)(I).

[118]42 C.F.R. §411.351 (1998).

[119]42 U.S.C.A. §1395nn(d)(1).

[120]42 U.S.C.A. §1395nn(d)(3).

[121]42 U.S.C.A. §1395nn(c).

[122]98 IRC §851(a).

[123]42 U.S.C.A. §1395nn(d)(2).

cannot come within this exception merely by moving to a location on the boundary of the rural area.

Exceptions to Compensation Arrangements

Bona Fide Employment Relationships.   The Stark laws' self-referral prohibitions do not apply to amounts paid by an employer to a physician or a member of his or her immediate family if the physician or family member has a bona fide employment relationship with the employer for provision of services.[124] This exception applies only if:

1. The employment is for identifiable services.
2. The remuneration is consistent with fair market value of the services and is not determined in any manner that takes into account volume or value of referrals made by the physician.
3. The remuneration is provided under an agreement that would be commercially reasonable even if no referrals were made to the employer.
4. The employment meets any other requirements the Secretary of Health and Human Services may impose by regulation as needed to protect against program or patient abuse.

Note that productivity bonuses are permitted under the bona fide employment relationship exception if the bonus is based on services performed personally by the physician or family member; however, for group practices, the productivity bonus cannot be tied to services provided under the referring physician's supervision and cannot include sharing in the group's profits.

De Minimus Remuneration.   In this exception, forgiveness of amounts owed for inaccurate tests or procedures or correction of minor billing errors is not considered remuneration. Similarly, the provision of materials used only to collect, transport, process, or store specimens of the entity performing the diagnostic tests or to order or communicate the results of these tests or procedures is not deemed remuneration under the Stark laws.[125]

Isolated Transactions.   One-time transactions, such as a sale of a physician's practice, also may be permitted under the Stark laws[126] if:

1. The amount of remuneration paid under the transaction is consistent with fair market value and is not based, directly or indirectly, on the volume or value of any referrals made by the referring physician.

2. The remuneration is provided under an agreement that would be commercially reasonable even if no referrals were made to the entity.
3. The arrangement meets any other requirements the Secretary of Health and Human Services may impose by regulation to protect against program or patient abuse.

Note that, in the final regulations for Stark I, the "isolated transactions" exception also includes the requirements that there be no financial relationship between the parties for six months after the isolated transaction, unless the new financial relationship itself qualifies for a separate exception and the transaction involves a single payment — installment or long-term payment arrangements are not acceptable.

Payments by a Physician for Items and Services.   The Stark self-referral prohibitions do not apply to payments made by a physician to a laboratory for the provision of clinical laboratory services or to an entity as compensation for other items or services if the prices of the goods or services are consistent with fair market value.[127] Because clinical laboratory services often are significantly discounted as standard practice in the industry, the general fair market value standard is not applicable to these services.

Personal Service Arrangements.   Appropriate remuneration by an entity for specific physician services is not a violation of the Stark laws.[128] Remuneration from an entity under an arrangement for physician services (including remuneration for specific physician services furnished to a nonprofit blood center) is permitted if:

1. The arrangement is in writing, signed by the parties, and specifies which services are covered.
2. The arrangement covers all services to be provided by the physician or immediate family member to the entity.
3. The aggregate services contracted for do not exceed those that are reasonable and necessary for the legitimate business purposes of the arrangement.
4. The term of the arrangement is for at least one year.
5. The compensation to be paid over the term of the arrangement is set in advance, does not exceed fair market value, and, with the exception of a physician incentive plan (PIP) (see below), is not determined in a manner that takes into account the volume or value of any referrals or other business generated between the parties.
6. The services to be performed under the arrangement do not involve the counseling or promotion of a busi-

---

[124]42 U.S.C.A. §1395nn(e)(2).

[125]42 U.S.C.A. §1395nn(h)(1)(c).

[126]42 U.S.C.A. §1395nn(e)(6).

[127]42 U.S.C.A. §1395nn(e)(8).

[128]42 U.S.C.A. §1395nn(e)(2).

ness arrangement or other activity that violates any state or federal law.

7. The arrangement meets any other requirements that the Secretary of Health and Human Services may impose as needed to protect against program or patient abuse.

Under this exception, PIPs are treated specifically. PIPs are any compensation arrangement between an entity and a physician or physician group that directly or indirectly may have the effect of reducing or limiting services provided to individuals enrolled in the entity.[129] PIPs may be based directly or indirectly on the volume or value of referrals or other business between the parties[130] if:

1. No specific payment is made directly or indirectly under the plan to a physician or physician group as an inducement to reduce or limit medically necessary services provided a specific individual enrolled with the entity.
2. A PIP that places a physician or a physician group at substantial financial risk as defined by law[131] complies with any requirements the Secretary of Health and Human Services may impose.
3. The entity provides the DHHS on request access to descriptive information regarding the PIP to permit the Secretary of the DHHS to determine whether it is in compliance with these requirements.

Physician Recruitment. A hospital may provide remuneration to a physician to induce that physician to relocate to the geographic area served by the hospital so that the physician may join the medical staff[132] if:

1. The physician is not required to refer patients to the hospital.
2. The amount of remuneration under the arrangement is not determined in a manner that takes into account, directly or indirectly, the volume or value of any referrals made by the referring physician.
3. The arrangement meets such other requirements as the Secretary of Health and Human Services may impose by regulation as needed to protect against program or patient abuse.

Note that this particular exception applies only to physicians outside the geographic area who have previously existing practices. It does *not* apply to arrangements in which the hospital attempts to retain physicians in the geographic area nor to arrangements with physicians who have no existing practice.

Remuneration Unrelated to Designated Services. Remuneration provided by a hospital to a physician is not subject to the Stark laws' prohibition if it does not relate to the provision of designated health services.[133]

Rental of Office Space and Equipment. Certain provisions for rental of office space and equipment also are permitted under the Stark laws.[134] Payments made by a lessee to a lessor for the use of an office space or equipment are not within the self-referral ban if:

1. The lease is in writing, is signed by the parties, and indicates the space or equipment subject to the lease.
2. The space or equipment rented or leased does not exceed what is reasonable and necessary for the legitimate business purposes of the lease or rental and is used exclusively by the lessee when being used by the lessee.
3. For office space rentals, the lessee's payments for the use of space consisting of common areas if the payments do not exceed the lessee's pro rata share of expenses for the space based on the ratio of space used exclusively by the lessee to the total amount of space, other than the common areas, occupied by all persons using such common areas.
4. The term of the lease is for at least one year.
5. The rental charges over the term of the lease are set in advance, consistent with fair market value, and not calculated in any way on the basis of the volume or value of referrals or other business between the parties.
6. The lease would be commercially reasonable even if no referrals were made between the parties.
7. The lease meets any other requirements that the Secretary of Health and Human Services may impose by regulation to protect against program or patient abuse.

Specific Group Practice Arrangements with a Hospital. An arrangement between a hospital and a group, through which designated health services are provided by the group but are billed for by the hospital, is permitted under the Stark laws[135] if:

1. The arrangement is pursuant to the provision of inpatient services as defined by law.[136]
2. The arrangement began before December 19, 1989, and has continued without interruption since its inception.
3. Substantially all of the designated health services covered by the arrangement furnished to patients of the hospital are furnished by the group under the arrangement.

[129]42 U.S.C.A. §1395nn(e)(3)(B)(ii).
[130]42 U.S.C.A. §1395nn(e)(3)(B)(i).
[131]42 U.S.C.A. §1395mm(i)(8)(A)(ii).
[132]42 U.S.C.A. §1395nn(e)(5).
[133]42 U.S.C.A. §1395nn(e)(4).
[134]42 U.S.C.A. §1395nn(e)(1).
[135]42 U.S.C.A. §1395nn(e)(7).
[136]42 U.S.C.A. §1395x(b)(3).

4. The arrangement is pursuant to an agreement in writing that specifies the services to be provided by the parties and the compensation for these services.

5. The compensation paid under the agreement is consistent with fair market value and compensation per unit of service, fixed in advance, and not determined in a manner that takes into account the volume or value of any referrals or other business generated between the parties.

6. The compensation is provided pursuant to an agreement that would be reasonable even if no referrals were made to the entity.

7. The agreement between the parties meets such other requirements as the Secretary of Health and Human Services may impose by regulation as needed to protect against program or patient abuse.

General Exceptions Applicable to All Financial Relationships

Both the in-office ancillary services exception and the physician services exception covered here depend on the technical definition of *group practice*. A group practice within the contemplation of the Stark laws is defined as follows:

1. A group of two or more physicians legally organized as a partnership, professional corporation, foundation, not-for-profit corporation, faculty practice plan, or similar association.

2. In which each physician who is a member of the group provides substantially the full range of services the physician routinely provides, including medical care, consultation, diagnosis or treatment, through the joint use of shared office space, facilities, equipment, and personnel.

3. For which substantially all services of the physicians who are members of the group are provided through the group and are billed under a billing number assigned to the group, and the amounts so received are treated as receipts of the group.

4. In which overhead expenses of and income derived from the practice are distributed in accordance with methods previously determined.

5. In which no physician who is a member of the group directly or indirectly receives compensation based on the volume or value of referrals by the physician except under special rules for profits and productivity bonuses (discussed below).

6. In which members of the group personally conduct no less than 75% of the patient–physician encounters of the group practice.

7. That meets such other standards as the Secretary of Health and Human Services may impose by regulation.

Members of a group practice include partners, full-time and part-time employees, and contract physicians.

Note that, under the Stark I final regulations,[137] *substantially all services* means that 75% of the total patient care services performed by the group practice members must be furnished, billed, and treated as for the group. Under these same regulations, *patient care services* are represented by any tasks performed by a group member that addresses the medical needs of specific patients, regardless of whether they involve patient encounters. This requirement does not apply to group practices located in health professional shortage areas defined in the Public Health Service Act.[138] The percentage of patient care services is to be measured on the basis of the total patient care time each member spends on these services. Therefore, if a ten-member physician group practice consists of eight devoting 100% of their total patient care time to the group practice, one devoting 80%, and one 10%, together, the ten physicians devote 890% of their total time to the group practice, meaning that the physicians in the group devote 89% of their combined patient care services to the group, thus satisfying the 75% requirement. Note that all group practices that meet the definition of group practice in the statute must submit an annual written statement to their Medicare carrier attesting that in the most recent 12-month period (on the basis of the fiscal year, calendar year, or immediate 12-month period), they have met the 75% patient care services requirement.

Special rules apply for profits and productivity bonuses in group practices. A physician in a group practice may be paid a share of the group's overall profits or a productivity bonus based on services personally performed or "incident to" such personally performed services so long as the share or bonus is not determined in any manner directly related to the volume or value of referrals by the physician.[139] In addition, special rules apply for faculty practice plans. Where a faculty practice plan is associated with a hospital, higher educational institution, or medical school with an approved medical residency training program in which physician members may provide a variety of different specialty services and professional services within and outside the group or perform other tasks such as research, the group practice exception applies only to the services provided within the faculty practice plan.[140]

In-Office Ancillary Services. Several types of ancillary service provision are permitted under the Stark laws.[141] In-office ancillary services are permitted to be provided if:

---

[137]42 C.F.R. §411.350 (1998).

[138]42 U.S.C.A. §§201 *et seq.*

[139]42 U.S.C.A. §1395nn(h)(4)(B)(i).

[140]42 U.S.C.A. §1395nn(e)(4)(B)(ii).

[141]42 U.S.C.A. §1395nn(b)(2).

1. They are other than durable medical equipment provision and parenteral or enteral nutrient provision (although the provision of infusion pumps is allowed).
2. They are furnished personally by the referring physician, a physician who is a member of the same group practice as the referring physician, or individuals who are directly supervised by the physician or by another physician in the group practice.
3. They are furnished in a building in which the referring physician or another physician who is a member of the same group practice furnishes physicians' services unrelated to the furnishing of designated health services or, in the case of a referring physician who is a member of a group practice, in another building that is used by the group practice for the provision of some or all of the group's clinical laboratory services or for the centralized provision of the group's designated health services other than clinical laboratory services.
4. They are billed by the physician performing or supervising their services, a group practice of which such physician is a member under a billing number assigned to the group practice, or an entity wholly owned by such physician or group practice.
5. The ownership or investment interest in such services meets such other requirements as the Secretary of Health and Human Services may impose by regulation as needed to protect against program or patient abuse.

Note that the Secretary of Health and Human Services may allow for other circumstances in the provision of ancillary services if they do not present a risk of program or patient abuse.[142] One contentious issue in this exception is whether laboratories shared between independent practitioners and groups could fall within the exception. In the preamble of the Stark I final regulations,[143] it would appear that individual physicians who set up a laboratory separate from their practices, share in its costs, and bill individually for services provided by the laboratory to their own patients alone would violate Stark I; the in-office ancillary exception could apply if each physician met the location, billing, and supervision requirements. Similarly, group practices that share a laboratory would not be within the exception; however, individual physicians in a group may bill for a test they refer to the shared laboratory if the physician personally performs or directly supervises the test. This interpretation by HCFA would seem problematic for most practitioners; and since shared laboratories are not expressly noted in the Stark I final regulations, attempts to fit these arrangements within the in-office ancillary exception would seem risky.

Physician Services. Self-referral prohibitions do not apply to physician services[144] provided personally by or under the personal supervision of another physician in the same group practice.[145]

Prepaid Plans. Physician self-referral prohibitions do not apply to federally qualified HMOs,[146] plans receiving payments on a prepaid basis in demonstration projects under specific statutory authority,[147] and prepayment plans providing services under other federal statutory authority or programs.[148]

Reporting Requirements

Under the Stark laws, every entity that provides covered services under the Medicare and Medicaid programs must provide the Secretary of Health and Human Services information regarding the entity's ownership, investment, and compensation arrangements,[149] including the covered items and services provided by the entity and the names and unique physician identification numbers of all physicians with an ownership or investment interest[150] or compensation arrangement[151] in the entity or whose immediate family members have such an ownership or investment interest or such a compensation relationship with the entity. This disclosure requirement does not apply to designated health services provided outside the United States or to entities that the Secretary of Health and Human Services determines provide services for which payment may be made very infrequently. Further, under the Stark I final regulations,[152] entities that provide 20 or fewer Medicare Part A and Part B items and services during a calendar year are not required to disclose this information. Under Stark I, an entity that is required to disclose must provide the information on the HCFA-prescribed form to its Medicare carrier or intermediary as well as provide updates regarding any change in the submitted information.[153] Failure to report this when required makes the entity subject to civil penalties of up to $10,000 for each day of the period following the deadline for submission of the information until the information finally is submitted.[154]

---

[142]42 U.S.C.A. §1395nn(b)(2)(A)(II).

[143]60 Fed. Reg. 41,914-41,982 (August 14, 1995).

[144]42 U.S.C.A. §1395x(q).

[145]42 U.S.C.A. §1395nn(h)(4).

[146]42 U.S.C.A. §300e-9(d).

[147]42 U.S.C.A. §§1395b-1(a), 1320a-1.

[148]42 U.S.C.A. §§1395mm, 1395l(a)(1)(A).

[149]42 U.S.C.A. §1395nn(f).

[150]42 U.S.C.A. §1395nn(a)(2)(A).

[151]42 U.S.C.A. §1395nn(a)(2)(B).

[152]42 C.F.R. §411.361(b) (1998).

[153]42 C.F.R. §411.361(e) (1998).

[154]42 C.F.R. §411.361(f) (1998).

Stark Advisory Opinions

Similar to steps taken under HIPAA for the Antikickback Statute, under the BBA, Congress has mandated the Secretary of Health and Human Services to issue advisory opinions for providers who wish information about whether their arrangements violate the Stark self-referral prohibitions.[155] Final regulations have been promulgated for Stark advisory opinions that mirror those provided under the Antikickback Statute.[156] Advisory opinions are binding on the Secretary of Health and Human Services and the parties that request such an opinion. However, it is important to note that information provided under these advisory opinions can and may be used later in enforcement actions against the requestor. Therefore, although potentially beneficial, seeking an advisory opinion may be highly risky in terms of inviting close scrutiny by the government.

HCFA-AO-98-001

This advisory opinion concerns whether investment in and ownership of an ambulatory surgical treatment center (ASTC) by physicians who would refer patients to ASTC and perform surgery there would violate the prohibition of self-referral. In addition, a request was made for the evaluation to determine whether the ASTC fulfilled the rural exception under the statute. The investors would be physicians who would refer patients to the ASTC, and some would perform medical and surgical procedures there. The HCFA determined that the interests involved did constitute ownership or investment interest within the meaning of the Stark laws. However, because the ASTC would be within a rural area, it met part one of the rural provider exception; the HCFA indicated that as long as "substantially all" (i.e., greater than 75%) the services are to be furnished by the ASTC in the rural area, it would meet the other requirement of the rural provider exception. But because the ASTC has not yet been built, on the basis of the applicant's certification that greater than 99% of the population who would use the facility reside in the rural area, HCFA concluded that the arrangement could fall within the rural provider exception.

HCFA-AO-98-002

This advisory opinion concerns whether partners and physician-employees of a proposed partnership, under the in-office ancillary services exception, may refer Medicare or Medicaid patients for eyeglass prescriptions filled subsequent to cataract surgery with the insertion of an intraocular lens without violating the prohibition against self-referral. The partnership would provide ophthalmology services for patients and eyeglasses and contact lenses for patients and nonpatients. All leases and employment contracts would be assigned to the partnership. The partnership would create an additional site for services, so that there would be a total of three locations. Each partner would contribute 50% of the assets of the partnership and receive 50% of the revenues after expenses. Each physician-owner and physician-employee would be paid a salary unrelated to referrals. HCFA indicated that there is a financial relationship for purposes of Medicare referrals, and the physicians involved could refer only if an exception applies. HCFA indicated that the in-office ancillary services exception applies. First, the partnership fulfilled the definition of group practice (each member of the group substantially provides the full range of services and all leases have been assigned to the partnership), substantially all the physician-members' services are provided through the group and billed by the group represented by the partnership, overhead expenses and income from the practice are distributed in accordance with previously determined methods, no physician-member will be compensated directly or indirectly based on volume or value of referrals, and members of the group provide at least 75% of the physician–patient encounters. The partnership as group practice fulfills the in-office ancillary services exception because services will be furnished or supervised by the referring physician or by a member of the same group practice, the services will be furnished in an appropriate location, and the services will be billed under the billing number assigned to the group practice.

Sanctions

Each fraud and abuse statute has sanctions for violations of its individual tenets. In addition, other statutes that target health care fraud have been used to punish offenders of the fraud and abuse laws. In addition, non–health care statutes such as the conspiracy laws,[157] false statements laws,[158] general false claim laws,[159] mail and wire fraud laws,[160] money laundering laws,[161] and racketeering laws[162] have been used with health care fraud and abuse laws. Sanctions include both criminal and civil penalties

---

[155]42 U.S.C. §1395nn(g)(6).

[156]63 Fed. Reg. 1646-1658 (January 9, 1998).

[157]18 U.S.C.A. §§2, 286, 287, 371.

[158]18 U.S.C.A. §1001; see also United States v. O'Brien, 14 F.3d 703 (1st Cir. 1994); United States v. Henry, 12 F.3d 215 (6th Cir. 1993); United States v. Alemany-Rivera, 781 F.2d 229 (1st Cir. 1985), *cert. denied* 475 U.S. 1086 (1986).

[159]18 U.S.C.A. §§287, 1001.

[160]18 U.S.C.A. §1341, 1343; see also United States v. Collins, 596 F.2d 166 (6th Cir. 1979); United States v. Weiss, 930 F.2d 185 (2d Cir. 1991).

[161]18 U.S.C.A. §§1956, 1957.

[162]18 U.S.C.A. §1962.

and represent a significant cost to providers. In addition, usually providers have limited ability to challenge such sanctions; therefore, they represent a powerful tool for the government to induce specific preferred behavior as well as an important funding mechanism for its activities. The various sanctions discussed in this section are based on federal law; in addition, states also impose sanctions specific to the particular state. Generally, the OIG has the authority to enforce civil penalties[163] whereas the Department of Justice has authority to enforce criminal fraud and abuse laws, with the assistance of the FBI.[164] States assist in the enforcement of fraud and abuse laws as related to Medicaid through Medicaid fraud control units.[165]

False Claims—Criminal Sanctions

A large proportion of fraud and abuse prosecutions and sanctions have been for false claims by providers. Under the Medicare and Medicaid laws, an action by a provider serving the Medicare or Medicaid program constitutes a felony and is criminally punishable by a fine of up to $25,000 and up to five years' imprisonment[166] if the provider:

1. Knowingly and willfully makes or causes to be made a false statement or representation of a material fact in a claim for a benefit or payment or for use in determining rights to such benefits or payment under Medicare, Medicaid, or a state health care program funded through a federal block grant.
2. Knowingly and willfully makes or causes to be made, or induces or causes to be induced, the making of any false statements of material facts with regard to an institution's compliance with conditions of participation.
3. Conceals or fails to disclose knowledge of the occurrence of an event affecting an individual's right to a benefit or payment with the intent to fraudulently secure the benefit or payment.
4. Converts a Medicare benefit or payment intended for the use of another.
5. Bills for a physician's services knowing that the individual who provided the service was not a physician.
6. Bills for services not provided.
7. Misrepresents services actually provided.
8. Falsely certifies that certain services were medical necessary.
9. Knowingly and with fraudulent intent retains Medicare and Medicaid funds improperly paid.

Fraudulently retaining Medicare or Medicaid funds also constitutes the felony of concealment under the U.S. criminal code;[167] conviction of this latter felony requires actual knowledge of falsity.[168] In addition, it is a misdemeanor offense for a person other than the one who furnishes medical items or services (such as a beneficiary, billing clerk, or secretary) to commit the listed offenses, which is punishable by a fine of up to $10,000 and up to a one-year imprisonment.[169] Beyond the Medicare and Medicaid programs, these criminal penalties now are applicable to all claims to federal health care programs under the provisions of the Health Insurance Portability and Accountability Act of 1996.[170]

In addition, under the FCA's criminal sanction provisions, conviction of presenting a claim that the claimant knows to be "false, fictitious, or fraudulent"[171] carries a mandated fine and prison sentence. The fine is determined through the general provisions in the U.S. criminal code and the maximum prison sentence is five years.[172] Generally, the provider must be shown to have made the actual physical presentation of the claim or caused another to present the claim.[173] Knowledge has been held to require actual knowledge of the falsity[174] as well as the less stringent standard of reckless disregard or conscious avoidance of the truth.[175]

Note that criminal conviction of a federal crime of fraud or false statements prevents the provider or individual convicted from denying the essential elements of the criminal offense for civil sanction purposes.[176]

Finally, note that specific criminal convictions can result in mandatory or permissive exclusion from federal and state health care programs (discussed below).

---

[163]50 Fed. Reg. 45,488–45,491 (October 31, 1985).

[164]63 Fed. Reg. 36,846–36,849 (July 8, 1998).

[165]42 U.S.C.A. §§1396a(a)(61), 1396b(q).

[166]42 U.S.C.A. §§1320a-7b(a), 1320a-7b(c).

[167]18 U.S.C.A. §4.

[168]See, e.g., United States v. Laughlin, 26 F.3d 1523 (10th Cir. 1994); Godwin v. Visiting Nurse Ass'n Home Health Serv., 831 F.Supp. 449 (E.D. Pa. 1993).

[169]42 U.S.C.A. §1320a-7b(a)(6).

[170]42 U.S.C.A. §1320a-7b(a)(1).

[171]18 U.S.C.A. §287.

[172]18 U.S.C.A. §287.

[173]See, e.g., United States v. Kline, 922 F.2d 610 (10th Cir. 1990); United States v. Catena, 500 F.2d 1319 (3d Cir.), cert. denied 419 U.S. 1047 (1974).

[174]See, e.g., United States v. Precision Med. Labs., Inc., 593 F.2d 434, 443 (2d Cir. 1978).

[175]See, e.g., United States v. Nazon, 940 F.2d 255, 259–260 (7th Cir. 1991); United States v. Campbell, 845 F.2d 1374 (6th Cir.), cert. denied 488 U.S. 908 (1988).

[176]42 U.S.C.A. §1320a-7a(c)(3).

False Claims—Civil Sanctions

Much more common is the imposition of civil sanctions against providers deemed to have presented false claims. The Medicare and Medicaid laws also include civil monetary sanctions (also known as the Civil Monetary Penalty Law, CMPL).[177] This provision grants the Secretary of Health and Human Services the authority to impose civil sanctions against providers who make false claims. HIPAA amended the CMPL, allowing for sanctions against providers for fraudulent actions relating to any federal health care program, increasing penalties from $2,000 to $10,000 for each fraudulent claim, and increasing the penalty assessment from two to three times the amount claimed.[178] HIPAA also allows for civil monetary penalties against providers or individuals who offer remuneration to individuals who are eligible for Medicare or Medicaid benefits if the person making such an offer knows or should know that the remuneration will influence the patient to obtain or receive goods or services from a particular provider.[179] This provision expressly incorporates Antikickback Statute activities into the HIPAA. HIPAA also provides for civil sanctions for upcoding or provision of medically unnecessary services if the provider acts with deliberate ignorance or reckless disregard for the truth.[180] HIPAA also allows for civil sanctions against Medicare HMOs if they fail to carry out their contract or carry out their contract in a manner inconsistent with the efficient administration of the program.[181]

In imposing civil sanctions, the Secretary of Health and Human Services is required to take into account the following:

1. The nature of the claims.
2. The circumstances under which they were presented.
3. The degree of culpability of the claimant.
4. The claimant's history of prior offenses.
5. The financial condition of the person presenting the claim.
6. Any other matters as justice may require.[182]

The Secretary of Health and Human Services has six years after the date on which the claim was presented to institute an action against the claimant.[183] The Secretary's final determination and sanctions are subject to judicial review; however, the findings of the Secretary regarding questions of fact are conclusive if supported by substantial evidence on the record.[184] In addition, the Secretary also may bring action against a provider in U.S. district court to enjoin future provider or individual activities, making the provider or individual subject to a civil monetary penalty.[185]

Criminal conviction before civil proceedings by the Secretary estops (i.e., bars) the convicted entity from denying the essential elements of the criminal offense.[186] In addition, because civil proceedings by themselves are administrative and not quasi-criminal, the Secretary is not required to establish the elements of the offense beyond a reasonable doubt.[187] Further, because these proceedings are civil, the penalties may be based on the amount claimed rather than the actual loss to the government and does not violate constitutional protections.[188] Therefore, providers and others may face significant liabilities under the civil sanction provisions, liabilities much greater than the amount claimed.

The FCA also has specific provisions for civil sanctions. Violations of the FCA subject the offender to a civil penalty for each claim of between $5,000 and $10,000 plus triple the damages sustained by the government.[189] Note that no proof of actual damages (such as actual payment of claim approval) is required to show a violation of the FCA.[190] Here, too, providers and others face significant penalties, far in excess of the billed amounts.[191] Actual knowledge is not required to be held liable under the civil FCA; acts in deliberate ignorance of the truth or falsity of the information or acts in reckless disregard of the truth or falsity of the information are sufficient,[192] although

---

[177]42 U.S.C.A. §1320a-7a; see also 63 Fed. Reg. 68,687 (December 14, 1998).

[178]42 U.S.C.A. §1320a-7a(a)(7).

[179]42 U.S.C.A. §1320a-7b.

[180]42 U.S.C.A. §1320a-7b.

[181]42 U.S.C.A. §1320a-7b.

[182]42 U.S.C.A. §1320a-7a(d)(3).

[183]42 U.S.C.A. §1320a-7a(c)(1).

[184]42 U.S.C.A. §1320a-7a(e).

[185]42 U.S.C.A. §1320a-7a(k).

[186]42 U.S.C.A. §1320a-7a(c)(3).

[187]See, e.g., Scott v. Bowen, 845 F.2d 856 (9th Cir. 1988).

[188]See, e.g., Mayers v. United States Dept. of Health and Human Servs., 806 F.2d 995 (11th Cir. 1986), *cert. denied* 484 U.S. 822 (1987); see also Chapman v. United States Dept. of Health and Human Servs., 821 F.2d 523 (10th Cir. 1987); Bernstein v. Sullivan, 914 F.2d 1395 (10th Cir. 1990).

[189]31 U.S.C.A. §3729(a).

[190]See, e.g., Hagood v. Sonoma Cty. Water Agency, 929 F.2d 1416 (9th Cir. 1991); United States v. Kensington Hosp., 760 F.Supp. 1120 (E.D. Pa. 1991).

[191]See, e.g., United States v. Lorenzo, 768 F.Supp. 1127 (E.D. Pa. 1991) (false claims for $130,719.10 resulted in FCA penalties of $18,807,157.30); but see United States v. Bajakajian, 118 S.Ct. 2028 (1998) (penalties that are excessive and disproportionate to damages to United States may violate Excessive Fines Clause of the Eighth Amendment).

[192]31 U.S.C.A. §3729(b); see also United States v. Oakwood Downriver Med. Ctr., 687 F.Supp. 302 (E.D. Mich. 1988); United States v. Children's Shelter, Inc., 604 F.Supp. 865 (W.D. Okla. 1985).

liability cannot be imposed based on innocent mistakes or negligence.[193]

Antikickback Statute—Criminal Sanctions

Violations of the Antikickback Statute are considered felonies and are punishable by criminal sanctions of fines up to $25,000 and imprisonment for up to five years.[194] In addition, exclusion from public health care programs also may result (discussed below).

Antikickback Statute—Civil Sanctions

Interestingly, the Antikickback Statute does not have provisions specifically for imposing civil monetary penalties for violations of the statute. The federal government therefore has relied on other statutes to impose civil sanctions on providers for its violation. Although the government has not been successful in using generic antikickback laws as an authority to impose civil sanctions,[195] the use of the civil FCA has been accepted by courts.[196] However, with the passage of the BBA, Antikickback Statute violations are subject to civil monetary penalties of $50,000 plus treble damages for each violation.[197] Note that these penalties apply not only to those parties engaged in the kickback arrangement but also to persons who arrange or contract for the provision of health care items or services, through employment or otherwise, with an individual or entity that the persons know or should know have been excluded from participation.[198]

Stark Sanctions

The Stark laws contain provisions only for civil sanctions. However, these civil sanctions are severe. Violations of the self-referral ban are subject to penalties of $15,000–$100,000 per claim. Generally, sanctions include:

1. Denial of payment for designated services rendered in violation of the Stark laws.

2. Refunds of the amounts that were paid for such designated services.
3. For persons who present or cause to be presented a bill or claim for a service that the person knows or should know is for a service for which payment may not be made or for which a refund has not been made, to civil monetary penalties of up to $15,000 per claim.
4. For physicians or entities that enter into arrangements or schemes that the physician or entity knows or should know has a principal purpose of ensuring referrals by the physician to a particular entity that, if the physician directly made referrals to the entity, would be a violation of the Stark laws, to civil monetary penalties of not more than $100,000 for each scheme.[199]

Program Exclusion

Exclusion from federal health care program participation (also known informally as the *death penalty*) is unquestionably the most severe criminal penalty that may be imposed on a provider. An exclusion sanction prohibits the provider from obtaining reimbursement for any items or services furnished by the provider to program beneficiaries on or after the effective date of the exclusion.[200] Indeed, no funds from Medicare, state health care programs, or any executive branch procurement or nonprocurement programs can be used to reimburse for any items or services ordered by the excluded provider. Under the HIPAA, mandatory exclusion must be imposed on providers and others convicted of a felony relating to health care fraud, theft, embezzlement, or other financial misconduct associated with the delivery of a health care item or service or in connection with an act or omission involving *any* health care program operated in whole or in part by the federal, state, or local governments.[201] The Federal Employee Health Benefit Program is not included within this set of health care programs.[202] In addition, mandatory exclusion applies to providers who have been convicted of criminal offenses relating to patient abuse as well as any felony conviction relating to the unlawful manufacture, distribution, prescription, or dispensing of a controlled substance.[203] Exclusion is for a minimum of five years unless the Secretary of Health and Human Services waives the exclusion because the individual or entity is the sole community physician or sole source of essential specialized care in the community; this waiver can occur only on request of a state.[204]

[193]See, e.g., Wang v. FMC Corp., 975 F.2d 1412 (9th Cir. 1992).
[194]42 U.S.C.A. §1320a-7b.
[195]United States v. Kensington Hosp., 760 F.Supp. 1120 (E.D. Pa. 1991) (rejecting government claims under generic antikickback statute for health care fraud under state Medicaid plan).
[196]See, e.g., Roy v. Anthony, 914 F.Supp. 1504 (S.D. Ohio 1996); Pogue v. American Healthcorp, 914 F.Supp. 1507 (M.D. Tenn. 1996).
[197]42 U.S.C.A. §1320a-7a(a)(7).
[198]42 U.S.C.A. §1320a-7a(a)(6).

[199]42 U.S.C.A. §1395nn(g)(4).
[200]42 C.F.R. §1001.1901(b)(1) (1998).
[201]42 U.S.C.A. §1320a-7(a)(3).
[202]42 U.S.C.A. §1320a-7b.
[203]42 U.S.C.A. §1320a-7(a).
[204]42 U.S.C.A. §1320a-7(c)(3)(B).

In addition, under the BBA,[205] other exclusion rules have been added. If a provider is mandatorily excluded on or after the date of the bill's enactment and that individual has been convicted of one or more offenses for which a mandatory exclusion may be imposed, the provider must be excluded from public health program participation for at least ten years.[206] Further, if the provider has been convicted on two or more occasions where mandatory exclusion may be imposed, the provider must be *permanently* excluded from public health care programs.[207]

The Secretary of Health and Human Services also has the authority to impose "permissive" exclusions against health care providers and entities.[208] Providers and others may be excluded if they have been convicted of a misdemeanor offense relating to fraud and convicted of an offense relating to the obstruction of an investigation.[209] In addition, exclusions may be imposed if the provider or entity is convicted of a misdemeanor offense relating to controlled substances, has had his or her license revoked or suspended, has been excluded or suspended from any federal or state health care program, has billed for excessive charges or unnecessary services or failed to provide medically necessary services, or has engaged in fraud, kickback, and other prohibited activities.[210] Further, an entity may be excluded if it is controlled by a sanctioned individual, if an individual or entity fails to disclose required information, or if an entity fails to take corrective action mandated by the HCFA.[211] Individuals may be excluded if they default on health education loans or scholarship obligations, violate the limitations on physician charges, or bill for services of an assistant for cataract surgery.[212] Finally, those who control a sanctioned entity may be excluded from public health care programs.[213] Note that the HIPAA has mandated that a three-year minimum exclusion is required for convictions of misdemeanor criminal health care offenses or convictions relating to any obstruction of an investigation,[214] a one-year minimum exclusion is mandated for activities relating to professional competence or financial integrity,[215] and a one-year minimum exclusion is mandated for providers who provide services or items that exceed a patient's needs or do not meet professionally recognized standards.[216] In addition to the permissive exclusion against persons who control a sanctioned entity, even officers and managing employees of the entity may be sanctioned without knowledge of the illegal activities and without having participated in the wrongful acts. In addition, investors in the entity may be subject to sanctions if the government can show that the investors acted in deliberate indifference to wrongful activities of the entity.

The BBA expanded permissive exclusions by allowing the Secretary of Health and Human Services to refuse to enter into an agreement, terminate an existing agreement, or refuse to renew an agreement with a physician or supplier that has been convicted of a felony under federal or state law for an offense that the Secretary of Health and Human Services deems "detrimental to the best interests of the program or program beneficiaries."[217] Note that this provision allows the Secretary of Health and Human Services to exclude providers from public health program participation for felony convictions that are not health care related. Further, the BBA also allows for exclusion of an entity if an individual transfers ownership or control of the entity to an immediate family member or to a member of the person's household in anticipation of or following a conviction, assessment, or exclusion against the person.[218] *Member of the household* includes "any person, any individual sharing a common abode as part of a single family unit with the person, including domestic employees and others who live together as a family unit, but not including a roomer or boarder."[219]

Note that mandatory exclusion and criminal conviction generally do not violate constitutional protections against double jeopardy. Since the mandatory exclusion provisions are considered remedial and not punitive, they are not considered to be punishing the wrongdoer twice.[220] In addition, assessment of both criminal and civil penalties for a particular action by the government does not violate the double jeopardy prohibition if the civil penalty is not overwhelmingly disproportionate to the damages caused to the government.[221] Indeed, no violation of the double

---

[205]Pub. L. No. 105-33, 111 Stat. 251 (1997).

[206]42 U.S.C.A. §1320a-7(c)(3)(G)(i).

[207]42 U.S.C.A. §1320a-7(c)(3)(G)(ii).

[208]42 C.F.R. §§1001.201 (1998) *et seq.*; 42 U.S.C.A. §§1320a-7(b) *et seq.*

[209]42 C.F.R. §§1001.201 (1998), 1001.301 (1998).

[210]42 C.F.R. §§1001.401 (1998), 1001.501 (1998), 1001.601 (1998), 1001.701 (1998), 1001.801 (1998), 1001.951 (1998).

[211]42 C.F.R. §§1001.1001 (1998), 1001.1101 (1998), 1001.1201 (1998), 1001.1301 (1998), 1001.1401 (1998).

[212]42 C.F.R. §§1001.1501 (1998), 1001.1601 (1998), 1001.1701 (1998).

[213]42 U.S.C.A. §1320a-7(b)(15).

[214]42 U.S.C.A. §1320a-7(c)(3)(D).

[215]42 U.S.C.A. §1320c-5(b)(1).

[216]42 U.S.C.A. §1320c-5(b)(1).

[217]42 U.S.C.A. §1320a-7.

[218]42 U.S.C.A. §1320a-7(b)(8)(A)(iii).

[219]42 U.S.C.A. §1320a-7(j)(2).

[220]See, e.g., Manocchio v. Kusserow, 961 F.2d 1539 (11th Cir. 1992); Kahn v. Inspector General of the U.S. Dept. of Health and Human Servs., 848 F.Supp. 432 (S.D. N.Y. 1994); Manocchio v. Sullivan, 768 F.Supp. 814 (S.D. Fla. 1991).

[221]United States v. Halper, 490 U.S. 435, 449 (1989); see also Hudson v. United States, 118 S.Ct. 488 (1997) (double jeopardy claim can be substantiated only when the defendant shows clear proof of the government ignoring the legislative intent when classifying a penalty as civil).

jeopardy prohibition occurs if two separate government sovereigns bring their actions; therefore, if a state government pursues a criminal action against a provider while the federal government pursues a civil action for the same acts, these two suits are not considered in violation of double jeopardy.[222]

The Secretary of Health and Human Services does have some discretion in imposing exclusion periods. Aggravating and mitigating circumstances can be used by the Secretary to determine an appropriate exclusion period.[223] Aggravating factors regarding the action include:

1. The acts produced a loss to Medicare and state health programs of $1500 or more.
2. The acts were committed over a period of one or more years.
3. The acts had a significant adverse physical, mental, or financial impact on one or more program beneficiaries or others.
4. The sentence for the crime included imprisonment.
5. The convicted individual or entity has a prior criminal, civil, or administrative sanction record.
6. The convicted individual or entity has been overpaid a total of $1500 or more by Medicare or state health care programs as a result of improper billing.

Mitigating factors include:

1. The individual or entity was convicted of three or fewer misdemeanor offenses, and the amount of loss to Medicare and the state health care programs was less than $1500.
2. The court determined that the individual had a mental, emotional, or physical condition before or during the commission of the offense.
3. The individual's or entity's cooperation with federal or state officials resulted in convictions or exclusions of others or the imposition of civil monetary penalties.

Mitigating factors are considered only when aggravating factors justify an exclusion of more than five years. Mitigating factors do not reduce the exclusionary period below the five-year minimum.

After the exclusion period, if a provider desires to serve in public health care programs, the entity or individual must submit a written request to OIG for reinstatement.[224] After the OIG receives the request, it will require that the requestor provide specific information and authorize the OIG to obtain information from sources such as private health insurers, peer review bodies, probation officers, and professional colleagues so that it may assess whether to grant the excluded provider's request.[225] The decision for reinstatement rests solely within the discretion of OIG; there is *no* administrative or judicial review for the OIG decision.[226]

Notes on Fraud and Abuse

Compliance Programs

Compliance programs are internal systems that provide controls to promote adherence to federal and state laws as well as ethical conduct. In the health care industry, adoption and implementation of an effective compliance plan is essential to avoiding and mitigating against potential liability under the fraud and abuse laws. Indeed, effective compliance plans are a requirement under settlements made with the OIG. Four major characteristics must be in place for any acceptable compliance program: the program must have true behavior objectives that decrease the risk of illegal conduct by individuals in the organization, it must reaffirm key organizational principles such as high-quality service, it must meet the requirements of the U.S. Sentencing Guidelines[227] both substantively and in form, and it must be compatible with the organization's culture for effective implementation. More specifically, the OIG has attempted to provide industry guidance by formulating and releasing compliance program guidance for hospitals, clinical laboratories, and home health agencies.[228] Close attention to these documents is essential as a risk management tool to minimize the potential penalties for violation of fraud and abuse laws.

Additional Reading. C. L. Basri, *The Office of Inspector General's Compliance Program Guideline for Hospitals,* pub. no. B0-001E (New York: Practising Law Institute — Corporate Law, June–July 1998); K. Boxer and H. Gregory, *Compliance Is Good for Your Corporate Health,* pub. no. B0-001E (New York: Practising Law Institute — Corporate Law, June–July 1998); College of American Pathologists, *Compliance Guidelines for*

[222]See, e.g., United States v. Bradford, 886 F.Supp. 744 (E.D. Wash. 1995); Health v. Alabama, 474 U.S. 82 (1985); United States v. Guzman, 85 F.3d 823 (1st Cir. 1996); United States v. Louisville Edible Oil Products, Inc., 926 F.2d 584 (6th Cir. 1991); United States v. Lane, 891 F.Supp. 8 (D. Me. 1995); United States v. Trammell, 133 F.3d 1343 (10th Cir. 1998); United States v. Leone, 78 F.3d 595 (9th Cir. 1996); Booth v. State, 903 P.2d 1079 (Alaska Ct. App. 1995); United States v. Pena, 918 F.Supp. 1431 (D. Kan. 1996); United States v. Scholz, 899 F.Supp. 484 (D. Nev. 1995).

[223]42 C.F.R. §1001.102 (1998).

[224]42 C.F.R. §1001.3001(a) (1998).

[225]42 C.F.R. §1001.3001(a)(3) (1998).

[226]42 C.F.R. §1001.3004(c) (1998).

[227]T. E. Bartrum and L. E. Bryant, "The Brave New World of Health Care Compliance Programs," *Annals Health Law* 6 (1997), pp. 51–75.

[228]Available at http://www.os.dhhs.gov/progorg/oig/modcomp.

Pathologists (Northfield, IL: College of American Pathologists, 1998); W. R. Hirsh, *Corporate Compliance Program Workbook* (San Francisco: Davis Wright Tremaine LLP, 1998); J. G. Sheehan, *The Office of Inspector General: Health Care Financing Administration Projects,* Pub. No. B4-7234 (New York: Practising Law Institute—Corporate Law, April 1998).

HIPAA Additional Provisions

A variety of provisions in the HIPAA have amended other statutes to strengthen efforts to combat fraud and abuse. In addition, the HIPAA created a new "federal health care offense,"[229] which is a violation of or a criminal conspiracy to violate provisions of the federal law that relate to a public or private "health care benefit program." A health care benefit program is

[a]ny public or private plan or contract, affecting commerce, under which any medical benefit, item, or service is provided to any individual and includes any individual or entity who is providing a medical benefit, item, or service for which payment may be made under the plan or contract.[230]

In addition, the HIPAA established the offense of "health care fraud," which is the knowing and willful execution of a scheme to defraud a health care benefit program or to obtain through false representations money or other property owned by a health care benefit program.[231] The sanctions for the health care fraud offense include fines and a maximum of ten years' imprisonment;[232] if the violation results in serious bodily injury, the maximum imprisonment is for life.[233] The HIPAA also established penalties for false statements relating to health care matters as well as obstruction of criminal investigations of health care offenses.[234] Also, physicians are expressly liable for civil monetary penalties for falsely certifying home health care services under the HIPAA.[235]

The HIPAA also establishes the Medicare Integrity Program, which contracts out to private organizations the responsibility for audits, medical and utilization reviews, and fraud reviews to external entities, replacing carriers and intermediaries who traditionally performed this role.[236] In addition, the statute authorizes the DHHS to pay individuals such as Medicare beneficiaries who report health care fraud to the OIG,[237] in an effort to integrate beneficiaries into the fraud detection process. This program will pay individuals if the information provided leads to the recovery of at least $100. The information must be specific to an individual or entity and time period. The amount of the award will be the lesser of 10% of the overpayments recovered or $1000.[238] A new health care fraud and abuse database is also authorized by the statute, the Healthcare Integrity and Protection Data Bank.[239] This database will archive information of final adverse actions against health care providers, suppliers, and practitioners, including health care–related information on civil judgments, criminal convictions, federal or state agency actions on licensure or certification, provider exclusion from health programs, and other relevant actions or decisions.

Additional Reading. A. M. Altschuler et al., "Health Care Fraud," *American Criminal Law Review* 35 (1998), pp. 857–59; C. M. Faddick, "Health Care Fraud and Abuse: New Weapons, New Penalties, and New Fears for Providers Created by the Health Insurance Portability and Accountability Act of 1996 (HIPAA)," *Annals Health Law* 6 (1997), pp. 77–103; W. S. Painter, "Recent Legislation, Cases and Other Developments Affecting Healthcare Providers and Integrated Delivery Systems," *American Law Institute–American Bar Association* 51 (1997), pp. 97–187.

Home Health Referrals Disclosure Requirements

The BBA establishes several rules regarding post–hospital discharge to home health providers.[240] If the patient is a Medicare beneficiary, on discharge, the hospital must notify the patient of the availability of home health services that participate in the Medicare program in the area where the patient resides and that has requested the hospital to list as available. In addition, if it has a financial interest in a home health care provider, the hospital must disclose to the Secretary of Health and Human Services information on the nature of the financial interest, the number of individuals discharged from the hospital and identified as needing home health services, and the percentage of these individuals who received such services from the home health provider.

Additional Reading. J. C. Render, "Health Care Law: A Survey of 1997 Developments," *Indiana Law Review*

[229]18 U.S.C.A. §§24, 669, 982, 1035, 1136, 1345, 1347, 1510, 1518, 1956, 3486.
[230]18 U.S.C.A. §24(b).
[231]18 U.S.C.A. §1347.
[232]18 U.S.C.A. §1347(2).
[233]18 U.S.C.A. §1347(2).
[234]18 U.S.C.A. §§1035, 1518.
[235]42 U.S.C.A. §1320a-7a(b)(3)(A)(ii).
[236]42 U.S.C.A. §1395b-5.
[237]42 U.S.C.A. §1395b-5.
[238]See 63 Fed. Reg. 31,123 (July 8, 1998); 42 C.F.R. Part 420.
[239]42 U.S.C.A. §1320a-7e(a); see 63 Fed. Reg. 58,341 (December 29, 1998); 64 Fed. Reg. 7653 (February 16, 1999).
[240]42 U.S.C.A. §1395x.

31 (1998), pp. 621–67; J. A. Rovner, "Balanced Budget Act Further Expands Health Care Fraud and Abuse Controls," *Health Law* 10, no. 2 (1997), pp. 1–4.

Medicare Carrier and Intermediary Suspension of Payments

Medicare carriers and intermediaries have authority to suspend part or all payments to a provider or supplier.[241] Carriers and intermediaries that desire to suspend payments generally must provide written notice of such an intent and a 15-day response period to the affected provider or supplier.[242] However, in the event that the carrier has reliable evidence of a provider's or supplier's billing that involves fraud or misrepresentation, the carrier or intermediary has no obligation to provide notice or a response period.[243] Providers cannot appeal the suspension of payments; they are permitted only to forward a written statement to the carrier or intermediary. However, if fraud or misrepresentation is involved, the provider may not be given even an opportunity to present a statement for consideration.[244]

Self-Disclosure Program

The DHHS and OIG have created a program to allow providers to voluntarily report fraudulent conduct in federal health care programs. This program is an expansion of a pilot program under Operation Restore Trust and is available to all providers. The program is aimed at correcting past fraudulent conduct and preventing future fraudulent conduct. The disclosure must be in writing, submitted to the Assistant Inspector General for Investigative Operations, contain a certification of truthfulness, and describe good faith efforts undertaken to bring the matter to the OIG's attention. The provider must conduct an internal investigation and self-assessment, with the results submitted to the OIG, including information relating to the identification of officers, employees, and agents who knew of, encouraged, or participated in detecting the fraudulent conduct. The internal investigation also must document how the fraudulent conduct was discovered and what has been done to address the problem and prevent future abuses. Financial analyses also must be performed to determine the amount of overpayment by federal health programs. Note that no immunity is provided to those named in the report to the OIG. Once the report is submitted, the OIG will conduct an independent verification; note that any fraudulent conduct outside the scope of that disclosed during the verification process is considered new matters subjecting the provider to sanctions. The major advantage of self-disclosure is early communication and cooperation with the OIG such that more onerous penalties and settlements may be avoided, including federal health program exclusion. However, the significant risk extant with allowing government access to provider internal materials may outweigh the benefits of self-disclosure.

Additional Reading. G. Aston, "Feds Unveil New Fraud Disclosure Policy," *American Medical News* (November 9, 1998), pp. 5–6; "Letting It All Hang Out: The OIG's Provider Self-Disclosure Protocol," *Focus on Fraud and Abuse* 2, no. 2 (1998), pp. 1–2.

Stark II Proposed Regulations

Proposed final regulations have been published by the HCFA that would amend the final Stark I regulations and apply them to all designated services under Stark II.[245] Of note, physicians may obtain some flexibility under certain referral relationships. For example, de minimus compensation allows a physician to accept gifts or services that do not exceed $50 (not to exceed $300 annually), discounts based on volume of referrals are exempt if the discounts are passed on to patients or their insurers, and the fair market value exception allows written compensation arrangements that cover all services that will be provided by the physician and set a term of less than one year, as long as the compensation is consistent with a fair market appraisal, is commercially reasonable, furthers a legitimate business purpose, and complies with the Antikickback Statute.

Additional Reading. L. E. Patrick, "A Complicate Prescription," *South Carolina Law* 10 (1999), pp. 22–26; L. A. Rinehart, "The Proposed Stark II Regulations: HCFA Debuts the 'New Rules'," *Legal Medicine Perspectives* 5, no. 2 (1998), pp. 2–4; A. B. Wachler and P. A. Avery, "Stark II Proposed Regulations: Rule Offers Additional Guidance While Regulators Seek More Input from Health Care Community," *Health Law* 1998 (1998), p. 60.

The Emergency Medical Treatment and Active Labor Act (EMTALA)

The Emergency Medical Treatment and Active Labor Act (EMTALA), also known as the *anti-patient dumping act,* was passed by Congress as part of the Consolidated Omnibus Budget Reconciliation Act of 1985 and took

---

[241]42 C.F.R. §405.370 (1998).

[242]42 C.F.R. §405.374(a) (1998).

[243]42 C.F.R. §405.374(b) (1998).

[244]42 C.F.R. §405.374(b) (1998).

[245]63 Fed. Reg. 1659–1728 (January 9, 1998).

effect August 1, 1986.[246] EMTALA was designed to address the perceived "dumping" of financially undesirable patients (e.g., indigent or without health insurance) who require emergency care to the public hospital system.[247] EMTALA governs all hospitals that participate in the Medicare program,[248] that is, virtually every hospital in the United States. However, the requirements of the statute indicate that any and all patients who come to the hospital's emergency room are protected by its provisions.[249] Although not strictly a fraud and abuse statute, it implicates similar governmental actor authority (i.e., HCFA, OIG) and imposes similar penalties (i.e., Medicare exclusion, civil monetary penalties) and thus, practically speaking, is reasonably considered a fraud and abuse statute.

Requirements

Any person who presents him- or herself to a hospital that participates in the Medicare program and requests emergency care or is in active labor is entitled by the statute to obtain an appropriate medical screening examination to assess whether an emergency medical condition is present.[250] As long as a hospital has an emergency department or offers emergency care (even without a formal emergency department), it is subject to EMTALA.[251] If an emergency medical condition is present, the patient cannot be transferred until the emergency medical condition is stabilized and, if necessary, definitive treatment is provided. Finally, transfer of an unstabilized patient is allowed if the patient or his or her representative makes a written request for the transfer after being informed of the risk of transfer and the transferring hospital's EMTALA obligation to provide additional examination or treatment or a physician or appropriate qualified medical person (if the physician is not present but has made the determination after consulting with the qualified medical person) signs a certification summarizing the risks and benefits of the transfer and that the benefits of the transfer are "reasonably expected to" outweigh its risks.[252] The requirement for stabilization or appropriate transfer is met if the patient refuses the hospital's offer for additional treatment or examination or refuses to consent to transfer after being informed of the risks and benefits from such a decision.[253] Transfer must be to an appropriate facility.

Note that physicians who are on-call to the emergency room must come to the hospital and provide the necessary services to the presenting patient. Further, hospitals must accept appropriate transfers from others if they have the capacity and capability to effectively treat the patient.[254]

Obviously, there are critical definitions within the statute. First, an *emergency medical condition* is

A. a medical condition manifesting itself by acute symptoms of sufficient severity (including severe pain) such that the absence of immediate medical attention could reasonably be expected to result in (I) placing the health of the individual (or, with respect to a pregnant woman, the health of the woman or her unborn child) in serious jeopardy, (II) serious impairment to bodily functions, or (III) serious dysfunction of any bodily organ or part; or
B. with respect to a pregnant woman who is having contractions (I) that there is inadequate time to effect a safe transfer to another hospital before delivery, or (II) that transfer may pose a threat to the health or safety of the woman or unborn child.[255]

An emergency medical condition includes psychiatric conditions and substance abuse circumstances.[256]

A *transfer* within the meaning of the statute is:

1. movement (including discharge) of a person;
2. from the hospital's facilities;
3. at the direction of any person employed by, affiliated or associated directly or indirectly with the hospital;
4. but does not include movement of a person who:
   (a) has been declared dead; or
   (b) leaves the facility without the permission of the person employed by, affiliated or associated directly or indirectly with the hospital.[257]

[246]42 U.S.C. §1395dd.

[247]See, e.g., D. U. Himmelstein et al., "Patient Transfers: Medical Practice as Social Triage," *American Journal of Public Health* 74 (1984), pp. 494–97; R. Schiff et al., "Transfers to a Public Hospital: A Prospective Study of 467 Patients," *New England Journal of Medicine* 314 (1986), pp. 552–57; but see D. A. Hyman, "Patient Dumping and EMTALA: Past Imperfect/Future Shock," *Health Matrix* 8 (1998), pp. 29–56 (criticizing studies and indicating patient dumping problems are overestimated).

[248]42 U.S.C.A. §1395dd(e)(2).

[249]42 U.S.C.A. §1395dd(a); see, e.g., Correa v. Hospital San Francisco, 69 F.3d 1184 (1st Cir. 1995), *cert. denied* 517 U.S. 1136 (1996); Power v. Arlington Hosp. Ass'n, 42 F.3d 851 (4th Cir. 1994); Collins v. DePaul Hosp., 963 F.2d 303 (10th Cir. 1992); Brooker v. Desert Hosp. Corp., 947 F.2d 412 (9th Cir. 1991); Burditt v. U.S. Dept. of Health and Human Services, 934 F.2d 1362 (5th Cir. 1991); Gatewood v. Washington Healthcare Corp., 933 F.2d 1037 (D.C. Cir. 1991); Cleland v. Bronson Health Care Group, Inc., 917 F.2d 266 (6th Cir. 1990).

[250]42 U.S.C.A. §§1395dd(a), 1395dd(b).

[251]See 59 Fed. Reg. 32,086, 32,101 (1994).

[252]42 U.S.C.A. §1395dd(c); 42 C.F.R. §489.24 (1998).

[253]42 U.S.C.A. §§1395dd(b)(2), 1395dd(b)(3).

[254]42 U.S.C.A. §§1395dd(c)(1)(A), 1395dd(c)(2); 42 C.F.R. §489.24(e) (1998).

[255]42 U.S.C.A. §1395dd(e)(1).

[256]42 C.F.R. §489.24(b) (1998).

[257]42 U.S.C.A. §1395dd(e)(4).

A patient is *stabilized* if "no material deterioration of the condition is likely, within reasonable medical probability, to result from or occur during the transfer of the individual from a facility."[258] For pregnant women undergoing contractions, *stabilized* means the complete delivery of the child and placenta.[259]

An *appropriate transfer* is one:

A. in which the transferring hospital provides the medical treatment within its capacity which minimizes risks to the individual's health and, in the case of a woman in labor, the health of the unborn child;

B. in which the receiving facility —
   (i) has the available space and qualified personnel for the treatment of the individual, and
   (ii) has agreed to accept the transfer of the individual and to provide appropriate medical treatment;

C. in which the transferring hospital sends to the receiving facility all medical records (or copies thereof), related to the emergency condition for which the individual has presented, available at the time of the transfer, including the name and address of any on-call physician . . . who has refused or failed to appear within a reasonable time to provide necessary stabilizing treatment;

D. in which the transfer is effected through qualified personnel and transportation equipment, as required, including the use of necessary and medically appropriate life support measures during the transfer; and

E. which meets such other requirements as the Secretary may find necessary in the interest of the health and safety of individuals transferred.[260]

Conspicuous by its absence, it is critical to note that regulations do not define the term *appropriate* with regard to *appropriate medical screening evaluation*.[261] Here, there is significant risk that this term would pose conflicting interpretation between providers and government authority. Prudence would dictate that providers err on the side of thoroughness as to patient examination in these circumstances.

Hospitals must maintain a log of all patients seen in their emergency rooms and report violations of EMTALA within 72 hours of their occurrence. Further, hospitals must post signs in their emergency departments, hospital entrances, admitting areas, waiting rooms, treatment areas, and elsewhere[262] notifying all individuals of the hospital's obligations under EMTALA, such as maintaining a list of on-call physicians for emergency care and providing notice as to whether the hospital participates in

Medicaid.[263] Further, the hospital is prohibited from delaying care to inquire about a patient's insurance status[264] and also is prohibited from retaliation against a physician who refuses to approve transfer of an unstable patient or "whistleblowers" who report EMTALA violations.[265] EMTALA further requires the hospital to specify in its bylaws or rules and regulations the specific medical personnel qualified to conduct medical screening examinations and sign certifications of transfer in the absence of a physician.[266]

Penalties

Penalties for violation of the statute are severe; hospitals that violate the statute may be excluded from the Medicare and Medicaid programs[267] and/or be fined up to $50,000 per violation;[268] this amount is limited to $25,000 per violation for hospitals with fewer than 100 beds.[269] Further, physicians also may be subject to similar exclusions and fines of up to $50,000 for violation of the statute's mandates if their violation is "gross and flagrant" or repeated.[270] Beyond penalties imposed by the federal government, patients adversely affected by EMTALA violations have a private right of action against the providers that violate the statute, including equitable relief and damages.[271] Further, any other hospital that suffers some financial loss because of a hospital's violation of EMTALA can recover damages or seek equitable relief against the violating hospital.[272] Indeed, hospitals receiving a transfer of an unstable patient that they believe is in violation of EMTALA *must* report this potential violation to the HCFA or face exclusion from Medicare themselves.[273] Therefore, the broad exposure from a violation of EMTALA on hospitals provides a strong financial incentive to scrupulously fulfill the requirements of the statute.

Enforcement

Overall, the enforcement of EMTALA is within the purview of the Department of Health and Human

---

[258]42 U.S.C.A. §1395dd(e)(3)(B).

[259]See, e.g., Burditt v. U.S. Dept. of Health and Human Services, 934 F.2d 1362, 1369–70 (5th Cir. 1991).

[260]42 U.S.C.A. §1395dd(c)(2).

[261]See, e.g., 42 C.F.R. Parts 405, 489 (1998).

[262]42 C.F.R. §489.20(q)(1) (1998).

[263]42 C.F.R. §489.20(q)(2) (1998).

[264]42 C.F.R. §489.24(c)(3) (1998).

[265]42 U.S.C.A. §§1395dd(f), 1395dd(i).

[266]42 C.F.R. §§489.24(a) (1998), 489(d)(1)(ii)(C) (1998).

[267]42 U.S.C.A. §1395cc(b)(2).

[268]42 U.S.C.A. §1395dd(d)(1)(A).

[269]Pub. L. No. 101-508, §4008(b)(2), 104 Stat. 1388 (1990).

[270]42 U.S.C.A. §1395dd(d)(1)(B).

[271]42 U.S.C.A. §1395dd(d)(2)(A).

[272]42 U.S.C.A. §1395dd(d)(2)(B).

[273]42 C.F.R. §489.20(m) (1998).

Services, which delegates its authority to two agencies within it: HCFA and OIG. HCFA assumes duties associated with terminating providers from Medicare, while OIG has the power to impose fines on these providers.

The mechanics of EMTALA enforcement begin with a complaint of an alleged EMTALA violation reported to one of the HCFA's ten regional offices. After obtaining such a complaint, the HCFA regional office refers the complaint to the state hospital licensing or other relevant authority to conduct an on-site investigation. This authority forwards the information back to the HCFA regional office.[274] HCFA then usually authorizes the state authority to conduct an unscheduled facilitywide survey of the hospital in question. If the information gathered leads the HCFA regional office to believe a violation has occurred, it sends a notification letter and a statement of deficiencies to the hospital. Within this letter, the hospital is informed of the findings of the state authority's survey and indicates that the hospital will be terminated from Medicare participation unless it submits an acceptable "plan of correction." To avoid termination, the hospital must submit to HCFA an acceptable plan of correction; if it does so effectively, HCFA will "rescind" the proposed Medicare termination.[275] HCFA then will refer the case to the OIG for its assessment as to whether civil monetary penalties are appropriate.

Two tracks are delineated with regard to the time period in which the hospital must act to avoid termination from federal health programs: a "fast track" 23-day schedule, or a "slow track" 90-day schedule.[276] If the provider EMTALA violation is deemed by HCFA to pose "immediate and serious jeopardy to the health and safety of individuals presenting themselves to the hospital for emergency services," the 23-day fast track schedule applies.[277] However, if the EMTALA violation does not pose such an immediate and serious threat, HCFA will utilize the 90-day slow track.

The OIG, to impose a fine, must first refer the action to a state PRO for its assessment as to whether the patient involved had an emergency medical condition that was appropriately stabilized in comport with the statute's requirements.[278] The PRO will meet with the hospital and physicians engaged in the care associated with the purported violation and provide written notice for review of the circumstances; the PRO must provide the physician or the hospital an opportunity to discuss the case before the PRO completes its report. The PRO must submit a written report to HCFA within 60 days of receiving an EMTALA case for review. It appears that the PRO must provide the OIG with a copy of the report, and it appears the PRO should provide a copy to the investigated physician or hospital.[279] The identity of the evaluating PRO physician is confidential unless he or she consents to its release.[280] The PRO may decide that there was no violation and report this information to the OIG, which then will close the case. On the other hand, the PRO review may indicate that there was an emergency medical circumstance that was not appropriately stabilized. If this is the case, the OIG will determine if monetary sanctions are appropriate. The amount of the sanctions depends on consideration of a variety of aggravating and mitigating factors, including the corrective action taken by the hospital, the financial condition of the hospital, culpability, and the nature and circumstances of the violation.[281] Generally, if a financial penalty is imposed, it is paid by the hospital as part of a settlement agreement with the OIG; the OIG has allowed clauses within the settlement agreement that indicate no admission of guilt by the provider.

The Matter of Baby K

In *The Matter of Baby K*,[282] the question was presented as to whether a hospital and its physicians were required under EMTALA to treat an anencephalic infant who presented to the emergency room, even though it believed such futile treatment was morally and ethically wrong. In the case, Baby K was born at the hospital anencephalic, with no cognitive abilities or awareness. After her birth, her physicians placed her on a mechanical ventilator to allow confirmation of her diagnosis and to apprise Baby K's mother of the infant's poor prognosis. Baby K was expected to die within a few days due to breathing difficulties and other complications. Since aggressive measures would provide no therapeutic or palliative benefit, her physicians recommended she be provided only supportive care. However, Baby K's mother disagreed and insisted on mechanical ventilation; the physicians and

[274]G. M. Luce, *Defending the Hospital Under EMTALA: New Requirements, New Liabilities* (Washington, DC: National Health Lawyers Association, 1995), p. 4.

[275]Health Care Financing Administration, U.S. Department of Health and Human Services, *Medicare/Medicaid State Operations Manual* (Washington, DC: Health Care Financing Administration, 1995), Part 3412.

[276]42 C.F.R. §489.53 (1998).

[277]42 C.F.R. §489.53(c)(2)(i)(A) (1998).

[278]42 U.S.C.A. §1395dd(d)(3); 42 C.F.R. §489.24(g) (1998).

[279]42 C.F.R. §§489.24(g)(2)(v) (1998), 489.24(h) (1998).

[280]42 C.F.R. §489.24(h) (1998).

[281]42 U.S.C.A. §1320a-7a(d), 1395dd(d)(1); 42 C.F.R. §§1003.106(a)(4) (1998), 1003.106(b)(5) (1998); Burditt v. U.S. Dept. of Health and Human Services, 934 F.2d 1362 (5th Cir. 1991) (affirming ALJ's assessments regarding aggravating and mitigating factors under regulations).

[282]16 F.3d 590 (4th Cir. 1994).

hospital objected to this treatment and attempted to transfer Baby K to another hospital. However, other hospitals would not accept the patient. Ultimately, she was transferred to a nearby nursing home after her acute respiratory distress was treated.

But because of her condition, Baby K required frequent readmissions to the hospital through the emergency room due to breathing difficulties. Each time, the hospital provided care, including ventilatory support. However, after the second presentation, the hospital, joined by Baby K's father, brought suit, claiming that all the hospital was required to provide was warmth, nutrition, and hydration, rather than life-supporting respiratory support. Baby K's mother resisted this action. On appellate review, the court held that the wording of the statute was clear and that the hospital was required to provide such stabilizing care each time Baby K presented to the emergency department. The court indicated that treatment was required even if futile, the patient's life expectancy was extremely limited, would exceed the prevailing standard of care, and be considered morally or ethically wrong. The statute simply did not allow for such exceptions, and therefore the court concluded that even in these circumstances, stabilizing care must be provided.

Notes on EMTALA

EMTALA and Medical Malpractice

It should be noted that EMTALA and medical malpractice are distinct legal concepts and causes of action. That is, EMTALA is not a federal medical malpractice statute.[283] EMTALA concerns access to care, whereas medical malpractice concerns quality of care provided. This means that patients may bring both suits against providers when injury occurs associated with emergency medical treatment.

Additional Reading. S. E. Hamm. "Power v. Arlington Hospital: A Federal Court End Run Around State Malpractice Limitations," *Brigham Young University Journal of Public Law* 7 (1993), pp. 335–50; A. J. McKitrick, "The Effect of State Medical Malpractice Caps on Damages Awarded Under the Emergency Medical

Treatment and Active Labor Act," *Cleveland State Law Review* 42 (1994), pp. 171–97.

EMTALA and Managed Care

Significant issues face providers when members of managed care organizations present to the emergency rooms and departments of non–managed care hospitals for care, do not obtain prior authorization from their managed care organizations, and the clinical circumstance was not a "true" emergency. Because these providers are not within the selected group or network of the managed care organization, managed care organizations have refused to pay for the care rendered, placing the patient in the unenviable position of paying for this care out of pocket or placing the provider in a similarly unenviable position of trying to collect for such costs of care. Interestingly enough, these circumstances fall outside the standard type of patient the EMTALA sought to protect — those without any form of insurance. Indeed, EMTALA's requirements force providers to treat patients who present to them with potential emergency medical conditions; hence, more brazen managed care organizations can err on the side of denying payment because there is little risk that this policy would result in denial of care and patient injury. It should be noted that Medicare-participating managed care plans must cover emergency care by non–plan providers without prior authorization.[284] This situation has spurred efforts to require managed care organizations to pay for this nonemergency care provided in the emergency setting by out-of-network providers if the patient can show that a "prudent layperson" would have sought this care. However, no federal legislation has provided a blanket application of this standard, although some states have done so.[285]

Additional Reading. G. L. Luke, J. E. Weber, and A. R. Derse, "Universal Emergency Access Under Managed Care: Universal Doubt or Mission Impossible?" *Cambridge Quarterly on Healthcare Ethics* 8 (1999), pp. 213–25; J. M. Stieber and L. J. Spar, "EMTALA in the 90's — Enforcement Challenges," *Health Matrix* 8 (1998), p. 70.

EMTALA Guidance—State Operations Manual

The HCFA publishes *The State Operations Manual* that, although not having the force and effect of law,

[283]See, e.g., Marshall v. East Carroll Parish Hosp. Serv. Dist., 134 F.3d 319 (5th Cir. 1998); Vickers v. Nash Gen. Hosp., Inc., 78 F.3d 139 (4th Cir. 1996); Gatewood v. Washington Healthcare Corp., 933 F.2d 1037 (D.C. Cir. 1991); Correa v. Hospital San Francisco, 69 F.3d 1184 (1st Cir. 1995), *cert. denied* 517 U.S. 1136 (1996); Summers v. Baptist Med. Ctr. Arkadelphia, 69 F.3d 902 (8th Cir. 1995); Eberhardt v. City of Los Angeles, 62 F.3d 1253 (9th Cir. 1995); Repp v. Anadarko Mun. Hosp., 43 F.3d 519 (10th Cir. 1994); Holcomb v. Monahan, 30 F.3d 116 (11th Cir. 1994).

[284]42 U.S.C.A. §1395mm(c)(4)(B); 42 C.F.R. §417.401 (1998).
[285]See, e.g., *Arkansas Code Annotated* §20-9-309(c)(1) (1997); *Maryland Code Annotated, Health — General* §19-701(d) (1998).

provides significant guidance as to the interpretation of key aspects of the statute as well as information on how the HCFA will assess particular hospital actions. This manual, available on the World Wide Web at http://www.hcfa.gov/pubforms/progman.htm, is a useful resource for those who seek specific guidance on a wide variety of EMTALA issues, including details on what constitutes an appropriate medical screening examination, the definition of *stabilization*, what constitutes coming to the emergency department and hospital, enforcement procedures, what situations constitute an immediate and serious threat to patients, and issues associated with managed care.

Liability of the Provider Under EMTALA— No Improper Motive

At one time, there was a split in legal authority as to whether a plaintiff-patient must show the provider had an "improper motive" when transferring him or her to succeed in an EMTALA action. The area is rife with confusion because motive considerations can be assessed at the medical screening examination, stabilization, and transfer decision-making points, as well as distinctions between private causes of action versus those brought by the Secretary of Health and Human Services.[286] However, the U.S. Supreme Court has addressed the issue and held that patients may succeed in an EMTALA action without proof that a transfer was based on an improper motive.[287]

Physical Presence in the Emergency Room

Physical presence in the emergency room or department is required to trigger the requirements of EMTALA. This requirement is true even if the patient is directed to another hospital because a physician in an emergency room communicates with an ambulance driver to take the patient to that other hospital,[288] where a hospital service directed paramedics to take the patient to a more distant hospital,[289] or when a request by telephone is made to admit a patient to the emergency department but the patient never arrives.[290] Note, however, that if a patient does enter the emergency room or department and then is transferred to another department and discharged inappropriately, that patient may still bring suit under EMTALA even though the discharge did not occur from the emergency room or department itself.[291] Similarly, if a patient presents in an emergent condition to a different department, such as being brought to a labor and delivery area, and then is discharged prematurely, EMTALA still applies.[292] Further, if the hospital owns and operates the ambulance in which the patient is being transported, the patient is considered to have come to the emergency room.[293]

Additional Reading. M. J. Fell, "The Emergency Medical Treatment and Active Labor Act of 1986: Providing Protection from Discrimination in Access to Emergency Medical Care," *Catholic University Law Review* 43 (1994), p. 628; B. R. Furrow, "An Overview and Analysis of the Impact of the Emergency Medical Treatment and Active Labor Act," *Journal of Legal Medicine* 16 (1995), pp. 325–55.

State Prelitigation Notification Requirements

Currently there is a conflict of authority as to whether patients may sue providers under EMTALA without fulfilling state requirements of notice before suit. Some authorities indicate that patients must fulfill state requirements or risk loss of the ability to sue.[294] Other courts indicated that noncompliance with state notification requirements is not fatal to plaintiffs who wish to sue providers under EMTALA.[295]

Additional Reading. "In First Time Ruling, Federal Court Finds Maine Notice Rule No Bar to EMTALA Suit," *BNA Health Law Reporter* 8 (1999), pp. 323–24; "New York's 90-Day Notice of Claim Rule Applies to EMTALA Suits, Second Circuit Holds," *BNA Health Law Reporter* 8 (1999), pp. 155–56.

---

[286]See, e.g., T. R. Shewchuk, "Must a Hospital Have Acted with an Improper Motive to Be Liable Under the Emergency Medical Treatment and Active Labor Act?" *Preview of U.S. Supreme Court Cases* 3 (1998), pp. 142–45.

[287]Roberts v. Galen of Virginia, Inc., 119 S.Ct. 685 (1999).

[288]Arrington v. Wong, 19 F.Supp.2d 1151 (D. Haw. 1998).

[289]Johnson v. University of Chicago Hosps., 982 F.2d 230 (7th Cir. 1992).

[290]Miller v. Medical Ctr. of Southwest La., 22 F.3d 626 (5th Cir. 1994).

[291]Thornton v. Southwest Detroit Hosp., 895 F.2d 1131 (6th Cir. 1990).

[292]McIntyre v. Schick, 795 F.Supp. 777 (E.D. Va. 1992).

[293]42 C.F.R. §489.24(b) (1998).

[294]See Hardy v. New York City Health & Hosp. Corp., 164 F.3d 789 (2d Cir. 1999).

[295]See, e.g., Power v. Arlington Hosp. Ass'n, 42 F.3d 851 (4th Cir. 1994); Hewitt v. Inland Hosp., No. 98-CV-206-B (D. Me. Feb. 3, 1999); Cooper v. Gulf Breeze Hosp., 893 F.Supp. 1538 (N.D. Fla. 1993); Bowen v. Mercy Mem. Hosp. Corp., 1995 WL 805189 (E.D. Mich. Dec. 8, 1995); Keating v. Tangipahoa Hosp., 1995 WL 91128 (E.D. La. Mar. 1, 1995); Reid v. Ind. Osteopathic Med. Hosp., 709 F.Supp. 853 (S.D. Ind. 1989).

Further Reading

Advisory Opinions

Faddick CM. Health Care Fraud and Abuse: New Weapons, New Penalties, and New Fears for Providers Created by the Health Insurance Portability and Accountability Act of 1996 (HIPAA). *Annals Health L* 1997;6:77–103.

Kelly SJ. The Health Insurance Portability and Accountability Act of 1996: A Medicare Fraud Advisory Opinion Mandate Sends the Inspector General "Shopping for Hats." *Ohio L J* 1998;59:303–37.

OIG Outlines Advisory Opinion Procedures. *Andrews Healthcare Fraud Litig Rep* 1997:23.

Antikickback Statute

Fabrikant R. *Health Care Reform: The Use of Anti-Kickback Statutes in Private Litigation, and the Need for an Anti-Trust Approach.* Pub. no. A4-4455. Practising Law Institute — Commercial Law, September–October 1994.

Kikkawa K. Medicare Fraud and Abuse and Qui Tam: The Dynamic Duo or the Odd Couple? *Health Matrix* 1998;8:83–123.

Kucera WR. Hanlester Network v Shalala: A Model Approach to the Medicare and Medicaid Kickback Problem. *Nw U L Rev* 1996;91:413–42.

Phelps LM. Calling Off the Bounty Hunters: Discrediting the Use of Alleged Anti-Kickback Violations to Support Civil False Claims Actions. *Vand L Rev* 1998;51:3–47.

Salcido R. Mixing Oil and Water: The Government's Mistaken Use of the Medicare Anti-Kickback Statute in False Claims Act Prosecutions. *Annals Health L* 1997;6:105–35.

Antikickback Statute—Civil Sanctions

Faddick CM. Health Care Fraud and Abuse: New Weapons, New Penalties, and New Fears for Providers Created by the Health Insurance Portability and Accountability Act of 1996 (HIPAA). *Annals Health L* 1997;6:77–103.

Kusserow RP. Civil Monetary Penalties Law of 1981: A New Effort to Confront Fraud and Abuse in Federal Health Care Programs. *Notre Dame L Rev* 1983;58:985–94.

Antikickback Statute—Criminal Sanctions

Faddick CM. Health Care Fraud and Abuse: New Weapons, New Penalties, and New Fears for Providers Created by the Health Insurance Portability and Accountability Act of 1996 (HIPAA). *Annals Health L* 1997;6:77–103.

Kirschenbaum AM, Kuhlik BN. Federal and State Laws Affecting Discounts, Rebates, and Other Marketing Practices for Drugs and Devices. *Food & Drug L J* 1992;47:533–62.

EMTALA

Bosler TH, Davis PM. Is EMTALA a Defanged COBRA? *J Mo B* 1995;51:165–69.

Chiles LM. Summers v. Baptist Medical Center Arkadelphia: A "Disparate" Application of EMTALA's Terms. *Ark L Rev* 1997;50:559–89.

Creswell CC. Power v. Arlington Hospital Association: Extending COBRA's Striking Distance While Weakening the Power of Its Venom. *Ga L Rev* 1995;29:1171–1204.

Dame LA. The Emergency Medical Treatment and Active Labor Act: The Anomalous Right to Health Care. *Health Matrix* 1998;8:3–28.

Dowdy AK et al. The Anatomy of EMTALA: A Litigator's Guide. *St Mary's L J* 1996;27:463–512.

Epp PK. In Defense of the Masses — An Interpretation of the Emergency Medical Treatment and Active Labor Act: In Re Baby K. *Creighton L Rev* 1995;28:1209–53.

Hamm SE. Power v. Arlington Hospital: A Federal Court End Run Around State Malpractice Limitations. *BYU J Pub L* 1993;7:335–50.

Health Care Financing Administration, Department of Health and Human Services. *State Operations Manual*, HCFA Pub. 7, Transmittal No. 2, June 1, 1998.

Hyman DA. Patient Dumping and EMTALA: Past Imperfect/Future Shock. *Health Matrix* 1998;8:29–56.

Kuettel AC. The Changing Role of Receiving Hospitals Under the Emergency Medical Treatment and Active Labor Act. *J Legal Med* 1998;19:351–75.

Larson EA. Did Congress Intend to Give Patients the Right to Demand and Receive Inappropriate Medical Treatments?: EMTALA Reexamined in Light of Baby K. *Wis L Rev* 1995:1425–59.

Luce GM. *Defending the Hospital Under EMTALA: New Requirements, New Liabilities.* Washington, DC: National Health Lawyers Association, 1995.

McKitrick AJ. The Effect of State Medical Malpractice Caps on Damages Awarded Under the Emergency Medical Treatment and Active Labor Act. *Clev St L Rev* 1994;42:171–97.

Myerberg DZ. The Fourth Circuit's Baby K Decision: "Plain Language" Does Not Make Good Law. *W Va L Rev* 1995;98:397–448.

Singer LE. Look What They've Done to My Law, Ma: COBRA's Implosion. *Hous L Rev* 1996;33:113–72.

Smith SB. The Critical Condition of the Emergency Medical Treatment and Active Labor Act: A Proposed Amendment to the Act After In the Matter of Baby K. *Vand L Rev* 1995;48:1491–1538.

Stieber JM, Spar LJ. EMTALA in the 90's — Enforcement Challenges. *Health Matrix* 1998;8:57–81.

Stricker TL. The Emergency Medical Treatment and Active Labor Act: Denial of Emergency Medical Care Because of Improper Economic Motives. *Notre Dame L Rev* 1992;67:1121–60.

False Claims Act

Meador P, Warren ES. The False Claims Act: A Civil War Relic Evolves into a Modern Weapon. *Tenn L Rev* 1998;65:455–83.

Phelps LM. Calling Off the Bounty Hunters: Discrediting the Use of Alleged Anti-Kickback Violations to Support Civil False Claims Actions. *Vand L Rev* 1998;51:1003–47.

Snyder AG. The False Claims Act Applied to Health Care Institutions: Gearing Up for Corporate Compliance. *DePaul J Health Care L* 1996;1:1–54.

Stewart DO. Recent Developments in the False Claims Act. *Pub Cont L J* 1991;20:386–98.

U.S. General Accounting Office. *Medicare: Application of the False Claims Act to Hospital Billing Practices.* Pub. no. GAO/HEHS-98-195. Washington, DC: U.S. General Accounting Office, 1998.

False Claims Act—Claims for Services Not Provided or Medically Unnecessary

Aussprung L. Fraud and Abuse. *J Legal Med* 1998;19:1–62.

Boxer K, Gregory H. *Compliance Is Good for Your Corporate Health.* Pub. no. B0-001E. Practising Law Institute—Corporate Law, June–July 1998.

O'Leary HE. Regulating Health Care Costs Through Fraud Enforcement. *Def Couns J* 1995;62:211–24.

False Claims Act—Coinsurance and Deductible Waivers

DeBry K et al. Health Care Fraud. *Am Crim L Rev* 1996;33:815.

McDowell TN. The Medicare-Medicaid Anti-Fraud and Abuse Amendments: Their Impact on the Present Health Care System. *Emory L J* 1987;36:691–754.

Valiant C, Hastings DA. New Managed Care Safe Harbor Regulations Don't Protect Many Mainstream Managed Care Activities. *Healthspan* 1993;10(2):10–14.

False Claims Act—DRG Creep and DRG Payment Window Claims

Frankford DM. The Complexity of Medicare's Hospital Reimbursement System: Paradoxes of Averaging. *Iowa L Rev* 1993;78:517–668.

Frankford DM. The Medicare DRG's: Efficiency and Organizational Rationality. *Yale J on Reg* 1993;10:273–346.

Krecke KA. Abusing the Patient: Medicare Fraud and Abuse and Hospital-Physician Incentive Plans. *Soc Sec Rep Ser* 1988;20:723–48.

Mariner WK. Prospective Payment for Hospital Services: Social Responsibility and the Limits of Legal Standards. *Cumb L Rev* 1987;17:379–415.

False Claims Act—False Cost Reporting

Bucy PH. Health Care Reform and Fraud by Health Care Providers. *Vill L Rev* 1993;38:1003–49.

Cooper NA. Third Party Liability or the False Claims Act: It Is Time for Consultants to Pay the Price for Their Bad Advice. *Marshall L Rev* 1996;29:923–55.

Ryan DJ. The False Claims Act: An Old Weapon with New Firepower Is Aimed at Health Care Fraud. *Annals Health L* 1995;4:127–50.

False Claims Act—Managed Care False Claims

Davies SL, Jost TS. Managed Care: Placebo or Wonder Drug for Health Care Fraud and Abuse? *Ga L Rev* 1997;31:373–417.

Krohn MD. The False Claims Act and Managed Care: Blowing the Whistle on Underutilization. *Cumb L Rev* 1998;28:443–72.

False Claims Act—Physicians at Teaching Hospitals (PATH)

Aussprung L. Fraud and Abuse. *J Legal Med* 1998; 19:1–62.

Boxer K, Gregory H. *Compliance Is Good for Your Corporate Health.* Pub. no. B0-001E. Practising Law Institute—Corporate Law, June–July 1998.

False Claims Act—Physician-Incentive Programs That Limit Necessary Services

Krecke KA. Abusing the Patient: Medicare Fraud and Abuse and Hospital-Physician Incentive Plans. *Soc Sec Rep Ser* 1988;20:723–48.

Latham SR. Regulation of Managed Care Incentive Payments to Physicians. *Am J L & Med* 1996;22:399–432.

Richards EP, Mclean TR. Physicians in Managed Care. *J Legal Med* 1997;18:443–73.

False Claims Act—Poor Quality of Care

Aussprung L. Fraud and Abuse. *J Legal Med* 1998; 19:1–62.

False Claims Act—Unbundling and Fragmenting Services

Teplitzky SV, DiAntonio JV. GAO Report Underscores Unjust Use of False Claims Act. *Andrews Gov't Cont Litig Rep* 1998;12(9):10.

See Also

Sheehan JG. *The Office of Inspector General: Health Care Financing Administration Projects.* Pub. no. B4-7234. Practising Law Institute — Corporate Law, April 1998.

False Claims—Civil Sanctions

Bucy PH. Civil Prosecution of Health Care Fraud. *Wake Forest L Rev* 1995;30:693–757.

Dougherty FM. Imposition of Civil Penalties, Under State Statute, upon Medical Practitioner for Fraud in Connection with Claims Under Medicaid, Medicare, or Similar Welfare Programs for Providing Medical Services. In: *American Law Reports,* 4th ed. Rochester, NY: Lawyers Cooperative Publishing Co., 1997; 32:671–77.

Jost TS. Medicare and Medicaid False Claims: Prohibitions and Sanctions. *Annals Health L* 1994;3:41–54.

Veilleux DR. Filing of False Insurance Claims for Medical Services as Grounds for Disciplinary Action Against Dentist, Physician, or Other Medical Practitioner. In: *American Law Reports,* 4th ed. Rochester, NY: Lawyers Cooperative Publishing Co., 1997;70:132–62.

False Claims—Criminal Sanctions

Harrington MP. Health Care Crimes: Avoiding Overenforcement. *Rutgers L J* 1994;26:111–53.

Jost TS. Medicare and Medicaid False Claims: Prohibitions and Sanctions. *Annals Health L* 1994;3:41–54.

OIG Special Fraud Alerts

Becker S. Health Care Joint Ventures. *ALI–ABA* 1998; 4:67–87.

Colborn C. *Fraud and Abuse: Anti-Kickback Developments and Practical Considerations.* Pub. no. A4-4428. Practising Law Institute — Corporate Law, September–October 1993.

Kucera WR. Hanlester Network v. Shalala: A Model Approach to the Medicare and Medicaid Kickback Problem. *NW U L Rev* 1996;91:413–52.

Lucas PH. The Service's Latest Attempt to Regulate Hospital-Physician Relationships: A Critical Analysis. *Akron Tax J* 1992;9:13–48.

Manger JA. Fraud Alert on Physicians Incentives Go Too Far. *Healthspan* 1992;9(5):2.

O'Conner DJ. Charitable Exemptions: Hospital-Physician Joint Ventures and Integrated Delivery Systems. *Colo Law* 1994;23:797–804.

Soltman RP. *Liabilities in Acquisitions of Healthcare Providers: A Practical Approach to Avoiding or Minimizing Liabilities for the Buyer.* Pub. no. B4-7234. Practising Law Institute — Commercial Law, April 1998.

Program Exclusions

Aussprung L. Fraud and Abuse. *J Legal Med* 1998; 19:1–62.

Bucy PH. Civil Prosecutions of Health Care Fraud. *Wake Forest L Rev* 1995;30:693–757.

Jost TS. Medicare and Medicaid False Claims: Prohibitions and Sanctions. *Annals Health L* 1994;3:41–54.

Morris L. *OIG Administrative Sanctions.* Pub. no. B7-6958. Practising Law Institute — Corporate Law, November 1996.

Qui Tam Suits

Beane D. Qui Tam Actions. *J Legal Med* 1993;14:279–99.

Blanch JT. The Constitutionality of the False Claims Act's Qui Tam Provision. *Harv J L & Pub Pol'y* 1993; 16:701–68.

Estrada L. An Assessment of Qui Tam Suits by Corporate Counsel Under the False Claims Act: United States ex rel. Doe v. X Corp. *Geo Mason L Rev* 1998; 7:163–89.

Forney GL. Qui Tam Suits: Defining the Rights and Rules of the Government and the Relator Under the False Claims Act. *Minn L Rev* 1998;82:1357–90.

Hamer S. Lincoln's Law: Constitutional and Policy Issues Posed by the Qui Tam Provisions of the False Claims Act. *Kan J L & Pol* 1997;6:89–102.

Raspanti MS, Laigaie DM. Current Practice and Procedure Under the Whistleblower Provisions of the Federal False Claims Act. *Temp L Rev* 1998;71:23–53.

Strader KD. Counterclaims Against Whistleblowers: Should Counterclaims Against Qui Tam Plaintiffs Be Allowed in False Claims Act Cases? *U Cin L Rev* 1993;62:713–64.

Safe Harbors

Aaron HE. Application of the Medicare and Medicaid Anti-Kickback Statute to Business Arrangements Between Hospitals and Hospital-Based Physicians. *Annals Health L* 1992;1:53–69.

DeBry K et al. Health Care Fraud. *Am Crim L Rev* 1996;33:815–38.

Kusserow RP. The Medicare and Medicaid Anti-Kickback Statute and the Safe Harbor Regulations — What's Next? *Health Matrix* 1992;2:49–70.

Valiant C, Hastings DA. New Managed Care Safe Harbor Regulations Don't Protect Many Mainstream Managed Care Activities. *Healthspan* 1993;10:10–14.

Safe Harbors—Discounts

Chanance SJ. Drug Discount Pricing Arrangement Does Not Violate Antikickback Statute. *NY Health Update* 1998;5(4):5

Kirschenbaum AM, Kuhlik BN. Federal and State Laws Affecting Discounts, Rebates and Other Marketing Practices for Drugs and Devices. *Food & Drug L J* 1992;47:533–62.

Sheller PM. *Fraud and Abuse: Implications for Purchasers and Suppliers of Drugs, Devices, and Medical Supplies.* Pub. no. A4-4455. Practising Law Institute — Commercial Law, September–October 1994.

Safe Harbors—Employees

Caldwell-Brown D. Additional Compensation Arrangement for Unionized Employees Not Subject to Sanctions. *NY Health Update* 1998;5(8):6.

Reisman GD. U.S. Court of Appeals Rejects Claim That Antikickback Statute Is Unconstitutionally Vague. *NY Health Update* 1998;5(11):5.

Safe Harbors—Group Purchasing Organizations

Altschuler AM et al. Health Care Fraud. *Am Crim L Rev* 1998;35:841–74.

Sheller PM. *Fraud and Abuse: Implications for Purchasers and Suppliers of Drugs, Devices, and Medical Suppliers.* Pub. no. A4-4455. Practising Law Institute — Commercial Law, September–October 1994.

Safe Harbors—Investment Interest

Altschuler AM et al. Health Care Fraud. *Am Crim L Rev* 1998;35:841–74.

Kusserow RP. The Medicare and Medicaid Anti-Kickback Statute and the Safe Harbor Regulations — What's Next? *Health Matrix* 1992;2:49–70.

Safe Harbors—Lease of Space and Equipment Rentals

Altschuler AM et al. Health Care Fraud. *Am Crim L Rev* 1998;35:841–74.

Ball DW. Medicare Fraud and Abuse Anti-Kickback Safe Harbor Regulations. *S C Law* 1991;3:34–7.

Kusserow RP. The Medicare and Medicaid Anti-Kickback Statute and the Safe Harbor Regulations — What's Next? *Health Matrix* 1992;2:49–70.

Safe Harbors—Managed Care

Altschuler AM et al. Health Care Fraud. *Am Crim L Rev* 1998;35:841–74.

Safe Harbors—Personal Services and Management Contracts

Yankowitz BJ. *Selected Topics in Non-Exempt Financing for Health Care Providers.* Pub. no. A4-4428. Practising Law Institute — Commercial Law, September–October 1993.

Safe Harbors—Referral Services

Kusserow RP. The Medicare and Medicaid Anti-Kickback Statute and the Safe Harbor Regulations — What's Next? *Health Matrix* 1992;2:49–70.

Safe Harbors—Sale of Practice

Ball DW. Medicare Fraud and Abuse Anti-Kickback Safe Harbor Regulations. *S C Law* 1991;3:34–7.

Kusserow RP. The Medicare and Medicaid Anti-Kickback Statute and the Safe Harbor Regulations — What's Next? *Health Matrix* 1992;2:49–70.

Temkin HL. Medicare Fraud and Abuse. *Wis Law* 1989;62:13–65.

Safe Harbors—Waiver of Beneficiary Cost Sharing

Altschuler AM et al. Health Care Fraud. *Am Crim L Rev* 1998;35:841–74.

Safe Harbors—Warranties

Altschuler AM et al. Health Care Fraud. *Am Crim L Rev* 1998;35:841–74.

Kusserow RP. The Medicare and Medicaid Anti-Kickback Statute and the Safe Harbor Regulations — What's Next? *Health Matrix* 1992;2:49–70.

Learn M. Applying Medicare and Medicaid Anti-Kickback Laws to Disease Management Programs: Ramifications for the Pharmaceutical Industry and a Regulatory Proposal. *Temp L Rev* 1996;69:245–74.

Sheller PM. *Fraud and Abuse: Implications for Purchasers and Suppliers of Drugs, Devices, and Medical Supplies.* Pub. no. A4-4455. Practising Law Institute — Commercial Law, September–October 1994.

Sanctions

Harrington MP. Health Care Crimes: Avoiding Overenforcement. *Rutgers L J* 1994;26:111–53.

Jost TS. Medicare and Medicaid False Claims: Prohibitions and Sanctions. *Annals Health L* 1994;3:41–54.

Nalven DS. Medicare and Medicaid Fraud: An Enforcement Priority for the 1990's. *Boston B J* 1994;38:9–17.

Stafford G. *Medicare and Medicaid Fraud and Abuse.* Pub. no. J4-3556. Practising Law Institute — Tax Law and Estate Planning, October 1984.

Stark II Advisory Opinions

Rovner JA. Balanced Budget Act Further Expands Healthcare Fraud and Abuse Controls. *Health Law* 1997;10(2):1–4.

Wachler AB, Avery PA. Stark II Proposed Regulations: Rule Offers Additional Guidance While Regulators Seek More Input From Health Care Community. *Health Law* 1998:1–62.

Wachler AB, Avery PA. Stark II Proposed Regulations: Rule Offers Additional Guidance While Regulations Seek More Input from Health Care Community. *Health Law* 1998;1:1–62.

Stark Laws

Barratt K et al. Stark Self Referral Rules Burdened with Complexities. *Wis Med J* 1995;94:697–701.

Beck S et al. Stark Self Referral Law. *Iowa Med* 1995;85:484–87.

Biggs SM. Stark I and II: Pitfalls in Medical Practice. *Hosp Phys* 1995;31(5):52–54.

Klein JS. The Stark Laws: Conquering Physician Conflicts of Interest. *Geo L J* 1998;87:499–529.

Patrick LE. A Complicated Prescription. *S C Law* 1999; 10:22–26.

Stark Laws—Exceptions

Patrick LE. A Complicated Prescription. *S C Law* 1999; 10:22–26.

Radinsky G. Defining a Group Practice: An Analysis of the Stark I Final Rule. *St Louis U L J* 1997;41:1119–56.

Reiss JB. Commenting on Payment and Reimbursement Issues Affecting the Marketing of Drugs, Medical Devices, and Biologicals with Emphasis on the Anti-Kickback Statute and Stark II. *Food & Drug L J* 1997;52:99–108.

Smith MH. Physician Ownership and Self-Referral Prohibition Expanded Under COBRA. *Colo Law* 1994; 23:1085–88.

Thomas JH. Stark II Limits on Physician Self-Referral. *Fla B J* 1994;68:75–78.

Tichon M. Compliance Issues Under the New Fraud and Abuse Rules. *Whittier L Rev* 1995;16:1085–1110.

Wachler AB, Avery PA. Final Stark Regulations Implement Self-Referral Prohibitions Impacting Health Care Providers. *Mich B J* 1995;74:1274–80.

Wachler AB, Avery PA. Stark II Proposed Regulations: Rule Offers Additional Guidance While Regulations Seek More Input from Health Care Community. *Health Law* 1998;1:1–62.

Wachler AB et al. Stark I Final Regulations: Implications for Health Care Providers and Supplies. *Health Law* 1995:1–29.

Stark Laws—Reporting Requirements

DiGiovanni L, Gibofsky A. Medicare Fraud and the Implications for Joint Ventures: Are We Working at Cross Purposes? *Leg Med* 1995:279–303.

Stark Laws—Stark I and II

Ivers D. Stark II: The Quagmire Thickens. *J Ark Med Soc* 1998;95:75–78.

Larios D et al. How the New Stark II Regulations Affect Group Practice. *Tenn Med* 1998;91:128–30.

Radinsky G. Defining a Group Practice: An Analysis of the Stark I Final Rule. *St Louis U L J* 1997;41:1119–56.

Vaughn TD. Stark II: New Restrictions on Referrals. *Mo Dent J* 1995;75:13–15.

Stark Sanctions

Klein JE. The Stark Laws: Conquering Physician Conflicts of Interest? *Geo L J* 1998;87:499–529.

Wachler AB, Avery PA. Final Stark Regulations Implement Self-Referral Prohibitions Impacting Health Care Providers. *Mich B J* 1995;74:1274–80.

Wachler AB et al. Stark I Final Regulations: Implications for Health Care Providers and Suppliers. *Health Law* 1995:1–29.

Other Reading

Aspen Health Law Center. *Health Care Fraud and Abuse.* Gaithersburg, MD: Aspen, 1998.

Aussprung L. Fraud and Abuse. *J Legal Med* 1998;19:1–62.

Beck S et al. Stark Self Referral Law. *Iowa Med* 1995; 85:484–87.

Kochman TJ, Meguerian G. False Claims. *Am Crim L Rev* 1994;31:525–38.

Kucera WR. Hanlester Network v. Shalala: A Model Approach to the Medicare and Medicaid Kickback Problem. *NW Univ L Rev* 1996;91:413–52.

Patrick LE. A Complicated Prescription. *S C Law* 1999; 10:22–26.

Web Sites

Advisory opinions: *http://www.hhs.gov/progorg/oig/advopn/index.htm*

Excluded providers: *http://www.jupiter.psc.gov/cgi-bin/oig_counter.pl*

False Claims Act home page: *http://www.falseclaim.com/*

False Claims Act Resource Center: *http://www.falseclaimsact.com*

Fighting fraud and abuse — Medicare's program integrity home page: *http://payerid.org/*

Fraud alerts: *http://www.dhhs.gov/progorg/oig/frdalert/index.htm* and *http://www.wellmedicine.com/fraud alert.htm*

Fraud self-disclosure protocols: *http://www.hhs.gov/progorg/oig*

HCFA model compliance program guides: *http://www.dhhs.gov/progorg/oig/modcomp*

HCFA State Operations Manual: *http://www.hcfa.gov/pubforms/progman.htm*

Health care compliance manager: *http://www.hcc manager.com/*

Health Care Financing Administration: *http://www.payerid.com/*

Health Services of America regulatory compliance corner: *http://www.hsca.com/regcorner.htm*

HIPAA: *http://jmrassociates.com/hipaa.htm*

The HIPAA wizard: *http://www.hipaawizard.com/*

Inspector general publishes proposal for new Medicare Anti-Kickback Law safe harbors: *http://www.arent-fox.com/alerts/safeharb.html*

Medicare and state health care programs — Fraud and abuse: *http://www.retreach.net/~wmanning/advopn.htm*

Medicare Program integrity home page: *http://www.hcfa.gov/medicare/fraud/default3.htm*

The qui tam information center: *http://www.quitam.com/*

Stark advisory opinions: *http://www.hcfa.gov/regs/aop/default.htm*

Stark II questions and answers: *http://www.eyeworld.org/november/1193.asp*

Taxpayers Against Fraud — The False Claims Act legal center: *http://www.taf.org/taf/*

13

Antitrust Law

Antitrust law is one of the most complex areas of the legal system. Its task is to establish the boundaries of acceptable activities of competitors in a free market. The fundamental goal of antitrust law is to protect fair competition for consumer benefit; but note that antitrust law does *not* protect individual competitors.[1] Antitrust law is applicable to health care generally[2] and to medicine as a "learned profession."[3] Further, these laws are extremely important in the current health delivery climate because the intensive competition between health care providers and the consolidation of the health care industry may put many business arrangements at antitrust risk. The key antitrust laws are the Sherman Act,[4] which prohibits arrangements that unreasonably restrain competition and monopolization; the Clayton Act,[5] which prohibits business mergers and related activities that present a reasonable probability of substantially decreasing competition; and the Federal Trade Commission Act,[6] which prohibits unfair modes of competition. These are federal statutes and the discussion within this chapter focuses on these laws, since state antitrust laws usually utilize the same analysis and prohibit the same types of activities.[7]

Sherman Act

Section 1. Agreements That Unreasonably Restrain Competition

Section 1 of the Sherman Act[8] is one of the most important and frequently used antitrust laws applied to health care. This provision of the Sherman Act prohibits (1) an agreement or conspiracy (2) that unreasonably restrains competition.

For the purposes of Section 1, for an agreement to be shown, the parties (1) must be legally capable of agreeing (i.e., conspiring) and (2) have actually agreed. As a preliminary matter, actions by a single party cannot be violations of Section 1.[9] Individual components of a single integrated enterprise are considered a single party and hence these individual components cannot be deemed to enter into an agreement with each other. For example, components treated as a single party are business entities wholly owned by the same owners;[10] a corporation, its directors, its officers, and its employees;[11] corporations and their unincorporated divisions;[12] corporations and their wholly owned subsidiaries;[13] sister

---

[1]See, e.g., Brown Shoe Co. v. United States, 370 U.S. 294, 320 (1962); Brunswick Corp. v. Pueblo Bowl-O-Mat, Inc., 429 U.S. 477 (1977).

[2]See, e.g., Arizona v. Maricopa Cty. Med. Soc'y, 457 U.S. 332 (1982); American Medical Ass'n v. United States, 317 U.S. 519 (1943).

[3]See Goldfarb v. Virginia State Bar, 421 U.S. 773 (1975).

[4]15 U.S.C.A. §§1, 2.

[5]15 U.S.C.A. §18.

[6]15 U.S.C.A. §45.

[7]See, e.g., 6 Trade Reg. Rep. (Chicago: Commerce Clearing House, 1993), ¶30,201–35,602 (listing state antitrust laws).

[8]15 U.S.C.A. §1.

[9]See, e.g., Fisher v. City of Berkeley, 475 U.S. 260 (1986); Copperweld Corp. v. Independence Tube Corp., 467 U.S. 752, 759 (1984).

[10]See, e.g., Century Oil Tool, Inc. v. Production Specialties, Inc., 737 F.2d 1316 (5th Cir. 1984).

[11]See, e.g., Nurse Midwifery Ass'n v. Hibbit, 918 F.2d 605 (6th Cir. 1990), *cert. denied* 112 S.Ct. 406 (1991).

[12]See, e.g., The Domed Stadium Hotel, Inc. v. Holiday Inns, Inc., 732 F.2d 480 (5th Cir. 1984).

[13]See, e.g., Copperweld Corp. v. Independence Tube Corp., 467 U.S. 752 (1984); Okusami v. Psychiatric Inst. of Wash., 959 F.2d 1062 (D.C. Cir. 1992).

corporations;[14] and sister corporations and their common parent.[15]

The definition of an agreement or conspiracy is quite expansive. There is no need for the parties to have entered into an express or formal agreement. The parties need merely to have reached some mutual understanding to take the particular action; an agreement arises when the parties "had a unity of purpose or a common design and understanding, or a meeting of the minds in an unlawful arrangement."[16] Such an agreement can be inferred using circumstantial evidence.[17]

If there is an agreement inducing a particular action, then the action will be subject to antitrust analysis to determine if it unreasonably restrains competition. Two standards exist to assess the competitive effects of the action: per se and rule of reason analysis.

Per se analyses are applied to anticompetitive agreements that are deemed to be "naked" restraints on competition; that is, they have no plausible procompetitive justification, have pernicious effects on competition, or lack any redeeming competitive virtue. Therefore, they are per se illegal.[18] Examples of such actions include competitor agreements for allocating markets,[19] group boycotts,[20] price fixing,[21] rigging competitive bidding processes,[22] and tying arrangements (where one product or service cannot be purchased

unless another is as well).[23] No actual anticompetitive effects of the agreement on competition need be shown.[24]

Much more frequent is the application of rule of reason analysis.[25] Under rule of reason analysis, the plaintiff challenging the purported actions first must establish what constitutes the relevant product market and the relevant geographic market that affect competition.[26] The plaintiff then must establish that the parties had market power, that is, "the ability to raise prices above the competitive level by restricting output"[27] of the product in question. The court assesses the procompetitive and anticompetitive effects of the parties' agreement to determine if there has been a violation of Section 1. If the balance weighs in favor of procompetitive effects, there is no violation. If the balance weighs in favor of antitcompetitive effects, the agreement is unlawful. Because of the fact-intensive nature of rule of reason analysis, litigation using this standard is extremely costly in terms of time and money, and court decisions regarding particular arrangements have limited applicability in other contexts.

Section 2. Monopolization and Attempted Monopolization

Section 2 of the Sherman Act[28] focuses on the actions of an individual party or entity with substantial market power that engages in exclusionary behavior toward other actual or potential competitors.

Section 2 prohibits monopolization. Plaintiffs alleging that a party has engaged in monopolization behavior in violation of this law must show all of the following:

1. The relevant product and geographic markets.[29]
2. That the party engaged in the behavior has monopoly power.
3. That the party's monopoly power was obtained, maintained, or extended by "predatory" or unreasonably anticompetitive conduct.[30]

[14]See, e.g., Advanced Health-Care Servs., Inc. v. Radford Comm. Hosp., 910 F.2d 139 (4th Cir. 1990).

[15]See, e.g., Carinha v. Action Crane Corp., 396 N.Y.S.2d 191 (N.Y. App. Div. 1977).

[16]American Tobacco Co. v. United States, 328 U.S. 781, 810 (1946); see also Monsanto Co. v. Spray-Rite Serv. Corp., 465 U.S. 752, 764 (1984) (noting a conspiracy is a conscious commitment to a common scheme designed to achieve an unlawful objective); FTC v. Indiana Fed'n of Dentists, 476 U.S. 447 (1986) (an agreement between a group of dentists to refuse to supply insurers with patients' X rays is an antitrust violation).

[17]See, e.g., Monsanto Co. v. Spray-Rite Serv. Corp., 465 U.S. 752, 764 (1984); In re Coordinated Pretrial Proceedings in Petroleum Prods, Antitrust Litigation, 906 F.2d 432 (9th Cir. 1990), cert. denied sub nom. Chevron Corp. v. Arizona, 500 U.S. 959 (1991); Edward J. Sweeney & Sons, Inc. v. Texaco, Inc., 637 F.2d 105, 111 (3d Cir. 1980), cert. denied 451 U.S. 911 (1981).

[18]See, e.g., Northern Pac. Ry. Co. v. United States, 356 U.S. 1, 5 (1958).

[19]See, e.g., United States v. Topco Assocs., 405 U.S. 596 (1972); Palmer v. BRG of Georgia, Inc., 498 U.S. 46 (1990); see also Ryco Mfg. Co. v. Eden Servs., 823 F.2d 1215 (8th Cir. 1987), cert. denied 484 U.S. 1026 (1988) (resale price maintenance agreements, where resell price is fixed, per se illegal).

[20]See, e.g., Radiant Burners, Inc. v. Peoples Gas Light & Coke Co., 364 U.S. 656 (1961).

[21]See, e.g., Palmer v. BRG of Georgia, Inc., 498 U.S. 46 (1990); Arizona v. Maricopa Cty. Med. Soc'y, 457 U.S. 332 (1982); United States v. A. Lanoy Alston, D.M.D., 974 F.2d 1206 (9th Cir. 1992).

[22]United States v. Misle Bus & Equip. Co., 967 F.2d 1227 (8th Cir. 1992).

[23]See, e.g., United States Steel Corp. v. Fortner Enterprises, Inc., 429 U.S. 610, 620 (1977); United States v. Loew's Inc., 371 U.S. 38, 45, 48 n. 5 (1962); Northern Pac. Ry. Co. v. United States, 356 U.S. 1, 6–7 (1956).

[24]See, e.g., Superior Ct. Trial Lawyers Ass'n v. FTC, 493 U.S. 411 (1990); National Soc'y of Professional Engineers v. United States, 435 U.S. 679, 692 (1978).

[25]See, e.g., Chicago Bd. of Trade v. United States, 246 U.S. 231 (1918); Continental TV, Inc. v. GTE Sylvania, Inc., 433 U.S. 36 (1977).

[26]See, e.g., Oksanen v. Page Mem. Hosp., 945 F.2d 696 (4th Cir. 1991), cert. denied 502 U.S. 1074 (1992).

[27]Wilk v. American Med. Ass'n, 895 F.2d 352, 359 (7th Cir.), cert. denied 496 U.S. 927 (1990).

[28]15 U.S.C.A. §2.

[29]See, e.g., Delaware & Hudson Ry. v. Consolidated Rail Corp., 902 F.2d 174 (2d Cir. 1990), cert. denied 500 U.S. 928 (1991).

[30]See, e.g., United States v. Grinnell Corp., 384 U.S. 563 (1966).

Note that simply because an organization is large or has significant economic power within a market does not, alone, constitute illegal monopolization behavior if that power is a result of a superior product, business acumen, or historic accident.[31]

Monopoly power is defined as the ability to control price or exclude competition.[32] Although the tests vary, generally monopoly power may be inferred if the party has a market share of 65% or more and some entry barriers deter other potential competitors from entering into the market.[33] The concept of predatory conduct is amorphous[34] but generally describes behavior that has significant exclusionary effects without resulting in or from substantive competition (e.g., low prices, high production efficiency, high quality, innovation).

Section 2 also prohibits efforts to monopolize by parties with market, but not monopoly, power that engage in activities likely to lead to monopoly power. For a plaintiff to prevail on an attempted monopolization claim requires a showing of all the following:

1. The relevant product and geographic markets.[35]
2. A specific intent to monopolize these market.
3. Predatory behavior engaged in to implement the specific intent.
4. A dangerous probability of success if the conduct continues.[36]

Often, specific attempts to monopolize are implied from the party's predatory conduct.[37] In addition, the dangerous probability of success requirement may be implied from the party's market share, even though no hard-and-fast rule specifies what market share, alone, indicates a dangerous probability of successful monopolization.[38]

Clayton Act

The Clayton Act, particularly Section 7,[39] governs business consolidations including mergers, joint ventures, and acquisitions of business assets. Section 7 prohibits such consolidations that would be reasonably expected to substantially decrease competition.[40] Mergers and other business consolidations are discussed extensively in the Federal Trade Commission (FTC) and Department of Justice's (DOJ) *Horizontal Merger Guidelines*.[41] As well, some business consolidations must be reported to the DOJ and FTC before completion.[42]

Section 7 of the Clayton Act prohibits business consolidations "in any line of commerce . . . in any section of the country [if] the effect of such acquisition may be substantially to lessen competition, or to tend to create a monopoly."[43] Therefore, traditional corporate mergers and joint ventures would be subject to scrutiny, as well as acquisition of stock or assets such as patents,[44] trademarks,[45] sales agreements,[46] leases,[47] and transactions that result in a transfer of decision-making control.[48] Indeed, note that the acquisition does not need to result in actual control;[49] influence, such as through seats on the acquired company's board of directors in contemplation of eventual control, brings the acquisition under Clayton Act scrutiny.[50] However, if stock acquisitions are not for control or future control and represent investments only, then the Clayton Act may not apply.[51]

---

[31]See, e.g., Berkey Photo, Inc. v. Eastman Kodak Co., 603 F.2d 263 (2d Cir. 1979), *cert. denied* 444 U.S. 1093 (1980); United States v. Grinnell Corp., 384 U.S. 563, 570–71 (1966).

[32]See, e.g., United States v. E.I. du Pont de Nemours & Co., 351 U.S. 377 (1956).

[33]See, e.g., MCI Communications Corp. v. American Tel. & Telegraph Co., 708 F.2d 1081 (7th Cir. 1982), *cert. denied* 464 U.S. 891 (1983).

[34]See, e.g., Cargill, Inc. v. Monfort of Colorado, Inc., 479 U.S. 104, 117 n.12 (1986).

[35]See, e.g., Smith v. Northern Mich. Hosps., 703 F.2d 942 (6th Cir. 1983).

[36]See, e.g., Spectrum Sports, Inc. v. McQuillan, 506 U.S. 447 (1993).

[37]See, e.g., McGahee v. Northern Propane Gas Co., 858 F.2d 1487 (11th Cir. 1988), *cert. denied* 490 U.S. 1084 (1989).

[38]See, e.g., United States v. Citizens & Southern Nat'l Bank, 422 U.S. 86, 120 (1975); United States v. Marine Bancorporation, Inc., 418 U.S. 602, 631 (1974); Twin Labs., Inc. v. Weider Health & Fitness, 900 F.2d 566 (2d Cir. 1990).

[39]15 U.S.C.A. §18.

[40]See, e.g., Brown Shoe Co. v. United States, 370 U.S. 294 (1962).

[41]56 Fed. Reg. 41,552–41,563 (September 10, 1992).

[42]15 U.S.C.A. §18a.

[43]15 U.S.C.A. §18.

[44]See, e.g., SCM Corp. v. Xerox Corp., 645 F.2d 1195, 1205 (2d Cir. 1981).

[45]See, e.g., United States v. Lever Bros. Co., 216 F.Supp. 887, 889 (S.D. N.Y. 1963).

[46]See, e.g., United States v. ITT Continental Baking Co., 485 F.2d 16, 21 (10th Cir. 1973).

[47]See, e.g., United States v. Archer Daniels Midland Co., 584 F.Supp. 1134, 1139 (S.D. Iowa 1984), *aff'd* 785 F.2d 206 (8th Cir. 1986), *cert. denied* 481 U.S. 1028 (1987).

[48]See, e.g., McTamney v. Stolt Tankers & Terminals, SA, 678 F.Supp. 118, 120 (E.D. Pa. 1987).

[49]See, e.g., Denver & Rio Grande W.R.R. v. United States, 387 U.S. 485, 501 (1967).

[50]See, e.g., American Crystal Sugar Co. v. Cuban-Am. Sugar Co., 152 F.Supp. 387, 392 (S.D. N.Y. 1957), *aff'd* 259 F.2d 524 (2d Cir. 1958); Gulf & Western Indus. v. Great Atlantic & Pacific Tea Co., 476 F.2d 687, 694 (2d Cir. 1973).

[51]See, e.g., Gulf & Western Indus v. Great Atlantic & Pacific Tea Co., 476 F.2d 687, 694 (2d Cir. 1973); United States v. Tracinda Inv. Corp., 477 F.Supp. 1093, 1100 (C.D. Cal. 1979).

The Clayton Act also requires that both parties in the acquisition either be engaged in interstate commerce or affect interstate commerce.[52] To engage in interstate commerce, an entity must produce or distribute its products across state lines.[53] Entities may affect interstate commerce if their actions affect goods or services that cross state lines. Generally, mergers within the health care field such as those between hospitals will fall within this latter categorization even if they do not fall within the former.[54]

Federal Trade Commission Act

The Federal Trade Commission Act,[55] specifically Section 5,[56] prohibits "unfair methods of competition" and thus encompasses activities subject to scrutiny under the Sherman and Clayton Acts.[57] In addition, because of the broad wording of the law,[58] actions that may not be reachable under the Sherman and Clayton Acts due to technical reasons or because the conduct has not yet resulted in an actual unreasonable restraint on trade (e.g., a mere invitation by one competitor to another to fix prices rather than actual fixing) still may be prosecuted under the Federal Trade Commission Act.[59] Indeed, the Supreme Court has interpreted the Federal Trade Commission Act in a much broader fashion than the Sherman or Clayton Act.[60] Overall, the Federal Trade Commission Act is a catchall statute that is expansive enough to cover virtually any anticompetitive activity.

Enforcement and Penalties

Antitrust laws are enforced by private parties, state attorneys general, the FTC, and the DOJ. The Federal Trade Commission Act is enforced only by the FTC.

Both criminal and civil penalties are available under the antitrust laws. Violations of the Sherman Act may be criminally prosecuted in federal district court by the Antitrust Division of the DOJ and result in significant penalties including corporate fines of up to $10 million or twice the pecuniary loss of the victims,[61] and individual fines of up to $350,000, twice the pecuniary gain the individual derived, or twice the pecuniary loss of the victims, whichever is greatest, and imprisonment of up to three years.[62] These penalties may and have been applied to health care providers.[63]

Clayton Act violations are subject to more limited penalties, including fines of up to $5000 and imprisonment of up to one year.[64] Civil action also may be taken by the government and result in injunctions, consent decrees, damages in the amount of the harm, or cease-and-desist orders against the offending party.[65]

Note that the Federal Trade Commission Act allows for only FTC enforcement; therefore, no private cause of action exists.[66] In addition, since the FTC is an executive branch agency, its adjudications are administrative. An administrative law judge hears the case, with a right of appeal to the full Federal Trade Commission, that is, the five appointed commissioners of the FTC. Commission decisions adverse to a party may be appealed to a federal court of appeals; however, decisions adverse to the FTC cannot be appealed. If the commission finds that an action is unlawful, a cease-and-desist order generally is entered and affirmative action by the offending party also may be required. Violations of cease-and-desist orders are subject to a $10,000 civil penalty for each day of the violation.[67] In place of a cease-and-desist order, the FTC may obtain a consent agreement with the offending party. The consent agreement is a settlement agreement and no admission of illegality is made under such an agreement by the party engaged in the challenged action; however, when issued in final form, these consent agreements have the force and effect of law.[68]

Private parties that suffer anticompetitive injury may bring civil actions for damages under the Sherman Act and the Clayton Act. These parties must demonstrate a

---

[52]15 U.S.C.A. §18; see also Summit Health, Ltd. v. Pinhas, 500 U.S. 322 (1991).

[53]See, e.g., United States v. American Bldg. Maintenance Industries, 422 U.S. 271 (1975).

[54]See, e.g., Hospital Bldg. Co. v. Trustees of Rex Hosp., 425 U.S. 738 (1976).

[55]15 U.S.C.A. §§41–51.

[56]15 U.S.C.A. §45.

[57]See, e.g., FTC v. Motion Picture Advertising Serv. Co., 344 U.S. 392 (1953).

[58]"Unfair methods of competition in or affecting commerce, and unfair or deceptive acts or practices in or affecting commerce, are hereby declared unlawful." 15 U.S.C.A. §45(a)(1).

[59]See, e.g., Rhinechem Corp., 93 F.T.C. 233 (1979); Dean Foods Co., 70 F.T.C. 1146, 1290–92 (1966).

[60]See, e.g., FTC v. Brown Shoe Co., 384 U.S. 316, 321 (1966).

[61]15 U.S.C.A. §1; 18 U.S.C.A. §3571.

[62]15 U.S.C.A. §§1, 2; 18 U.S.C.A. §3571.

[63]See, e.g., United States v. A. Lanoy Allston, D.M.D., 974 F.2d 1206 (9th Cir. 1992).

[64]15 U.S.C.A. §§13(a), 24.

[65]See 15 U.S.C.A. §§1311–14.

[66]See, e.g., Holloway v. Bristol-Meyers Corp., 485 F.2d 986 (D.C. Cir. 1973); Valet Apartment Servs. v. Atlanta Journal & Const., 865 F.Supp. 828 (N.D. Ga. 1994).

[67]15 U.S.C.A. §45(m).

[68]16 C.F.R. §2.32 (1998).

violation of the antitrust laws, an injury to the parties' business or property (or threatened injury for injunctive suits), and a causal relationship between the antitrust violation and the injury. If successful, damages are three times actual damages and attorneys' fees[69] or an injunction,[70] whichever is relevant.

Antitrust Enforcement Policies

Recognizing the tremendous changes in health care delivery, the FTC and DOJ have issued some formal guidance with regard to specific activities and their antitrust risk. This guidance is indicated in the *Statements of Enforcement Policy and Analytical Principles Relating to Health Care and Antitrust*[71] (1994 guidelines) and in the *Statements of Antitrust Enforcement Policy in Health Care*[72] (1996 guidelines). In these publications, the FTC and DOJ have indicated specific activities deemed suspect as well as safe harbors that will not draw these agencies' antitrust challenge. These are extremely important documents, ushering in the modern health care era and providing physicians and health care institutions with significant insight as to how particular business activities will be viewed by the FTC and the DOJ.

The 1994 guidelines cover the areas of (1) hospital mergers, (2) hospital joint ventures involving high-technology equipment, (3) hospital joint ventures involving specialized clinical or other expensive health care services, (4) providers' collective provision of non-fee-related information to purchasers of health care services, (5) providers' collective provision of fee-related information to purchasers of health care services, (6) provider participation in exchanges of price and cost information, (7) joint purchasing arrangements among health care providers, (8) physician network joint ventures, and (9) analytic principles relating to multiprovider networks. The 1996 guidelines update and expand analysis of items 8 and 9. Examples of the application of the analyses from the guidelines are listed in the appendix to this chapter. These examples, in combination with consent decrees, business review letters, and advisory opinions, provide important insight as to how business relationships may be structured to avoid violating antitrust laws.

---

[69]15 U.S.C.A. §45(a).

[70]See, e.g., 15 U.S.C.A. §26.

[71]U.S. Department of Justice and the Federal Trade Commission, *Statements of Enforcement Policy and Analytical Principles Relating to Health Care and Antitrust* (Washington, DC: DOJ and FTC, September 1994).

[72]U.S. Department of Justice and the Federal Trade Commission, *Statements of Antitrust Enforcement Policy in Health Care* (Washington, DC: DOJ and FTC, August 1996).

1994 Guidelines

Statement 1. Enforcement Policies on Hospital Mergers — Rural Hospital Safety Zone

Statement 1 relates to hospital mergers for rural hospitals that are less than five years old. The FTC and DOJ will not challenge mergers between two general acute-care hospitals where one of the hospitals has an average of fewer than 100 licensed beds over the three most recent years and a daily inpatient census of fewer than 40 patients over the three most recent years, absent extraordinary circumstances. This statement notes that if the hospital merger is not within the safety zone, it can still pass antitrust muster if the merger would not increase the likelihood of illegal market power exercise, either because of the existence, postmerger, of strong competitors or because the merging hospitals are sufficiently differentiated; the merger would allow the hospitals to realize significant cost savings that otherwise would not be realized; or the merger would eliminate a hospital that likely would fail, with its assets subsequently exiting the market.

Statement 2. Enforcement Policy on Hospital Joint Ventures Involving High-Technology or Other Expensive Health Care Equipment

Absent extraordinary circumstances, the DOJ and FTC indicate in this statement that they will not challenge joint ventures among hospitals to purchase or otherwise share the cost, operation, and marketing of high-technology or other expensive equipment and their related services if the joint venture includes only the number of hospitals necessary to support the equipment. Equipment support in this context includes an assessment of equipment cost, expected useful life, minimum number of procedures that must be done to meet its financial breakeven point, the expected number of procedures the equipment will be used for given the patient population served by the joint venture, and the expected price to be charged for the use of the equipment, based on objective evidence (e.g., similar technologies and similar markets).

The equipment in this safety zone can be either new or existing. Note, however, that if one of the hospitals could support the equipment independently and enters into a joint venture agreement with other hospitals, this arrangement would not fall within the safety zone.

Joint venture arrangements that do not fall within this safety zone will be assessed under a rule of reason analysis. The analysis will assess whether there are competitive reductions and, if so, whether any procompetitive efficiencies will outweigh these reductions. The analysis employed uses a four-step process:

1. Define the relevant market.
2. Evaluate any reduction in competition due to the venture.
3. Evaluate the impact of procompetitive efficiencies.
4. Evaluate collateral agreements that may unreasonably restrict competition.

The greater the amount of competition reduction, the greater amount of procompetitive efficiencies that must be shown.

Statement 3. Enforcement Policy on Hospital Joint Ventures Involving Specialized Clinical or Other Expensive Health Care Services

This statement provides information on how the agencies will evaluate joint ventures involving specialized or expensive health care services. The agencies indicate that no safety zone is provided for service agreements because of their need to obtain additional expertise in evaluating the cost of, demand for, and potential benefits from such ventures.

Effectively, the analysis for joint venture service agreements is the same as that for ventures involving equipment that do not fall within the safety zone. The DOJ and FTC will use a rule of reason analysis and the four-step process: defining the relevant market, evaluating any reduction in competition due to the venture, evaluating the impact of procompetitive efficiencies, and evaluating collateral agreements. Like the policy statement for joint ventures in equipment, greater reductions of competition require greater efficiencies from the venture to pass antitrust muster.

Statement 4. Providers' Collective Provision of Non–Fee-Related Information to Purchasers of Health Care Services

Multiple providers' collective provision of medical data that may improve purchasers' assessment of the mode, quality, or efficiency of treatment will not be challenged by the FTC or DOJ, absent extraordinary circumstances. Examples of information provision that will not be challenged include a medical society's collection of outcome data from its members for a particular procedure that they believe should be covered by a purchaser and providers' development of suggested clinical practice guidelines for patient management developed to assist providers in clinical decision making that also may provide useful information to purchasers, providers, and patients.

This statement notes explicitly that the agencies recognize that, in the course of providing underlying medical data to purchasers, providers may collectively engage in discussions with purchasers about the scientific merit of the data; this collective discussion is acceptable. However, the safety zone does not protect efforts by providers to coerce a purchaser's decision making by implying or actually threatening a boycott of plans that do not follow the providers' joint recommendations or accept the providers' clinical practice guidelines. In addition, the safety zone does not apply to any actions by providers that collectively threaten to or refuse to deal with a purchaser because they object to the purchaser's administrative, clinical, or other requirements relating to the provision of services.

Statement 5. Providers' Collective Provision of Fee-Related Information to Purchasers of Health Care Services

This statement provides a safety zone for providers' collective provision to purchasers of the providers' current or historical fees or other aspects of reimbursement (e.g., discounts, alternative modes accepted such as capitation, risk-withhold fee arrangements, all-inclusive fees) if the following conditions are met:

1. The collection is managed by a third party such as a purchaser, government agency, health care consultant, academic institution, or trade association.
2. Any information shared *between the competitors furnishing data* is at least three months old, although the information regarding current fee-related information may be provided to purchasers.
3. For any information available to the providers furnishing data, there are at least five providers reporting data on which each disseminated statistic is based, no individual provider's data may represent more than 25% on a weighted basis for that statistic, and any information disseminated must be sufficiently aggregated so that it does not allow recipients to identify the prices charged by any individual provider.

Generally, the agencies in promulgating these conditions wish to ensure that an exchange of price or cost information is not used by competing providers for discussion or coordination of provider prices or costs.

The FTC and DOJ indicate that the safety zone does not apply to collective negotiations between providers and unintegrated purchasers in contemplation or furtherance of any agreement among the providers on fees or other terms of reimbursement. The safety zone also does not apply to any agreement among unintegrated providers to deal with purchasers only on agreed-on terms. These considerations apply both to current fees and prospective fees. Of course, integrated providers that collectively threaten or actually engage either implicitly or explicitly to boycott or engage in similar conduct to coerce a purchaser to accept collectively determined fees or other terms of reimbursement would not be protected by this safety zone and, indeed, may be engaging in per se illegal activities.

In assessing the appropriateness of fee-related provision of information to purchasers, the agencies will make an assessment that includes the nature of the information provided, the nature and extent of the communication among the providers and between the providers and the purchaser, the rationale for providing the information, and the nature of the market in which the information is provided.

Statement 6. Provider Participation in Exchanges of Price and Cost Information

Absent extraordinary circumstances, the DOJ and FTC will not challenge provider participation in written surveys of prices for health care services or wages, salaries, or benefits of health care personnel if:

1. The survey is managed by a third party such as a purchaser, government agency, health care consultant, academic institution, or trade association.
2. The information provided by the survey participants is based on data more than three months old.
3. At least five providers are reporting the data on which each disseminated statistic is based, no individual provider's data represents greater than 25% on a weighted basis of that statistic, and any information disseminated is sufficiently aggregated that it would not allow recipients to identify prices charged or compensation paid by any particular provider.

Again, like the policy stated in Statement 5, these conditions are set forth to ensure that an exchange of price or cost data is not used by competing providers for discussion or coordination of provider prices or costs.

This statement notes that exchanges that fall outside the safety zone will be evaluated to determine whether the information exchange may have anticompetitive effects that outweigh any procompetitive aspects that would justify the exchange of information. However, exchange of data relating to future prices for provider services or future compensation for employees very likely would be considered anticompetitive.

Statement 7. Joint Purchasing Arrangements Among Health Care Providers

This statement indicates that, absent extraordinary circumstances, the FTC and the DOJ will not challenge joint purchasing arrangements among health care providers if the purchases account for less than 35% of the total sales of the purchased product or service in the relevant market and the cost of the products and services purchased jointly accounts for less than 20% of the total revenues from all products or services sold by each competing participant in the joint purchasing agreement.

These conditions are imposed in an effort to avoid the potential reduction in competition when an arrangement accounts for such a large portion of the purchases in a market such that the parties can exercise anticompetitive market power, and situations where the products or services being jointly purchased account for such a large proportion of the total cost of the services being sold by the participants that the joint purchasing arrangement may facilitate price fixing.

The agencies note that joint purchasing arrangements falling outside the safety zone still may be appropriate. Several mitigating factors will reduce the risk that the joint purchasing arrangement will be found unacceptable:

1. If members of the purchasing group are not required to purchase all of a particular product or service through the purchasing arrangement.
2. Negotiations for the joint purchasing arrangement are performed by an independent employee or agent who is not also an employee or participant in the joint purchasing arrangement.
3. Communications between the purchasing group and each individual participant are kept confidential and not discussed with or disseminated to other participants.

The agencies indicate that these three safeguards will substantially reduce, if not eliminate, the purchasing arrangement as a method for discussing and coordinating prices of health care services in violation of antitrust laws.

Statements 8 (physician network joint ventures) and 9 (multiprovider networks) are elaborated and expanded by the 1996 guidelines, which follow.

1996 Guidelines

In response to the continuing change in health delivery infrastructures and business arrangements, the FTC and DOJ issued the 1996 guidelines, addressing physician network joint ventures and multiprovider networks. In these guidelines, the agencies continue to use the statement numbers of the 1994 guidelines.

Statement 8. Physician Network Joint Ventures

This statement first describes a safety zone under which physician network joint ventures will not be challenged by the agencies absent extraordinary circumstances.

First, the FTC and DOJ will not challenge an exclusive physician network joint venture whose physician-participants share substantial financial risk and constitute 20% or less of the physicians in each physician specialty with active hospital staff privileges practicing in the relevant geographic market. In an "exclusive" venture, the physician-participants do not individually contract or affiliate with other network joint ventures or health plans. The statement notes that in relevant markets where there are fewer than five physicians in a particular specialty, an exclusive physician network joint venture otherwise qualifying for this antitrust safety zone may include one physician from that specialty on a nonexclusive basis, even though this inclusion would result in the venture having greater than 20% of the physicians in that specialty.

Second, the FTC and DOJ will not challenge a nonexclusive physician network joint venture whose physician-participants share substantial financial risk and constitute 30% or less of the physicians in each physician specialty with active hospital staff privileges who practice in the relevant geographic market. In a "nonexclusive" venture, the physician-participants either do or can affiliate with other networks or contract individually with health plans. The agencies indicate that, in relevant markets with fewer than four physicians in a particular specialty, a nonexclusive network joint venture otherwise qualifying for this safety zone may include one physician from that specialty even though this inclusion would result in the venture having greater than 30% of the physicians in that specialty.

For the purposes of these safety zones, the FTC and DOJ expressly review aspects of nonexclusivity and sharing financial risk. With regard to exclusivity, the policy statement notes that nonexclusivity must be substantively true, not merely based on the form of the contractual agreement. On this issue, the agencies will assess whether the "indicia of nonexclusivity" exist:

1. Viable competing networks or managed care plans with adequate physician participation exist in the market.
2. Physicians in the network actually individually participate in, or contract with, other networks or managed care plans, or there is other evidence of their willingness to do so.
3. Physicians in the network earn substantial revenue from other networks or through individual contracts with managed care plans.
4. The absence of any indications of significant departicipation from other networks or managed care plans in the market.
5. The absence of any indication of coordination among the physicians in the network regarding price or other competitively significant terms of participation in other networks or managed care plans.

The agencies note that networks may limit or condition physician-participants' freedom to contract outside the network in a manner that may fall short of a commitment to full exclusivity; however, if these provisions significantly restrict the ability or willingness of a network's physicians to join other networks or contract individually with managed care plans, the network will be considered exclusive for the purpose of the safety zones.

Substantial sharing of financial risk also is of major concern to the FTC and DOJ. Sharing risk is considered to be a reliable indicator of sufficient integration of the physician network that provides incentives for physicians to cooperate in controlling costs and improving quality.

Examples of substantial financial risk provided by the policy statement include the following:

1. Agreement by the venture to provide services to a health plan using capitation.
2. Agreement by the venture to provide designated services or classes of services to a health plan on a percentage of premium or percentage of revenue basis.
3. Use of the venture of significant financial incentives for the physicians as a group to achieve specified cost-containment goals (e.g., withhold arrangements with distribution based on group performance in meeting cost-containment goals or overall cost or utilization targets established so that physicians are subject to substantial financial rewards or penalties based on group performance in meeting the targets).
4. Agreement by the venture to provide a complex or extended course of treatment that requires the substantial coordination of care by physicians in different specialties offering a complementary combination of services for a fixed, predetermined payment, where the costs of that course of treatment for any individual patient can vary greatly due to the individual patient's condition, the choice, complexity, or length of treatment, or other factors (i.e., global fee or all-inclusive case rate arrangements).

Note that physician network arrangements that contain both risk-sharing and non–risk-sharing arrangements are not covered by the safety zone. However, physician-participants in the network may be paid using different acceptable risk-sharing arrangements (e.g., primary care physicians being paid capitation while specialist physicians being paid on the basis of withhold arrangements).

Physician network joint ventures that do not come within the safety zones still may be acceptable under antitrust analysis. Indeed, "[t]he Agencies emphasize that merely because a physician network joint venture does not come within a safety zone in no way indicates that it is unlawful under antitrust laws."[73]

The FTC and DOJ indicate that physician network joint ventures that do not fall within the safety zones will be analyzed using a rule of reason if the physicians' integration through the network is likely to produce significant efficiencies that benefit consumers and any price agreements or other agreements that otherwise would be per se illegal by the network physicians are reasonably necessary to realize those efficiencies. Rule of reason analysis, like in other policy statements, is a four-step process, assessing the definition of the relevant market, evaluating any reduction of competition of the physician joint venture, evaluating the impact of procompetitive efficiencies, and evaluating collateral agreements.

---

[73]Ibid., p. 63.

Sharing substantive financial risk generally establishes both the overall efficiency goal and requirement for the venture. However, physician network arrangements that do not involve risk sharing may obtain the necessary efficiencies through adequate integration. Integration may be shown through the network implementing an active and ongoing program to evaluate and modify practice patterns by the network's physicians. Such a program could include:

1. Establishing mechanisms to monitor and control utilization of health care services that are designed to control costs and ensure quality of care.
2. Selectively choosing network physicians who are likely to further these efficiency objectives.
3. The significant investment of both monetary and human capital in the necessary infrastructure with the capability to realize the claimed efficiencies.

The agencies note that programs with these characteristics are not the only ones capable of showing integration. However, substantive analysis will focus on the network's likelihood of producing significant efficiencies.

The FTC and DOJ have indicated that several factors point to a network's activities as anticompetitive:

1. Statements evidencing an anticompetitive purpose.
2. A recent history of anticompetitive behavior or collusion in the market, including efforts to obstruct or undermine the development of managed care.
3. Obvious anticompetitive structures in the network (e.g., an exclusive network with a very high percentage of local area physicians without any plausible business or efficiency justification).
4. The absence of any mechanisms with the potential for generating significant efficiencies or otherwise increasing competition through the network.
5. The presence of anticompetitive collateral agreements.
6. The absence of mechanisms to prevent the network's operation from having anticompetitive spillover effects outside the network.

The presence of these characteristics may lead to the agencies' determination that the venture is merely a vehicle for fixing prices or engaging in naked anticompetitive conduct, risking an assessment under a per se rather than rule of reason analysis.

Statement 9. Multiprovider Networks

In this statement, the agencies indicate how multiprovider networks will be assessed. *Multiprovider arrangements* are defined as ventures among providers that jointly market their health care services to health plans and other purchasers. Multiprovider networks are much more heterogeneous than physician networks and may render services beyond physician services, have differing contractual relationships between providers, and provide different efficiencies in the relevant market. Standard physician networks are a subset of multiprovider networks. However, because multiprovider networks are so heterogeneous, the FTC and DOJ did not promulgate a safe harbor in this statement.

Analysis of multiprovider network agreements is very similar to that of physician network joint ventures. Multiprovider networks will be evaluated under the rule of reason analysis if the providers' integration through the network is likely to produce significant efficiencies that benefit consumers and any price agreements or other agreements that would otherwise be per se illegal by the network providers are reasonably necessary to realize those efficiencies. Like physician networks, efficiencies may be realized through agreement by the participating providers to share substantial financial risk for the services provided through the network. Examples of substantial financial risk provided by the policy statement are identical to those given for physician network joint ventures. Similarly, multiprovider networks that do not involve sharing substantial financial risk may obtain adequate efficiencies through integration. However, because of the wide range of providers involved in multiprovider networks, specific types of clinical integration will be evaluated on a case-by-case basis in assessing whether the integration is sufficient to warrant rule of reason analysis.

Note, however, some multiprovider networks are not substantially integrated and use a "messenger model" arrangement to make contracting between providers and payers easier. Messenger models can be organized and operated in a variety of ways. For example, network providers may use an agent or third party to convey to purchasers information obtained individually from providers about prices or price-related information that the providers are willing to accept. The agent in some cases may convey to the providers all contract offers made by purchasers, with each provider making an independent, unilateral decision to accept or reject the contract offer. In others, the agent may have received some authority from individual providers to accept contract offers on their behalf. The agent also may help providers understand the contracts offered, through, for example, providing objective or empirical data regarding the terms of an offer (e.g., comparison of the offered terms to other contracts agreed to by network participants).

The key issue in all messenger model arrangements is whether the arrangement creates or facilitates an agreement among competitors on prices or price-related terms, making it illegal. Determining whether there is such an agreement is a factual question in each case. The FTC and DOJ will examine whether the agent facilitates collective decision making by network providers, rather than independent, unilateral, decisions. In particular, the agencies examine whether the agent coordinates the providers, coordinates responses to a particular proposal, disseminates to network providers the views or intentions of other network providers as to the proposal, expresses an opinion on the terms offered, collectively negotiates for the providers, or determines whether or not to convey an offer based on the agent's judgment about the attractiveness of the prices or price-related terms. If the agent engages in such activities, the arrangement may amount to a per se illegal price-fixing agreement. Note, however, that arrangements designed to simply minimize costs associated with the contracting process and that do not result in competitors collectively obtaining prices or price-related information are not per se illegal price fixing.

Rule of reason analysis for multiprovider network agreements is somewhat different from that for physician networks primarily because of the broad array of providers that may be involved. Although the standard four-step test applies, certain specific differences arise. The first step continues to be determining the relevant market. However, the second step (assessing competitive effects and reductions in competition) is more extensive. For multiprovider networks, evaluation requires an assessment of "horizontal" versus "vertical" effects. Agreements between or among *competitors* are considered horizontal; agreements between or among entities that are *not* competitors are considered vertical.

When considering horizontal effects, the FTC and DOJ will assess the multiprovider's likely overall competitive effects, considering all the market conditions, including market share for services provided and concentration of competitors in the relevant market. They will be particularly attentive to the factors affecting the ability and willingness of health plans and other purchasers of health care services to switch among different health care providers or networks in response to price increases.

The agencies also examine the incentives faced by providers in the network and whether different groups of providers in a multiprovider network may have significantly different incentives that would reduce the likelihood of anticompetitive conduct. For example, if health plans and other purchasers can contract on competitive terms with other networks or individual providers while obtaining a similar quality and range of services, the multiprovider network is less likely to be anticompetitive.

Another area of importance in evaluating multiprovider networks' competitive effects is whether competing providers in the network have agreed among themselves to offer services exclusively through the network. In assessing whether the exclusivity raises antitrust concerns, the FTC and DOJ review:

1. The market share of the providers subject to the exclusivity agreement.
2. The terms of the exclusive agreement, including the duration and providers' ability and financial incentives to withdraw from the arrangement.
3. The number of providers that need to be included for the network and potentially competing networks to compete effectively.
4. The justification for the exclusivity agreement.

Vertical analysis by the agencies focuses around competitive concerns when a network's power in one market allows it to limit competition in another. Exclusivity or nonexclusivity is an important aspect in this analysis, as it is in horizontal agreements, and relevant factors assessed in horizontal agreements would be assessed for vertical ones. Further, the agencies will determine whether the multiprovider network is truly nonexclusive by considering at least the following factors, which are similar to those indicated for physician networks:

1. Viable competing networks or managed care plans with adequate provider participation currently exist in the market.
2. Providers in the network actually individually participate in, or contract with, other networks or managed care plans, or there is other evidence of their willingness and incentive to do so.
3. Providers in the network earn substantial revenue from other networks or through individual contracts with managed care plans.
4. The absence of any indications of substantial departicipation from other networks or managed care plans in the market.
5. The absence of any indications of coordination among providers in the network regarding price or other competitively significant terms of participation in other networks or managed care plans.

The policy statement also notes that truly exclusive arrangements, whether horizontal or vertical, may not be explicit. Consequently, substantive analysis is performed; the agencies do not merely rely on the label that the multiprovider network uses deeming itself nonexclusive.

The exclusion of providers is assessed, too. Because multiprovider networks will contract with some, but not all, providers in an area, there is a risk of an anticompetitive effect as well as procompetitive efficiencies. The agencies apply a rule of reason analysis in determining the legality of multiprovider network exclusion of providers as well as its policies regarding referrals of enrollees to network providers. If other networks offering the same types of services exist or could be formed or exclusion or referral policies do not affect competition, it is unlikely that significant competitive harm is associated with an exclusion of particular providers.

The third step (assessing procompetitive efficiencies) then is performed. As usual, the greater are the anticompetitive effects, the greater the procompetitive efficiencies must be. And the fourth step (evaluating collateral agreements) also is performed.

Business Review and Advisory Opinions

The DOJ and the FTC issue business review or advisory opinions regarding the antitrust legality of business activities.[74] Generally, the agencies respond to business review or advisory opinion requests within 90 days after all necessary information is submitted, except requests relating to hospital mergers outside the antitrust safety zone and multiprovider networks. Business review or advisory opinion requests regarding multiprovider networks or other nonmerger health care matters generally are provided within 120 days after all necessary information is received. Also, consent decrees through administrative law actions provide effective guidance about the acceptability of provider agreements as to antitrust.

Beyond the broad antitrust guidelines, these business review, advisory opinions, and consent decrees are extremely helpful in assessing the kinds of activities deemed legal by the agencies in their analysis of business relationships. It cannot be emphasized strongly enough that these sources should be reviewed and accessed for all agreements that have the potential for antitrust scrutiny. Summaries of several recent substantive assessments follow. An up-to-date list is available at the FTC web site.

In Re Institutional Pharmacy Network (1998) (Consent Order)[75]

Five pharmacies that provide prescription drugs to patients in long-term care institutions such as nursing homes, foster homes, and assisted living facilities (institutional pharmacies) formed the Institutional Pharmacy Network (IPN). IPN was formed to offer services jointly to MCOs that provide health care for Medicaid recipients and other medically needy persons in Oregon. IPN provided no new or more efficient services and the member pharmacies did not share risk. The five institutional pharmacies provided pharmacy services to approximately 80% of the patients receiving institutional pharmacy services in Oregon. IPN members agreed to allow IPN to collectively negotiate on behalf of each of them and fix the fees charged. IPN negotiated with four MCOs and each MCO paid IPN members a higher rate than to other institutional pharmacies. The FTC brought suit claiming the arrangement was anticompetitive; the parties settled. Under the consent decree, IPN and its member pharmacies were required to cease its joint price negotiations and agreements. However, the pharmacies were allowed to engage in conduct reasonably necessary to operate any qualified risk-sharing joint arrangement or any qualified clinically integrated joint arrangement. The pharmacies also had to distribute the consent order and file compliance

reports indicating that corporate decision makers are aware of the consent decree and are complying with it under penalty of criminal contempt.

In Re M.D. Physicians of Southwest La., Inc. (1998) (Consent Order)[76]

M.D. Physicians of Southwest La., Inc. (MDP) is a physician group that includes a majority of the physicians in and around Lake Charles, Louisiana, in Calcasieu Parish. MDP was formed in 1987 to deal with MCOs entering into the market. According to the FTC, until 1994, MDP refused to participate in health care plans offered by Blue Cross and Blue Shield of Louisiana, the Louisiana State Employee Benefits Program, the Louisiana State Employees Group Benefits Program, Aetna Insurance Company, Healthcare Advantage, Inc., and other payers attempting to do business in Calcasieu Parish. During this period, the physicians in MDP dealt with payers only through MDP. However, these physicians had not integrated their practices in any economically significant manner and had not created any efficiencies that might have justified their concerted actions; formation of MDP appeared to be for the purpose of fixing prices and other terms under which MDP physicians would deal with payers and to prevent or delay entry of managed care into the market. The FTC challenged MDP actions as anticompetitive and the parties settled. MDP agreed to stop its anticompetitive activities, including not engaging in collective negotiations about price or fixing prices for its members. MDP was allowed to engage in conduct that is reasonably necessary to operate any qualified risk-sharing joint arrangement or qualified clinically integrated joint arrangement (the latter with prior notice to the FTC). MDP also had to distribute copies of the consent order and file compliance reports to the FTC.

In Re Mesa County Physicians Independent Practice Association, Inc. (1998) (Consent Order)[77]

Mesa County Physicians Independent Practice Association (Mesa IPA), formed in 1987, included more than 180 physicians, representing at least 85% of all physician and at least 90% of the primary care physicians in private practice in Mesa County, Colorado. Mesa IPA was formed to protect the economic interests of Mesa County physicians in their dealings with managed care organizations. Mesa IPA contracted with Rocky Moun-

---

[74]28 C.F.R. §50.6 (1998); 16 C.F.R. §§1.1–1.4 (1998).

[75]In re Institutional Pharmacy Network, FTC File No. 9610005 (FTC May 21, 1998).

[76]In re M.D. Physicians of Southwest La., Inc., File No. 9410095 (FTC June 19, 1998).

[77]In re Mesa County Physicians Indep. Practice Ass'n, Inc., Docket No. 9284 (FTC February 19, 1998).

tain HMO, a payer based in Mesa County, whose enrollees accounted for at least 50% of the total patient volume of Mesa IPA's physician members. In 1993, Mesa IPA began negotiating on behalf of its members with several payers that sought to enter Mesa County. Mesa IPA encouraged its members to refuse to deal individually with the payers or do so only on terms approved by Mesa IPA's Contract Review Committee. Mesa IPA's Board of Directors approved a set of guidelines and a fee schedule conversion factor to be used to review contract offers. The conversion factors resulted in significantly higher prices for physicians' services for several payers than would have been the case absent the agreement among Mesa IPA members. As a result of these activities, PPOs, HMOs, and employer health care purchasing cooperatives were precluded from doing business in Mesa County. The FTC challenged Mesa IPA's activities as anticompetitive, and the parties settled. The FTC concluded that Mesa IPA members had not integrated their medical practices to create efficiencies that justified their collective contract negotiations and other anticompetitive activity. The consent order prohibited Mesa IPA from engaging in collective negotiations for its members, collectively refusing to contract with payers, acting as an exclusive bargaining agent for its members, restricting its members from dealing with payers through an entity other than Mesa IPA, exchanging information among its physician members about the terms on which physicians are willing to deal with payers, and encouraging or pressuring others to engage in any activities prohibited by the consent order. Mesa IPA also was required to notify its members and third parties about the consent order, amend its physicians' manual to bring it in compliance with the consent order, abolish its Contract Review Committee, provide payers the option to terminate any existing contracts with the IPA that do not comply with the order, and for the next five years, publish and distribute copies of the complaint and order to its members. Mesa IPA was allowed to engage in legitimate activities that are reasonably necessary for Mesa IPA to operate any qualified risk-sharing joint arrangement or any qualified clinically integrated joint arrangement.

Phoenix Medical Network, Inc. (1998)[78]

Phoenix Medical Network (PMN) proposed to form a for-profit company owned by its physician members, most of whom would be the providers for the network, in northwestern Pennsylvania. PMN would be formed to enter into provider contracts with payers on behalf of

its physician members. The network would be nonexclusive; PMN physicians would share financial risk through a percentage of premium methodology and participate in utilization review, quality assurance programs, and credentialing programs. PMN would have approximately 18% of primary care physicians and approximately 40% of specialist physicians in the anticipated market. The proposal was not challenged by the FTC as anticompetitive because, although some of the levels of physician participation were high, there are plausible business reasons for such inclusion; payers in the area did not express concern that the formation of PMN would directly impede competition; and PMN's structure for risk sharing had the potential to inject a new type of competition into the market. However, antitrust concerns would be raised if the physician-participants refused to participate in other managed care plans, if they agreed to participate only on terms comparable to PMN, or they otherwise used PMN as a vehicle for coordinating their pricing.

CVT Surgical Center (1997)[79]

Two groups of peripheral vascular surgeons in the Baton Rouge, Louisiana, area proposed to merge into a single integrated practice to contract more efficiently with managed care and other payers. The proposed market was a large geographic area that extended to New Orleans. The proposal was not challenged by the DOJ as anticompetitive. Even though the DOJ did not accept the market definition provided by the physician groups, it still allowed the merger. The DOJ defined the market as Baton Rouge, so that the merged entity would have approximately 50% of the vascular surgeons in the area. However, even with this market definition, several factors influenced the DOJ to allow the merger. The DOJ noted that a New Orleans–based clinic had opened a facility in Baton Rouge, and peripheral vascular surgeons affiliated with this clinic either already practiced in Baton Rouge or would do so in response to any price increases by the merged entity; other types of specialists such as cardiologists could perform many of the procedures; payers required as few as only one peripheral vascular surgeon in a network to adequately serve the needs of their enrollees; payers indicated to the DOJ that they believed there were other market substitutes available or recruitable if the merged entities raised prices anticompetitively; and significant efficiencies could result, including improved patient care due to increased patient volume.

---

[78]"Phoenix Medical Network, Inc.," *FTC Staff Advisory Letter* (May 19, 1998).

[79]"CVT Surgical Center," *DOJ Business Review Letter* (Antitrust Div., April 16, 1997).

First Priority Health System (1997)[80]

First Priority Health (FPH), an HMO, and NEPPO Ltd. (NEPPO), a limited partnership of 166 primary care and specialist physicians, proposed a joint venture to form First Priority Health System (FPHS), a risk-bearing health delivery organization that would provide and manage health care services for HMO enrollees in Scranton, Pennsylvania, and surrounding counties. NEPPO agreed that FPHS would be the exclusive managed care plan for most of its primary care physicians, who would serve as gatekeepers; however, all NEPPO primary care physicians would be able to contract with non–gatekeeper-type plans. All specialists contracting with FPHS and all primary care physicians not in NEPPO would be allowed to contract with other payers. Prices for all physicians in FPHS would be determined by the Reimbursement Committee of FPHS, which was made up entirely of members of the FPHS Board of Directors appointed by FPH, the payer. No physicians would be involved in setting prices paid by FPHS for physician services. The proposed agreement was not challenged by the DOJ as anticompetitive because it represented an innovative and potentially procompetitive venture, nearly 70% of the area's primary care physicians would be available to contract with other health plans to provide primary care services, and the venture would not likely foreclose other area managed care plans from competing for enrollees in the area.

FTC v. College of Physicians-Surgeons of Puerto Rico (1997) (Consent Order)[81]

The College of Physicians-Surgeons of Puerto Rico (College) and three physician groups collectively demanded that the Puerto Rican government recognize the College as the exclusive bargaining agent for all the physicians of Puerto Rico, allow the College to collectively negotiate contracts for the physicians, provide more control to the physicians over the distribution of funds, and decrease the financial risk borne by the physicians. The College indicated that if its demands were not met, it would boycott Puerto Rican health care programs. The demands were not met and the College and three physician groups boycotted the programs. The FTC and the Attorney General of Puerto Rico claimed the College and the physician groups violated antitrust laws by harming consumers through denying them access to health care services, restraining competition among physicians, fixing prices, raising costs to consumers and payers, and depriving con-

sumers of independently determined reimbursement policies and prices. The parties settled, and the College and physician groups agreed not to boycott or refuse to deal with payers, not to refuse to provide services to individuals covered by payers, and not to negotiate or fix prices charged for physician services. The settlement also required the defendants to pay $300,000 in restitution to the catastrophic fund of the government of Puerto Rico and publish in the College's official newsletter the consent order and distribute copies of the consent order to payers. The settlement did not prevent the defendants from engaging in qualifying, integrated joint ventures that produce procompetitive efficiencies.

Vermont Physicians Clinic (1997)[82]

Approximately 40 physicians practicing several specialties in the Rutland, Vermont, area proposed to form a joint venture, the Vermont Physicians Clinic (Clinic), to offer their services as a group to health care payers. Clinic would negotiate risk contracts with payers, provide utilization review, quality improvement, and administrative services. These activities would provide significant efficiencies that would benefit payers and their enrollees. The joint venture would include no more than 30% of the physicians in most of physician specialties. The proposal was not challenged by the DOJ as anticompetitive because local area managed care plans and other payers expressed no concerns that the Clinic would lessen competition substantially and the joint venture would provide competition to the only other managed care entity in the area.

Yellowstone Physicians, L.L.C. (1997)[83]

Several groups of physicians proposed to form Yellowstone Physicians, L.L.C. (Yellowstone), a multispecialty physician network joint venture for the Billings, Montana, market. The market includes two HMOs, two hospitals, several PPOs, and a public/private employer-based purchasing cooperative that is organizing an effort to contract with provider-sponsored networks. The proposed arrangement would be nonexclusive, with approximately 39% of Billings's area physicians, including 33% of primary care physicians, 64% of the area's general surgeons, and 53% of the obstetricians–gynecologists. These physicians would share financial risk through either capitation or fee for service with withholds. A medical services discounted internal fee schedule would determine payments to participating

---

[80]"First Priority Health System," *DOJ Business Review Letter* (Antitrust Div., November 3, 1997).

[81]FTC v. College of Physicians-Surgeons of P.R., FTC File No. 9710011 (D.P.R. Oct. 2, 1997).

[82]"Vermont Physicians Clinic," *DOJ Business Review Letter* (Antitrust Div., July 30, 1997).

[83]"Yellowstone Physicians, L.L.C.," *FTC Staff Advisory Letter* (May 14, 1997).

physicians, with surpluses and withholds allocated based on physician performance against predetermined quality assurance and cost-containment goals. Financial risk would be managed through implementation of utilization review, quality assurance activities, and credentialing standards and procedures. The proposal was not challenged by the FTC as anticompetitive. Yellowstone's structure was seen to involve provider sharing of substantial financial risk through its medical management protocols and financial incentives. However, the FTC expressed concern with regard to the high percentage of specialists that would participate in the venture because the market contained a large multispecialty clinic; therefore, when Yellowstone would enter the market, payers most likely would have to contract with Yellowstone or the large clinic. This situation would have the danger of Yellowstone physicians either refusing to participate in other managed care plans or conditioning their participation on obtaining terms similar to Yellowstone's. Yellowstone responded that: the provider panel was structured in this manner because, in some circumstances, participation of particular group practices was necessary to ensure adequate coverage for that specialty at each Billings hospital; some groups had members in which one or more physicians were unusually qualified in particular specialties, thus requiring their inclusion in Yellowstone for quality of care purposes; it was impossible or impractical for Yellowstone to offer participation to some but not all members of a group practice; and some of the physicians already practiced together in integrated groups, and including them in Yellowstone's provider panel would not reduce competition between these group members because they already do not compete with each other. These justifications were accepted by the FTC as valid business reasons for its provider panel structure. Finally, no payers expressed concern over Yellowstone's formulation or operational plan and the FTC noted that Yellowstone's entry into the market would introduce a type of competition into the Billings market that had not existed before.

Allied Colon and Rectal Specialists (1996)[84]

Seven of nine dedicated colon and rectal specialists in Maricopa County, Arizona, who also represented seven of ten of these specialists statewide, proposed to form a nonexclusive physician network of colon and rectal surgical specialists in the Phoenix area that would negotiate and contract with health benefit plans to provide colon and rectal surgical and related services. The venture would be called Allied Colon and Rectal Specialists (Allied). Allied physician-participants would be paid on the basis of capitation or a discounted fee-for-service system with a 20% withhold. The

withhold amounts would be distributed on the basis of reaching preestablished efficiency and quality parameters. Allied also would establish safeguards on information flow among its members to eliminate anticompetitive sharing of information. The proposed arrangement was not challenged by the DOJ as anticompetitive. The DOJ indicated that the arrangement involved significant risk sharing and had the potential to benefit MCOs and their enrollees through efficiencies that could result from the payers' ability to contract with a group of providers through a single entity and from utilization review and quality assurance activities. Finally, the high percentage of providers in Allied would not raise concerns because many other types of surgeons, including general surgeons and osteopathic surgeons, routinely performed similar procedures; this perspective was verified by payers in the market.

Children's Healthcare, P.A. (1996)[85]

Sixty-five to 70 pediatricians, representing approximately 50–75% of the pediatricians in several important local markets in southern New Jersey, proposed to form a nonexclusive joint venture network. The network would have been formed for the purpose of negotiating and contracting with managed care plans to provide children's health care. Members of the network would have maintained independent practices and generally would have been allowed to participate in other networks or contract individually with payers. The proposed network was challenged by the DOJ as anticompetitive. The DOJ noted that basic health care for children was provided in local markets; this was verified by discussions with payers, hospitals, employers, and physicians. Further, family practitioners and other physicians were not effective substitutes for pediatricians in managed care plans. Because of these factors, the network would have achieved substantial market power in several significant local markets, which would have allowed it to increase prices and reduce competition in those markets; consumers would have faced a high risk of anticompetitive action and harm if the network were formed as proposed.

Cincinnati Regional Orthopedic and Sports Medicine Associates, Inc. (1996)[86]

Of the 158 orthopedic surgeons in the greater Cincinnati, Ohio, metropolitan area, 56 (35% of the special-

[84]"Allied Colon and Rectal Specialists," *DOJ Business Review Letter* (Antitrust Div., July 1, 1996).

[85]"Children's Healthcare, P.A.," *DOJ Business Review Letter* (Antitrust Div., March 1, 1996).

[86]"Cincinnati Regional Orthopedic and Sports Medicine Assocs., Inc.," *DOJ Business Review Letter* (Antitrust Div., October 4, 1996).

ists in the market) proposed to form a nonexclusive physician joint venture network, the Cincinnati Regional Orthopedic Sports Medicine Association (CROSMA). CROSMA would be formed to negotiate and contract with MCOs and other payers. CROSMA would contract with payers using capitation and, at a later time, could expand to the use of discounted fee for service with a withhold of at least 20%. CROSMA would establish safeguards to prevent flow of competitively related information among its physicians. The withhold would be distributed only if the physicians as a group met preestablished efficiency and quality goals. CROSMA also would engage in utilization review and quality assurance monitoring. The proposed arrangement was not challenged by the DOJ as anticompetitive because there was substantial sharing of risk, it was nonexclusive, it potentially would benefit managed care plans and their enrollees through efficiencies that could result from the payers' ability to contract with a group of providers through a single entity, and utilization review and quality assurance measures could improve the quality of care.

Home Care Alliance, Inc. (1996)[87]

Three home health providers in Mississippi proposed to form a nonexclusive network, Home Care Alliance, Inc. (Alliance), to contract with managed care plans, employers, and other payers to provide statewide home health care coverage. The Alliance would use a messenger model for contracting by providing each payer with each home health provider's fee schedule and transmitting any payer contract offers to the providers for their consideration. Each payer could accept or reject each contract as well as contract independently with any payer as well as join any other network. The Alliance would engage in utilization review, quality assurance, and credentialing of its members but would not attempt to impose any standards for these activities on payers. In Mississippi, home health providers serve in state-designated territories beyond which the providers may not market. The three home health providers forming Alliance served completely separate parts of the state with the exception of one county. The proposal was not challenged by the DOJ as anticompetitive because the use of the messenger model would preclude any sharing of each home health provider's contract terms, would allow other home health care providers to join the network without harming competition, and would not result in price agreements among competitors.

Mayo Medical Laboratories (1996)[88]

Mayo Medical Laboratories (Mayo) proposed to establish two networks of hospital labs to perform services for outpatients who are members of managed care plans. One network was a statewide network in Michigan and the other was a regional network in the San Francisco Bay area. Mayo indicated that HMOs and other payers increasingly preferred regional, statewide, or national laboratory service contracts. The proposed networks would provide a great majority of laboratory services using capitation or withhold arrangements. Mayo indicated that since some of the payers would request the use of discounted fee for service, in these situations the networks would use an independent agent that would develop an initial offer based on a price survey of network members. Individual network members would make independent decisions with regard to accepting the payer's offer. Mayo's members also would work with payers and their physician panels to create integrated laboratory delivery systems. The proposal was not challenged by the FTC as anticompetitive. The FTC noted that Mayo's proposed use of an agent did result in a price agreement among the members of the network. However, because the networks would involve substantial integration among their members that was likely to produce significant efficiencies, the price agreements were reasonably necessary for the networks to achieve this efficiency, and the networks intended to apply the types of coordination and integration among the network laboratories to manage costs under the risk contracts to their services provided under the nonrisk contracts, it was permissible. Finally, the FTC noted that neither planned network involved a large percentage of hospitals in its service area, and Mayo faced significant competition from commercial laboratories; therefore, the two networks posed no significant risk to competition in the areas where they would operate.

Southwest Florida Oral Surgery Associates (1996)[89]

Southwest Florida Oral Surgery Associates (SFOSA), comprising three oral and maxillofacial surgery practices in different cities in southwest Florida, proposed to form a cooperative (the Cooperative) to jointly market their members' services to employers, MCOs, and other payers. The Cooperative's activities would include group purchasing, joint marketing, and sharing of medical information systems. Membership would be nonexclusive, with members allowed to join other networks and market their practices independently. There would be no

---

[87]"Home Care Alliance, Inc.," *DOJ Business Review Letter* (Antitrust Div., October 4, 1996).

[88]"Mayo Med. Labs.," *FTC Staff Advisory Letter* (July 17, 1996).
[89]"Southwest Florida Oral Surgery Associates," *FTC Staff Advisory Letter* (December 2, 1996).

requirement that all practices enter into any particular service agreement, and no members would be barred from entering into other arrangements not offered through the Cooperative. Each of the member practices would continue to operate individually and perform its own claims processing and administrative functions. The Cooperative would designate one employee from one of the practices to serve as a "marketing representative," responsible for all communication between the member practices and payers. The marketing representative would not negotiate with payers or enter into contracts on behalf of the practices and would circulate any proposed contracts to member practices only individually. Each practice would be free to accept or reject these offers or negotiate terms directly with the payer. Member practices would not discuss among themselves any terms of any contract offers. The proposal was not challenged by the FTC as anticompetitive because there was no issue of a horizontal agreement on prices and it appeared that the parties would not enter into other potentially anticompetitive agreements in dealing with payers in the market.

United States v. Woman's Hospital Foundation (1996) (Consent Order)[90]

Woman's Hospital is a specialty hospital that delivers approximately 94% of the privately insured newborns in Baton Rouge, Louisiana. Woman's Hospital also has on staff virtually every obstetrician and gynecologist in Baton Rouge. In 1993, Woman's Hospital formed an alliance with almost all the obstetricians and gynecologists in Baton Rouge serving privately insured patients to maintain its monopoly in inpatient hospitalization obstetrical services. Further, Woman's Hospital persuaded these physicians not to admit their patients to other hospitals and attempted to get a competitor to agree not to provide inpatient obstetrical services at its health center. The alliance established a minimum fee schedule for physician services and jointly negotiated with managed care plans for hospital and physician services. The resulting fees were substantially higher than fees these physicians had obtained previously, when they individually contracted with the largest MCO in Baton Rouge. The DOJ brought suit against the parties to the alliance and a settlement resulted. The settlement stopped the hospital and the physicians from preventing other medical facilities in Baton Rouge from providing inpatient obstetrical services and from colluding to drive up costs for obstetrical care in Baton Rouge; it was designed to foster the development of lower-cost managed care plans in Baton Rouge.

In Re RxCare of Tennessee, Inc. (1996) (Consent Order)[91]

RxCare was created by the Tennessee Pharmacists Association, the largest professional pharmacist association in the state. RxCare runs a pharmacy network that includes greater than 95% of all chain and independent pharmacies in Tennessee. RxCare member pharmacies fill prescriptions for patients covered by Blue Cross/Blue Shield of Tennessee and several MCOs providing services in public and private health care plans and are reimbursed by these payers. RxCare required that all its member pharmacies agree to a "most favored nation" (MFN) clause, indicating that if a member pharmacy accepted a reimbursement from a payer that was lower than the RxCare rate, the pharmacy would have to accept that lower rate for all RxCare business as well. RxCare enforced the MFN clause and urged pharmacies to refrain from participating in networks that offered reimbursement rates lower than that of RxCare. The MFN clause resulted in a price floor because pharmacies were reluctant to have to accept reimbursement rates for all their RxCare's business lower than RxCare's levels, resulting in payers paying higher pharmacy reimbursement rates in Tennessee than in other states. Further, other entities had not been able to establish lower-priced pharmacy networks in Tennessee. The FTC challenged RxCare's MFN clause and actions as anticompetitive; the parties settled. The FTC noted that the MFN clause discouraged network pharmacies from discounting and thus limited price competition among pharmacies in their contracts with pharmacy benefits managers and payers, particularly since RxCare represented such a large proportion of each pharmacy's business. In addition, because of RxCare's significant presence in the market, pharmacies would incur financially unacceptable revenue loss if they accepted rates below RxCare's reimbursement rate for all their RxCare business. The consent order required RxCare to eliminate the MFN clause from its contracts with participating pharmacies and to show compliance with the order by periodic reporting to the FTC.

United States v. Classic Care Network (1995) (Consent Order)[92]

Eight hospitals created the Classic Care Corporation to negotiate managed care contracts. The hospitals entered into agreement that each hospital would not enter into contracts with any managed care organizations without the

---

[90]United States v. Woman's Hosp. Found., No. 96-389-B-M2 (M.D. La. April 23, 1996).

[91]In re RxCare of Tenn., Inc., FTC File No. 951-0059 (FTC Dec. 21, 1995).

[92]United States v. Classic Care Network, 1995-1 Trade Cas. (CCH) ¶70,997, No. 94-5566 (E.D. N.Y. May 1, 1995).

approval of every other hospital in the network, that the network would be the sole bargaining agent for each hospital regarding managed care contracts, that no discounts would be permitted from its inpatient hospital rates in managed care contracts, and that outpatient discounts for the network hospital were to be limited to no more than 10% off regular rates. The DOJ challenged the agreement as anticompetitive, indicating that it unreasonably restrained trade and price competition. The parties settled; the hospitals agreed to not enter into contracts with any other hospital in the area with terms regarding the negotiation of or refusal to accept any contracts with managed care or other payers, not to communicate the amount of any negotiated fee or discounts, to have each hospital file annually for five years certification that it is abiding by the settlement, and to have each hospital certify that its directors and officers had read the settlement agreement and were aware that noncompliance with it could result in conviction for criminal contempt, imprisonment, and fines.

ACMG, Inc. (1994)[93]

ACMG proposed to the Montana State Medical Society to form a statewide PPO. At the time, only one managed care program was operating in the state. ACMG planned to have the PPO market only to self-funded employers. The PPO would have been sponsored by the medical association and operated by ACMG. Physicians would have agreed to adopt a compensation schedule that set a maximum payment for each service; physicians would have been required to submit current fees for each service for review by ACMG, and ACMG would have notified each physician of any fees exceeding the maximum allowable charge. Physicians also would have agreed to subject themselves to a 15% risk pool for each payer in the program. It was estimated that approximately 50% of the physicians in the state would have participated and that the PPO would have few, if any, competitors. The agreement was challenged by the FTC as anticompetitive because the arrangement involved a horizontal agreement among competing physicians that could not be justified as ancillary to partial integration of the physicians' practices and there was a substantial possibility that the PPO would obtain market power.

Bay Area Business Group on Health (1994)[94]

The Bay Area Business Group on Health (BBGH), a San Francisco nonprofit organization, solicited business membership for which 16 businesses expressed interest. BBGH proposed to ask several HMOs to bid on two standard benefit plans and to negotiate prices with those HMOs. BBGH-participating companies could negotiate separately from the group with HMOs not involved with or approved by BBGH. The proposed arrangement was not challenged by the DOJ as anticompetitive because a substantial majority of all potential HMO customers were not to be represented by BBGH and BBGH had the potential to create efficiencies in the delivery of HMO services that could result in lower health care costs in the market. Even though some current BBGH members were direct competitors, the members' costs of purchasing HMO health benefits accounted for only a small percentage of the selling price of their products and services.

Birmingham Cooperative Clinical Benchmarking Demonstration Project (1994)[95]

Ten hospitals and 24 businesses in the Birmingham area proposed to collect information on clinical effectiveness and costs of obstetrical delivery, pneumonia treatment, and acute myocardial infarction treatment as well as to compare outcomes between Birmingham averages, national averages, and national "benchmark" averages. The information would be collected by an independent corporation, and each report would be based on data more than three months old. This proposal was not challenged by the DOJ as anticompetitive because this collaboration between purchasers and providers had the potential for allowing businesses to make better informed health care purchasing decisions and promoting hospital effectiveness and efficiency in delivery of these services.

Collaborative Provider Organization, Inc. (1994)[96]

Des Moines General Hospital and 177 physicians located in south-central Iowa proposed to form a PHO to offer a health care plan to businesses in a 25-county area that were seeking new ways to cover their workers' health care needs. The PHO providers would contract with payers using capitation and discounted fee for service with a 20% withhold. The Collaborative Provider Organization (CPO) would not be directly involved in setting fees but would retain a third-party administrator who would survey CPO providers and compile aggregate fee information to be used in negotiating contracts with purchasers

[93]"ACMG, Inc.," *FTC Staff Advisory Opinion* (July 5, 1994).

[94]"Bay Area Business Group," *DOJ Business Review Letter* (Antitrust Div., February 18, 1994).

[95]"Birmingham Cooperative Clinical Benchmarking Demonstration Project," *DOJ Business Review Letter* (Antitrust Div., June 20, 1994).

[96]"Collaborative Provider Organization," *DOJ Business Review Letter* (Antitrust Div., July 6, 1994).

for health care services. In the most populous county, less than 20% of all licensed physicians would join CPO, and less than 20% of primary care physicians in the county would participate. In addition, in 18 to 30 identified specialties, CPO would have less than 20% of the providers; however, in 12 specialties, CPO would have greater than 20%. No CPO provider would have access to another CPO provider's fees, pricing data, or financial information. The proposal was not challenged by the DOJ as anticompetitive since the providers participating in CPO would share risk through both capitation and a withhold agreement. Further, the proposal would provide an additional, alternative health care system in the market and thus could increase competition and lower costs for consumers in that market.

Houston Health Care Coalition (1994)[97]

Several Houston, Texas, area businesses proposed to join together as the Houston Health Care Coalition (Coalition) and form the Group Purchasing Association (Association). No Coalition member would be required to join the Association. Any person, business association, or organization meeting the Association's membership criteria could join the Association by paying a membership fee. The Association would be formed to seek lower health care costs and to contract with health care providers to provide health care services to Coalition member employees. The Association would be a nonprofit corporation and would contract with any health care provider that accepted the Association's reimbursement schedule and met its objective quality criteria. Each Association member would be able to contract with a provider at the price negotiated by the Association or could negotiate its own agreement with the provider or any non-Association provider. The Association would have no control over any member's design, implementation, or operation of its benefits package. The Coalition would set reimbursement rates by having a consultant compile data from approximately 65 providers for services associated with specified DRGs. No provider would have access to the data submitted by any other provider, and only Association members would have access to the information. These aggregated rates would be the basis of the fee schedule. No more than 20% of any health care specialist providers in any market would be Association members. In addition, no provider who was also an Association member would be allowed to negotiate or set reimbursement rates for the Association. The proposed arrangement was not challenged by the DOJ as anticompetitive because the group purchasing concern had the potential for reduced costs for health care services in the market and appropriate safeguards against potential provider collusion.

New Jersey Hospital Association (1994)[98]

The New Jersey Hospital Association proposed to perform a survey and report on wages and salaries paid by hospitals in New Jersey in aggregated form and at least three months old. This proposal was not challenged by the DOJ as anticompetitive because the survey and report would be compiled and published by an independent third party on the basis of information at least three months old and would provide information solely on an aggregated basis so that individual hospital responses would not be discernable.

Physician Care, Inc. (1994)[99]

More than 100 of the 276 physicians in south-central Kentucky proposed to form a nonexclusive provider network, Physician Care, Inc. (PCI), to offer services to self-insured employers and other payers in the area. Providers would be paid using capitation or discounted fee for services with a 20% withhold. PCI would establish utilization standards and other measures to contain costs. In some markets, as much as 37% or more of the primary care providers would be in PCI. No PCI provider would have access to another provider's fees, pricing data, or other financial information. The proposal was not challenged by the DOJ as anticompetitive because the venture was nonexclusive, the providers share no significant financial risk, financial data would not be shared, and the venture would provide an alternative health care service to consumers. Although high percentages of providers in certain markets would be participating in PCI, in the largely rural areas where the network would operate, the percentages are necessary to provide adequate coverage for enrollees.

Preferred Podiatric Network, Inc. (1994)[100]

Preferred Podiatric Network, Inc. (PPN), a subsidiary of the New York State Podiatric Medical Association, proposed to act as a nonexclusive intermediary to facilitate communication between unintegrated groups of podia-

---

[97]"Houston Health Care Coalition," *DOJ Business Review Letter* (Antitrust Div., March 23, 1994).

[98]"New Jersey Hospital Association," *DOJ Business Review Letter* (Antitrust Div., February 18, 1994).

[99]"Physician Care, Inc.," *DOJ Business Review Letter* (Antitrust Div., October 28, 1994).

[100]"Preferred Podiatric Network, Inc.," *DOJ Business Review Letter* (Antitrust Div., September 14, 1994).

trists who are members of the association and managed care plans. PPN would not negotiate with payers and fee information would not be shared with or among members; PPN would merely gather and provide to payers generalized price information. Each member would be free to accept or reject any offer. This proposed arrangement was not challenged by the DOJ as anticompetitive because the fee information would not be shared, PPN would be a bona fide intermediary and not a negotiator for competing podiatrists, PPN was nonexclusive, and PPN would not impede the participation of its members as providers in other managed care networks.

Pulmonary Associates Ltd. and Albuquerque Pulmonary Consultants P.A. (1994)[101]

Two pulmonary specialist groups in Albuquerque, New Mexico, proposed to merge their practices. Each group had four full-time and one part-time physician. The merged entity would compete with at least 100 physicians offering similar services in the market. The proposal was not challenged by the DOJ as anticompetitive because the pulmonologists were not the exclusive providers of the services they rendered; indeed, they faced competition from general, cardiac, and thoracic surgeons as well as internal medicine and family practice physicians. Further, because HMOs and other payers in the area employed, contracted with, or reimbursed many nonpulmonologists for the same services that were offered by pulmonologists and staff privileges in market hospitals were extended to nonpulmonologists to perform these services, the merged entity would not be able to exert market power.

Notes on Antitrust

Clayton Act and Nonprofits

Because of the unique wording of the Clayton Act, it has been questioned as to whether activities relating to the acquisitions of nonprofit entities such as hospitals fall within the statute. Most courts have come to the conclusion that, notwithstanding the wording of the statute, the Clayton Act does encompass nonprofit asset acquisitions and the FTC therefore can challenge these business consolidations.[102]

Additional Reading. D. L. Glazer, "Clayton Act Scrutiny of Nonprofit Hospital Mergers: The Wrong Rx for Ailing Institutions," *Washington Law Review* 66 (1991), pp. 1041–60; P. A. Jorissen, "Antitrust Challenges to Nonprofit Hospital Mergers Under Section 7 of the Clayton Act," *Loyola University of Chicago Law Journal* 21 (1990), 1231–68; L. L. Stephens, "Nonprofit Hospital Mergers and Section 7 of the Clayton Act: Closing an Antitrust Loophole," *Boston University Law Review* 75 (1995), pp. 477–503.

"Essential Facility"

An essential facility is one that, in practical terms, cannot be reproduced by competitors. An entity or individual who controls an essential facility may be liable under antitrust laws if the entity or the individual refuses to allow access to that facility on fair terms. However, for providers that wish access to a hospital, it has been held that the essential facility doctrine is inapplicable to hospitals and physician staff.[103] Therefore, even if the hospital is the only one in the community, providers have no right of access under antitrust laws.

Additional Reading. M. L. Azcuenaga, "Essential Facilities and Regulation: Court or Agency Jurisdiction?" *Antitrust Law Journal* 58 (1989), pp. 879–86; A. Kezsbom and A. V. Goldman, "No Shortcut to Antitrust Analysis: The Twisted Journey of the 'Essential Facilities' Doctrine," *Columbia Business Law Review* (1996), pp. 1–36; S. D. Makar, "The Essential Facility Doctrine and the Health Care Industry," *Florida State University Law Review* 21 (1994), pp. 913–43; C. M. Seelan, "The Essential Facilities Doctrine: What Does It Mean to Be Essential?" *Marquette Law Review* 80 (1997), pp. 1117–33.

Exclusion of a Class of Provider

Hospitals may attempt to exclude certain types of providers from their staffs. These actions are subject to antitrust laws. Overall, if the exclusion results in higher-quality services, thus making the excluding entity more competitive, then the exclusions are not illegal. Therefore, exclusion of nurse anesthetists[104] and podiatrists[105] has

---

[101]"Pulmonary Association, Ltd.," *DOJ Business Review Letter* (Antitrust Div., October 31, 1994).

[102]See, e.g., FTC v. Freeman Hosp., 69 F.3d 260 (8th Cir. 1995); FTC v. University Health, Inc., 938 F.2d 1206, 1217 (11th Cir. 1991); United States v. Rockford Mem. Corp., 898 F.2d 1278, 1281 (7th Cir. 1990); cf. United States v. Carilion Health Sys., 707 F.Supp. 840, 841 n.1 (W.D. Va.) (Clayton Act does not apply to nonprofit acquisitions), *aff'd per curiam without published opinion* 892 F.2d 1042 (4th Cir. 1989).

[103]See, e.g., Pontius v. Children's Hosp., 552 F.Supp. 1352, 1370 (W.D. Pa. 1982); Castelli v. Meadville Med. Ctr., 702 F.Supp. 1201, 1209 (W.D. Pa. 1988).

[104]See, e.g., Bhan v. NME Hosp. Inc., 929 F.2d 1404 (1991).

[105]See, e.g., Cameron v. New Hanover Mem. Hosp., Inc., 293 S.E.2d 901 (N.C. Ct. App. 1982).

been held to be valid under antitrust laws.[106] However, discrimination of osteopathic physicians by allopathic physicians in staff decisions has been held to violate antitrust laws when different standards were applied to one versus the other.[107] However, if the same standards are applied, there is no antitrust violation.[108] Further, exclusive contracts with a physician or group of physicians or other providers are not illegal under antitrust laws if the decision is to promote high-quality care.[109] This concept applies to insurance companies that selectively contract with institutional providers such as hospitals.[110]

Additional Reading. B. A. Liang, "An Overview and Analysis of Challenges to Medical Exclusive Contracts," *Journal of Legal Medicine* 18 (1997), pp. 1–45; G. Reindl, "Denying Hospital Privileges to Non-Physicians: Does Quality Justify a Potential Restraint of Trade?" *Indiana Law Review* 19 (1986), pp. 1219–51; D. Ruder, "Antitrust and the Credentialing and Decredentialing of Physicians," *Northern Kentucky Law Review* 19 (1992), pp. 351–64.

Failing Firm Defense

Section 7 of the Clayton Act[111] is not violated if the only alternative to a business consolidation is elimination of one of the merging firms from the market.[112] This defense has been held by the Supreme Court to require that the firm alleged to be failing must be subject to "the grave probability of a business failure" and the acquiring firm be the only available purchaser.[113] The DOJ and the FTC have refined the Supreme Court analysis by indicating that:

1. The purportedly failing entity must be unable to meet its financial obligations in the near future.
2. The entity must be unable to reorganize under Chapter 11 of the Bankruptcy Act.
3. The entity must have made an unsuccessful good faith effort to obtain reasonable alternative offers for the acquisition of its assets that would have kept those assets in the relevant markets.
4. Without the acquisition, the assets of the failing entity would exit the relevant market.[114]

The primary difficulty of this defense is the definition of a *reasonable alternative offer*. The FTC and DOJ have indicated that offers to purchase the assets at a price greater than the liquidation value of the assets is considered reasonable.[115]

Additional Reading. E. O. Correia, "Re-Examining the Failing Company Defense," *Antitrust Law Journal* 64 (1996), pp. 683–701; R. D. Friedman, "Untangling the Failing Company Doctrine," *Texas Law Review* 64 (1986), pp. 1375–1426; T. Paredes, "Turning the Failing Firm Defense into a Success: A Proposal to Revise the Horizontal Merger Guidelines," *Yale Journal on Regulation* 13 (1996), pp. 347–90.

Health Care Quality Improvement Act and Peer Review

The Health Care Quality Improvement Act[116] (HCQIA) was enacted in response to antitrust suits against providers that participated in peer review activities that resulted in sanctions against the reviewed providers.[117] To encourage participation in peer review activities, HCQIA provides for limited immunity from damages that may arise due to adverse decisions that affect a provider's privileges. HCQIA applies to hospitals, other health care entities, and professional societies if they engage in formal peer review activities intended to promote a high quality of care. The peer review actions are subject to the statute's immunity provisions if:

---

[106]See also Capital Imaging Assocs., P.C. v. Mohawk Valley Med. Assocs., Inc., 996 F.2d 537 (2d Cir. 1993), *cert. denied* 510 U.S. 947 (1993) (radiology group challenging exclusive contract granted by IPA HMO to another group under antitrust laws did not state an actionable claim).

[107]Weiss v. York Hosp., 548 F.Supp. 1048 (M.D. Pa. 1982).

[108]See, e.g., Flegel v. Christian Hosp. Northeast-Northwest, 1992-2 Trade Cas. (CCH) ¶70,355 (1992), *aff'd* 4 F.3d 682 (8th Cir. 1993).

[109]See, e.g., Dos Santos v. Columbus-Cuneo-Cabrini Med. Ctr., 684 F.2d 1346 (7th Cir. 1982); Capili v. Shott, 620 F.2d 438 (4th Cir. 1980); Balaklaw v. Lovell, 14 F.3d 793 (2d Cir. 1994).

[110]See, e.g., Ball Mem. Hosp., Ind. v. Mutual Hosp. Ins., Inc., 784 F.2d 1325 (7th Cir. 1986), *reh'g denied* 788 F.2d 1223 (7th Cir. 1986); but see St. Bernard Gen. Hosp., Inc. v. Hospital Serv. Ass'n of New Orleans, Inc., 712 F.2d 978 (5th Cir. 1983), *cert. denied* 466 U.S. 970 (1984) (Blue Cross and an association of hospitals' program to providing different reimbursement amounts to participating and nonparticipating hospitals and the refusal to admit certain hospitals to participating status stated a prima facie case of per se illegal price fixing and refusal to deal).

[111]18 U.S.C.A. §18.

[112]See, e.g., International Shoe Co. v. FTC, 280 U.S. 291, 302–303 (1930).

[113]Citizen Publishing Co. v. United States, 394 U.S. 131, 137 (1969).

[114]U.S. Department of Justice and Federal Trade Commission, *Horizontal Merger Guidelines* (1992), section 5; 57 Fed. Reg. 41,552–41,563 (September 10, 1992).

[115]DOJ and FTC, ibid., section 5.1, note 36; 57 Fed. Reg., ibid.

[116]42 U.S.C.A. §§11101–11152.

[117]See Patrick v. Burget, 486 U.S. 94 (1988) (peer review activities subject to antitrust laws if no adequate supervision by the state).

1. The challenged peer review action has been taken in the reasonable belief that the action was in furtherance of high-quality health care.
2. The action was taken after reasonable efforts to obtain the facts of the matter.
3. The entity gave the affected provider adequate notice and hearing procedures.
4. There was a reasonable belief that the action was warranted.[118]

Additional Reading. J. Darricades, "Medical Peer Review: How Is It Protected by the Health Care Quality Improvement Act of 1986?" *Journal of Contemporary Law* 18 (1992), pp. 263–83; M. Frazer, "Patrick v. Burget and the Health Care Quality Improvement Act: The Future Scope of Peer Review," *Wayne Law Review* 35 (1989), pp. 1181–1201; S. L. Horner, "The Health Care Quality Improvement Act of 1986: Its History, Provisions, Applications and Implications," *American Journal of Law and Medicine* 16 (1990), pp. 453–96; C. S. Morter, "The Health Care Quality Improvement Act of 1986: Will Physicians Find Peer Review More Inviting?" *Virginia Law Review* 74 (1988), pp. 1115–40.

Hospital-Based Physicians and Tying Arrangement Claims

Hospital-based physicians such as radiologists, anesthesiologists, and pathologists provide services through the hospital. It might be argued that such arrangements, if exclusive and resulting in the exclusion of other providers from rendering these services, are per se illegal tying arrangements. However, the courts generally have not accepted this assertion. Exclusive contracts between hospitals and radiologists,[119] anesthesiologists,[120] and pathologists[121] have all survived antitrust scrutiny.

Additional Reading. D. W. Clark, "Ties That May Bind: Antitrust Liability for Exclusive Hospital-Physician Contracts After Jefferson Parish Hospital District v. Hyde," *Mississippi Law Journal* 54 (1984), pp. 1–42; K. Laurence, "Antitrust Laws, Health Care Providers, and Managed Care," *American Law Institute–American Bar*

Association C653 (1991), pp. 279–467; B. A. Liang, "An Overview and Analysis of Challenges to Medical Exclusive Contracts," *Journal of Legal Medicine* 18 (1997), pp. 1–45.

Premerger Notification Requirements

Under Section 7A of the Clayton Act,[122] also known as the Hart-Scott-Rodino Act, proposed mergers must be reported to the FTC and the Department of Justice if:

1. either party of the merger engages in or activities affect interstate commerce;
2. the transaction fulfills the "size of the parties test," i.e., the transaction concerns the acquisition of assets or voting securities where:
   a. the entity being acquired is engaged in manufacturing and has total assets or annual net sales of $10 million or more; or is not engaged in manufacturing and has assets totaling $10 million or more and the acquiring firm has annual net sales or total assets of $100 million or more; or
   b. the acquired entity has total assets or annual net sales of $100 million or more, and the acquiring firm has total assets or annual net sales of $10 million or more; and
3. the transaction fulfills the "size of the transaction test," i.e., due to the transaction, the acquiring party would obtain 15 percent or more of the voting securities or assets of the acquired entity or would obtain voting securities or assets of the acquired party exceeding $15 million.[123]

If the transaction falls within these parameters, the parties must file the appropriate fee and submit their transaction for review. The parties are then subject to waiting periods before they may consummate their transaction so that the DOJ and the FTC may review the legality of their actions.[124] Noncompliance with the premerger notification requirements is punishable by civil penalties of up to $10,000 per day, which can result in tremendous fines.[125] Note that generally the information submitted under Section 7A is confidential.[126] If the agencies do not enjoin a transaction, it is important to

---

[118]See, e.g., Austin v. McNamara, 979 F.2d 728 (9th Cir. 1992); Smith v. Ricks, 31 F.3d 1478 (9th Cir. 1994).

[119]See, e.g., Beard v. Parkview Hosp., 912 F.2d 138 (6th Cir. 1990); Mays v. Hospital Auth. of Henry Cty., 582 F.Supp. 425 (N.D. Ga. 1984).

[120]See, e.g., Jefferson Parish Hosp. Dist. No. 2 v. Hyde, 466 U.S. 2 (1984).

[121]See, e.g., Collins v. Associated Pathologists, Ltd., 844 F.2d 473 (7th Cir.), *cert. denied* 488 U.S. 852 (1988); Steuer v. National Medical Enterprises, Inc., 846 F.2d 70 (4th Cir. 1988).

[122]15 U.S.C.A. §18a.

[123]15 U.S.C.A. §18a(a)(1)–(3); 16 C.F.R. §§801–803 (1998).

[124]15 U.S.C.A. §§18a(b), 18(e)(1)–(2).

[125]See, e.g., United States v. Beazer PLC, 1992-2 Trade Cas. (CCH) ¶69,923 (D.D.C. 1992) ($760,000); United States v. General Cinema Corp., 1992-1 Trade Cas. (CCH) ¶69,681 (D.D.C. 1992) ($950,000); United States v. Cox Enters., 1991-2 Trade Cas. (CCH) ¶69,540 (D.D.C. 1991) ($1.75 million); United States v. Aero Ltd. Partnership, 1991-1 Trade Cas. (CCH) ¶69,451 (D.D.C. 1991) ($1.125 million).

[126]15 U.S.C.A. §18a(h); see also Lieberman v. FTC, 771 F.2d 32 (2d Cir. 1985); Mattox v. FTC, 752 F.2d 116 (5th Cir. 1985).

note that this does not preclude later government challenge and requests to obtain divestiture or rescission of the consolidation.[127]

Additional Reading. M. A. Head and T. M. Murphey, *Premerger Notification Requirements of the Hart-Scott-Rodino Antitrust Improvements Act of 1976,* pub. no. B4-6688 (New York: Practising Law Institute — Corporate Law, September 1984); J. F. Rill and V. R. Metallo, "Convergence of Premerger Notification and Review: A Case Study," *Wake Forest Law Review* 28 (1993), pp. 35–50; H. I. Saferstein, *Hart-Scott-Rodino Act Compliance and Enforcement: Recent Developments,* pub. no. B4-6807 (New York: Practising Law Institute — Corporate Law, December 1987).

Price Setting by Insurance Companies

It might be thought that price setting by insurance companies would be price fixing in violation of antitrust laws. However, generally this would not be considered a restraint on trade since these provisions are simply contractual terms between the buyer and seller of medical services.[128]

Professional and Nonprofessional Codes and Standards

Professional organizations such as the American Medical Association and the American Dental Association at one time prohibited advertising, particularly of prices. However, this prohibition was found to be in violation of antitrust laws as unlawful restrictions on price competition.[129] Similarly, an American Medical Association standard to avoid association with chiropractors was deemed illegal under antitrust law.[130] However, other limitations that protect consumers[131] such as advertising only providers who have met certain standards of education and

---

[127]15 U.S.C.A. §18a(i).

[128]See, e.g., Kartell v. Blue Shield of Mass., Inc., 749 F.2d 922 (1st Cir. 1984), *cert. denied* 471 U.S. 1029 (1985); Brillhart v. Mutual Med. Ins., 768 F.2d 196 (7th Cir. 1985).

[129]American Medical Ass'n, 94 F.T.C. 701 (1979), *aff'd as modified* American Medical Ass'n v. FTC, 638 F.2d 443 (2d Cir. 1980), *aff'd by an equally divided Court* 455 U.S. 676 (1982); American Dental Ass'n Letter, 111 F.T.C. 735 (1988).

[130]Wilk v. American Medical Ass'n, 895 F.2d 352 (7th Cir.), *cert. denied* 496 U.S. 927 (1990).

[131]See, e.g., Sanjuan v. American Bd. of Psychiatry, 40 F.3d 247 (7th Cir. 1994) (rejecting a foreign physician's challenge to the denial of board certification and therefore the ability to charge higher price, noting that antitrust laws are designed to protect patients).

training[132] and restricting membership in a professional society that does not have an effect on the ability to practice[133] generally are not considered violations of antitrust laws.

Additional Reading. D. Burda, "AMA Conspiracy Case Comes to an End," *Modern Healthcare* (December 3, 1990), p. 14; P. C. Kissam, "Antitrust Law and Professional Behavior," *Texas Law Review* 62 (1983), pp. 1–66; C. D. Weller, "Antitrust, Joint Ventures and the End of the AMA's Contract Practice Ethics: New Ways of Thinking About the Health Care Industry," *North Carolina Central Law Journal* 14 (1983), pp. T3–32.

"Qualified Risk-Sharing Joint Arrangement" and "Qualified Clinically Integrated Joint Arrangement"

In many recent consent orders, the FTC has indicated that parties may not engage in anticompetitive activities but may engage in activities that are reasonably necessary to operate a "qualified risk-sharing joint arrangement" and "qualified clinically integrated joint arrangement." A qualified risk-sharing joint arrangement must satisfy two conditions: First, participating entities must share financial risk; and second, the arrangements must be nonexclusive in both form and substance. A qualified clinically integrated joint arrangement includes nonexclusive arrangements where the entities undertake cooperative activities to obtain efficiencies in the delivery of clinical services without necessarily sharing substantial financial risk. Generally, the FTC requires that entities that have been subject to consent decrees notify the FTC if they contemplate forming clinically integrated arrangements without risk sharing because of the significant variation of efficiencies that these arrangements may or may not generate.[134]

Additional Reading. "Colorado Physician Group to Settle FTC Charges That They Conspired to Raise Prices," *National Association of Attorneys General Antitrust Report* 25, no. 1 (1998), p. 22; "Louisiana Group of Doctors to Settle FTC Charges That It Fixed Prices," *National Association of Attorneys General Antitrust Report* 25, no. 3 (1998), p. 21; "Oregon Group of Institutional Pharmacies to Settle FTC Charges That It Fixed Prices," *National Association of Attorneys General Antitrust Report* 25, no. 3 (1998), p. 19.

---

[132]See, e.g., MacHovec v. Council for the Nat'l Register of Health Servs. Providers in Psychology, Inc., 616 F.Supp. 258 (E.D. Va. 1985).

[133]See, e.g., Marrese v. Am. Acad. Orthopaedic Surgeons, 1991 WL 5827 (N.D. Ill. 1991), *aff'd without opinion* 977 F.2d 585 (7th Cir. 1992).

[134]See, e.g., In re M.D. Physicians of Southwest La., Inc., File No. 9410095 (FTC June 19, 1998).

Staff Privileges and MCO Panel Membership

Generally, providers denied staff privileges at a hospital because of existing contracts for the denied provider's services cannot successfully seek relief under antitrust laws. The Supreme Court has noted that as long as the market as a whole is unaffected by the contract, there is no restraint on trade.[135] In addition, even revocation of staff privileges due to new provider contracts is not considered an antitrust violation;[136] this includes circumstances where the physician remains on the medical staff but cannot practice.[137] Also, loss of staff privileges and denial of membership as an HMO provider have not served as a basis for a successful antitrust claim.[138] Exclusion of providers from participation in a closed-panel HMO also does not generally constitute an antitrust violation.[139] However, if providers exclude a competitor by requiring the hospital to terminate that competitor's privileges and, as a result, obtain an appreciable increase in income, these providers have shown a power to exclude and the ability to raise prices and thus have violated antitrust laws.[140] Note, however, that it generally has been held that the medical staffs and a hospital are legally incapable of conspiring under antitrust laws in peer review activities and are considered part of the hospital's management structure.[141]

---

[135]Jefferson Parish Hosp. Dist. No. 2 v. Hyde, 466 U.S. 2, 31–32 (1984).

[136]See, e.g., Beard v. Parkview Hosp., 912 F.2d 138 (6th Cir. 1990); Coffey v. Healthtrust, Inc., 955 F.2d 1388 (10th Cir. 1992); Belmar v. Cipolla, 475 A.2d 533 (N.J. 1984).

[137]See, e.g., Collins v. Associated Pathologists, Ltd., 844 F.2d 473 (7th Cir. 1988); Coffey v. Healthtrust, Inc., 955 F.2d 1388 (10th Cir. 1992); Jackson v. Radcliffe, 795 F.Supp. 197 (S.D. Tex. 1992).

[138]See, e.g., Levine v. Central Fla. Med. Affiliates, Inc., 864 F.Supp. 1175 (M.D. Fla. 1994); Capital Imaging Assocs., P.C. v. Mohawk Valley Med. Ass'n, 996 F.2d 537 (2d Cir. 1993), cert. denied 510 U.S. 947 (1993); Leak v. Grant Med. Ctr., 893 F.Supp. 757 (S.D. Ohio 1995).

[139]See, e.g., Northwest Med. Labs., Inc. v. Blue Cross and Blue Shield of Oregon, Inc., 775 P.2d 863 (Or. Ct. App. 1989), aff'd 794 P.2d 428 (Or. 1990).

[140]See, e.g., Oltz v. St. Peter's Comm. Hosp., 861 F.2d 1440 (9th Cir. 1988).

[141]See, e.g., Pudlo v. Adamski, 2 F.3d 1153 (7th Cir. 1993); Cohn v. Bond, 953 F.2d 154 (4th Cir. 1991), cert. denied 505 U.S. 1230 (1992); Oksanen v. Page Mem. Hosp., 945 F.2d 696 (4th Cir. 1991), cert. denied 502 U.S. 1074 (1992); Nurse Midwifery Assocs. v. Hibbett, 689 F.Supp. 799 (M.D. Tenn. 1988), aff'd in part and rev'd in part 918 F.2d 605 (6th Cir. 1990), modified on reh'g 927 F.2d 904 (6th Cir. 1991); but see Bolt v. Halifax Hosp. Med. Ctr., 891 F.2d 810 (11th Cir.), cert. denied 495 U.S. 924 (1990) (hospital can conspire with members of medical staff since actions are not unilateral).

Additional Reading.   A. R. Gough, "Quality of Care, Staff Privileges, and Antitrust Law," *University of Detroit Law Review* 64 (1987), pp. 505–28; B. A. Liang, "An Overview and Analysis of Challenges to Medical Exclusive Contracts," *Journal of Legal Medicine* 18 (1997), pp. 1–45; J. Neff, "Physician Staff Privilege Cases: Antitrust Liability and the Health Care Quality Improvement Act," *William and Mary Law Review* 29 (1988), pp. 609–33; K. Oltrogge, "An Ounce of Prevention Is Worth a Pound of Cure: The Need for States to Legislate in the Area of Hospital Professional Review Committee Proceedings," *Washington and Lee Law Review* 46 (1989), pp. 961–1002.

State Action Immunity

Certain mergers may be immune from antitrust laws on the basis of the state action doctrine exemption. If a government entity acts in a manner that, although the actions could be construed as suspect under antitrust laws, is clearly articulated as state policy, these actions are immune from antitrust scrutiny.[142] Similarly, private entities may avail themselves of state action antitrust immunity if their conduct is clearly articulated in line with state action and is actively supervised by the state itself.[143] However, note that there must be adequate supervision for the immunity to attach; otherwise, the immunity is lost.[144] It would appear that mergers in the health care industry, as a general rule, would not fall within these parameters[145] unless the acquiring entity, such as a hospital, is owned or controlled by a government unit and a statute provides the government entity the authority to acquire other facilities or expand.[146] Also, peer review

---

[142]See, e.g., Parker v. Brown, 317 U.S. 341 (1943); Town of Hallie v. City of Eau Claire, 471 U.S. 34 (1985); California Retail Liquor Dealers Ass'n v. Midcal Aluminum, Inc., 445 U.S. 97 (1980); Martin v. Mem. Hosp. at Gulfport, 86 F.3d 1391 (5th Cir. 1996); Martin v. Mem. Hosp., 86 F.3d 1391 (5th Cir. 1996); Bloom v. Hennepin Cty., 783 F.Supp. 418 (D. Minn. 1992); Local Government Antitrust Act, 15 U.S.C.A. §35(a).

[143]See, e.g., California Retail Liquor Dealers Ass'n v. Midcal Aluminum, Inc., 445 U.S. 97, 105 (1980); Drs. Steuer and Latham v. Nat'l Med. Enters., Inc., 672 F.Supp. 1489 (D.S.C. 1987); Coastal Neuro-Psychiatric Assocs., P.A. v. Onslow Mem. Hosp., Inc., 795 F.2d 340 (4th Cir. 1986).

[144]See, e.g., Patrick v. Burget, 486 U.S. 94 (1988), reh'g denied 487 U.S. 1243 (1988) (state action exemption did not apply for peer review activities not adequately supervised by the state); FTC v. Ticor Title Ins. Co., 504 U.S. 621 (1992), cert. denied 510 U.S. 1190 (1994) (mere potential for state supervision was inadequate for state action exemption).

[145]See, e.g., North Carolina v. P.I.A. Asheville, 740 F.2d 274 (4th Cir. 1984), cert. denied 471 U.S. 1003 (1985).

[146]See, e.g., FTC v. Hospital Bd. of Directors, 38 F.3d 1184 (11th Cir. 1994); Askew v. DCH Regional Health Care Auth., 995 F.2d 1033 (11th Cir.), cert. denied 510 U.S. 1012 (1993).

activities, at least on the basis of state law, would appear not to be amenable to state action immunity due to inadequate supervision[147] (although the Health Care Quality Improvement Act may confer immunity on the basis of its statutory provisions).

Additional Reading. R. K. Campbell, "Hospital Collaboration Laws, Antitrust, and State Action Immunity:

---

[147]See, e.g., Shahawy v. Harrison, 875 F.2d 1529 (11th Cir. 1989); Miller v. Indiana Hosp., 930 F.2d 334 (3d Cir. 1991).

Will These Statutes Pass Muster?" *Emory Law Journal* 47 (1998), pp. 1003–39; S. D. Makar, "Local Government, Privatization, and Antitrust Immunity," *Florida Bar Journal* 68 (1994), pp. 38–45; J. F. Ponsoldt, "Immunity Doctrine, Efficiency Promotion, and the Applicability of Federal Antitrust Law to State Approved Hospital Acquisitions," *Journal of Corporate Law* 12 (1986), pp. 37–72; J. Rosenstein, "Active Supervision of Health Care Cooperative Ventures Seeking State Action Antitrust Immunity," *Seattle University Law Review* 18 (1995), pp. 29–55.

Appendix: FTC and DOJ Guideline Examples[148]

1. Statement of Department of Justice and Federal Trade Commission Enforcement Policy on Mergers Among Hospitals

No examples are provided for this policy statement.

2. Statement of Department of Justice and Federal Trade Commission Enforcement Policy on Hospital Joint Ventures Involving High-Technology or Other Expensive Health Care Equipment

Examples of Hospital High-Technology Joint Ventures

The following are examples of hospital joint ventures that are unlikely to raise significant antitrust concerns. Each is intended to demonstrate an aspect of the analysis that would be used to evaluate the venture.

1. New Equipment That Can Be Offered Only by a Joint Venture. All the hospitals in a relevant market agree that they jointly will purchase, operate, and market a helicopter to provide emergency transportation for patients. The community's need for the helicopter is not great enough to justify having more than one helicopter operating in the area and studies of similarly sized communities indicate that a second helicopter service could

---

[148]This appendix is quoted from the U.S. Department of Justice and the Federal Trade Commission. *Statements of Antitrust Enforcement Policy in Health Care* (Washington, DC: DOJ and FTC, August 1996). Note that the 1996 guidelines repeated statements 1–7 without change from the 1994 guidelines.

not be supported. This joint venture falls within the antitrust safety zone. It would make available a service that would not otherwise be available, and for which duplication would be inefficient.

2. Joint Venture to Purchase Expensive Equipment. All five hospitals in a relevant market agree to jointly purchase a mobile health care device that provides a service for which consumers have no reasonable alternatives. The hospitals will share equally in the cost of maintaining the equipment, and the equipment will travel from one hospital to another and be available one day each week at each hospital. The hospitals' agreement contains no provisions for joint marketing of, and protects against exchanges of competitively sensitive information regarding, the equipment. There are also no limitations on the prices that each hospital will charge for use of the equipment, on the number of procedures that each hospital can perform, or on each hospital's ability to purchase the equipment on its own. Although any combination of two of the hospitals could afford to purchase the equipment and recover their costs within the equipment's useful life, patient volume from all five hospitals is required to maximize the efficient use of the equipment and lead to significant cost savings. In addition, patient demand would be satisfied by provision of the equipment one day each week at each hospital. The joint venture would result in higher use of the equipment, thus lowering the cost per patient and potentially improving quality.

This joint venture does not fall within the antitrust safety zone because smaller groups of hospitals could afford to purchase and operate the equipment and recover their costs. Therefore, the joint venture would be analyzed under the rule of reason. The first step is to define the relevant market. In this example, the relevant market consists of the services provided by the equipment, and the five hospitals all potentially compete against each other for patients requiring this service.

The second step in the analysis is to determine the competitive effects of the joint venture. Because the joint venture is likely to reduce the number of these health care devices in the market, there is a potential restraint on competition. The restraint would not be substantial, however, for several reasons. First, the joint venture is limited to the purchase of the equipment and would not eliminate competition among the hospitals in the provision of the services. The hospitals will market the services independently and will not exchange competitively sensitive information. In addition, the venture does not preclude a hospital from purchasing another unit should the demand for these services increase.

Because the joint venture raises some competitive concerns, however, it is necessary to examine the potential efficiencies associated with the venture. As noted above, by sharing the equipment among the five hospitals significant cost savings can be achieved. The joint venture would produce substantial efficiencies while providing access to high quality care. Thus, this joint venture would on balance benefit consumers since it would not lessen competition substantially, and it would allow the hospitals to serve the community's need in a more efficient manner. Finally, in this example the joint venture does not involve any collateral agreements that raise competitive concerns. On these facts, the joint venture would not be challenged by the Agencies.

3. Joint Venture of Existing Expensive Equipment Where One of the Hospitals in the Venture Already Owns the Equipment.

Metropolis has three hospitals and a population of 300,000. Mercy and University Hospitals each own and operate their own magnetic resonance imaging device ("MRI"). General Hospital does not. Three independent physician clinics also own and operate MRIs. All of the existing MRIs have similar capabilities. The acquisition of an MRI is not subject to review under a certificate of need law in the state in which Metropolis is located.

Managed care plans have told General Hospital that unless it can provide MRI services, it will be a less attractive contracting partner than the other two hospitals in town. The five existing MRIs are slightly underutilized — that is, the average cost per scan could be reduced if utilization of the machines increased. There is insufficient demand in Metropolis for six fully-utilized MRIs.

General has considered purchasing its own MRI so that it can compete on equal terms with Mercy and University Hospitals. However, it has decided based on its analysis of demand for MRI services and the cost of acquiring and operating the equipment that it would be better to share the equipment with another hospital. General proposes forming a joint venture in which it will pur-

chase a 50% share in Mercy's MRI, and the two hospitals will work out an arrangement by which each hospital has equal access to the MRI. Each hospital in the joint venture will independently market and set prices for those MRI services, and the joint venture agreement protects against exchanges of competitively sensitive information among the hospitals. There is no restriction on the ability of each hospital to purchase its own equipment.

The proposed joint venture does not fall within the antitrust safety zone because General apparently could independently support the purchase and operation of its own MRI. Accordingly, the Agencies would analyze the joint venture under a rule of reason.

The first step of the rule of reason analysis is defining the relevant product and geographic markets. Assuming there are no good substitutes for MRI services, the relevant product market in this case is MRI services. Most patients currently receiving MRI services are unwilling to travel outside of Metropolis for those services, so the relevant geographic market is Metropolis. Mercy, University, and the three physician clinics are already offering MRI services in this market. Because General intends to offer MRI services within the next year, even if there is no joint venture, it is viewed as a market participant.

The second step is determining the competitive impact of the joint venture. Absent the joint venture, there would have been six independent MRIs in the market. This raises some competitive concerns with the joint venture. The fact that the joint venture will not entail joint price setting or marketing of MRI services to purchasers reduces the venture's potential anticompetitive effect. The competitive analysis would also consider the likelihood of additional entry in the market. If, for example, another physician clinic is likely to purchase an MRI in the event that the price of MRI services were to increase, any anticompetitive effect from the joint venture becomes less likely. Entry may be more likely in Metropolis than other areas because new entrants are not required to obtain certificates of need.

The third step of the analysis is assessing the likely efficiencies associated with the joint venture. The magnitude of any likely anticompetitive effects associated with the joint venture is important; the greater the venture's likely anticompetitive effects, the greater must be the venture's likely efficiencies. In this instance, the joint venture will avoid the costly duplication associated with General purchasing an MRI, and will allow Mercy to reduce the average cost of operating its MRI by increasing the number of procedures done. The competition between the Mercy/General venture and the other MRI providers in the market will provide some incentive for the joint venture to operate the MRI in as low-cost a manner as possible. Thus, there are efficiencies associated with the joint venture that could not be achieved in a less restrictive manner.

The final step of the analysis is determining whether the joint venture has any collateral agreements or conditions that reduce competition and are not reasonably necessary to achieve the efficiencies sought by the venture. For example, if the joint venture required managed care plans desiring MRI services to contract with both joint venture participants for those services, that condition would be viewed as anticompetitive and unnecessary to achieve the legitimate procompetitive goals of the joint venture. This example does not include any unnecessary collateral restraints.

On balance, when weighing the likelihood that the joint venture will significantly reduce competition for these services against its potential to result in efficiencies, the Agencies would view this joint venture favorably under a rule of reason analysis.

4. Joint Venture of Existing Equipment Where Both Hospitals in the Venture Already Own the Equipment. Valley Town has a population of 30,000 and is located in a valley surrounded by mountains. The closest urbanized area is over 75 miles away. There are two hospitals in Valley Town: Valley Medical Center and St. Mary's. Valley Medical Center offers a full range of primary and secondary services. St. Mary's offers primary and some secondary services. Although both hospitals have a CT scanner, Valley Medical Center's scanner is more sophisticated. Because of its greater sophistication, Valley Medical Center's scanner is more expensive to operate and can conduct fewer scans in a day. A physician clinic in Valley Town operates a third CT scanner that is comparable to St. Mary's scanner and is not fully utilized.

Valley Medical Center has found that many of the scans that it conducts do not require the sophisticated features of its scanner. Because scans on its machine take so long, and so many patients require scans, Valley Medical Center also is experiencing significant scheduling problems. St. Mary's scanner, on the other hand, is underutilized, partially because many individuals go to Valley Medical Center because they need the more sophisticated scans that only Valley Medical Center's scanner can provide. Despite the underutilization of St. Mary's scanner, and the higher costs of Valley Medical Center's scanner, neither hospital has any intention of discontinuing its CT services. Valley Medical Center and St. Mary's are proposing a joint venture that would own and operate both hospitals' CT scanners. The two hospitals will then independently market and set the prices they charge for those services, and the joint venture agreement protects against exchanges of competitively sensitive information between the hospitals. There is no restriction on the ability of each hospital to purchase its own equipment.

The proposed joint venture does not qualify under the Agencies' safety zone because the participating hospitals can independently support their own equipment. Accordingly, the Agencies would analyze the joint venture under a rule of reason. The first step of the analysis is to determine the relevant product and geographic markets. As long as other diagnostic services such as conventional X-rays or MRI scans are not viewed as a good substitute for CT scans, the relevant product market is CT scans. If patients currently receiving CT scans in Valley Town would be unlikely to switch to providers offering CT scans outside of Valley Town in the event that the price of CT scans in Valley Town increased by a small but significant amount, the relevant geographic market is Valley Town. There are three participants in this relevant market: Valley Medical Center, St. Mary's, and the physician clinic.

The second step of the analysis is determining the competitive effect of the joint venture. Because the joint venture does not entail joint pricing or marketing of CT services, the joint venture does not effectively reduce the number of market participants. This reduces the venture's potential anticompetitive effect. In fact, by increasing the scope of the CT services that each hospital can provide, the joint venture may increase competition between Valley Medical Center and St. Mary's since now both hospitals can provide sophisticated scans. Competitive concerns with this joint venture would be further ameliorated if other health care providers were likely to acquire CT scanners in response to a price increase following the formation of the joint venture.

The third step is assessing whether the efficiencies associated with the joint venture outweigh any anticompetitive effect associated with the joint venture. This joint venture will allow both hospitals to make either the sophisticated CT scanner or the less sophisticated, but less costly, CT scanner available to patients at those hospitals.

Thus, the joint venture should increase quality of care by allowing for better utilization and scheduling of the equipment, while also reducing the cost of providing that care, thereby benefiting the community. The joint venture may also increase quality of care by making more capacity available to Valley Medical Center; while Valley Medical Center faced capacity constraints prior to the joint venture, it can now take advantage of St. Mary's underutilized CT scanner. The joint venture will also improve access by allowing patients requiring routine scans to be moved from the sophisticated scanner at Valley Medical Center to St. Mary's scanner where the scans can be performed more quickly.

The last step of the analysis is to determine whether there are any collateral agreements or conditions associated with the joint venture that reduce competition and are not reasonably necessary to achieve the efficiencies sought by the joint venture. Assuming there are no such agreements or conditions, the Agencies would view this joint venture favorably under a rule of reason analysis.

As noted in the previous example, excluding price setting and marketing from the scope of the joint venture reduces the probability and magnitude of any anticompetitive effect of the joint venture, and thus reduces the likelihood that the Agencies will find the joint venture to be anticompetitive. If joint price setting and marketing were, however, a part of that joint venture, the Agencies would have to determine whether the cost savings and quality improvements associated with the joint venture offset the loss of competition between the two hospitals. Also, if neither of the hospitals in Valley Town had a CT scanner, and they proposed a similar joint venture for the purchase of two CT scanners, one sophisticated and one less sophisticated, the Agencies would be unlikely to view that joint venture as anticompetitive, even though each hospital could independently support the purchase of its own CT scanner. This conclusion would be based upon a rule of reason analysis that was virtually identical to the one described above.

3. Statement of Department of Justice and Federal Trade Commission Enforcement Policy on Hospital Joint Ventures Involving Specialized Clinical or Other Expensive Health Care Services

Example — Hospital Joint Venture for New Specialized Clinical Service Not Involving Purchase of High-Technology or Other Expensive Health Care Equipment

Midvale has a population of about 75,000 and is geographically isolated in a rural part of its state. Midvale has two general acute care hospitals, Community Hospital and Religious Hospital, each of which performs a mix of basic primary, secondary, and some tertiary care services. The two hospitals have largely non-overlapping medical staffs. Neither hospital currently offers open-heart surgery services, nor has plans to do so on its own. Local residents, physicians, employers, and hospital managers all believe that Midvale has sufficient demand to support one local open-heart surgery unit.

The two hospitals in Midvale propose a joint venture whereby they will share the costs of recruiting a cardiac surgery team and establishing an open-heart surgery program, to be located at one of the hospitals. Patients will be referred to the program from both hospitals, which will share expenses and revenues of the program. The hospitals' agreement protects against exchanges of competitively sensitive information.

As stated above, the Agencies would analyze such a joint venture under a rule of reason. The first step of the rule of reason analysis is defining the relevant product and geographic markets. The relevant product market in this case is open-heart surgery services because there are no reasonable alternatives for patients needing such surgery. The relevant geographic market may be limited to Midvale. Although patients now travel to distant hospitals for open-heart surgery, it is significantly more costly for patients to obtain surgery from them than from a provider located in Midvale. Physicians, patients, and purchasers believe that after the open-heart surgery pro-

gram is operational, most Midvale residents will choose to receive these services locally.

The second step is determining the competitive impact of the joint venture. Here, the joint venture does not eliminate any existing competition because neither of the two hospitals previously was providing open-heart surgery. Nor does the joint venture eliminate any potential competition because there is insufficient patient volume for more than one viable open-heart surgery program. Thus, only one such program could exist in Midvale, regardless of whether it was established unilaterally or through a joint venture.

Normally, the third step in the rule of reason analysis would be to assess the procompetitive effects of, and likely efficiencies associated with, the joint venture. In this instance, this step is unnecessary, since the analysis has concluded under step two that the joint venture will not result in any significant anticompetitive effects.

The final step of the analysis is to determine whether the joint venture has any collateral agreements or conditions that reduce competition and are not reasonably necessary to achieve the efficiencies sought by the venture. The joint venture does not appear to involve any such agreements or conditions; it does not eliminate or reduce competition between the two hospitals for any other services or impose any conditions on use of the open-heart surgery program that would affect other competition.

Because the joint venture described above is unlikely significantly to reduce competition among hospitals for open-heart surgery services, and will in fact increase the services available to consumers, the Agencies would view this joint venture favorably under a rule of reason analysis.

4. Statement of Department of Justice and Federal Trade Commission Enforcement Policy on Providers' Collective Provision of Non-Fee-Related Information to Purchasers of Health Care Services

No examples are provided for this policy statement.

5. Statement of Department of Justice and Federal Trade Commission Enforcement Policy on Providers' Collective Provision of Fee-Related Information to Purchasers of Health Care Services

No examples are provided for this policy statement.

6. Statement of Department of Justice and Federal Trade Commission Enforcement Policy on Provider Participation in Exchanges of Price and Cost Information

No examples are provided for this policy statement.

7. Statement of Department of Justice and Federal Trade Commission Enforcement Policy on Joint Purchasing Arrangements Among Health Care Providers

Example — Joint Purchasing Arrangement Involving Both Hospitals in Rural Community That the Agencies Would Not Challenge

Smalltown is the county seat of Rural County. There are two general acute care hospitals, County Hospital ("County") and Smalltown Medical Center ("SMC"), both located in Smalltown. The nearest other hospitals are located in Big City, about 100 miles from Smalltown.

County and SMC propose to join a joint venture being formed by several of the hospitals in Big City through which they will purchase various hospital supplies — such as bandages, antiseptics, surgical gowns, and masks. The joint venture will likely be the vehicle for the purchase of most such products by the Smalltown hospitals, but under the joint venture agreement, both retain the option to purchase supplies independently.

The joint venture will be an independent corporation, jointly owned by the participating hospitals. It will purchase the supplies needed by the hospitals and then resell them to the hospitals at average variable cost plus a reasonable return on capital. The joint venture will periodically solicit from each participating hospital its expected needs for various hospital supplies, and negotiate the best terms possible for the combined purchases. It will also purchase supplies for its member hospitals on an ad hoc basis.

Competitive Analysis. The first issue is whether the proposed joint purchasing arrangement would fall within the safety zone set forth in this policy statement. In order to make this determination, the Agencies would first inquire whether the joint purchases would account for less than 35% of the total sales of the purchased products in the relevant markets for the sales of those products. Here, the relevant hospital supply markets are likely to be national or at least regional in scope. Thus, while County and SMC might well account for more than 35% of the total sales of many hospital supplies in Smalltown or Rural County, they and the other hospitals in Big City that will participate in the arrangement together would likely not account for significant percentages of sales in the actual relevant markets. Thus, the first criterion for inclusion in the safety zone is likely to be satisfied.

The Agencies would then inquire whether the supplies to be purchased jointly account for less than 20% of the total revenues from all products and services sold by each of the competing hospitals that participates in the arrangement. In this case, County and SMC are competing hospitals, but this second criterion for inclusion in the safety zone is also likely to be satisfied, and the Agencies would not challenge the joint purchasing arrangement.

8. Statement of Department of Justice and Federal Trade Commission Enforcement Policy on Physician Network Joint Ventures

Examples of Physician Network Joint Ventures

The following are examples of how the Agencies would apply the principles set forth in this statement to specific physician network joint ventures. The first three are new examples: 1) a network involving substantial clinical integration, that is unlikely to raise significant competitive concerns under the rule of reason; 2) a network involving both substantial financial risk-sharing and non-risk-sharing arrangements, which would be analyzed under the rule of reason; and 3) a network involving neither substantial financial risk-sharing nor substantial clinical integration, and whose price agreements likely would be challenged as per se unlawful. The last four examples involve networks that operate in a variety of market settings and with different levels of physician participants; three are networks that involve substantial financial risk-sharing and one is a network in which the physician participants do not jointly agree on, or negotiate, price.

1. Physician Network Joint Venture Involving Clinical Integration. Charlestown is a relatively isolated, medium-sized city. For the purposes of this example, the services provided by primary care physicians and those provided by the different physician specialties each constitute a relevant product market; and the relevant geographic market for each of them is Charlestown.

Several HMOs and other significant managed care plans operate in Charlestown. A substantial proportion of insured individuals are enrolled in these plans, and enrollment in managed care is expected to increase. Many physicians in each of the specialties participate in more than one of these plans. There is no significant overlap among the participants on the physician panels of many of these plans.

A group of Charlestown physicians establishes an IPA to assume greater responsibility for managing the cost and quality of care rendered to Charlestown residents who are members of health plans. They hope to reduce costs while maintaining or improving the quality of care, and thus to attract more managed care patients to their practices.

The IPA will implement systems to establish goals relating to quality and appropriate utilization of services by IPA participants, regularly evaluate both individual participants' and the network's aggregate performance with respect to those goals, and modify individual participants' actual practices, where necessary, based on those evaluations. The IPA will engage in case management, preauthorization of some services, and concurrent and retrospective review of inpatient stays. In addition, the

IPA is developing practice standards and protocols to govern treatment and utilization of services, and it will actively review the care rendered by each doctor in light of these standards and protocols.

There is a significant investment of capital to purchase the information systems necessary to gather aggregate and individual data on the cost, quantity, and nature of services provided or ordered by the IPA physicians; to measure performance of the group and the individual doctors against cost and quality benchmarks; and to monitor patient satisfaction. The IPA will provide payers with detailed reports on the cost and quantity of services provided, and on the network's success in meeting its goals.

The IPA will hire a medical director and a support staff to perform the above functions and to coordinate patient care in specific cases. The doctors also have invested appreciable time in developing the practice standards and protocols, and will continue actively to monitor care provided through the IPA. Network participants who fail to adhere to the network's standards and protocols will be subject to remedial action, including the possibility of expulsion from the network.

The IPA physicians will be paid by health plans on a fee-for-service basis; the physicians will not share substantial financial risk for the cost of services rendered to covered individuals through the network. The IPA will retain an agent to develop a fee schedule, negotiate fees, and contract with payers on behalf of the venture. Information about what participating doctors charge non-network patients will not be disseminated to participants in the IPA, and the doctors will not agree on the prices they will charge patients not covered by IPA contracts.

The IPA is built around three geographically dispersed primary care group practices that together account for 25% of the primary care doctors in Charlestown. A number of specialists to whom the primary care doctors most often refer their patients also are invited to participate in the IPA. These specialists are selected based on their established referral relationships with the primary care doctors, the quality of care provided by the doctors, their willingness to cooperate with the goals of the IPA, and the need to provide convenient referral services to patients of the primary care doctors. Specialist services that are needed less frequently will be provided by doctors who are not IPA participants. Participating specialists constitute from 20% to 35% of the specialists in each relevant market, depending on the specialty. Physician participation in the IPA is non-exclusive. Many IPA participants already do and are expected to continue to participate in other managed care plans and earn substantial income from those plans.

Competitive Analysis. Although the IPA does not fall within the antitrust safety zone because the physicians do not share substantial financial risk, the Agencies would analyze the IPA under the rule of reason because it offers the potential for creating significant efficiencies and the price agreement is reasonably necessary to realize those efficiencies. Prior to contracting on behalf of competing doctors, the IPA will develop and invest in mechanisms to provide cost-effective quality care, including standards and protocols to govern treatment and utilization of services, information systems to measure and monitor individual physician and aggregate network performance, and procedures to modify physician behavior and assure adherence to network standards and protocols. The network is structured to achieve its efficiencies through a high degree of interdependence and cooperation among its physician participants. The price agreement, under these circumstances, is subordinate to and reasonably necessary to achieve these objectives.

Furthermore, the Agencies would not challenge under the rule of reason the doctors' agreement to establish and operate the IPA. In conducting the rule of reason analysis, the Agencies would evaluate the likely competitive effects of the venture in each relevant market. In this case, the IPA does not appear likely to limit competition in any relevant market either by hampering the ability of health plans to contract individually with area physicians or with other physician network joint ventures, or by enabling the physicians to raise prices above competitive levels. The IPA does not appear to be overinclusive: many primary care physicians and specialists are available to other plans, and the doctors in the IPA have been selected to achieve the network's procompetitive potential. Many IPA participants also participate in other managed care plans and are expected to continue to do so in the future. Moreover, several significant managed care plans are not dependent on the IPA participants to offer their products to consumers. Finally, the venture is structured so that physician participants do not share competitively sensitive information, thus reducing the likelihood of anticompetitive spillover effects outside the network where the physicians still compete, and the venture avoids any anticompetitive collateral agreements.

Since the venture is not likely to be anticompetitive, there is no need for further detailed evaluation of the venture's potential for generating procompetitive efficiencies. For these reasons, the Agencies would not challenge the joint venture. However, they would reexamine this conclusion and do a more complete analysis of the procompetitive efficiencies if evidence of actual anticompetitive effects were to develop.

2. Physician Network Joint Venture Involving Risk-Sharing and Non–Risk-Sharing Contracts.

An IPA has capitation contracts with three insurer-developed HMOs. Under its contracts with the HMOs, the IPA receives a set fee per member per month for all covered services required by enrollees in a particular health plan. Physician-participants in the IPA are paid on a fee-for-service basis, pursuant to a fee schedule developed by the

IPA. Physicians participate in the IPA on a non-exclusive basis. Many of the IPA's physicians participate in managed care plans outside the IPA, and earn substantial income from those plans.

The IPA uses a variety of mechanisms to assure appropriate use of services under its capitation contracts so that it can provide contract services within its capitation budgets. In part because the IPA has managed the provision of care effectively, enrollment in the HMOs has grown to the point where HMO patients are a significant share of the IPA doctors' patients.

The three insurers that offer the HMOs also offer PPO options in response to the request of employers who want to give their employees greater choice of plans. Although the capitation contracts are a substantial majority of the IPA's business, it also contracts with the insurers to provide services to the PPO programs on a fee-for-service basis. The physicians are paid according to the same fee schedule used to pay them under the IPA's capitated contracts. The IPA uses the same panel of providers and the same utilization management mechanisms that are involved in the HMO contracts. The IPA has tracked utilization for HMO and PPO patients, which shows similar utilization patterns for both types of patients.

Competitive Analysis.   Because the IPA negotiates and enters into both capitated and fee-for-service contracts on behalf on its physicians, the venture is not within a safety zone. However, the IPA's HMO contracts are analyzed under the rule of reason because they involve substantial financial risk-sharing. The PPO contracts also are analyzed under the rule of reason because there are significant efficiencies from the capitated arrangements that carry over to the fee-for-service business. The IPA's procedures for managing the provision of care under its capitation contracts and its related fee schedules produce significant efficiencies; and since those same procedures and fees are used for the PPO contracts and result in similar utilization patterns, they will likely result in significant efficiencies for the PPO arrangements as well.

3. Physician Network That Is Per Se Unlawful.   A group of physicians in Clarksville forms an IPA to contract with managed care plans. There is some limited managed care presence in the area, and new plans have announced their interest in entering. The physicians agree that the only way they can effectively combat the power of the plans and protect themselves from low fees and intrusive utilization review is to organize and negotiate with the plans collectively through the IPA, rather than individually.

Membership in the IPA is open to any licensed physician in Clarksville. Members contribute $2,000 each to fund the legal fees associated with incorporating the IPA and its operating expenses, including the salary of an executive director who will negotiate contracts on behalf of the

IPA. The IPA will enter only into fee-for-service contracts. The doctors will not share substantial financial risk under the contracts. The Contracting Committee, in consultation with the executive director, develops a fee schedule.

The IPA establishes a Quality Assurance and Utilization Review Committee. Upon recommendation of this committee, the members vote to have the IPA adopt two basic utilization review parameters: strict limits on documentation to be provided by physicians to the payers, and arbitration of disputes regarding plan utilization review decisions by a committee of the local medical society. The IPA refuses to contract with plans that do not accept these utilization review parameters. The IPA claims to have its own utilization review/quality assurance programs in development but has taken very few steps to create such a program. It decides to rely instead on the hospital's established peer review mechanisms.

Although there is no formal exclusivity agreement, IPA physicians who are approached by managed care plans seeking contracts refer the plans to the IPA. Except for some contracts predating the formation of the IPA, the physicians do not contract individually with managed care plans on terms other than those set by the IPA.

Competitive Analysis.   This IPA is merely a vehicle for collective decisions by its physicians on price and other significant terms of dealing. The physicians' purpose in forming the IPA is to increase their bargaining power with payers. The IPA makes no effort to selectively choose physicians who are likely to further the network's achievement of efficiencies, and the IPA involves no significant integration, financial or otherwise. IPA physicians' participation in the hospital's general peer review procedures does not evidence integration by those physicians that is likely to result in significant efficiencies in the provision of services through the IPA. The IPA does not manage the provision of care or offer any substantial potential for significant procompetitive efficiencies. The physicians are merely collectively agreeing on prices they will receive for services rendered under IPA contracts and not to accept certain aspects of utilization review that they do not like.

The physicians' contribution of capital to form the IPA does not make it a legitimate joint venture. In some circumstances, capital contributions by an IPA's participants can indicate that the participants have made a significant commitment to the creation of an efficiency-producing competitive entity in the market. Capital contributions, however, can also be used to fund a cartel. The key inquiry is whether the contributed capital is being used to further the network's capability to achieve substantial efficiencies. In this case, the funds are being used primarily to support the joint negotiation, and not to achieve substantial procompetitive efficiencies. Thus, the physicians' agreement to bargain through the joint venture will be treated as per se illegal price fixing.

4. Exclusive Physician Network Joint Venture with Financial Risk-Sharing and Comprising More Than Twenty Percent of Physicians with Active Admitting Privileges at a Hospital. County Seat is a relatively isolated, medium-sized community of about 350,000 residents. The closest town is 50 miles away. County Seat has five general acute care hospitals that offer a mix of basic primary, secondary, and tertiary care services.

Five hundred physicians have medical practices based in County Seat, and all maintain active admitting privileges at one or more of County Seat's hospitals. No physician from outside County Seat has any type of admitting privileges at a County Seat hospital. The physicians represent ten different specialties and are distributed evenly among the specialties, with 50 doctors practicing each specialty.

One hundred physicians (also distributed evenly among specialties) maintain active admitting privileges at County Seat Medical Center. County Seat's other 400 physicians maintain active admitting privileges at other County Seat hospitals.

Half of County Seat Medical Center's 100 active admitting physicians propose to form an IPA to market their services to purchasers of health care services. The physicians are divided evenly among the specialties. Under the proposed arrangement, the physicians in the network joint venture would agree to meaningful cost containment and quality goals, including utilization review, quality assurance, and other measures designed to reduce the provision of unnecessary care to the plan's subscribers, and a substantial amount (in this example 20%) of the compensation due to the network's physician participants would be withheld and distributed only if these measures are successfully met. This physician network joint venture would be exclusive: Its physician participants would not be free to contract individually with health plans or to join other physician joint ventures.

A number of health plans that contract selectively with hospitals and physicians already operate in County Seat. These plans and local employers agree that other County Seat physicians, and the hospitals to which they admit, are good substitutes for the active admitting physicians and the inpatient services provided at County Seat Medical Center. Physicians with medical practices based outside County Seat, however, are not good substitutes for area physicians because such physicians would find it inconvenient to practice at County Seat hospitals due to the distance between their practice locations and County Seat.

Competitive Analysis. A key issue is whether a physician network joint venture, such as this IPA, comprising 50% of the physicians in each specialty with active privileges at one of five comparable hospitals in County Seat would fall within the antitrust safety zone. The physicians within the joint venture represent less than 20% of all the physicians in each specialty in County Seat.

County Seat is the relevant geographic market for purposes of analyzing the competitive effects of this proposed physician joint venture. Within each specialty, physicians with admitting privileges at area hospitals are good substitutes for one another. However, physicians with practices based elsewhere are not considered good substitutes.

For purposes of analyzing the effects of the venture, all of the physicians in County Seat should be considered market participants. Purchasers of health care services consider all physicians within each specialty, and the hospitals at which they have admitting privileges, to be relatively interchangeable. Thus, in this example, any attempt by the joint venture's physician participants collectively to increase the price of physician services above competitive levels would likely lead third-party purchasers to recruit non-network physicians at County Seat Medical Center or other area hospitals.

Because physician network joint venture participants constitute less than 20% of each group of specialists in County Seat and agree to share substantial financial risk, this proposed joint venture would fall within the antitrust safety zone.

5. Physician Network Joint Venture with Financial Risk-Sharing and a Large Percentage of Physicians in a Relatively Small Community. Smalltown has a population of 25,000, a single hospital, and 50 physicians, most of whom are family practitioners. All of the physicians practice exclusively in Smalltown and have active admitting privileges at the Smalltown hospital. The closest urban area, Big City, is located some 35 miles away and has a population of 500,000. A little more than half of Smalltown's working adults commute to work in Big City. Some of the health plans used by employers in Big City are interested in extending their network of providers to Smalltown to provide coverage for subscribers who live in Smalltown but commute to work in Big City (coverage is to include the families of commuting subscribers). However, the number of commuting Smalltown subscribers is a small fraction of the Big City employers' total workforce.

Responding to these employers' needs, a few health plans have asked physicians in Smalltown to organize a non-exclusive IPA large enough to provide a reasonable choice to subscribers who reside in Smalltown but commute to work in Big City. Because of the relatively small number of potential enrollees in Smalltown, the plans prefer to contract with such a physician network joint venture rather than engage in what may prove to be a time-consuming series of negotiations with individual Smalltown physicians to establish a panel of physician providers there.

A number of Smalltown physicians have agreed to form a physician network joint venture. The joint venture will contract with health plans to provide physician services to subscribers of the plans in exchange for a monthly capitation fee paid for each of the plan's subscribers. The physicians forming this joint venture would constitute about half of the total number of physicians in Smalltown. They would represent about 35% of the town's family practitioners, but higher percentages of the town's general surgeons (50%), pediatricians (50%), and obstetricians (67%). The health plans that serve Big City employers say that the IPA must have a large percentage of Smalltown physicians to provide adequate coverage for employees and their families in Smalltown and in a few scattered rural communities in the immediate area and to allow the doctors to provide coverage for each other.

In this example, other health plans already have entered Smalltown and contracted with individual physicians. They have made substantial inroads with Smalltown employers, signing up a large number of enrollees. None of these plans has had any difficulty contracting with individual physicians, including many who would participate in the proposed joint venture.

Finally, the evidence indicates that Smalltown is the relevant geographic market for all physician services. Physicians in Big City are not good substitutes for a significant number of Smalltown residents.

Competitive Analysis. This proposed physician network joint venture would not fall within the antitrust safety zone because it would comprise over 30% of the physicians in a number of relevant specialties in the geographic market. However, the Agencies would not challenge the joint venture because a rule of reason analysis indicates that its formation would not likely hamper the ability of health plans to contract individually with area physicians or with other physician network joint ventures, or enable the physicians to raise prices above competitive levels. In addition, the joint venture's agreement to accept capitated fees creates incentives for its physicians to achieve cost savings.

That health plans have requested formation of this venture also is significant, for it suggests that the joint venture would offer additional efficiencies. In this instance, it appears to be a low-cost method for plans to enter an area without investing in costly negotiations to identify and contract with individual physicians.

Moreover, in small markets such as Smalltown, it may be necessary for purchasers of health care services to contract with a relatively large number of physicians to provide adequate coverage and choice for enrollees. For instance, if there were only three obstetricians in Smalltown, it would not be possible for a physician network joint venture offering obstetrical services to have less than 33% of the obstetricians in the relevant area. Furthermore, it may be impractical to have less than 67% in the plan because two obstetricians may be needed in the venture to provide coverage for each other.

Although the joint venture has a relatively large percentage of some specialties, it appears unlikely to present

competitive concerns under the rule of reason because of three factors: (1) the demonstrated ability of health plans to contract with physicians individually; (2) the possibility that other physician network joint ventures could be formed; and (3) the potential benefits from the coverage to be provided by this physician network joint venture. Therefore, the Agencies would not challenge the joint venture.

6. Physician Network Joint Venture with Financial Risk-Sharing and a Large Percentage of Physicians in a Small, Rural County. Rural County has a population of 15,000, a small primary care hospital, and ten physicians, including seven general and family practitioners, an obstetrician, a pediatrician, and a general surgeon. All of the physicians are solo practitioners. The nearest urban area is about 60 miles away in Big City, which has a population of 300,000, and three major hospitals to which patients from Rural County are referred or transferred for higher levels of hospital care. However, Big City is too far away for most residents of Rural County routinely to use its physicians for services available in Rural County.

Insurance Company, which operates throughout the state, is attempting to offer managed care programs in all areas of the state and has asked the local physicians in Rural County to form an IPA to provide services under the program to covered persons living in the County. No other managed care plan has attempted to enter the County previously.

Initially, two of the general practitioners and two of the specialists express interest in forming a network, but Insurance Company says that it intends to market its plan to the larger local employers, who need broader geographic and specialty coverage for their employees. Consequently, Insurance Company needs more of the local general practitioners and the one remaining specialist in the IPA to provide adequate geographic, specialty, and backup coverage to subscribers in Rural County. Eventually, four of the seven general practitioners and the one remaining specialist join the IPA and agree to provide services to Insurance Company's subscribers, under contracts providing for capitation. While the physicians' participation in the IPA is structured to be non-exclusive, no other managed care plan has yet entered the local market or approached any of the physicians about joining a different provider panel. In discussing the formation of the IPA with Insurance Company, a number of the physicians have made clear their intention to continue to practice outside the IPA and have indicated they would be interested in contracting individually with other managed care plans when those plans expand into Rural County.

Competitive Analysis. This proposed physician network joint venture would not fall within the antitrust safety zone because it would comprise over 30% of the general practitioners in the geographic market. Under the circumstances, a rule of reason analysis indicates that the

Agencies would not challenge the formation of the joint venture, for the reasons discussed below.

For purposes of this analysis, Rural County is considered the relevant geographic market. Generally, the Agencies will closely examine joint ventures that comprise a large percentage of physicians in the relevant market. However, in this case, the establishment of the IPA and its inclusion of more than half of the general practitioners and all of the specialists in the network are the results of the payer's expressed need to have more of the local physicians in its network to sell its product in the market. Thus, the level of physician participation in the network does not appear to be overinclusive, but rather appears to be the minimum necessary to meet the employers' needs.

Although the IPA has more than half of the general practitioners and all of the specialists in it, under the particular circumstances this does not, by itself, raise sufficient concerns of possible foreclosure of entry by other managed care plans, or of the collective ability to raise prices above competitive levels, to warrant antitrust challenge to the joint venture by the Agencies. Because it is the first such joint venture in the county, there is no way absolutely to verify at the outset that the joint venture in fact will be non-exclusive. However, the physicians' participation in the IPA is formally non-exclusive, and they have expressed a willingness to consider joining other managed care programs if they begin operating in the area. Moreover, the three general practitioners who are not members of the IPA are available to contract with other managed care plans. The IPA also was established with participation by the local area physicians at the request of Insurance Company, indicating that this structure was not undertaken as a means for the physicians to increase prices or prevent entry of managed care plans.

Finally, the joint venture can benefit consumers in Rural County through the creation of efficiencies. The physicians have jointly put themselves at financial risk to control the use and cost of health care services through capitation. To make the capitation arrangement financially viable, the physicians will have to control the use and cost of health care services they provide under Insurance Company's program. Through the physicians' network joint venture, Rural County residents will be offered a beneficial product, while competition among the physicians outside the network will continue.

Given these facts, the Agencies would not challenge the joint venture. If, however, it later became apparent that the physicians' participation in the joint venture in fact was exclusive, and consequently other managed care plans that wanted to enter the market and contract with some or all of the physicians at competitive terms were unable to do so, the Agencies would re-examine the joint venture's legality. The joint venture also would raise antitrust concerns if it appeared that participation by most of the local physicians in the joint venture resulted in anticompetitive effects in markets outside the joint venture, such as uniformity of fees charged by the physicians in their solo medical practices.

7. Physician Network Joint Venture with No Price Agreement and Involving All of the Physicians in a Small, Rural County.

Rural County has a population of 10,000, a small primary care hospital, and six physicians, consisting of a group practice of three family practitioners, a general practitioner, an obstetrician, and a general surgeon. The nearest urban area is about 75 miles away in Big City, which has a population of 200,000, and two major hospitals to which patients from Rural County are referred or transferred for higher levels of hospital care. Big City is too far away, however, for most residents of Rural County to use for services available in Rural County.

HealthCare, a managed care plan headquartered in another state, is thinking of marketing a plan to the larger employers in Rural County. However, it finds that the cost of contracting individually with providers, administering the system, and overseeing the quality of care in Rural County is too high on a per capita basis to allow it to convince employers to switch from indemnity plans to its plan. HealthCare believes its plan would be more successful if it offered higher quality and better access to care by opening a clinic in the northern part of the county where no physicians currently practice.

All of the local physicians approach HealthCare about contracting with their recently formed, non-exclusive, IPA. The physicians are willing to agree through their IPA to provide services at the new clinic that HealthCare will establish in the northern part of the county and to implement the utilization review procedures that HealthCare has adopted in other parts of the state.

HealthCare wants to negotiate with the new IPA. It believes that the local physicians collectively can operate the new clinic more efficiently than it can from its distant headquarters, but HealthCare also believes that collectively negotiating with all of the physicians will result in it having to pay higher fees or capitation rates. Thus, it encourages the IPA to appoint an agent to negotiate the non-fee-related aspects of the contracts and to facilitate fee negotiations with the group practice and the individual doctors. The group practice and the individual physicians each will sign and negotiate their own individual contracts regarding fees and will unilaterally determine whether to contract with HealthCare, but will agree through the IPA to provide physician, administrative, and utilization review services. The agent will facilitate these individual fee negotiations by discussing separately and confidentially with each physician the physician's fee demands and presenting the information to HealthCare. No fee information will be shared among the physicians.

Competitive Analysis.   For purposes of this analysis, Rural County is considered the relevant geographic market. Generally, the Agencies are concerned with joint ventures that comprise all or a large percentage of the physicians in the relevant market. In this case, however, the joint venture appears on balance to be procompetitive. The potential for competitive harm from the venture is not great and is outweighed by the efficiencies likely to be generated by the arrangement.

The physicians are not jointly negotiating fees or engaging in other activities that would be viewed as per se antitrust violations. Therefore, the IPA would be evaluated under the rule of reason. Any possible competitive harm would be balanced against any likely efficiencies to be realized by the venture to see whether, on balance, the IPA is anticompetitive or procompetitive.

Because the IPA is non-exclusive, the potential for competitive harm from foreclosure of competition is reduced. Its physicians are free to contract with other managed care plans or individually with HealthCare if they desire. In addition, potential concerns over anticompetitive pricing are minimized because physicians will continue to negotiate prices individually. Although the physicians are jointly negotiating non-price terms of the contract, agreement on these terms appears to be necessary to the successful operation of the joint venture.

The small risk of anticompetitive harm from this venture is outweighed by the substantial procompetitive benefits of improved quality of care and access to physician services that the venture will engender. The new clinic in the northern part of the county will make it easier for residents of that area to receive the care they need. Given these facts, the Agencies would not challenge the joint venture.

9. Statement of Department of Justice and Federal Trade Commission Enforcement Policy on Multiprovider Networks

Examples of Multiprovider Network Joint Ventures

The following are four examples of how the Agencies would apply the principles set forth in this statement to specific multiprovider network joint ventures, including: 1) a PHO involving substantial clinical integration, that does not raise significant competitive concerns under the rule of reason; 2) a PHO providing services on a per case basis, that would be analyzed under the rule of reason; 3) a PHO involving substantial financial risk sharing and including all the physicians in a small rural county, that does not raise competitive concerns under the rule of reason; and 4) a PHO that does not involve horizontal agreements on price.

1. PHO Involving Substantial Clinical Integration. Roxbury is a relatively isolated, medium-sized city. For the purposes of this example, the services provided by primary care physicians and those provided by the different physician specialists each constitute a relevant product market; and the relevant geographic market for each of them is Roxbury.

Several HMOs and other significant managed care plans operate in Roxbury. A substantial proportion of insured individuals are enrolled in these plans, and enrollment in managed care is expected to increase. Many physicians in each of the specialties and Roxbury's four hospitals participate in more than one of these plans. There is no significant overlap among the participants on the physician panels of many of these plans, nor among the active medical staffs of the hospitals, except in a few specialties. Most plans include only two or three of Roxbury's hospitals, and each hospital is a substitute for any other.

One of Roxbury's hospitals and the physicians on its active medical staff establish a PHO to assume greater responsibility for managing the cost and quality of care rendered to Roxbury residents who are members of health plans. They hope to reduce costs while maintaining or improving the quality of care, and thus to attract more managed care patients to the hospital and their practices.

The PHO will implement systems to establish goals relating to quality and appropriate utilization of services by PHO participants, regularly evaluate both the hospital's and each individual doctor's and the network's aggregate performance concerning those goals, and modify the hospital's and individual participants' actual practices, where necessary, based on those evaluations. The PHO will engage in case management, preadmission authorization of some services, and concurrent and retrospective review of inpatient stays. In addition, the PHO is developing practice standards and protocols to govern treatment and utilization of services, and it will actively review the care rendered by each doctor in light of these standards and protocols.

There is a significant investment of capital to purchase the information systems necessary to gather aggregate and individual data on the cost, quantity, and nature of services provided or ordered by the hospital and PHO physicians; to measure performance of the PHO, the hospital, and the individual doctors against cost and quality benchmarks; and to monitor patient satisfaction. The PHO will provide payers with detailed reports on the cost and quantity of services provided, and on the network's success in meeting its goals.

The PHO will hire a medical director and support staff to perform the above functions and to coordinate patient care in specific cases. The doctors and the hospital's administrative staff also have invested appreciable time in developing the practice standards and protocols and will continue actively to monitor care provided through the PHO. PHO physicians who fail to adhere to the network's standards and protocols will be subject to remedial action, including the possibility of expulsion from the network.

Under PHO contracts, physicians will be paid by health plans on a fee-for-service basis; the hospital will be paid a set amount for each day a covered patient is in the hospital and will be paid on a fee-for-service basis for other services. The physicians will not share substantial financial risk for the cost of services rendered to covered individuals through the network. The PHO will retain an agent to develop a fee schedule, negotiate fees, and contract with payers. Information about what participating doctors charge non-network patients will not be disseminated to participants of the PHO, and the doctors will not agree on the prices they will charge patients not covered by PHO contracts.

All members of the hospital's medical staff join the PHO, including its three geographically dispersed primary care group practices that together account for about 25% of the primary care doctors in Roxbury. These primary care doctors generally refer their patients to specialists on the hospital's active medical staff. The PHO includes all primary care doctors and specialists on the hospital's medical staff because of those established referral relationships with the primary care doctors, the admitting privileges all have at the hospital, the quality of care provided by the medical staff, their commitment to cooperate with the goals of the PHO, and the need to provide convenient referral services to patients of the primary care doctors. Participating specialists include from 20% to 35% of specialists in each relevant market, depending on the specialty. Hospital and physician participation in the PHO is non-exclusive. Many PHO participants, including the hospital, already do and are expected to continue to participate in other managed care plans and earn substantial income from those plans.

Competitive Analysis.   The Agencies would analyze the PHO under the rule of reason because it offers the potential for creating significant efficiencies and the price agreement among the physicians is reasonably necessary to realize those efficiencies. Prior to contracting on behalf of competing physicians, the PHO will develop mechanisms to provide cost-effective, quality care, including standards and protocols to govern treatment and utilization of services, information systems to measure and monitor both the individual performance of the hospital and physicians and aggregate network performance, and procedures to modify hospital and physician behavior and assure adherence to network standards and protocols. The network is structured to achieve its efficiencies through a high degree of interdependence and cooperation among its participants. The price agreement for physician services, under these circumstances, is subordinate to and reasonably necessary to achieve these objectives.

Furthermore, the Agencies would not challenge establishment and operation of the PHO under the rule of reason. In conducting the rule of reason analysis, the Agencies would evaluate the likely competitive effects of the venture in each relevant market. In this case, the PHO does not appear likely to limit competition in any relevant market either by hampering the ability of health plans to contract individually with area hospitals or physicians or with other network joint ventures, or by enabling the hospital or physicians to raise prices above competitive levels. The PHO does not appear to be overinclusive: many primary care physicians as well as specialists are available to other plans, and the doctors in the PHO have been included to achieve the network's procompetitive potential. Many PHO doctors also participate in other managed care plans and are expected to continue to do so in the future. Moreover, several significant managed care plans are not dependent on the PHO doctors to offer their products to consumers. Finally, the venture is structured so that physician participants do not share competitively sensitive information, thus reducing the likelihood of anticompetitive spillover effects outside the network where the physicians still compete, and the venture avoids any anticompetitive collateral agreements.

Since the venture is not likely to be anticompetitive, there is no need for further detailed evaluation of the venture's potential for generating procompetitive efficiencies. For these reasons, the Agencies would not challenge the joint venture. They would reexamine this conclusion, however, and do a more complete analysis of the procompetitive efficiencies if evidence of actual anticompetitive effects were to develop.

2. PHO That Provides Services on a Per Case Basis.

Goodville is a large city with a number of hospitals. One of Goodville's hospitals, together with its oncologists and other relevant health care providers, establishes a joint venture to contract with health plans and other payers of health care services to provide bone marrow transplants and related cancer care for certain types of cancers based on an all-inclusive per case payment. Under these contracts, the venture will receive a single payment for all hospital, physician, and ancillary services rendered to covered patients requiring bone marrow transplants. The venture will be responsible for paying for and coordinating the various forms of care provided. At first, it will pay its providers using a fee schedule with a withhold to cover unanticipated losses on the case rate. Based on its operational experience, the venture intends to explore other payment methodologies that may most effectively provide the venture's providers with financial incentives to allocate resources efficiently in their treatment of patients.

Competitive Analysis.   The joint venture is a multi-provider network in which competitors share substantial financial risk, and the price agreement among members of the venture will be analyzed under the rule of reason. The per case payment arrangement involves the sharing of substantial financial risk because the venture will receive a single, predetermined payment for a course of treatment that requires the substantial coordination of care by different types of providers and can vary significantly in cost and complexity from patient to patient. The venture will pay its provider participants in a way that gives them incentives to allocate resources efficiently and that spreads among the participants the risk of loss and the possibility of gain on any particular case. The venture adds to the market another contracting option for health plans and other payers that is likely to result in cost savings because of its use of a per case payment method. Establishment of the case rate is an integral part of the risk-sharing arrangement.

3. PHO with All the Physicians in a Small, Rural County.   Frederick County has a population of 15,000, and a 50-bed hospital that offers primary and some secondary services. There are 12 physicians on the active medical staff of the hospital (6 general and family practitioners, 1 internist, 2 pediatricians, 1 otolaryngologist, and 2 general surgeons) as well as a part-time pathologist, anesthesiologist, and radiologist. Outside of Frederick County, the nearest hospitals are in Big City, 25 miles away. Most Frederick County residents receive basic physician and hospital care in Frederick County and are referred or transferred to the Big City physician specialists and hospitals for higher levels of care.

No managed care plans currently operate in Frederick County. Nor are there any large employers who selectively contract with Frederick County physicians. Increasingly, Frederick County residents who work for employers in Big City are covered under managed care contracts that direct Frederick County residents to hospitals and to numerous primary care and specialty physicians in Big City. Providers in Frederick County who are losing patients to hospitals and doctors in Big City want to contract with payers and employers so that they can retain these patients. However, the Frederick County hospital and doctors have been unsuccessful in their efforts to obtain contracts individually; too few potential enrollees are involved to justify payers' undertaking the expense and effort of individually contracting with Frederick County providers and administering a utilization review and quality assurance program for a provider network in Frederick County.

The hospital and all the physicians in Frederick County want to establish a PHO to contract with managed care plans and employers operating in Big City. Managed care plans have expressed interest in contracting with all Frederick County physicians under a single risk-sharing contract. The PHO also will offer its network to employers operating in Frederick County.

The PHO will market the services of the hospital on a per diem basis, and physician services on the basis of a fee schedule that is significantly discounted from the doctors' current charges. The PHO will be eligible for a bonus of up to 20% of the total payments made to it, depending on the PHO's success in meeting utilization targets agreed to with the payers. An employee of the hospital will develop a fee schedule, negotiate fees, and contract with payers on behalf of the PHO. Information about what participating doctors charge non-PHO patients will not be disseminated to the doctors, and they will not agree on the prices they will charge patients not covered by PHO contracts.

Physicians' participation in the PHO is structured to be non-exclusive. Because no other managed care plans operate in the area, PHO physicians do not now participate in other plans and have not been approached by other plans. The PHO physicians have made clear their intention to continue to practice outside the PHO and to be available to contract individually with any other managed care plans that expand into Frederick County.

Competitive Analysis.   The agreement of the physicians on the prices they will charge through the PHO would be analyzed under the rule of reason because they share substantial financial risk through the use of a pricing arrangement that provides significant financial incentives for the physicians, as a group, to achieve specified cost-containment goals. The venture thus has the potential for creating significant efficiencies, and the setting of price promotes the venture's use of the risk-sharing arrangement.

The Agencies would not challenge formation and operation of the PHO under the rule of reason. Under the rule of reason analysis, the Agencies would evaluate the likely competitive effects of the venture. The venture does not appear likely to limit competition in any relevant market. Managed care plans' current practice of directing patients from Frederick County to Big City suggests that the physicians in the PHO face significant competition from providers and managed care plans that operate in Big City. Moreover, the absence of managed care contracting in Frederick County, either now or in the foreseeable future, indicates that the network is not likely to reduce any actual or likely competition for patients who do not travel to Big City for care.

While the venture involves all of the doctors in Frederick County, this was necessary to respond to competition from Big City providers. It is not possible to verify at the outset that the venture will in fact be non-exclusive, but the physicians' participation in the venture is structured to be non-exclusive, and the doctors have expressed a willingness to consider joining other managed care plans if they begin operating in the area.

For these reasons, the Agencies would not challenge the joint venture. However, if it later became apparent that the physicians' participation in the PHO was exclusive in fact, and consequently managed care plans or employers that wanted to contract with some or all of the physicians at competitive terms were unable to do so, or that the PHO doctors entered into collateral agreements that restrained competition for services furnished outside the PHO, the Agencies likely would challenge the joint venture.

4. PHO That Does Not Involve Horizontal Agreements on Price.

A hospital and doctors and other health care providers on its medical staff have established a PHO to market their services to payers, including employers with self-funded health benefits plans. The PHO contracts on a fee-for-service basis. The physicians and other health care providers who are participants in the PHO do not share substantial financial risk or otherwise integrate their services so as to provide significant efficiencies. The payers prefer to continue to use their existing third-party administrators for contract administration and utilization management, or to do it in-house.

There is no agreement among the PHO's participants to deal only through the PHO, and many of them participate in other networks and HMOs on a variety of terms. Some payers have chosen to contract with the hospital and some or all of the PHO physicians and other providers without going through the PHO, and a significant proportion of the PHO's participants contract with payers in this manner.

In an effort to avoid horizontal price agreements among competing participants in the PHO while facilitating the contracting process, the PHO considers using the following mechanisms:

A. An agent of the PHO, not otherwise affiliated with any PHO participant, will obtain from each participant a fee schedule or conversion factor that represents the minimum payment that participant will accept from a payer. The agent is authorized to contract on the participant's behalf with payers offering prices at this level or better. The agent does not negotiate pricing terms with the payer and does not share pricing information among competing participants. Price offers that do not meet the authorized fee are conveyed to the individual participant.

B. The same as option A, with the added feature that the agent is authorized, for a specified time, to bind the participant to any contract offers with prices equal to, or better than, those in a contract that the participant has already approved.

C. The same as option A, except that in order to assist payers in developing contract offers, the agent takes the fee authorizations of the various participants and develops a schedule that can be presented to a payer showing the percentages of participants in the network who have authorized contracts at various price levels.

D. The venture hires an agent to negotiate prices with payers on behalf of the PHO's participants. The agent does not disclose to the payer the prices the participants are willing to accept, as in option C, but attempts to obtain the best possible prices for all the participants. The resulting contract offer then is relayed to each participant for acceptance or rejection.

Competitive Analysis. In the circumstances described in options A through D, the Agencies would determine whether there was a horizontal agreement on price or any other competitively significant terms among PHO participants. The Agencies would determine whether such agreements were subject to the per se rule or the rule of reason and evaluate them accordingly.

The existence of an agreement is a factual question. The PHO's use of options A through C does not establish the existence of a horizontal price agreement. Nor is there sharing of price information or other evidence of explicit or implicit agreements among network participants on price. The agent does not inform PHO participants about others' acceptance or rejection of contract offers; there is no agreement or understanding that PHO participants will only contract through the PHO; and participants deal outside the network on competitive terms.

The PHO's use of option D amounts to a per se unlawful price agreement. The participants' joint negotiation through a common agent confronts the payer with the combined bargaining power of the PHO participants, even though they ultimately have to agree individually to the contract negotiated on their behalf.

Further Reading

Antitrust Enforcement Policies

Balto DA. Cooperating to Compete: Antitrust Analysis of Health Care Joint Ventures. *St Louis U L J* 1998; 42:191–241.

Copland GH, Hepp PE. Government Antitrust Enforcement in the Health Care Markets: The Regulators Need Update. *W Va L Rev* 1996;99:107–53.

Hirshfeld E. Interpreting the 1996 Federal Antitrust Guidelines for Physician Joint Venture Networks. *Annals Health L* 1997;6:1–49.

Horoschak MJ. The New Statements of Antitrust Enforcement Policy in Health Care: Antitrust Guidance for Health Care Providers Enters a New Phase. *Antitrust* 1996;11:28–32.

Lifland WT. *Monopolies and Joint Ventures.* Pub. no. B4-7128. New York: Practising Law Institute—Corporate Law, May–July 1996, Appendix B. (Complete reprint of 1994 and 1996 guidelines.)

Marjancik N. Risky Business: Proposed Reform of the Antitrust Laws as Applied to Health Care Provider Networks. *Am J L & Med* 1998;24:59–87.

Miles JJ. Joint Venture Analysis and Provider-Controlled Health Care Networks. *Antitrust L J* 1997;66:127–66.

Squeri SJ. *Government Investigation and Enforcement.* Pub. no. B0-0023. New York: Practising Law Institute — Corporate Law, April–July 1998.

Business Review and Advisory Opinions

Briggs JD. Mergers and Acquisitions: An Outline of General Principles, Current Enforcement Practices, and Recent Contested Cases. *Antitrust L J* 1988;56:675–737.

DeSanti SJ, Nagata EA. Competitor Communications: Facilitating Practices or Invitations to Collude? An Application of Theories to Proposed Horizontal Agreements Submitted for Antitrust Review. *Antitrust L J* 1994; 63:93–131.

Kirkpatrick MW. Report of the American Bar Association Section of Antitrust Law Special Committee to Study the Role of the Federal Trade Commission. *Antitrust L J* 1989;58:43–178.

Roeder KH. The 1996 Antitrust Policy Statements: Balancing Flexibility and Certainty. *Ga L Rev* 1997;31:649–713.

Squeri SJ. *Government Investigation and Enforcement.* Pub. no. B0-0023. New York: Practising Law Institute — Corporate Law, April–July 1998.

Clayton Act

Ashdjian AM. Competitor Standing Under Cargill, Inc. v. Monfort of Colorado, Inc.: An Erosion of the Clayton Act. *Am U L Rev* 1987;37:259–84.

Devill EJ. Section 7 of the Clayton Act — Essential Elements. In: *Federal Jury Practice and Instructions.* St. Paul, MN: West Publishing Co., 1987;§90.49.

Graff GA. Target Standing Under Section 16 of the Clayton Act: When Your Antitrust Injury Hurts, Standing Can Be a Problem. *U Ill L Rev* 1991:219–50.

Halverson JT. Report to the House Delegates on Proposed Amendments to Section 7 of the Clayton Act. *Antitrust L J* 1986;55:673–89.

Hinshaw T et al. Federal Antitrust Laws: Clayton Act. In: *American Jurisprudence,* 2d ed. Rochester, NY: Lawyers Cooperative Publishing Co., 1998;§155–89.

Enforcement and Penalties

Cavanagh ED. Detrebling Antitrust Damages: An Idea Whose Time Has Come? *Tul L Rev* 1987;61:777–848.

Clark NE. Antitrust Comes Full Circle: The Return to the Cartelization Standard. *Vand L Rev* 1985;38:1125–97.

Hobbs CO. *FTC Enforcement: Antitrust Unfair and Deceptive Trade Practices.* Pub. no. B4-6755. New York: Practising Law Institute — Corporate Law, May 1986.

Squeri SJ. *Government Investigation and Enforcement: Antitrust Division and the Federal Trade Commission.* Pub. no. B4-7128. New York: Practising Law Institute — Corporate Law, May–July 1996.

Federal Trade Commission Act

Hobbs CO. *FTC Enforcement: Antitrust Unfair and Deceptive Trade Practices.* Pub. no. B4-6755. New York: Practising Law Institute — Corporate Law, May 1986.

Schechter RE. Letting the Right Hand Know What the Left Hand's Doing: The Clash of the FTC's False Advertising and Antitrust Policies. *B U L Rev* 1984;64:265–323.

Ward PC. Restitution for Consumers Under the Federal Trade Commission Act: Good Intentions or Congressional Intentions? *Am U L Rev* 1992;41:1139–97.

Sherman Act

Bowlus LA. Summit Health, LTD. v Pinhas: The Supreme Court's Eye-Opening Decision to Allow Sherman Act Jurisdiction in a Hospital-Exclusion Case. *U Tol L Rev* 1992;23:793–822.

Breer KJ. Systemcare v. Wang: A Look at Contracts Between Buyer and Seller and the "Concerted Action" Requirement Under §1 of the Sherman Antitrust Act. *Washburn L J* 1998;37:409–39.

Clark NE. Antitrust Comes Full Circle: The Return to the Cartelization Standard. *Vand L Rev* 1985;38:1125–97.

Erskine K. Square Pegs and Round Holes: Antitrust Law and Privileging Decision. *U Kan L Rev* 1996;44:399–421.

Huss MM. Eighth Circuit Extends McCarran Ferguson to Shield Alleged Monopolization of the Health Insurance Industry from Antitrust Scrutiny. *Wm Mitchell L Rev* 1989;15:713–38.

Jerry RH, Knebel DE. Antitrust and Employer Restraints in Labor Markets. *Indus Rel L J* 1984;6:173–254.

Pronger PA. Application of the Sherman Act to Health Care: New Developments and New Directions. *Antitrust L J* 1990;59:173–90.

Other Reading

Bork RH. *The Antitrust Paradox: A Policy at War with Itself.* New York: The Free Press, 1995.

Breit W, Elzinga KG. *The Antitrust Casebook: Milestones in Economic Regulation,* 3d ed. Ft. Worth, TX: Dryden Press, 1997.

Gellhorn E, Kovacic WE. *Antitrust Law and Economics in a Nutshell,* 4th ed. St. Paul, MN: West Publishing Co., 1994.

Kovaleff TP. *The Antitrust Impulse: An Economic, Historical, and Legal Analysis.* Armonk, NY: M. E. Sharpe, 1994.

Letwin W. *Law and Economic Policy in America: The Evolution of the Sherman Antitrust Act.* Chicago: University of Chicago Press, 1981.

Liang BA. The Anticompetitive Nature of Brand-Name Firm Introduction of Generics Before Patent Expiration. *Antitrust Bull* 1996;41:599–635.

MacEy JR, Miller GP. *Costly Policies: State Regulation and Antitrust Exemption in Insurance Markets.* Washington, DC: AEI Press, 1993.

McChesney FS, Shughart WF. *The Causes and Consequences of Antitrust: The Public-Choice Perspective.* Chicago: University of Chicago Press, 1995.

Peritz RJR. *Competition Policy in America, 1888–1992: History, Rhetoric, Law.* New York: Oxford University Press, 1996.

Posner RA. *Antitrust Law: An Economic Perspective.* Chicago: University of Chicago Press, 1978.

Shenefield JH, Stelzer IM. *The Antitrust Laws: A Primer*, 3d ed. Washington, DC: AEI Press, 1995.

Web Sites

ABA's antitrust page: *http://www.abanet.org/antitrust/home.html*

Antitrust law: *http://www.wtp.net/~moulton/antitrust.htm*

Antitrust law materials: *http://www.law.cornell.edu/topics/archive/antitrust.html*

Antitrust litigation, antimonopoly, and commercial litigation: *http://www.lawmall.com/index.html*

Antitrust and trade regulation: *http://www.nocall.org/antitrust.html*

Clayton Act of 1914: *http://ecolan.sbs.ohio-state.edu/aly/classes/powerpoint/ch16/tsld012.htm*

Federal Trade Commission (with advisory opinions): *http://www.ftc.gov*

Harvard's antitrust page: *http://roscoe.law.harvard.edu/courses/techseminar96/antitrust/antitrust.html*

Sherman Act: *http://www.cba.uga.edu/*

Sherman Antitrust Act: *http://encarta.msn.com/*

U.S. Department of Justice: *http://www.usdoj.gov/*

U.S. Department of Justice — Antitrust Division: *http://www.usdoj.gov/atr/index.html*

U.S. Department of Justice — Office of the Inspector General: *http://www.usdoj.gov/oig/ighp01.htm*

14

Alternative Dispute Resolution

Conflicts and disputes in health care are as common as in other industries and social circumstances. However, resolving medical disputes using the formal adjudication process of court litigation is time-consuming, is expensive, and often does not suit the parties' needs. Over the past three decades, however, the alternative dispute resolution (ADR) movement has recognized these limitations and formulated other mechanisms by which conflicts may be resolved. Each has important strengths and limitations; and ADR, in combination with formal adjudication, offers a broad array of tools to address the concomitantly broad array of conflicts that may arise in health care.

This chapter reviews the main ADR methods and indicates the type of circumstances that would appear most beneficial for each method's use. Note that each ADR method may vary when used in specific circumstances to resolve disputes, and the descriptions of the methods discussed here represent only basic ones.

Generally, the binding or nonbinding nature of any ADR process is based on a contract. Therefore, the terms of the agreement will dictate whether and which specific ADR process must be followed in an effort to resolve a dispute and whether the assessment is simply advisory or legally binding on both parties.

Formal Adjudication

Formal adjudication is the use of the well-recognized court system to resolve disputes, that is, litigation. Generally, the important characteristics of the formal adjudicatory system include the involuntary nature of the process (i.e., parties may be forced into adjudication by another party); a decision imposed by a third-party neutral decision maker with no specialized knowledge of the subject of the dispute; a very formal process as determined by rigid rules; an adversarial system where each party presents proofs and arguments, in a vast majority of

cases using attorneys, and where each party attempts to discount or discredit the other party's proofs and arguments; and a public forum where the dispute process is held and decided. The decision generally is rendered for one party or the other; that is, the resolution is mutually exclusive — one party wins, and one party loses.

Formal adjudication is most appropriate for circumstances where resolution of novel legal issues, party vindication, declaration of activities that are illegal, and establishment of formal legal precedent are of paramount importance. For example, cases that involve the civil rights of parties such as discrimination actions, present difficult issues of law that have not been resolved (such as antitrust assessments of new and unique business associations), or require a public policy stance (such as the legality of proposed regulations or orders) are appropriate for the court system to resolve.

Mediation

Mediation is a process by which a neutral third party is used to assist the parties to negotiate a resolution of their dispute. Note that the mediator merely assists the parties but has no power to impose any outcome on them.

Mediation is a voluntary process entered into by the parties in an effort to resolve their dispute. Generally, the enforceability of these mediated resolutions is a function of private contract law; any agreement to mediate, as well as an agreement to abide by the mediated decision, is enforceable according to the terms of a valid contract. The mediator generally is selected by the parties as a facilitator of communication. The process usually is informal, with no set rules except those imposed by the parties or the mediator in an effort to further productive communication (e.g., no interruptions when one party is speaking).

The major advantages of mediation are that the method is private and results are confidential; and the process focuses on an improvement of communication between the parties so that the interests, goals, and needs of each are identified and communicated to the other so as to lead to a mutually acceptable resolution to the conflict for the parties. Because the parties control the process without the constraint of rigid legal rules, creative and flexible solutions that address the parties' concerns regarding their dispute may be proposed and implemented. This process also allows the parties an opportunity to express a productive amount of emotion (in or outside the presence of the other party), shift the focus of the conflict from the past to the future, learn about interests that are important to the parties but that each is reluctant to disclose to the other, and provide new information that may be helpful in resolving the dispute.

Arbitration

Arbitration is a formalized system of dispute resolution where parties provide proofs and arguments to a neutral third party who has the power to impose a binding decision on the parties. A common variation includes the use of multiple arbitrators, for example, one selected by each party with the chosen arbitrators choosing a third. Arbitration is very similar to formal adjudication except that there is no or limited pretrial discovery by the parties, the hearing is more informal, and the rules of evidence are not applied as rigidly in an arbitration proceeding.

Arbitration has been used voluntarily by some parties to resolve private disputes and has been mandated by law for certain other conflicts. When private parties agree to use arbitration, they must decide on how to select the arbitrator(s), stipulate who will pay for these services, set an objective standard by which the arbitrator(s) will assess the conflict and claims of the parties (e.g., the law, trade or industry customs, or some combination), and specify the procedural rules that will be followed by the arbitrator. Unless otherwise indicated in the terms of the arbitration, arbitration does not allow for pretrial discovery. Generally, arbitration is considered a final, binding procedure.

The potential major advantages of arbitration are significant, including the ability to draw on arbitrators with specialized expertise relating directly to the conflict, the finality of the arbitrator's decision, the relative privacy of the dispute proceedings and the decision itself, party choice of procedural rules, and the relatively low cost (in terms of time and money) as compared with formal adjudication. Of course, whether these advantages actually result depends on the specific conflict, parties, and arbitrators involved.

Significantly, a strong public policy favors arbitration, and state and federal law make agreements to arbitrate specifically enforceable.[1] Courts have agreed with the broad enforceability of arbitration[2] and have specifically held that the Federal Arbitration Act preempts state law to the extent state law conflicts with the goals or policies of the statute.[3]

Unlike formal adjudication, once an arbitration decision has been made, there is no default mechanism by which the decision is enforced. However, the arbitration decision may be judicially confirmed by bringing the decision to a court; failure to abide by the arbitration at that point constitutes contempt of court. Both the Federal Arbitration Act and the Uniform Arbitration Act give courts jurisdiction to confirm (or refuse to confirm) an arbitration decision. The Federal Arbitration Act indicates that, generally, the court must confirm an arbitration award except under the following circumstances:[4]

(a) Where the award was procured by corruption, fraud, or undue means . . .

(b) Where there was evident partiality or corruption in the arbitrators . . .

---

[1]See, e.g., Federal Arbitration Act, 9 U.S.C.A. §§2 *et seq.*; see also Administrative Dispute Resolution Act, 5 U.S.C.A. §§5581–5593; *Arizona Revised Statutes Annotated* (St. Paul, MN: West, 1994), sections 12-1501–12-1518; *Arkansas Code Annotated* (Charlottesville, VA: Michie, 1995), sections 16-108-201–16-108-224; *Delaware Code Annotated* tit.10 §§5701–5725 (1996); *Florida Statutes* ch. 682.01–682.22 (1990); *Idaho Code* §§7-901–7-922 (1990); *Iowa Code Annotated* §§679A.1–679A.19 (1987); *Kansas Statutes Annotated* §§5-401–5-422 (1995); *Kentucky Revised Statutes Annotated* (Charlottesville, VA: Michie, 1996), sections 417.145–417.240; *Minnesota Statutes* §§572.08–572.30 (1996); *Montana Code Annotated* §§27-5-111–27-5-324 (1996); *Nevada Revised Statutes* §§38.015–38.360 (1995); *New Jersey Statutes Annotated* (St. Paul, MN: West, 1996), sections 2A:23A-1–2A:23A-19; *Ohio Revised Code Annotated* (St. Paul, MN: West, 1992), sections 2711.01–2711.16; *Pennsylvania Consolidated Statutes* §§7301–7320 (1982); *Rhode Island General Laws* §§10-3-1–10-3-21 (1996); *South Dakota Codified Laws* (Charlottesville, VA: Michie, 1996), sections 21-25A-1–21-5A-38; *Tennessee Code Annotated* §§29-5-301–29-5-320 (1996); *Utah Code Annotated* §§78-31a-1–78-31a-20 (1996); *Vermont Statutes Annotated* tit. 12, §§5651–5681 (1996); *Wyoming Statutes Annotated* (Charlottesville, VA: Michie, 1986), sections 1-36-101–1-36-119.

[2]See, e.g., United Steelworkers of Am. v. Warrior & Gulf Navigation Co., 363 U.S. 574 (1960); Shearson/American Express v. McMahon, 482 U.S. 220 (1987); Mitsubishi Motors Corp. v. Soler Chrysler-Plymouth, 473 U.S. 614 (1985); Rodriguez De Quijas v. Shearson/American Express, Inc., 490 U.S. 477 (1989); Gilmer v. Interstate/Johnson Lane Corp., 111 S.Ct. 1647 (1991); Madden v. Kaiser Found. Hosps., 131 Cal.Rptr. 882 (Cal. 1976).

[3]See, e.g., Southland Corp. v. Keating, 465 U.S. 1 (1984); Volt Information Sciences, Inc. v. Stanford Univ., 489 U.S. 468 (1989).

[4]Federal Arbitration Act, 9 U.S.C.A. §§2, 10.

(c) Where the arbitrators were guilty of misconduct in refusing to postpone the hearing, on sufficient cause shown, or in refusing to hear evidence pertinent and material to the controversy; or of any other misbehavior by which the rights of any party have been prejudiced.

(d) Where the arbitrators exceeded their powers, or so imperfectly executed them that a mutual, final, and definite award upon the subject matter was not made.

Arbitration may be mandated before formal adjudication. Generally, this "court-annexed arbitration" is provided for in state law and requires that a certain class of cases (e.g., automobile torts) or a certain monetary amount be at issue.[5] This requirement to use ADR before accessing the formal adjudication system also applies to other ADR methods.[6]

Hybrid Methods

Med-Arb

As might be expected from its label, med-arb is a combination of mediation and arbitration. In this ADR process, initially the parties agree to mediate their dispute using the neutral third party as a mediator. If mediation does not result in an agreement or settlement, then the mediator changes roles to an arbitrator with the power to issue a final and binding decision on the parties. The primary advantage of using this hybrid method is that it is potentially more efficient: The same neutral third party is used in both processes so that there is no need to educate a new one regarding the facts and interests involved in the dispute. However, a significant disadvantage of med-arb is that the parties may not be very open in the mediation stage because sensitive disclosures may be used against them if and when the neutral evaluator becomes an arbitrator. Thus, the third neutral party as mediator will have less to work with when attempting to help the parties craft a creative solution to their conflict. Indeed, the dispute resolution framework may be significantly altered by the specter of arbitration, which focuses on a rights-based decision; parties therefore may spend all their time trying to convince the mediator that each is "right" in anticipation of an arbitration decision.

An alternative is med-arb that results in only an advisory arbitration decision. This process attempts to mitigate the identified problems with binding arbitration. Because the mediator has no binding power to arbitrate a final decision, the parties have an increased incentive to substantively use the mediation process to resolve their dispute. It also allows the mediator as an advisory arbitrator to merely indicate what he or she believes the ultimate result would be at arbitration. The clear disadvantage of this process is its potential length, since it requires an extra step of binding arbitration. However, it appears that, at least in labor disputes, approximately 85% of cases do settle using this ADR method.[7]

Mini-Trial

The mini-trial is an evaluative process, most often used in business disputes. Summary presentations are made by each party's attorneys to a panel composed of a neutral advisor and high-level executives of each party who have the power to accept a settlement. After the presentations, the executives try to settle the dispute through negotiation. If negotiation fails to result in a settlement, the neutral advisor provides an assessment as to the probable outcome of the dispute. The major characteristics of a mini-trial are that the process is voluntary and confidential; the parties agree to follow certain protocols or procedures; before the mini-trial, the parties agree to informally exchange important documents, provide summaries of witness testimony, and provide short statements regarding the dispute (and often provide that this information is confidential and inadmissible in any future proceeding); and a neutral third party is chosen by consent of the parties (e.g., a former judge or an individual who has expertise in the subject matter, who may take a passive role in the process or act as a mediator). Some mini-trials include no third-party neutral advisor. At the presentation itself, the attorneys for each side attempt to provide a brief, cogent summary of their best case, usually with a time limit. Rigid rules of formal adjudication do not apply and rebuttal and questions and answers are asked and provided.

The basic dynamic involved in the mini-trial is that both parties' executive representatives are provided with the appropriate information to assess the merits of each party's position regarding the dispute. With this information, the parties may come up with a solution that makes business sense from their own perspectives, while taking into account unique business needs.

---

[5]See, e.g., *California Health and Safety Code* §1373.19 (indicating that a single arbitrator may assess claims for health services claim up to $200,000); *Hawaii Arbitration Rules* (Charlottesville, VA: Michie, 1995), rule 8 (monetary claims below $150,000 must go to court-annexed arbitration except under certain circumstances).

[6]See, e.g., *California Civil Code* §4607 (contested custody cases must go to mediation); *Texas Code Annotated, Civil Practice and Remediation Code* §154.021 (court given discretion to send certain cases to ADR); *Florida Statutes Annotated* ch. 44 (same).

[7]S. B. Goldberg, "Grievance Mediation: A Successful Alternative to Labor Arbitration," *Negotiation Journal* 5 (1989), pp. 9–15.

Summary Jury Trial

The summary jury trial is an evaluative process like a mini-trial but differing in several important ways. These differences stem from the goal of the process: determining what a jury might decide in the case. Hence, instead of a third-party neutral with corporate executives, an actual judge and advisory jury drawn from the actual jury pool are used. Jurors are not told that their role is advisory until after they return to give their verdict. Attorneys for each side make summary presentations as in the mini-trial; however, the presentations usually are based on information that has been the subject of discovery and would be admissible at trial. Once the advisory jury has announced its decision, it answers questions regarding the verdict and its assessment and reaction to particular evidence and arguments. The attorneys, and their respective executive representatives, then attend a mandatory settlement conference to discuss settlement. If no settlement occurs, the advisory jury verdict is not admissible in future final adjudications.

A summary jury trial takes significant time and resources because it is similar to formal adjudication. This method therefore is most useful in circumstances where the dispute is unique or novel, precludes an easy prediction of what a jury would decide, and such unpredictability is what is preventing settlement.

ADR and Medical Malpractice Claims

Although a wide variety of medical disputes are amenable to ADR methods, one that has drawn significant attention is using ADR for medical malpractice dispute resolution. Arguments in favor of such ADR use include reducing litigation costs, having a more informed decision maker rather than a lay jury, reducing the significant emotional trauma from a lawsuit, allowing more plaintiffs with "minor" injuries to have their claims heard, and reducing the amount of frivolous litigation. State law often dictates how these contractual agreements must appear and the conditions under which they are valid,[8] subject to federal law.[9]

The difficulty with applying ADR to medical malpractice disputes is twofold. First, any voluntary process will require participation by all parties and their attorneys. This participation may not occur due to the desire, for example, of plaintiffs for a trial by jury in an effort to increase their perceived chance at success and of defen-

dants for full vindication because they face reports to the National Practitioner Data Bank if any amount is paid to end the dispute. Second, the vagaries of a malpractice case involve complex issues of fact and law that require extensive time and effort to fully assess. Nonbinding, summary facilitative processes such as mediation and its variants therefore are not well suited for application to malpractice disputes. Mandatory, binding arbitration is one method that can solve the voluntary party and attorney participation problem as well as provide for appropriate technical expertise; however, it too is limited by the summary nature of the assessment.

Although arbitration has its limitations, many institutional health care providers and managed care organizations now use mandatory arbitration in their contractual agreements to resolve any patient care dispute with the provider. Use of binding arbitration was pioneered on a broad scale by Kaiser-Permanente in California and has spread throughout the U.S. medical delivery system. Challenges to mandatory arbitration clauses by patients generally, but not always, have been rejected by the courts.[10] Significantly, the Federal Arbitration Act[11] as well as a plethora of laws in at least 40 states provide a basis for enforcing these provisions.[12] However, because of potential advantages for repeat player providers such as managed care organizations, significant requirements have been placed on providers and arbitrators in malpractice dispute resolutions. California has been particularly active in this area and has held that arbitrators must exercise good faith in all adjudications, including disclosure of previous relationships with parties,[13] and that providers

[8]See, e.g., *California Civil Procedure Code* §1295 (describing wording, font, and color of enforceable medical malpractice arbitration agreement).

[9]See, e.g., Perry v. Thomas, 482 U.S. 483 (1987) (state laws that are unique to arbitration agreements are preempted by federal law governing arbitration).

[10]See, e.g., Coon v. Nicola, 21 Cal.Rptr.2d 846 (Cal. Ct. App. 1993); Buraczynski v. Eyring, 919 S.W.2d 314 (Tenn. 1996); Broemmer v. Otto, 821 P.2d 204 (Ariz. 1991); Wilson v. Kaiser Found. Hosps., 190 Cal.Rptr. 649 (Cal. Ct. App. 1983); Dinong v. Kaiser Found. Hosp., 162 Cal.Rptr. 606 (Cal. Ct. App. 1980); Madden v. Kaiser Found. Hosps., 131 Cal.Rptr. 882 (Cal. 1976) (all upholding the use of ADR); but see Colorado Permanente Med. Group v. Evans, 926 P.2d 1218 (Colo. 1996); Saika v. Gold, 56 Cal.Rptr.2d 922 (Cal. Ct. App. 1996); Beynon v. Garden Grove Med. Group, 161 Cal.Rptr. 146 (Cal. Ct. App. 1980); but see Rosenfield v. Sup. Ct. 143 Cal.App.3d 198 (Cal. 1983); Graham v. Scissor-Tail, Inc., 28 Cal.3d 807 (Cal. 1990); Cheng-Canindin v. Renaissance Hotel Assocs., 50 Cal.App.4th 676 (Cal. Ct. App. 1996).

[11]9 U.S.C.A. §2.

[12]P. I. Carter, "Binding Arbitration in Malpractice Disputes: The Right Prescription for HMO Patients?" *Hamline Journal of Public Law and Policy* 18 (1997), pp. 423–51.

[13]See, e.g., Neaman v. Kaiser Found. Hosp., 11 Cal.Rptr.2d 879 (Cal. Ct. App. 1992) (overturning an arbitration decision on the basis of arbitrator nondisclosure of 5 cases out of 300 where he acted as Kaiser Foundation Hospital's chosen arbitrator); see also *California Civil Procedure Code* §1281.9 (1998) (requiring arbitrator disclosure concerning previous experience with parties).

may not unduly delay arbitration in malpractice cases.[14] Further, some states exclude certain types of claims from arbitration, such as those involving personal injury, tort, or insurance contracts.[15]

Because of the potentially controversial nature surrounding binding arbitration in malpractice disputes, the largest arbitration association in the United States, the American Arbitration Association (AAA), in association with the American Medical Association (AMA) and American Bar Association (ABA), has indicated that it no longer will participate in arbitration of medical malpractice under mandatory binding arbitration clauses in managed care contracts with patients. AAA will participate in such arbitration only if the patient asks for or agrees to arbitration for dispute resolution after the dispute arises.[16] With regard to the use of ADR in medical disputes, AAA, AMA, and ABA indicated that:

- Alternative dispute resolution can and should be used to resolve disputes over health care coverage and access arising out of the relationship between patients and private health plans and managed care organizations.
- Alternative dispute resolution can and should be used to resolve disputes over health care coverage and access arising out of the relationship between health care providers and private health plans and managed care organizations.
- In disputes involving patients, binding forms of dispute resolution should be used only where the parties agree to do so after a dispute arises.
- It is essential that due process protections be afforded to all participants in the ADR process.
- Review of managed health care decisions through alternative dispute resolution complements the concept of internal review of determinations made by private managed health care organizations.[17]

However, it is not yet clear as to whether this policy proposal will substantively affect the use of arbitration in malpractice disputes due to the significant number of non-AAA arbitrators available and the standard nature of these clauses in patient care contracts.

---

[14]See, e.g., Engalla v. Permanente Med. Group, Inc., 64 Cal.Rptr.2d 843 (Cal. 1997) (remanding case after holding that managed care organizations may not unduly delay selection of arbitrators in medical malpractice cases).

[15]See, e.g., *Arkansas Code Annotated* (Charlottesville, VA: Michie, 1997), section 16-108-201(b); *Kansas Statutes Annotated* §5-401(c) (1997); *Montana Code Annotated* §27-5-114 (2) (1997); *South Carolina Code Annotated* §15-48-10 (1998); *Texas Civil Practice Code Annotated* §171.001 (1997).

[16]"Arbitrators Oppose Binding Rulings on Patient Rights Disputes," *Managed Care Week* 8, no. 2 (1998), p. 1.

[17]G. H. Friedman, "AAA, ABA and AMA Issue Joint Resolution: Recommendations for Health Care Dispute Resolution," *Medical Malpractice Law and Strategy* 15, no. 10 (1998), p. 1.

Other Medical Disputes

A large number of potential disputes in the health care arena are amenable to ADR processes outside the medical malpractice realm. Because health care has become increasingly commercial in nature, commercial disputes over contracts between facilities or between facilities and medical providers can be addressed by ADR processes in the same way as other commercial disputes. However, unique aspects such as provider reputation, the health of a party, and the emotional concerns attendant to illness, disease, and treatment also make disputes in the health care arena unique among social relationships. The interface between the needs and capacities of the parties, whether they are to continue their relationship, third-party involvement, and the legal rights of the parties all play important roles in deciding which particular ADR method or combination of methods is relevant for a particular health care dispute. Of course, some circumstances are not well suited for ADR or formal adjudication, such as end-of-life situations. However, by assessing the needs of the parties in the context of their social and medical circumstances as well as their underlying incentives, an appropriate resolution strategy usually can be ascertained.

Examples of voluntary applications to several modern medical disputes outside the malpractice context follow.[18] These examples are designed to illustrate what types of ADR methods are appropriate for specific disputes rather than to be definitive statements on health law or policy.

Example 1. An Interfacility Dispute: St. Francis Hospital and Johnson City Hospital

Background

In the current health care climate, cost control has been a predominant consideration in the allocation of medical resources. As a result, federal, state, and local governments have attempted to utilize various strategies to minimize health care costs. One strategy has been to limit potential demand for expensive diagnostic technology by limiting its availability through requiring prior state-level approval before purchase of this type of capital. However, if a health care facility can demonstrate to the state authority that there is sufficient patient need, no overlap between this form of capital and the services derived from it, and available money to purchase and support the equipment, then the facility may be granted a so-called certificate of need (CON), which is a permit that allows

---

[18]These examples are abstracted from B. A. Liang, "Understanding and Applying Alternative Dispute Resolution Methods in Modern Medical Conflicts," *Journal of Legal Medicine* 19 (1998), pp. 397–430. Used with permission.

the facility to acquire such equipment. It is apparent that such a grant is valuable because of the highly exclusive nature of the grant and the concomitant income arising from it.

Case Scenario

In a local city, St. Francis Hospital has merged with Johnson City Hospital. Each hospital was under pressure to expand services and improve reimbursements obtained from their patients' insurance. Both are located in the same urban area but in different neighborhoods. St. Francis is a nonprofit, private facility that caters primarily to middle-class patients in its neighborhood. Johnson City Hospital is a nonprofit, private, inner-city facility, established during the forgone days of prosperity in its community. However, its current clientele consists of significantly poor and disenfranchised patients who primarily are Medicaid program participants or have no insurance at all. However, Johnson City Hospital does have one plus — it is a teaching hospital for the prestigious Physicians and Surgeons Medical School (P & S), located in the city. It therefore is staffed with outstanding resident physicians (house staff) who supplement the hospital's retained attending physicians.

St. Francis–Johnson City Hospital (the Hospital) merged just over one year ago. Subsequent to the merger, the Hospital obtained a CON for a new magnetic resonance imaging machine that would significantly enhance physicians' ability to diagnose disorders in emergency and other clinical situations. The Hospital was granted the CON on the basis of Johnson City's locale, which has limited health care resources, and St. Francis's fiscal soundness, which would allow it to buy and maintain the machinery.

The current dispute is over where to locate the MRI. Johnson City contends that the MRI should be located at its facility because CON approval was based on its patients' medical needs. St. Francis, on the other hand, indicates that the machine could not even have been purchased without its funds and so should be located at St. Francis. The state authority has expressed no opinion on the matter. There is vague talk of legal action by the parties. How can this dispute be settled?

From an ADR standpoint, the choice of methodology requires that the goals of the parties first be ascertained. Johnson City wishes the MRI to be located on its site primarily for financial reasons. It is no secret that reimbursement for MRI procedures is relatively high compared with their operational costs and that Johnson City has lost significant revenue by not having such services available. Second, if Johnson City had the MRI, then P & S likely would send more of its house staff to Johnson City. This would reduce certain staff costs because P & S will pay the salary of the house staff, whose presence will reduce the need for other health care providers. Finally, Johnson City's patient population will be better served by having advanced diagnostic equipment, such as an MRI, available on site. When referred elsewhere for an MRI procedure by Johnson City physicians, patients often do not follow through with the referral and never obtain the scan.

St. Francis has similar goals. It, too, wants to take advantage of the high reimbursement for MRI services. However, it also wishes to use the MRI as a marketing tool: "St. Francis and the 21st Century: Bringing Advanced Health Care to the Community" is an event envisioned by the marketing department.

What problems appear to be inhibiting settlement? First, that this issue was not addressed in the original CON application (or inadequately so) may indicate poor communication at the outset of the process. Another interpretation could be that the parties had some differences in their conceptions of the joint CON application. Each party could have interpreted its role as determinative in obtaining the MRI CON. Further, St. Francis's idea of marketing may make its interests as an organization subject to some opposing internal pressures. Note that both parties are in a continuing relationship with each other and other joint programs are contemplated.

ADR Assessment

At the outset, the continuing relationship between St. Francis and Johnson City makes the desirability of formal adjudication quite low. Further, the nature of the dispute (not involving novel legal issues or the desire to establish precedent) also makes formal adjudication inappropriate.

Arbitration is a possibility. Its advantages include a jointly chosen arbiter who can issue a final decision. The arbiter will have expertise in the area, thus ensuring that more technical arguments can be made. Additional advantages include confidentiality, relatively low cost, and more rapid resolution than with the formal adjudication. Most likely, all these characteristics are factors that both parties would find agreeable. However, arbiters' decisions usually are based on objective standards because arbitration is a rights-based procedure. Here, there is no clear-cut, single objective standard: The CON application apparently does not decide the issue; the state authority has expressed no opinion; the law does not seem to apply; and a rights-based process may sully the future relationship between the parties. Further, the possibility of either party withdrawing its support (Johnson City's patient base, St. Francis's money) would likely preclude acquisition of the MRI. Finally, arbitration does not fare as well as other ADR methods in terms of relative cost, speed, and ability to improve the parties' relationship by focusing on their joint interests. Hence, there appear to be some significant disadvantages in using arbitration to settle this dispute.

Mediation seems to provide a much better fit. There is a potential for clarifying communication lines and allowing for a creative resolution of the dispute without the necessity of revisiting the divergent CON application interpretations. The mediator also can take into account the possible internal pressures from the marketing department at St. Francis. Because the emphasis of the mediation process can be to focus on the future of the relationship and the joint interests of the parties, it can provide a foundation for building consensus between the hospitals. Also, because these parties are relatively new partners, a creative solution could spur additional, innovative joint ventures while simultaneously providing for and integrating in the process a communication pattern that takes into account the important allocative decisions that affect an organizational entity with separate and distinct sites. Further, an evaluative process could be integrated into the process to provide both parties the opportunity for reflection and feedback for each joint project so as to learn important lessons from each effort. These lessons, of course, could and should be applied to future projects. Therefore, mediation has many advantages in this situation.

Within this purview, it appears that evaluative hybrids methods would not be appropriate. Evaluative hybrids are ADR methods that are variants on primary processes such as mediation and formal adjudication. For example, summary jury trial, best for disputes involving a disparate view of the facts and law by opposing parties, would be inappropriate here because the parties do not disagree on the governing law. In addition, early neutral evaluation, also strong in law questions due to its adjudicatory nature, has similar limitations.

Therefore, in this interfacility dispute, a mediation process might be proposed by appropriate representatives of the two hospitals. The mediation process fits best with the underlying sources of the dispute and addresses these issues from the perspective of an ongoing relationship with much promise for the future. It allows for the application of creative, mutually beneficial solutions. Because both parties must have a strong incentive to come to the bargaining (or mediation) table due to the valuable property interest they jointly own (the CON), there is an enhanced likelihood for a successfully mediated settlement. Mediation also provides for retrospective analysis of the conflict that can teach important lessons to be applied in the future.

Arbitration, while meeting some of the needs to clarify past miscommunication, has some problems because it does not look to the parties' future relationship. Moreover, it requires some relatively objective standard for dispute resolution that does not appear to be clearly available here. Finally, law-based processes (evaluative hybrids) as well as formal adjudication seem inapplicable in this type of case because of the repeat player status of the parties and the ambiguity of applicable legal rules, which do not indicate a single appropriate winning party.

Example 2. An Intrafacility Conflict: Exclusive Contracts and Provider Termination

Background

To procure necessary health care services, an extremely common arrangement used by health care facilities is to contract for these services with either a single physician or physician groups as independent contractors. This contractual arrangement allows the health care facility to offer 24-hour physician service in the particular specialty and avoids the necessity and the expense of providing health, retirement, and other benefits to these individuals.

In this regard, the predominant contractual agreement mode used by hospitals when contracting for hospital-based physician services is the exclusive contract. Hospitals typically will contract with physicians for a specified time period with the stipulation that, if given the specified notice in the agreement, either the hospital or independent contractor physician may terminate the contract without cause.

Thus, these contracts are dual-edged swords. On the one hand, within the time period for which the exclusive contract is applicable, the physician or physician group has the right and power to charge for all physician services in the specialty, to the exclusion of other, nonexclusive contract physician(s). On the other hand, the hospital has the power to terminate the relationship for any or no reason at all after giving the requisite notice as indicated in the contract.

Case Scenario

Drake Hospital (the Hospital) is a relatively large (450 beds) community hospital located in an affluent suburb. It serves primarily middle- to upper-class patients in the area and has available all of the major medical specialty services. Virtually no patients who come to the Hospital are Medicaid patients. Those who have received care from the Hospital uniformly report satisfaction with its services. Patients generally find the new physical plant, available parking, and courteous staff quite pleasing. The cafeteria also is modern and its food edible. It therefore is no surprise that private physicians enjoy the amicable atmosphere and tolerable food as well as the private patients in the facility.

Dr. Smith is a board-certified radiologist at the Hospital. He graduated from P & S Medical School. Dr. Smith did residency training and entered private practice at the Hospital, working at the Hospital for the past 21 years under an exclusive contractual arrangement. Under the terms of the contract, the Hospital pays Dr. Smith a small salary, which is supplemented by charges to the Hospital or referred patients' third-party insurers for rendered radiology services, as is normal practice. Dr. Smith also sees several of his own patients, who come in for specific radiological procedures. For example, he performs and interprets chest X rays for a patient who was diagnosed several years ago with Hodgkin's disease and cured by radiation therapy but requires annual radiological films to check for any recurrence. There have never been any allegations of poor quality of care against Dr. Smith. In fact, two years ago, Dr. Smith was awarded the Hospital's Community Service Award for distinguished, long-term service to the Hospital and its patients.

One month ago, Dr. Smith was in the Radiology Department reading room interpreting some MRI scans when the Hospital administrator asked to see Dr. Smith privately. When both were in Dr. Smith's office, the administrator told him, "As you know, in about three months your contract is up for renewal. Now don't get me wrong; we on the board have been happy with all the work you've done. But we are not going to renew your contract; we just think it's time for some new blood."

After the administrator left, Dr. Smith sat alone and thought: "Why is this happening? This place is more than a workplace for me; this can't be happening. What can an older physician do for money? This shouldn't be happening; they don't have the right to sully my reputation. Should I contact a lawyer? I'm going to challenge this somehow." Dr. Smith then finished up the MRI readings for the day and left for home.

ADR Assessment

The goals of the parties in this situation are not entirely clear. The Hospital has terminated Dr. Smith's employment, and this action appears to be well within its contractual and legal rights. A question is raised regarding why the Hospital wants to fire Dr. Smith, particularly in light of his service to the facility and its satisfaction with his work.

From Dr. Smith's perspective, the termination results in the prospect of unemployment. Further, concerns regarding reputation are evident. It is clear that Dr. Smith would wish to stay at the Hospital if possible. He apparently has significant emotional ties there. However, it also is clear that Dr. Smith is contemplating legal action.

Because the goals of the Hospital are unclear, or unexpressed, there may be a lack of good communication between the parties. Perhaps the Hospital was not comfortable explaining to Dr. Smith that it felt he was getting on in years and could not maintain the rigors of a full-time practice. Or, although happy with Dr. Smith's services, the Hospital may have been offered a lower contract price by another radiologist or radiology group. Therefore, a method of dispute resolution that addresses this communication problem would be best.

From this assessment, mediation most likely would be an appropriate choice. The nature of the dispute seems to require more exchange of information (or the disclosure of new information). The parties must learn more about

their respective interests. Given the apparent difficulty in communication, mediation may provide a sensitive and reasonable forum to resolve the dispute.

Dr. Smith, however, appears to have conflicting goals that affect the appropriate choice of forum. On the one hand, Dr. Smith wishes to keep his radiology position at the Hospital. So, a continuing relationship is desired. However, it also appears that Dr. Smith has strong feelings that the termination was inappropriate. Further, there is a concern that his reputation will suffer.

In contract disputes involving physicians, the potential effect on the doctor's reputation is a very important concern. In few other professions does this concept apply so broadly and to such a great degree. For Dr. Smith, his reputation relates not only to patients but to other physicians. If other physicians attempt to refer patients to Dr. Smith and he is required to tell them he no longer has privileges at the Hospital, then there may be some implication of questionable competence or poor quality of care. Further, if Dr. Smith attempts to find other work, then the same shadow on his reputation may arise. Although Dr. Smith sees some private patients at the Hospital, the majority of his income derives from his Hospital practice and referrals from other physicians. Accordingly, his reputation becomes a significant concern to Dr. Smith as he considers actions involving (and possibly against) the Hospital.

Therefore, on one hand, a clearer understanding of the issues ("why is this happening?"), the desire to continue as the radiologist at the Hospital, and emotional ties might point toward a mediation approach. On the other hand, Dr. Smith's desire to maintain his reputation in the community (and with respect to other potential employers) would point to some other form of dispute resolution.

In this case, a combination of mediation and arbitration might be optimal. Perhaps the best fit would be mediation-advisory arbitration rather than a mediation-binding arbitration because the latter has some significant disadvantages as applied to this situation. First, there is a high probability that the Hospital would not want to be completely candid in discussing its decision not to renew Dr. Smith's contract if it knew that a binding decision could follow. The mediator therefore would have relatively less information with which to work when attempting to help the parties craft a jointly creative and beneficial solution. Further, because subsequent arbitration may focus on whether one party is "right," changing the dynamic to divert the dispute resolution process away from interest-based solutions to the conflict, there may be less tendency for the parties to try to resolve the problem at the mediation stage. Indeed, there may be a significant amount of game playing by the parties in an effort to convince the mediator that one or the other is deserving of a favorable decision.

The Hospital most likely would not wish to enter into a binding process and risk losing when it has a favorable legal position. Nevertheless, it may wish to enter into an ADR procedure to avoid the legal costs of formal adjudication and eschew negative publicity. Moreover, certain "emotional" considerations may be inducing the Hospital to treat Dr. Smith in a fair manner.

Mediation-advisory arbitration could address the disadvantages of mediation-binding arbitration. First, it bears emphasizing that advisory arbitration is just that — only advisory. This would preserve the creative solution emphasis and restore the mediation dynamic to the process, rather than focus on a determination of who is "right." More open communication between the parties, perhaps through the mediator, could occur and would allow the parties to participate actively in the dispute resolution process. If mediation fails, then an advisory position (an evaluative process) could give Dr. Smith and the Hospital an objective assessment regarding the conflict, should the matter proceed to formal adjudication.

This process also could serve Dr. Smith's need to address his professional reputation concern: The settlement or possibly an acceptable advisory opinion could expressly state that the Hospital's actions regarding Dr. Smith were not based on any quality of care concerns or similar language to that effect. This would give Dr. Smith the ability to go to other providers in search of employment and show that a neutral third party had found (and the Hospital had stated) that no quality of care issues triggered Dr. Smith's change in status at the Hospital.

Note, however, that a possible disadvantage of mediation-advisory arbitration is the potential length of the process. With both mediation and advisory arbitration, time may be spent on adjudicatory arbitration or formal court activity in addition to the extra step of advisory arbitration. However, empirical data suggests a significant probability that the dispute could be resolved without resorting to formal adjudication.

Therefore, in this scenario, mediation-advisory arbitration appears to be appropriate. Pure evaluative procedures, such as summary jury trial and early neutral evaluation, could be helpful if there is a different view of the legal rights of the parties. Here, it seems the Hospital has the authority not to renew Dr. Smith's contract. Arbitration, although possibly favorable to the Hospital, would not serve Dr. Smith's interest-based concerns very well and, as a single method, most likely would be inappropriate.

Example 3. Provider–Family End-of-Life Treatment Conflicts: Dr. Franklin–Jones Family Dispute

Background

The Patient Self-Determination Act of 1990 mandates that patients admitted to a hospital be given information regarding end-of-life directives and proxy decision making in the event that the patient cannot personally make these decisions. In this capacity, patients can make preauthorized treatment choices regarding the types of medical care to be provided in the event of a terminal health condition. For example, a patient can elect do not resuscitate (DNR) status for all incurable disorders. Further, an individual patient can elect to transfer this decision-making capacity to another person (for example, a family member or personal physician) in the event the patient loses the ability to make these decisions.

Case Scenario

Mrs. Jones is an 89-year-old woman with many of the conditions associated with being elderly. She has hypertension that is poorly controlled, non-insulin-dependent diabetes, renal disease, and a medical history that includes two heart attacks. She has been admitted to various hospitals many times, most recently (before the current admission) four months ago, when she was diagnosed with pneumonia and spent four weeks in the intensive care unit. She recovered from the event but was weakened considerably by it.

Following discharge, Mrs. Jones was cared for in her son's home. Her son and his family refused to send her to a nursing home. They believed that sending her to a nursing home "would be like saying we didn't want her." Mrs. Jones enjoyed living with her son's family and has a good relationship with them, particularly her grandchildren. She believes that her role in life is to "spoil my wonderful grandchildren as much as possible."

During past hospitalizations, Mrs. Jones told her family and Dr. Franklin, her personal family physician, that she did not want "heroic efforts" used in the event she loses her cogency. She signed an admission statement to that effect in accordance with the Patient Self-Determination Act when she was hospitalized four months ago. She also designated her son as proxy in the event she could not make end-of-life decisions. Moreover, she refused to be placed on a ventilator in the intensive care unit, stating: "If I can't live without that thing, I don't want to live; just give me antibiotics and if that isn't enough, so be it." The hospital staff complied with her wishes and she subsequently recovered. She also stated that, "If I don't know my family, I don't want to live; I mean, what would be the point?" The refusal of ventilator support was recorded on the medical chart; the latter statement was not.

Approximately two weeks ago, Mrs. Jones was hospitalized again. She was brought by her family to the emergency room at the hospital where she had been admitted for pneumonia treatment four months earlier. Her current medical illness stems directly from her renal disease and she was confused on admission, a normal medical finding in such clinical circumstances. She was admitted directly to the intensive care unit, where treatment was begun that focused on addressing her renal condition. Initially, the treatment appeared to be working. Mrs. Jones became mentally clearer and recognized her family. She joked with her grandchildren and introduced the house staff to her family. However, within a week of admission, her condition worsened significantly, to the point where she no longer recognized her family and was somnolent and unreactive.

Dr. Franklin, who was seeing her on a daily basis, noted that, over the past two days, Mrs. Jones entered into total renal failure and, despite 100% oxygen therapy, her blood oxygen levels dropped so far as to be providing her brain with inadequate oxygenation. After obtaining a scan of her brain function, it appeared that Mrs. Jones no longer had any brain activity. Dr. Franklin checked Mrs. Jones's medical chart and found that she did not sign a new DNR or proxy agreement. Dr. Franklin therefore went to Mrs. Jones's son to discuss the DNR status and withdrawal of life-support measures. Mrs. Jones's son, distraught over her condition, angrily stated that all efforts should be pursued, no DNR status was to be given, and that "I'll sue you for everything you've got and this hospital, too, if you let her die." Dr. Franklin believed Mrs. Jones's status should be DNR and that efforts to discontinue life-support measures should be undertaken in accordance with his knowledge of her wishes.

ADR Assessment

This is a significantly difficult (and, sadly, common) conflict to address. Aside from the ethical dilemmas presented, it is obvious that the dispute is rife with emotional issues associated with the death of a family member. The goal of Mrs. Jones's son, it appears, is currently short term. He wants her to live, or more accurately, he wants her to live, with her previous quality of life. Because of the nature of the conflict — the tragedy of the end of life of a loved one — he is beginning to experience the traditional psychological stages of those affected by human illness: denial, anger, bargaining, depression, and acceptance. He currently is denying her condition and is angry about it; his emotions are blotting out his mother's own ideal as to what is appropriate treatment in this clinical situation. Therefore, his goals (and his lack of flexibility) are not likely to change until he passes through the other psychological stages leading to acceptance.

Dr. Franklin's goals are more focused on Mrs. Jones's desires. Because Mrs. Jones made clear to her family and to Dr. Franklin that she would not want life-support treatment in the event of loss of cogency, Dr. Franklin raised this issue with the family. Moreover, Dr. Franklin believes that in the unlikely event Mrs. Jones survives her present illness, she will not leave the intensive care unit with any cogency or personality because of her lack of brain function and significant medical problems. Hence, Dr. Franklin is attempting to follow the directions provided orally by Mrs. Jones regarding her choice of care in such a circumstance.

An ADR procedure that addresses these parties' needs is not immediately apparent. Although the emotional barriers that exist might be handled through mediation, efforts to gain the parties' trust, particularly that of Mrs. Jones's son, are likely to fail at this stage. Any attempt to consider cessation of treatment would alienate Mrs. Jones's son from the process. Aside from Mrs. Jones's son, the hospital also might be unwilling to participate because of a perceived liability risk if it allows termination of life support.

An arbitration process suffers from the same weaknesses. Certainly, voluntary arbitration would not be acceptable to Mrs. Jones's son in his current state. Further, a mediation-arbitration procedure would not be acceptable, due to the weaknesses of mediation already noted. An evaluative procedure such as a mini-trial or summary jury trial has potential advantages through use of, and evaluation by, a neutral third party. The process would include an analysis of the law in the area and a clarification and objective assessment of the relevant facts (including Mrs. Jones's previous communication to her son and Dr. Franklin). But again, in his emotional state, this process also is likely to be futile because Mrs. Jones's son would not agree to the process. Further, even if he did engage in the process, any decision or proposal would be rejected by him if it involved the cessation of medical treatment for his mother. In addition, the process likely would take some time due to the necessary evidentiary and other requirements that need to be addressed, as well as the pragmatic concern of obtaining an appropriate adjudicator or jury.

Another possibility is to use an ombudsman, perhaps with psychological training, to allow Mrs. Jones's son to vent his frustrations and help him accept the reality of his mother's situation. However, once again, any consideration of a reduction of Mrs. Jones's care would result in her son rejecting this process. Anecdotal evidence also indicates that this method has a significant probability of failure.

This highly charged, emotional situation, which results in a single party with a focused and inflexible (and perhaps unrealistic) goal, presents significant problems for using any ADR process. It appears that, in this medical context, the only reasonable solution would be for the hospital and Dr. Franklin to access the formal adjudication system. This solution, albeit weak, may be the only one available. To bring an emotionally torn individual to court because of the impending death of a loved one certainly will not help in that individual's progression through the grieving process. Further, the position of the hospital and physician could appear to be draconian and lacking in compassion, although this generally would not be the case. Indeed, because of this perception, it may be necessary to allow the patient to stay in the intensive care unit until he or she dies. Such a solution is costly (in terms of dollars), inequitable (in terms of the patient's own directive), painful (in terms of the extended family grieving), and potentially unfair (for other patients who would benefit more from the concentrated resources provided in an intensive care unit).

Notes on ADR

Early Neutral Evaluation

Early neutral evaluation usually is a court-annexed process that requires the parties to have their dispute assessed by an experienced third-party neutral evaluator on the basis of short presentations by both parties. It thus is a rights-based procedure like arbitration and formal adjudication. Usually the third-party neutral is a volunteer attorney chosen by the court. Once the presentations are made, the parties negotiate in an effort at settlement. If they do not settle, the neutral evaluator assists the parties to simplify and clarify the case so that it will be more amenable to formal adjudication. This process was pioneered by the U.S. district court for northern California.

Additional Reading. M. A. Buckstein, "An Introductory Primer on Pre-Litigation ADR Counseling for the Outside Lawyer," *Dispute Resolution Journal* 52 (1997), pp. 35–42; E. S. Strong, "A User's Guide to Alternative Dispute Resolution in Business Cases," *Practical Lawyer* 43, no. 4 (1997), pp. 15–26.

Ethics of Summary Jury Trial

Summary jury trials utilize actual jurors taken from the jury pool to obtain advisory jury verdicts. However, these jurors are not told that they are not participating in an actual jury trial. This raises significant ethical issues associated with deceiving individuals as to their role in formal adjudication — none — while the parties and the judge retain this knowledge for their own personal benefit (e.g., reduction of court dockets, assessment of the potential for high jury award verdicts).

Additional Reading. C. W. Hatfield, "The Summary Jury Trial: Who Will Speak for the Jurors?" *Journal of Dispute Resolution* (1991), pp. 151–59; L. M. Ponte, "Putting Mandatory Summary Jury Trial Back on the Docket: Recommendations on the Exercise of Judicial Authority," *Fordham Law Review* 63 (1995), pp. 1069–98.

Incentives and Game Playing in Mediation

Generally, mediation looks to joint benefits to craft solutions to disputes between parties. Therefore, the focus of, for example, the mediator is to identify such joint bene-

fits. However, often this identification process becomes the paramount goal; once joint goals are identified, it is assumed that the parties will settle. Yet, even in circumstances where joint benefits are identified, no resolution of the dispute occurs or the dispute finally is resolved using formal adjudication. These situations can be explained in part because even though one party may have some interests in common with the other, unique interests are valued higher such that no resolution to the dispute is preferable for that party. The party can play games with the system by appearing cooperative and identifying joint benefits with the other party. If the mediator does not recognize that unique party goals and interests are greater than the joint benefits identified, the process may be frustrating and waste the time and resources of the party and mediator.

Additional Reading. B. A. Liang, "Understanding and Applying Alternative Dispute Resolution Methods in Modern Medical Conflicts," *Journal of Legal Medicine* 19 (1998), pp. 397–430.

Private Judging

With the advent and growth of ADR, a significant private market has sprouted to render adjudicative services and decisions. Private judging (also known as *rent a judge*) is a reflection of this growth. Many of these participants are retired judges who provide adjudication or engage in other ADR processes. In California, these private judges are paid by the parties and are empowered by state statute to enter final judgments, which have precedential value and can be appealed to appellate courts just like formal adjudications.[19] Similarly, Florida and Texas have statutory provisions that require referral of certain court cases to private ADR providers paid for by the parties.[20]

Additional Reading. H. I. Bendix and R. Chernick, "Renting the Judge," *Litigation* 21, no. 1 (1994), pp. 33–35.

"Rights-Based" Mediation

Generally, traditional mediation (also known as *interest-based mediation*) focuses on creating a mutually accept-

---

[19]See Assami v. Assami, 872 P.2d 1190 (Cal. 1994); Estate of Kent, 57 P.2d 901 (Cal. 1936); Solorzano v. Sup. Ct., 22 Cal.Rptr.2d 401 (Cal. App. 1993).

[20]See, e.g., *Texas Alcoholic Beverage Code* §102.77 (parties must pay for arbitration costs); *Florida Statutes Annotated* §44.103; *Florida Alternative Dispute Resolution* §718.1255 (mandating voluntary mediation and mandatory nonbinding arbitration).

able solution to resolve the dispute and does not involve an evaluation of the strengths and weaknesses of each party's case. However, rights-based mediation focuses on the legal rights of the parties, and thus the process is more akin to evaluative processes such as early neutral evaluation. Of course, often the line between rights-based mediation and interest-based mediation may be blurred because the third-party neutral mediator, in his or her effort to assist the parties in creating a solution, may assess the legal rights of the parties.

Additional Reading. M. D. Young, *The Mediation of Investor-Broker Disputes: A Fair and Cost-Effective Non-Binding Alternative to Arbitration or Litigation*, pub. no. B4-6932 (New York: Practising Law Institute — Corporate Law, July 1990).

Screening Panels

Screening panels usually perform state-mandated pretrial assessments. Plaintiffs, before submitting their medical malpractice claims for trial, are required to have their case assessed by a special panel; this panel usually is composed of physicians, other medical professionals, attorneys, and laypersons. These panels hear the plaintiff's case and issue a nonbinding opinion. Usually, either party can bring these cases to court, regardless of the panel's assessment. However, some states allow the panel's findings to be introduced into court. Results appear to be mixed, and their use has not become widespread. Difficulties have centered about the administrative burdens these panels represent and their associated delays; further, they may make assessments too early in the process, before either party has made significant inroads into investigating the claims.

Additional Reading. R. Boyle, "Medical Malpractice Screening Panels: A Judicial Evaluation of Their Practical Effect," *University of Pittsburgh Law Review* 42 (1991), pp. 939–60; J. A. Macchioroli, "Medical Malpractice Screening Panels: Proposed Model Legislation to Cure Judicial Ills," *George Washington Law Review* 50 (1990), pp. 181–260; D. J. Rasor, "Mandatory Medical Malpractice Screening Panels: A Need to Reevaluate," *Ohio State Journal on Dispute Resolution* 9 (1993), pp. 115–42.

Settlement Conference

Another form of ADR, the settlement conference (also known as the *voluntary settlement conference*), is a method by which a judge, a set of attorneys, or a "settlement master" (an independent party who assesses such conflicts) reads briefs and materials as well as hears pre-

sentations from both sides of a dispute, then actively seeks to craft a settlement package for the parties. The active nature of the intermediary (as opposed to other forms of ADR such as mediation where the mediator is merely a facilitator) includes asking questions of the parties and providing opinions to each party as to the relative strength of its case. Often, after reading the submitted documents and hearing each side, the intermediary may hold a caucus with each party individually and move between the parties in an effort to fashion a settlement. Settlement conferences are used by courts before formal adjudication in an attempt to have parties settle cases before they go to trial. Indeed, some courts will not set a case for trial unless some settlement conference has been held. The major complaint of this form of ADR is that they are considered by some to be coercive, and at times parties feel pressured to settle, do so, and later are dissatisfied with the result.

Additional Reading. J. E. Grenig, "Judicially Hosted Settlement Conferences," in *Alternative Dispute Resolution with Forms,* 2d ed. (St. Paul, MN: West Publishing Co., 1997), section 17.40; J. E. Grenig, "Voluntary Settlement Conference," in *Alternative Dispute Resolution with Forms,* 2d ed. (St. Paul, MN: West Publishing Co., 1997), section 18.42; B. E. Witkin, *California Procedure,* 4th ed. (St. Paul, MN: West Publishing Co., 1997), section 60.

Further Reading

ADR Agreement Drafting

American Arbitration Association. *Drafting Dispute Resolution Clauses: A Practical Guide.* Washington, DC: American Arbitration Association, 1992.

Center for Public Resources. *Dispute Resolution Clauses for Business Agreements.* New York: Center for Public Resources, 1992.

Committee on Dispute Resolution, Center for Public Resources. *Drafting Dispute Resolution Clauses: The State of the Art.* New York: Center for Public Resources, 1993.

Meyerson BE, Cooper C. *A Drafter's Guide to Alternative Dispute Resolution.* Chicago: American Bar Association, 1991.

ADR and Medical Malpractice Claims

Bartholomew L. The Realities of Medical Malpractice Mediation. *Addressing the Medical, Legal and Ethical Dilemmas in Modern Health Care: Proceedings of the 39th Annual Conference of the American College of Legal Medicine*, New Orleans, March 11–13, 1999. Milwaukee: American College of Legal Medicine, 1999;393–408.

Few Medical Malpractice Cases Submitted to ADR, Says GAO. *Alternatives to High Cost Litig* 1992;10:82–89.

Metzloff TB. Alternative Dispute Resolution Strategies in Medical Malpractice. *Alaska L Rev* 1992;9:429–55.

Stevens CM. The Benefits of ADR for Medical Malpractice. *Disp Resol J* 1995;50:65–69.

Arbitration

Buckner F. Arbitration Clauses in Contracts Between Providers and Patients. *Med Prac Management* 1998; Sept.–Oct.:98–101.

Horvath LM. Tenth Circuit Arbitration. *Denv U L Rev* 1996; 73:637–56.

Pertcheck KM. Arbitration Survey. *Denv U L Rev* 1995; 72:571–92.

Shell R. ERISA and Other Federal Employment Statutes: When Is Commercial Arbitration an "Adequate Substitute" for the Courts? *Tex L Rev* 1990;68:509–73.

Formal Adjudication

Dore LK. Secrecy by Consent: The Use and Limits of Confidentiality in the Pursuit of Settlement. *Notre Dame L Rev* 1999;74:283–402.

Liang BA. Understanding and Applying ADR Methods in Modern Medical Conflicts. *J Legal Med* 1998;19:397–430.

Med-Arb

Ravin RL. Y2K and ADR: Get Ready for Midnight. *Disp Resol J* 1998;53:8–15.

Sabatino JM. ADR as "Litigation Lite": Procedural and Evidentiary Norms Embedded Within Alternative Dispute Resolution. *Emory L J* 1997;47:1289–1349.

Mediation

Center for Dispute Settlement. *Mediation for the Professional*. Washington, DC: Center for Dispute Settlement, 1991.

Davidson JE. Successful Mediation: The Do's and Don't's. *Disp Resol J* 1998;53:26–29.

Litowitz DE. Internal versus External Perspectives on Law: Toward Mediation. *Fla St U L Rev* 1998;26:127–50.

Mini-Trial

Arnold T et al. Minitrials: Opportunities for Compromise. *Tex B J* 1988;51:34–49.

Grenig JE. Advantages and Disadvantages of Minitrials. In: *Alternative Dispute Resolution with Forms,* 2d ed. St. Paul, MN: West Publishing Co., 1997:§8.2.

Summary Jury Trial

Harges BM. The Promise of the Mandatory Summary Jury Trial. *Temp L Rev* 1990;63:799–827.

Newman G. The Summary Jury Trial as a Method of Dispute Resolution in the Federal Courts. *U Ill L Rev* 1990:177–205.

Other Reading

Fisher R, Ury W. *Getting to Yes: Negotiating Agreement Without Giving In,* 2d ed. New York: Penguin Books, 1991.

Goldberg SB et al. *Dispute Resolution: Negotiation, Mediation, and Other Processes,* 2d ed. Gaithersburg, MD: Aspen, 1992.

Liang BA. Understanding and Applying Alternative Dispute Resolution Methods in Modern Medical Conflicts. *J Legal Med* 1998;19:397–430.

Metzloff TB. Alternative Dispute Resolution Strategies in Medical Malpractice. *Alaska L Rev* 1992; 9:429–55.

Metzloff TB. The Unrealized Potential of Malpractice Arbitration. *Wake Forest L Rev* 1996; 31:203–30.

Rasor DJ. Mandatory Medical Malpractice Screening Panels: A Need to Reevaluate. *Ohio State J Disp Resol* 1993;9:115–42.

Simmons WO. An Economic Analysis of Mandatory Mediation and the Disposition of Medical Malpractice Claims. *J Legal Econ* 1996;6:41–75.

Stevens CM. The Benefits of ADR for Medical Malpractice: Adopting Contract Rather Than Tort Law. *Disp Resol J* 1995;50:65–69.

Weiler PC. *Medical Malpractice on Trial.* Cambridge, MA: Harvard University Press, 1991.

Web Sites

ABA net — Section of dispute resolution: *http://www.abanet.org/dispute*

Alternative dispute resolution: *http://www.state.nj.us/lps/ca/adr/htm*

Alternate dispute resolution resources: *http://adrr.com*

American Arbitration Association: *http://www.adr.org*

Chartered Institute of Arbitrators: *http://www.arbitrators.org*

Conflict Research Consortium: *http://www.colorado.edu/conflict*

CPR Institute for Dispute Resolution: *http://www.cpradr.org*

Georgetown University ADR resources page: *http://www//georgetown.edu/lr/rs/dispute.html*

Guide to alternate dispute resolution: *http://hg.org/adr.html*

Institute for Conflict Analysis and Resolution: *http://web.gmu.edu/departments/ICAR/*

JAMS-Endispute: *http://www.jams-endispute.com*

Law forum–ADR: *http://www.lawforum.net/services/alternative.htm*

Legal Information Institute — ADR: *http://www.cornell.edu/topics/adr.html*

Mediation information and resource center: *http://www.mediate.com*

Program on negotiation at Harvard Law School: *http://www.pon.harvard.edu*

Self-administered ADR: *http://wwwcpradr.org/selfadm.htm*

State Bar of Texas Alternative Dispute Section: *http://www.texasadr.org/index.html*

PART IV
End-of-Life Considerations

15

Advance Directives

Patients under the U.S. Constitution and the common law have the fundamental right to direct their medical care, even if such decision making results in their death (sometimes known as *the right to die*).[1] The right to die has an analysis similar to the basis for informed consent;[2] the patient has the right to determine which, if any, medical care he or she chooses to accept on the basis of his or her individual autonomy. These decisions must be respected by medical providers on this basis.

Advance directives are documents that provide medical care professionals with information regarding a patient's wishes as to the extent and nature of desired medical care if the patient loses decision-making capacity. Legal enforcement and liability may attach if health care professionals act beyond the sphere of patient-executed advance directives. Every state has some form of advance directive (also known as *natural death*) legislation specifying characteristics of these legal pronouncements. State legislation generally focuses on the characteristics of the two most common forms of the advance directive: the living will and the durable power

of attorney. These directives, and related issues, are discussed here.

Living Will

A living will is a written advance directive that indicates the clinical circumstances under which the patient would or would not want to have his or her life sustained through specific medical treatments. As can be seen by this definition, the living will can be as broad or as narrow as the executing individual wishes to make it. However, almost every state has a living will statute that may indicate the acceptable form of the living will for that state as well as specify certain conditions under which the living will is applicable (e.g., only if two or more physicians certify that the patient's condition is "terminal"; inapplicability to pregnant patients). In addition, as a general rule, once a living will is provided to a physician, that physician must either accede to its directives or transfer the patient to another physician who will. Generally, state laws also provide physicians with immunity from liability for complying with a properly executed living will.

The major difficulty with the living will is that it may have limited use clinically. Because every clinical circumstance cannot be determined *ex ante*, the living will may be too specific (e.g., listing only specific conditions or disease states when it applies, and only specific medical interventions to be forgone in these disease states) or too ambiguous (e.g., using ambiguous language such as "no heroic efforts should be provided if my condition is hopeless"). In these circumstances, the only recourse for a provider to avoid potential *ex post* lawsuits for inappropriate application of the living will is to bring the case to a court to ascertain whether specific withdrawals of medical intervention are contemplated by the living will in question.

---

[1]See, e.g., In re Quinlan, 355 A.2d 647 (N.J.), *cert. denied* Garger v. New Jersey, 429 U.S. 922 (1976); Cruzan v. Director, Missouri Dept. of Health, 497 U.S. 261 (1990); Washington v. Glucksberg, 521 U.S. 702 (1997); McKay v. Bergstedt, 801 P.2d 617 (Nev. 1990); In re Conroy, 486 A.2d 1209 (N.J. 1985); Union Pacific Ry. Co. v. Botsford, 141 U.S. 250 (1891); Pratt v. Davis, 79 N.E.562 (Ill. 1906); Mohr v. Williams, 104 N.W. 12 (Minn. 1905); see Chapter 3, "Informed Consent."

[2]See, e.g., Bouvia v. Superior Ct., 225 Cal.Rptr. 297 (Cal. Ct. App. 1986); Superintendent of Belchertown State School v. Saikewicz, 370 N.E.2d 417 (Mass. 1977); Foody v. Manchester Mem. Hosp., 482 A.2d 713 (Conn. Super. Ct. 1984); In re Fiori, 652 A.2d 1350 (Pa. Super. Ct. 1995); In re Westchester County Med. Ctr., 534 N.Y.S.2d 886 (N.Y. 1988).

Durable Power of Attorney

The durable power of attorney or health care proxy is another written advance directive. This document designates a specific person (or persons or institution) to make health care decisions for the patient if he or she is mentally incapacitated. The patient also may designate an alternate party if the specified person is unavailable or unwilling to serve in this capacity. The designated person, also known as the *attorney-in-fact*, will be a surrogate decision maker for the patient (known as the *principal*) in health care circumstances. No medical circumstances (other than mental incapacity), medical treatments, or proof of the attorney-in-fact's actual knowledge of the patient's wishes need to be in the document to make the document legally valid. Of course, such information may be specified if desired; however, this specification (or ambiguity) raises the same difficulties as with the living will. As is evident by the broad nature of a durable power of attorney, an individual named as attorney-in-fact has tremendous discretion in issuing a valid, binding decision with regard to the health care of the incapacitated patient. This characteristic alone makes the durable power of attorney more useful than the living will, which, as indicated earlier, could be too narrow or too broad for practical, clinical use. It is important to note, however, that this form of advance directive also is subject to state law, which may restrict the power of the attorney-in-fact beyond requiring that the patient be mentally incompetent (e.g., health care proxy decision making requires patient to be in a permanent coma or have a terminal condition).

The general concept behind the use of a durable power of attorney is that of "substituted judgment"; that is, the attorney-in-fact will make the decision that the patient, if he or she were competent, would make.[3] Of course, this is an ideal to which rarely, if ever, a proxy decision maker could reach. In most cases, and in cases where the patient was never competent, the general principle that is followed is to make the decision that would be in the best interests of the patient,[4] in the context of any relevant information the proxy decision maker has with regard to the preferences of the patient.

Because of the broad discretion given to the attorney-in-fact, it is essential that this individual be close to and discuss deeply the desires and wishes of the patient with regard to health care in various situations. Particularly if the patient's wishes are not within "traditional" socially accepted norms, the patient should choose an attorney-in-fact who understands and can articulate such wishes. In these circumstances, such information may be best included within the durable power of attorney document itself.

Patient Self-Determination Act

The Patient Self-Determination Act[5] is a federal statute passed by Congress in 1990 in an effort to allow patients to avoid unwanted life-sustaining medical intervention. The act requires that all facilities that receive Medicare or Medicaid reimbursement (home health agencies, hospices, hospitals, skilled nursing facilities, and health maintenance organizations) provide patients with information regarding the state's advance directive policies. Specifically, facilities are mandated to:

1. Provide all adult patients, residents, and enrollees with written information on their rights under state law (both statutory and common law) to make decisions regarding their health care, including the right to execute an advance directive.
2. Maintain the policies of the provider with respect to implementation of advance directives.
3. Document in the medical record whether the person has an advance directive.
4. Educate the facility's staff and the community about advance directives.
5. Ensure compliance with state law regarding advance directives.

Providers such as hospitals and nursing facilities must give this information to patients on admission, home health and hospice providers must indicate the statutory requirements before rendering care, and HMOs must provide this information at the time membership becomes effective. In addition, the Department of Health and Human Services is required to provide public education regarding advance directives and oversee provider compliance with the act. Note, however, that the act imposes these requirements institutionally; individual health care professionals and emergency medical teams have no obligations under the act. Similar advance directive requirements are mandated for hospitals and other health care organizations by JCAHO as a condition for accredi-

---

[3]See, e.g., In re Eichner, 420 N.E.2d 64 (N.Y.), *cert. denied* 454 U.S. 858 (1981); Foody v. Manchester Mem. Hosp., 482 A.2d 713 (Conn. 1984); In re Severns, 425 A.2d 156 (Del. 1980); In re Estate of Longeway, 549 N.E.2d 292 (Ill. 1989); In re Gardner, 534 A.2d 947 (Me. 1987); Superintendent of Belchertown State School v. Saikewicz, 370 N.E.2d 417 (Mass. 1977); In re Peter, 529 A.2d 419 (N.J. 1987); Leach v. Akron Gen. Med. Ctr., 426 N.E.2d 809 (Ohio 1980); In re Rosebush, 491 N.W.2d 633 (Mich. Ct. App. 1992); In re Hughes, 611 A.2d 1148 (N.J. Super. Ct. App. Div. 1992); In re Guardianship of Browning, 543 So.2d 258 (Fla. Dist. Ct. App. 1989); In re Estate of Austwick, 656 N.E.2d 773 (Ill. App. Ct. 1995); Lenz v. L.E. Phillips Career Development Ctr., 482 N.W.2d 60 (Wisc. 1992); In re Edna, 563 N.W.2d 485 (Wisc. 1997).

[4]See, e.g., Rasmussen v. Fleming, 741 P.2d 674 (Ariz. 1987); Conservatorship of Drabick, 245 Cal.Rptr. 840 (Cal. Ct. App. 1988); Conservatorship of Torres, 357 N.W.2d 332 (Minn. 1984); In re Colyer, 660 P.2d 738 (Wash. 1983).

[5]42 U.S.C.A. §§1395cc(f), 1396a(w).

tation. Failure of institutional health care providers to adhere to the provisions of the act by providing the Department of Health and Human Services formal notice of compliance *requires* the Secretary of the DHHS to impose the health finance "death penalty" (exclusion of the institution from the Medicare and Medicaid programs).[6]

Although laudable in its goals, it appears that the Act has not had its intended effect of broadening knowledge and execution of advance directives.[7] Institutional providers appear to be fulfilling most of their substantive responsibilities under the act;[8] yet only approximately 5–25% of the adult population has been estimated to have completed any form of an advance directive. This low percentage has been attributed to poor communication among patients, physicians, and family members.[9] Percentages also appear to be a function of the type and location of patients, with older, nursing home patients having the greatest completion rate; generally, these percentages for the elderly and nursing home residents represent completion by approximately one-third to one-half of the patients who are aware of these instruments.[10]

---

[6]42 U.S.C.A. §1395cc(b). See Chapter 12.

[7]See, e.g., E. J. Larson and T. A. Eaton, "The Limits of Advance Directives: A History and Assessment of the Patient Self-Determination Act," *Wake Forest Law Review* 32 (1997), pp. 249–93; U.S. General Accounting Office, *Patient Self-Determination Act — Providers Offer Information on Advance Directives But Effectiveness Uncertain*, pub. no. HEHS-95-135 (Washington, DC: U.S. General Accounting Office, 1995); J. S. Janofsky and B. W. Rovner, "Prevalence of Advance Directives and Guardianship in Nursing Home Patients," *Journal of Geriatric Psychiatry and Neurology* 6 (1994), pp. 214–16.

[8]U.S. Department of Health and Human Services, Office of Inspector General, *Patient Advance Directives: Early Implementation Experience*, pub. no. OEI 06-91-01130 (Washington, DC: Department of Health and Human Services, 1993).

[9]General Accounting Office, *Patient Self-Determination Act*, section 4; J. LaPuma et al., "Advance Directives on Admission: Clinical Implications and Analysis of the Patient Self-Determination Act," *JAMA* 266 (1991), pp. 402–405.

[10]See, e.g., J. M. Teno et al., "Do Formal Advance Directives Affect Resuscitation Decisions and the Use of Resources for Seriously Ill Patients," *Journal of Clinical Ethics* 5 (1994), pp. 23–30; Janofsky and Rovner, "Prevalence of Advance Directives"; E. H. Elpern et al., "A Preliminary Investigation of Opinions and Behaviors Regarding Advance Directives for Medical Care," *American Journal Critical Care* 2 (1993), pp. 161–67; M. P. Daly and J. Sobal, "Advance Directives Among Patients in a House Call Program," *Journal of the American Board of Family Practitioners* 5 (1992), pp. 11–15; L. L. Emanuel, M. J. Barry, and J. D. Stoeckle, "Advance Directives for Medical Care — A Case for Greater Use," *New England Journal of Medicine* 324 (1991), pp. 889–95; J. Cohen-Mansfield et al., "The Utilization of the Durable Power of Attorney for Health Care Among Hospitalized Elderly Patients," *Journal of the American Geriatrics Society* 39 (1991), pp. 1174–78.

Oral Directives

If an individual loses the capacity to make health care decisions but has not executed either a living will or health care proxy, oral directives may be used to assess what the patient would have wanted in the particular disease and illness circumstance. Oral directives are statements made by the patient to others expressing some form of preference with regard to health care treatment and nontreatment.

The standard by which these statements will be judged, and followed, once again is a function of state law. Generally, there is a high presumption for life, and the patient's statements must meet the "clear and convincing evidence" standard indicating the patient's true preferences in order to be followed.[11] Of course, the most important statements that engender controversy are those that would result in discontinuation of treatment. Again, it bears emphasizing that state law governs just what facts and circumstances would meet such a standard and, indeed, what such a standard would entail. Some courts are relatively strict in their assessment, so that the patient's previous statements must directly address with specificity the clinical situation at hand;[12] others allow for less strict evidence in allowing substituted decision making.[13]

However, a major issue arising from the "clear and convincing evidence" standard associated with oral directives is just how clear and how convincing the evidence need be. This is a difficult assessment to make, and, as might be expected, the results depend highly on the facts and circumstances of each case. Oral statements have been analyzed on a continuum between "casual remarks" and "solemn pronouncements," the latter of which constitutes clear and convincing evidence. Therefore, when a brother of a Catholic religious order repeatedly indicated to other members of his order that he would not want to have his life sustained if in a persistent vegetative state and such a state did occur several years later, the court found that the brother's statement was a solemn pronouncement and met the clear and convincing evidence standard, allowing for termination of life support.[14]

---

[11]See, e.g., Cruzan v. Director, Missouri Dept. of Health, 497 U.S. 261 (1990); In re Westchester Cty. Med. Ctr., 531 N.E.2d 607 (N.Y. 1988); Elbaum v. Grace Plaza of Great Neck, Inc., 544 N.Y.S.2d 840 (N.Y. App. Div. 1989); In re Eichner, 420 N.E.2d 64 (N.Y.), *cert. denied* 454 U.S. 858 (1981); In re Martin, 538 N.W.2d 399 (Mich. 1995).

[12]See, e.g., In re Eichner, 420 N.E.2d 64 (N.Y. 1981); In re Westchester Cty. Med. Ctr., 531 N.E.2d 607 (N.Y. 1988); Cruzan v. Harmon, 760 S.W.2d 408 (Mo. 1988).

[13]See, e.g., Conservatorship of Drabick, 245 Cal.Rptr. 840 (Cal. Ct. App. 1988); McConnell v. Beverly Enterprises — Conn., Inc., 553 A.2d 596 (Conn. 1989); In re Lawrance, 579 N.E.2d 32 (Ind. 1991); Gray v. Romeo, 697 F.Supp. 580 (D.R.I. 1988); In re Grant, 747 P.2d 445 (Wash. 1987).

[14]In re Eichner, 420 N.E.2d 64 (N.Y. 1981), *cert. denied* 454 U.S. 858 (1981).

Similarly, when a patient indicated over approximately one decade that she did not wish respirators, feeding tubes, or antibiotics if she were to become comatose without hope of regaining consciousness, the court held that these pronouncements constituted clear and convincing evidence when she suffered a subarachnoid hemorrhage that resulted in a persistent vegetative state and allowed for these wishes to be fulfilled.[15] Of particular note was that the patient repeatedly told her closest family members of these preferences and obtained promises from her spouse, sister, and son that they would exert every effort to prevent her from being kept alive if she were permanently unconscious.

However, absent a specific statement with regard to a specific medical circumstance, courts may not consider such statements as clear and convincing evidence. For example, statements indicating the patient would not want to be kept alive by artificial means if the patient's medical condition were hopeless have been held too ambiguous to justify termination of life support. Hence, a woman who previously made such statements and was demented after a series of strokes, rather than being in a coma or persistent vegetative state, did not meet the clear and convincing evidence standard for termination of life support, specifically blocking the insertion of a feeding tube for nutrition. In addition to not being in a coma or persistent vegetative state, the patient's condition was not considered terminal if she received artificial nutrition. The patient had never made statements *specifically* regarding the withholding of feeding and hydration.[16] The court therefore concluded that the statements made by the patient previously were mere reactions to hearing of others' prolonged death and not solemn pronouncements and so did not support efforts to block insertion of the feeding tube. Indeed, in another case, even when statements were made repeatedly by a patient to his spouse regarding the patient's preferences for withdrawal of life-sustaining treatment, it was held that if these statements did not rise to the level of specific, solemn pronouncements rather than general, vague, and casual remarks instituted by witnessing an agonizing death of another, the court would not find that these statements meet the standard of clear and convincing evidence.[17]

Finally, one court has articulated the standards to be used in determining when to terminate life-support treatment on the basis of external evidence. The New Jersey Supreme Court indicated that three standards should apply: a subjective standard, an objective standard, and a combination.[18] The subjective standard that fulfills the patient's wishes is appropriate when it is "clear"[19] that the patient would have refused the treatment in the present circumstances. However, when the desire of the patient is not clear, the "limited objective test" (i.e., a combination objective and subjective test) is applicable. Under circumstances where there is some trustworthy (but not clear or unequivocal) evidence that the patient would have refused the treatment and the burden of treatment is "markedly"[20] greater than the benefit of life to the patient, the medical interventions may be withdrawn. Finally, the "pure objective" test (i.e., a best interests of the patient assessment) is applicable when there is no reliable evidence of the patient's preferences. Under these circumstances, when no evidence is extant and the burdens of the patient's life with the medical interventions are "clearly and markedly"[21] greater than the benefits the patient obtains from life, and "the recurring, unavoidable and severe pain of the patient's life with the treatment [is] such that the effect of administering life sustaining treatment would be inhumane,"[22] then termination of life-supporting treatment is permitted.

The varying standards and uncertain nature of court assessment in these cases emphasize the importance of executing appropriate advance directives, preferably a health care proxy, for the patient's true desires to be effectuated or at least for a viable decision regarding the patient's disposition to be enforced.

Potential Reasons for Limited Advance Directive Use

As indicated previously, most of the potential difficulties surrounding the use of advance directives appear centered about the communications process. Patients may not wish to approach physicians on this topic because a patient may believe he or she has not established a personal relationship with a physician or that this kind of discussion may put the physician in a conflict-of-interest situation. The reticence of patients approaching physicians on this topic apparently is based to some extent on the expectation that

[15]Elbaum v. Grace Plaza of Great Neck, Inc., 544 N.Y.S.2d 840 (N.Y. App. Div. 1989).

[16]In re Westchester Cty. Med. Ctr., 531 N.E.2d 607 (N.Y. 1988); see also In re Martin, 538 N.W.2d 399 (Mich. 1995) (after conflict between spouse versus mother and daughter regarding guardianship, oral statements by patient based on wife's testimony and affidavit indicating he would not want to receive life-sustaining treatment in event of serious accident, terminal illness, or "dying by old age" was not clear and convincing evidence to show patient did not wish life-sustaining treatment when incompetent but conscious).

[17]In re Martin, 538 N.W.2d 399 (Mich. 1995).

[18]See In re Conroy, 486 A.2d 1209 (N.J. 1985); In re Jobes, 529 A.2d 434 (N.J. 1987); In re Peter, 529 A.2d 419 (N.J. 1987); In re Farrell, 529 A.2d 404 (N.J. 1987).

[19]In re Conroy, 486 A.2d 1209, 1229 (N.J. 1985).

[20]In re Conroy, 486 A.2d 1209, 1232 (N.J. 1985).

[21]In re Conroy, 486 A.2d 1209, 1232 (N.J. 1985).

[22]In re Conroy, 486 A.2d 1209, 1232 (N.J. 1985).

the physician will begin the dialogue on advance directives.[23] This also may occur because patients may misunderstand advance directives, assuming they are relevant only to those in poor health or at the end of life; other misperceptions may arise because some patients may believe that since care is allowed to be limited in certain circumstances, this preference may be extended to other circumstances as well. Further, some patients may be reticent to discuss these issues if they will involve a third party such as proxy decision maker, the latter of whom may be upset regarding the discussion of issues of death and dying.

When physicians take the initiative and discuss advance directives with patients, there is a significant increase in completion of these documents, at least in the home health care and nursing home settings.[24] Indeed, it appears that most patients want information on advance directives and are willing to discuss them.[25] However, physicians in general may be reluctant to discuss the topic of advance directives because of lack of knowledge, a misperception that such directives are inappropriate or unnecessary for younger, healthier patients,[26] the lack of pecuniary benefit from such discussions, and ethical concerns that setting an outcome of care as death is inappropriate. Another legally created issue is that the Patient Self-Determination Act mandates that discussions of advance directives be held on admission—simply not a good time to bring up such issues since patients are likely "ill, traumatized, or simply overwhelmed."[27]

Beyond low participation rates in patient formulation of advance directives, advance directives are not always followed by medical professionals.[28] A variety of factors appear to partially explain this result. The documents themselves may not express either the specific condition and action that the patient has indicated in his or her advance directive or they are hence too ambiguous for interpretation and hence implementation. This is particularly true when patients have not discussed the acceptable or unacceptable medical interventions with providers and proxy decision makers, a common phenomenon.[29] This problem is exacerbated by reports that physician and proxy decision makers do not fare well in their predictions of patient preferences.[30] Further, these documents may not be available; if members of the patient's family or his or her provider lacks actual knowledge of or access to these documents (e.g., they are stowed in a safety deposit box[31] or lost in transfer), there simply is no opportunity for their implementation. Aside from these formal issues, personal and social issues that arise from the end-of-life situation may impede implementation. Family wishes may override the terms of the patient's advance directive.[32] Although there are legal bases for the physician to fulfill the patient's wishes, direct contravention of a family member's opposition may invite legal proceedings, poor external relations, and very bad press—all of which have financial ramifications, do not assist the family member in his or her grieving process, and do not assist the patient in implementing his or her wishes. Finally, a physician's personal values and ethics may result in patient advance directives not being implemented, even without the consent or knowledge of the family.[33]

[23]Emanuel et al., "Advance Directives for Medical Care."

[24]L. J. Markson, J. Fanale, and K. Steel, "Implementing Advance Directives in the Primary Care Setting," *Archives of Internal Medicine* 154 (1994), pp. 2321–27.

[25]Emanuel et al., "Advance Directives for Medical Care."

[26]R. S. Morrison, W. E. Morrison, and D. F. Glickman, "Physician Reluctance to Discuss Advance Directives," *Archives of Internal Medicine* 154 (1994), pp. 2311–18.

[27] General Accounting Office, *Patient Self-Determination Act,* section 4.2.

[28]See, e.g., M. Danis, L. I. Southerland, and J. M. Garrett, "A Prospective Study of Advance Directives for Life-Sustaining Care," *New England Journal of Medicine* 324 (1991), pp. 882–88; The SUPPORT Principle Investigators, "A Controlled Trial to Improve Care for Seriously Ill Hospital Patients," *JAMA* 274 (1995), pp. 1591–98.

[29]E. J. Emmanuel, D. S. Weinberg, and R. G. Gonin, "How Well Is the Patient Self-Determination Act Working?: An Early Assessment," *American Journal of Medicine* 95 (1993), pp. 619–28.

[30]J. Suhl, P. Simons, and T. Reedy, "Myth of Substituted Judgment: Surrogate Decision Making Regarding Life Support Is Unreliable," *Archives of Internal Medicine* 154 (1994), pp. 90–96; A. B. Seckler et al., "Substituted Judgment: How Accurate Are Proxy Predictions?" *Annals of Internal Medicine* 115 (1991), pp. 92–98; P. M. Layde et al., "Surrogates' Predictions of Seriously Ill Patients' Resuscitation Preferences," *Archives of Family Medicine* 4 (1995), pp. 518–23; R. F. Uhlmann et al., "Physicians' and Spouses' Predictions of Elderly Patients' Resuscitation Preferences," *Journal of Gerontology* 43 (1988), pp. 115–21; N. R. Zweibel and C. K. Cassel, "Treatment Choices at the End of Life: A Comparison of Decisions by Older Patients and Their Physician-Selected Proxies," *Gerontologist* 29 (1989), pp. 615–29.

[31]A. W. Broadwell et al., "Advance Directives on Hospital Admission: A Survey of Patient Attitudes," *Southern Medical Journal* 86 (1993), pp. 165–68.

[32]J. W. Ely et al., "The Physician's Decision to Use Tube Feedings: The Role of the Family, the Living Will, and the Cruzan Decision," *Journal of the American Geriatric Society* 40 (1992), pp. 471–75.

[33]See, e.g., D. A. Asch et al., "Decisions to Limit or Continue Life-Sustaining Treatment by Critical Care Physicians in the United States: Conflicts Between Physicians' Practices and Patients' Wishes," *American Journal of Respiratory Critical Care Medicine* 151 (1995), pp. 288–92; SUPPORT Principle Investigators, "A Controlled Trial"; see also M. Z. Solomon et al., "Decisions Near the End of Life: Professional Views on Life-Sustaining Treatments," *American Journal of Public Health* 83 (1993), pp. 14–23 (medical professionals may be more willing to withhold or withdraw life-sustaining treatment than family members in contrast to public opinion perspective that medical professionals want to provide more rather than less care).

Objections to the Use of Advance Directives

Advance directives do not enjoy universal support by patient advocates or health care professionals. Some patient care advocates believe that advance directives and mandates under the Patient Self-Determination Act may result in a lower standard of care for patients who execute such agreements, that full efforts will not be provided these patients in the event of a medical emergency, that advance directives amount to active euthanasia, and that there is a significant potential for discrimination against the disabled or others with shorter life expectancy. However, no empirical data has shown support for these argued negative consequences. Some health care providers object to advance directives because their decision-making spectrum is reduced by patients who are not informed about the relative prognosis and treatment modalities available in clinical medicine, advance directives may preclude use of experimental treatment or participation in clinical trials, executing these documents may result in an adversarial patient–physician relationship, and advance directives inappropriately extend legal intrusions on medical practice. Empirical data refuting or supporting these objections is not extant to effectively analyze these concerns.

There also have been objections from a moral imperative ideal. Generally, these concerns focus on the need for physicians to ignore advance directives if and when limiting or withdrawing treatment is not in the best interests of the patient. The foundation of this belief centers around the observation that the ill patient does not have the nexus of psychological continuity and connectedness with the person who executed the advance directive. What a person wishes when he or she is healthy may be very different from that which he or she may wish when faced with the specter of death. Therefore, no moral authority requires physicians to adhere to such pronouncements for limiting or withholding care since the patient is now different.[34]

Other, more practical problems lead to an objection to advance directives. Advance directives in the context of emergency care and emergency circumstances may not be amenable to a calm, full review of a patient's advance directive, discussions with family members, or consultation with a proxy decision maker debating the pros and cons of each potential medical intervention — possibilities amenable to judicial decision making, perhaps, but not actual medical decision making. The question also arises as to the breadth of informed consent and the breadth of informed refusal. In addition, an individual patient's condition may not be stable in the course of treatment. It may change his or her preferences as to the scope of treatment and interventions acceptable or unacceptable and significantly muddy the interpretation of a previous advance directive, even assuming that the patient desires strict adherence to the directive. This latter desire appears to be a dubious assumption according to some of the medical literature.[35] This difficulty is particularly true if the patient is in significant pain, is fearful, or is under the influence of previous and new medications.

Wrongful Living and Other Causes of Action Involving Advance Directives

Very few courts have assessed liabilities that would attach for not following or following an advance directive. Generally, but not always, providers have escaped civil and criminal liability for good faith efforts in either case. However, there is the disturbing possibility that providers may be liable for civil battery if they do not fulfill the patient's advance directive or that they may be subject to criminal prosecution for homicide. These areas of the law are in significant flux and await further development in the courts. Some examples from the courts follow.

With regard to a cause of action for not fulfilling an advance directive, in *Anderson v. St. Francis-St. George Hospital*,[36] the patient, 82-year-old Edward Winter, was admitted to the hospital complaining of chest pains and then admitted into the CCU. After admission, the patient indicated to his physician that he did not want to be resuscitated because he did not wish to suffer the fate of his wife, who deteriorated after an emergency resuscitation. "No Code Blue" was indicated in his chart (i.e., any cardiac arrest should not be treated with resuscitation). Several days after the conversation, the patient experienced life-threatening ventricular tachycardia, which was successfully treated with defibrillation. After becoming conscious, the patient thanked the nurse for saving his life. Two hours later, the patient again experienced a similar tachycardia, which was successfully treated with intravenous lidocaine. Two days later, the patient experienced a stroke that partially paralyzed his right side. He remained in this condition until his death two years later.

---

[34]See, e.g., R. Dresser, "Missing Persons: Legal Perceptions of Incompetent Patients," *Rutgers Law Review* 46 (1994), pp. 609–719; R. Dresser, "Relitigating Life and Death," *Ohio State Law Journal* 51 (1990), pp. 425–37; R. Dresser, "Life, Death, and Incompetent Patients: Conceptual Infirmities and Hidden Values in the Law," *Arizona Law Review* 28 (1986), pp. 373–405.

[35]See, e.g., A. Sehgal et al., "How Strictly Do Dialysis Patients Want Their Directives Followed?" *JAMA* 267 (1992), pp. 59–63; R. M. Walker et al., "Living Wills and Resuscitation Preferences in an Elderly Population," *Archives of Internal Medcine* 155 (1995), pp. 171–75; A. B. Seckler et al., "Substituted Judgment: How Accurate Are Proxy Predictions?" *Annals of Internal Medicine* 115 (1991), pp. 92–98.

[36]671 N.E.2d 225 (Ohio 1996).

During this period, he continued to have family visits and engaged in family activities. Before his death, the patient brought a wrongful living suit against the hospital, indicating that the nurse's action was against his express wishes and prevented his natural death. After being heard on three levels, the Supreme Court of Ohio held that although patients have a right to limit their treatment to that desired, good faith, innocent actions that are in error should not lead to liability and courts may deter unwanted medical treatment by allowing for an action against a provider for battery. In this case, the court took note that the patient thanked the nurse for saving his life and the hedonic value of his remaining years. In addition, although the nurse's action was a technical battery, the battery was physically harmless (the stroke was not directly caused by this action). The court indicated that although it would recognize the battery cause of action, it would award only nominal damages for the battery due to its harmlessness. It then dismissed the case.

Therefore, the court did not hold that a viable cause of action existed for "wrongful living"; however, the important holding was that the court allowed the battery action against the health care provider. If this decision is accepted by more courts, it may lead to significant problems with regard to what kinds of actions providers will undertake in end-of-life circumstances, since a battery cause of action is accompanied by the possibility of punitive damages, whereas malpractice and other negligence-based causes of action generally are not. The incentive under pecuniary standards then always would be to avoid care so as to avoid the potential of punitive damages. Indeed, malpractice insurance specifically limits coverage to negligence-based claims and generally excludes all intentional torts such as battery.

Another court held that a battery cause of action should be allowed only if a physician contravenes the direct, express wishes of a patient, and only when there is a contemporaneous refusal of treatment by the fully informed, competent adult patient.[37] Further, battery claims have been allowed against providers when they provide unwanted treatment to prolong the patient's life.[38] Indeed, a jury in Michigan awarded a patient and her mother as proxy decision maker $16.5 million for medical battery when providers ignored the proxy's request to honor the patient's advance directive and to terminate life-support systems.[39]

Several suits have been filed in this area;[40] and this likely will be an important medical-legal issue in the foreseeable future as the population of this country continues to age.[41]

Criminal prosecution against a physician for terminating a patient's life support has occurred and ultimately resulted in vindication of the physician.[42] For example, in *Barber v. Superior Court*,[43] patient Clarence Herbert suffered a cardiopulmonary arrest after surgery to close an ileostomy. He was resuscitated and immediately placed on life support. However, it was determined that the arrest resulted in significant hypoxia and therefore a persistent vegetative state. The physicians in the case indicated to the family that the prognosis was extremely poor; at that juncture, the patient's family (spouse and eight of his children) executed a written request for the hospital to withdraw life-sustaining interventions. After being extubated, the patient continued to breathe on his own but without clinical improvement. After two days, physicians in consultation with the family terminated hydration and nutrition. He subsequently died after these actions. The state of California then brought charges of murder and conspiracy to commit murder against the physicians for their actions. However, although the actions by the physicians were premeditated and the physicians knew their actions would result in death, the murder statute in the state required that the actions be "unlawful." The appellate court determined that they were not. Because the patient had expressed previously that he did not wish to become "another Karen Ann Quinlan" and the physicians acted through the decision of the appropriate proxy decision makers, the family, the physicians could not be held for murder and conspiracy to commit murder. It then dismissed the case.

Notes on Advance Directives

Assisted Suicide

Assisted suicide has become a significant policy issue for those patients who wish to exercise "the right to

[37]See, e.g., Werth v. Taylor, 475 N.W.2d 426 (Mich. Ct. App. 1991); In re Spring, 405 N.E.2d 115 (Mass. 1980).

[38]See, e.g., Bartling v. Superior Ct., 209 Cal.Rptr. 220 (Cal. Ct. App. 1984), *dismissed after remand* 229 Cal.Rptr. 360 (Cal. Ct. App. 1986); Estate of Leach v. Shapiro, 469 N.E.2d 1047 (Ohio Ct. App. 1984).

[39]Editorial, "Death and Dying, a Series: The Right to Die," *Detroit News* (July 2, 1997), p. A8 (noting $16.5 million judgment and subsequent reduction on legal grounds to $1.4 million and settlement between the parties).

[40]See T. Lewin, "Ignoring End-of-Life Directives Begins to Cost; Lawsuits Increase Against Doctors, Hospitals, for Unwanted Life Saving Acts," *Sunday Tacoma Morning News Tribune* (June 9, 1996), p. G2.

[41]But see Causey v. St. Francis Med. Ctr., 719 So.2d 1072 (La. App. 1998) (family that desired to have medical treatment provided to patient in conflict with provider wishes could resolve its claim only as malpractice and not an intentional tort).

[42]Barber v. Superior Ct., 195 Cal.Rptr. 484 (Cal. Ct. App. 1983).

[43]Barber v. Superior Ct., 195 Cal.Rptr. 484 (Cal. Ct. App. 1983); see also Rosebush v. Oakland Cty. Prosecutor, 491 N.W.2d 633 (Mich. Ct. App. 1992) (termination of life-support treatment of minor in persistent vegetative state does not subject parents or physicians to criminal liability for homicide).

die." The issue has come into the public eye largely through the actions of Dr. Jack Kevorkian, who employs a "suicide machine" that provides patients the ability to take their own lives. Notwithstanding numerous legislative and prosecutorial efforts to make Kevorkian's action homicide, Kevorkian was only recently found guilty of murder for an assisted suicide that was broadcast on *60 Minutes*. The jury found that he had crossed the line by directly administering a lethal injection to a patient suffering from Lou Gehrig's disease rather than merely providing the patient with the knowledge and means to end his own life.[44] Assisted suicide has been the subject of legislative action legalizing the process. In a formal public action, Oregon in 1994 passed a citizen initiative, the "Death with Dignity" Measure 16, legally allowing for assisted suicide. This law provides that terminally ill adult patients who are residents of the state and are likely to die within six months (as found by two physicians), under certain conditions, may commit suicide by lethal injection with the assistance of medical providers. After legal challenges[45] and efforts to repeal the initiative, the law went into effect in 1997. It should be noted, however, that state statutes that prohibit assisted suicide are legally sound; the Supreme Court has held that there is no constitutional right requiring a state to allow for, and patients to have access to, assisted suicide.[46]

Additional Reading.   C. L. Bjorck, "Physician-Assisted Suicide: Whose Life Is It Anyway?" *Southern Methodist University Law Review* 47 (1994), pp. 371–97; M. T. CeloCruz, "Aid-in-Dying: Should We Decriminalize Physician-Assisted Suicide and Physician-Committed Euthanasia?" *American Journal of Law and Medicine* 18 (1992), pp. 369–94; L. L. Mangini, "To Help or Not to Help: Assisted Suicide and Its Moral, Ethical, and Legal Ramifications," *Seton Hall Legislative Journal* 18 (1994), pp. 728–78; C. K. Smith, "What About Legalized Assisted Suicide?" *Issues of Law and Medicine* 8 (1993), pp. 503–19; A. P. Tsarouhas, "The Case Against Legal Assisted Suicide," *Ohio Northern University Law Review* 20 (1994), pp. 793–814.

Children

As a general proposition, parents have decision-making authority regarding medical treatment for their children.

This proposition is based on the premise that parents have knowledge of the interests and values and will act in the best interests of their children.[47] However, as with informed consent situations, children may be able to override their parents' decisions under the "mature minor" exception.[48] Further, parents are limited by child abuse and child neglect statutes, which mandate that parents provide children with the basic requirements of daily living, including medical care. If parents do not fulfill this responsibility, the state may exercise its authority and take custody of the children to ensure that basic needs, including health care, are provided. As well, the state may bring criminal charges against these parents.[49] With regard to parental decisions that would cease life-sustaining treatments, some courts have indicated that any decision by parents to terminate treatments that would maintain the child's life, by definition, is neglect;[50] other courts have applied a balancing test to determine whether such denial is neglect.[51] Generally, the balancing test requires an assessment of three major issues: the prognosis for the child without treatment; the prognosis for the child with treatment; and the invasiveness of and pain associated with the treatment. The first two are intimately related to parental wishes since they must support the treatment modality. As is usual with balancing tests, the nature of the result is contingent on the actual facts and circumstances of the case. However, it would appear that as long-term benefits and prognosis for the child with the treatment decrease relative to nontreatment prognosis, courts concomitantly will decrease the pain associated with treatment they will sanction. Therefore, it has been held that chemotherapy for children that would involve significant long-term, painful, and debilitating treatment will not be ordered over the objections of parents even if such treatment is the only treatment that possibly could

[44]J. Hyde, "Kevorkian Upbraided at Sentencing: He Gets 10 to 25 Years in Michigan," *The Boston Globe*, April 14, 1999, A3.

[45]Lee v. Oregon, 107 F.3d 1382 (9th Cir.), *cert. denied* 118 S.Ct. 328 (1997).

[46]See Vacco v. Quill, 521 U.S. 793 (1997); Washington v. Glucksberg, 521 U.S. 702 (1997).

[47]See, e.g., Prince v. Commonwealth of Mass., 321 U.S. 158 (1944); Wisconsin v. Yoder, 406 U.S. 205 (1972); Parham v. J.R., 442 U.S. 584 (1979); Newmark v. Williams, 588 A.2d 1108 (Del. 1991).

[48]See Chapter 1; see also In re E.G., 549 N.E.2d 322 (Ill. 1989); In re Application of Long Island Jewish Med. Ctr., 557 N.Y.S.2d 239 (N.Y. 1990); Bellotti v. Baird, 443 U.S. 622 (1979); see also Poole v. South Plainfield Bd. of Education, 490 F.Supp. 948 (D. N.J. 1980).

[49]See, e.g., Walker v. Superior Ct., 763 P.2d 852 (Cal. 1988), *cert. denied* 491 U.S. 905 (1989); Funkhouser v. State, 763 P.2d 695 (Okla. Ct. App. 1988), *cert. denied* 490 U.S. 1066 (1989); Hall v. State, 493 N.E.2d 433 (Ind. 1986); see also Hermanson v. State, 604 So.2d 775 (Fla. 1992); State v. McKown, 475 N.W.2d 63 (Minn. 1991).

[50]See, e.g., In re Hamilton, 657 S.W.2d 425 (Tenn. Ct. App. 1983); In re Willmann, 493 N.E.2d 1380 (Ohio Ct. App. 1986); see also Newmark v. Williams, 588 A.2d 1108 (Del. 1990).

[51]See, e.g., Custody of a Minor, 379 N.E.2d 1053 (Mass. 1978); Newmark v. Williams, 588 A.2d 1108 (Del. 1991).

help the child.[52] It bears emphasizing once again that the ultimate determination is a function of state law.

Additional Reading. M. S. Feigenbaum, "Minors, Medical Treatment, and Interspousal Disagreement: Should Solomon Split the Child?" *DePaul Law Review* 41 (1992), pp. 841–84; L. A. Hawkins, "Living-Will Statutes: A Minor Oversight," *Virginia Law Review* 78 (1992), pp. 1581–1615; L. M. Kopelman, "Children and Bioethics: Uses and Abuses of the Best-Interests Standard," *Journal of Medical Philosophy* 22, no. 3 (1997), pp. 213–17; J. M. Kun, "Rejecting the Adage 'Children Should Be Seen and Not Heard' — The Mature Minor Doctrine," *Pace Law Review* 16 (1996), pp. 423–62; A. M. Massie, "Withdrawal of Treatment for Minors in a Persistent Vegetative State: Parents Should Decide," *Arizona Law Review* 35 (1993), pp. 173–218; J. A. Penkower, "The Potential Right of Chronically Ill Adolescents to Refuse Life-Saving Medical Treatment — Fatal Misuse of the Mature Minor Doctrine," *DePaul Law Review* 45 (1996), pp. 1165–1216; J. L. Rosato, "The Ultimate Test of Autonomy: Should Minors Have a Right to Make Decisions Regarding Life-Sustaining Treatment?" *Rutgers Law Review* 49 (1996), pp. 1–103.

Cruzan v. Director, Department of Health

The case of *Cruzan v. Director, Missouri Department of Health*[53] began the significant move toward a policy discussion of advance directives; indeed, the Patient Self-Determination Act was passed in the same year the Supreme Court issued its decision in the case. *Cruzan* involved a patient, Nancy Cruzan, who was in a persistent vegetative state after a motor vehicle accident. She did not require a ventilator; therefore, it was possible for her to live for an extended period with appropriate hydration and nutrition. Six years after the accident, her parents, her legal guardians, desired to have artificial nutrition and hydration removed; however, the hospital refused without a court order. The U.S. Supreme Court held that citizens have the right to refuse life-sustaining treatment. This right

may be exercised in limited circumstances by others in place of the patient him- or herself. However, the Supreme Court noted that states have a valid interest in protecting and preserving life. This interest justifies allowing states to prescribe procedures to ensure that the patient's wishes are being fulfilled, such as requiring clear and convincing evidence of the patient's wishes before permitting withdrawal of life-sustaining measures. Therefore, as in most advance directive situations, state law provides the primary guidance as to when and under what conditions termination of life support can occur.

Additional Reading. K. Daar, "The Right to Die After Cruzan," *Health Law* 4 (1991), pp. 1–11; S. R. Martyn, "Coming to Terms with Death: The Cruzan Case," *Hastings Law Journal* 42 (1991), pp. 817–58; R. W. Morales, "The Twilight Zone of Nancy Beth Cruzan: A Case Study of Nancy Beth Cruzan v. Director, Missouri Department of Health," *Howard Law Journal* 34 (1991), pp. 201–27; J. N. Suhr, "Cruzan v. Director, Missouri Department of Health: A Clear and Convincing Call for Comprehensive Legislation to Protect Incompetent Patients' Rights," *American University Law Review* 40 (1991), pp. 1477–1519.

DNR Orders

DNR (Do Not Resuscitate) orders, generally, are advance directives indicating the patient (or his or her family if the patient is incompetent) has decided that, at a minimum, cardiopulmonary resuscitation (CPR) is not to be provided. However, the DNR order, standing alone, suffers from problems of interpretation; the question remains as to what the term *resuscitate* actually means. For example, there may be potential differing expectations of physicians and patients as to this term. To a patient, resuscitation may mean CPR only; to the physician, resuscitation may involve CPR, electrical conversion of abnormal heart rhythms, tracheal intubation, intravenous medications, oxygen use, and other interventions. Discussions and communication with patients are imperative to clarify the limits of the order.

Additional Reading. K. M. Boozang, "Death Wish: Resuscitating Self-Determination for the Critically Ill," *Arizona Law Review* 35 (1993), pp. 23–85; V. A. Lonchyna, "To Resuscitate or Not . . . In the Operating Room: The Need for Hospital Policies for Surrogates Regarding DNR Orders," *Annals of Health Law* 6 (1997), pp. 209–27; M. E. Rosen, "The Do Not Resuscitate Policy Jurisdiction over Policy and the Therapeutic Privileges," *Health Law* 4 (1990), pp. 3–9; L. W. Vernaglia, "Propriety and Liability Related to Issuance or Enforcement of Do Not Resuscitate (DNR) Orders," in *American Law Reports,* 5th ed. (Rochester, NY: Lawyers Cooperative Publishing Co., 1998), vol. 46, pp. 793–811.

---

[52]Newmark v. Williams, 588 A.2d 1108 (Del. 1991); see also In re Guardianship of Barry, 445 So.2d 365 (Fla. Dist. Ct. App. 1984) (parents' decision to terminate life support for 10-month-old son with incurable and irreversible disease overrides any interests of the state); In re LHR, 321 S.E.2d 716 (Ga. 1984) (parents' decision to remove life-support systems from their child in an irreversible chronic vegetative state does not implicate state interest in maintaining life once diagnosis is made); Rosebush v. Oakland Cty. Prosecutor, 491 N.W.2d 633 (Mich. Ct. App. 1992) (termination of life-support treatment of a minor in a persistent vegetative state does not subject parents or physicians to criminal liability for homicide).
[53]497 U.S. 261 (1990).

Ethics Committees

Hospital and organizational ethics committees, which usually include members of the medical and legal professions, clergy, and laypersons, may provide useful guidance regarding end-of-life decision making through formulation of hospital policies, staff education, and internal and external conferences. However, it is exceedingly important to note that these committees have no formal standing under the law. Therefore, actions by a health care provider under recommendation by the ethics committee do not insulate that provider from suits for malpractice, wrongful death, or other civil (and criminal, if applicable) wrongs. Physicians and other health care professionals themselves must assess individual patient circumstances and be comfortable with any decision, since accountability ultimately rests with them.

Additional Reading. D. E. Hoffmann, "Regulating Ethics Committees in Health Care Institutions — Is It Time?" *Maryland Law Review* 50 (1991), pp. 746–97; A. L. Merritt, "The Tort Liability of Hospital Ethics Committees," *Southern California Law Review* 60 (1987), pp. 1239–97; R. F. Wilson, "Hospital Ethics Committees as the Forum of Last Resort: An Idea Whose Time Has Not Come," *North Carolina Law Review* 76 (1998), pp. 353–406.

Family Hierarchy of Decision Makers

In most states, in the absence of written advance directives, state law (sometimes known as *family consent statutes*) generally will govern the hierarchy of family members who may act as the patient's health care decision maker if the patient loses capacity. Usually, like the informal process with which most providers adhere, the patient's guardian is first in the hierarchy, then his or her spouse, and then others in an order similar to that of inheritance absent a will under the state's probate laws. These state statutes often specify that powers to make these medical decisions are applicable only when the patient becomes incompetent. It should be noted, however, that in some states family members have no legal right to make such decisions absent an express power giving these individuals that right; other states indicate that the patient's physician, with consultation of the patient's family, has this decision-making power. Therefore, it is imperative that providers and others understand who and in what order persons may exercise proxy decision-making rights for patients who lack capacity. It bears emphasizing that a written, valid advance directive always prevails over a family consent statute.

Additional Reading. A. A. Hamann, "Family Surrogate Laws: A Necessary Supplement to Living Wills and Durable Power of Attorney," *Villanova Law Review* 38 (1993), pp. 103–77; E. B. Krasik, "The Role of the Family in Medical Decision-Making for Incompetent Adult Patients: A Historical Perspective and Case Analysis," *University of Pittsburgh Law Review* 48 (1987), pp. 539–618; P. J. Vest, "Saying Yes or No to Life Sustaining Treatment, Who Decides? In Ohio: The Patient, Family, and Physician," *Capital University Law Review* 21 (1992), pp. 647–83.

In Re Quinlan

In re Quinlan,[54] another famous case involving end-of-life decision making, involved an assessment of whether physicians could intentionally withdraw or withhold life-sustaining treatment from Karen Ann Quinlan, a 22-year-old patient in a persistent vegetative state. Ms. Quinlan still maintained some brainstem function but was not expected to ever regain consciousness and she never executed an advance directive. Joseph Quinlan, the patient's father, requested that he be made the patient's guardian and that life support be discontinued and providers terminate "all extraordinary medical procedures." The Supreme Court of New Jersey held that the patient's father could withdraw medical intervention with confirmation of the patient's poor prognosis by a hospital committee.

Additional Reading. P. G. Peters, "The State's Interest in the Preservation of Life: From Quinlan to Cruzan," *Ohio State Law Journal* 50 (1989), pp. 891–977; G. U. Scharff, "In Re Quinlan Revisited: The Judicial Role in Protecting the Privacy Right of Dying Incompetents," *Hastings Constitutional Law Quarterly* 15 (1988), pp. 479–512; M. L. Stevens, "The Quinlan Case Revisited: A History of the Cultural Politics of Medicine and the Law," *Journal of Health Politics Policy and Law* 21 (1996), pp. 347–66.

In Re Wanglie

The *Wanglie* case[55] involved a "reverse" right to die situation: where the patient's family seek to continue life-sustaining treatment and the providers wish to discontinue it. Helga Wanglie was an 86-year-old, intubated patient in a persistent vegetative state. Physicians indicated that continued ventilatory support was "nonbeneficial" to the patient and indicated that it should be

---

[54]355 A.2d 647 (N.J.), *cert. denied sub nom.* Garger v. New Jersey, 429 U.S. 922 (1976).

[55]See M. Angell, "The Case of Helga Wanglie: A New Kind of Right to Die Case," *New England Journal of Medicine* 325 (1991), pp. 511–12.

removed, causing her death. Her spouse, an attorney, and her two children opposed the removal, indicating that "physicians should not play God, that the patient could not be better off dead, that removing life support showed moral decay of our civilization, and that a miracle could occur."[56] These sentiments or similar ones have been heard by many individuals who have worked in an ICU or other high-level critical care unit. Further, the spouse indicated that although initially he expressed that the patient had never indicated a preference regarding life-sustaining treatment, later he maintained that the patient had consistently indicated she desired respiratory support for her condition. The hospital requested that the court appoint an independent conservator for the patient to decide the issue; the court appointed the conservator but declined to rule on the issue of whether the hospital could remove life support from the patient. Because of the uncertain nature of the hospital's legal rights and obligations, it indicated that it would not discontinue life-sustaining intervention. Three days after this announcement, the patient died, ending the controversy. The result is one that often attends end-of-life circumstances: When there is conflict between the hospital and the patient's family, the hospital will be reluctant to act absent clear legal authority. However, in this case, it is far from clear whether the actions of the family or ultimately the decision to maintain the status quo was in the best interests or reflected the desires of the patient.

Additional Reading. M. Angell, "The Case of Helga Wanglie: A New Kind of Right to Die Case," *New England Journal of Medicine* 325 (1991), pp. 511–12; J. F. Daar, "A Clash at the Bedside: Patient Autonomy v. a Physician's Professional Conscience," *Hastings Law Journal* 44 (1993), pp. 1241–89; D. W. Pimley, "Patients' Final Days May Pit Family Against Providers," *BNA Health Care Policy Report* 7 (1999), pp. 29–32; C. A. Roach, "Paradox and Pandora's Box: The Tragedy of Current Right-to-Die Jurisprudence," *University of Michigan Journal of Law Reform* 25 (1991), pp. 133–90.

The Profoundly Disabled from Birth and Other Patients Who Never Have Been Competent

Patients who never have been competent to engage in medical decision making proffer difficult cases to determine whether life-sustaining treatment can or should be withheld or withdrawn. Clearly, a substituted judgment standard is impossible in these circumstances. Courts are split on this issue; and again, state law will dictate what

method is to be used in the particular jurisdiction. For example, courts have indicated that the decision to forgo treatment should be determined by the patient's choice if the patient were competent while taking into account his or her present and future incompetence as a factor,[57] on the basis of substituted judgment concepts derived from the state's family consent statute,[58] and by treating incompetent patients like children and using the best interests standard.[59]

State Interests Allowing for Limitations on Patient's Right to Die

The patient's power to forgo medical intervention is extensive but not absolute. Certain state interests are compelling enough to override the patient's (or a surrogate's) decision. Traditionally, these state interests are framed as (1) the preservation of life, (2) the protection of innocent third parties, (3) the prevention of suicide, and (4) the maintenance of the ethical integrity of the medical profession and other medical professionals.[60] However, in more modern jurisprudence, these factors have become less persuasive to courts and the patient's choice is much more frequently held to be viable. Only very special circumstances such as patient incompetence, parental refusal of treatment for a child on religious grounds, refusal by a child, and other circumstances (such as the patient is a prisoner[61]) may justify overriding the patient's wishes.

Additional Reading. R. L. Lapointe, "The Removal of Feeding Tubes: Has the Right to Die Reached Its Limit?" *New England Law Review* 24 (1989), pp. 185–223; P. G. Peters, "The State's Interest in the Preservation of Life:

---

[56]S. H. Miles, "Informed Demand for 'Non-Beneficial' Medical Treatment," *New England Journal of Medicine* 325 (1991), p. 513.

[57]See, e.g., Superintendent of Belchertown State School v. Saikewicz, 370 N.E.2d 417 (Mass. 1977).

[58]In re Lawrance, 579 N.E.2d 32 (Ind. 1991).

[59]In re Eichner, 420 N.E.2d 64 (N.Y. 1981) *cert. denied* 454 U.S. 858 (1981).

[60]See, e.g., Superintendent of Belchertown State School v. Saikewicz, 370 N.E.2d 417 (Mass. 1977); Rasmussen v. Fleming, 741 P.2d 674 (Ariz. 1987); Bartling v. Superior Ct., 209 Cal.Rptr. 220 (Cal. Ct. App. 1984); Satz v. Perlmutter, 362 So.2d 160 (Fla. Dist. Ct. App. 1978), *aff'd* 379 So.2d 359 (Fla. 1980); In re Conroy, 486 A.2d 1209 (N.J. 1985); In re Colyer, 660 P.2d 738 (Wash. 1983); Thor v. Superior Ct., 21 Cal.Rptr.2d 357 (Cal. 1993); John F. Kennedy Mem. Hosp. v. Heston, 279 A.2d 670 (N.J. 1971); In re President and Directors of Georgetown College, Inc., 331 F.2d 1000 (D.C. Cir. 1964).

[61]See, e.g., Commissioner of Correction v. Myers, 399 N.E.2d 452 (Mass. 1979); cf. Woodland v. Angus, 820 F.Supp. 1497 (D. Utah 1993) (pretrial "detainee" has right to refuse antipsychotic medication that would have allowed the patient to become cogent and competent to stand trial for murder).

From Quinlan to Cruzan," *Ohio State Law Journal* 50 (1989), pp. 891–977; D. L. Sloss, "The Right to Choose How to Die: Constitutional Analysis of State Laws Prohibiting Physician-Assisted Suicide," *Stanford Law Review* 48 (1996), pp. 937–73.

Values History

A values history is a document that seeks to ascertain a patient's personal beliefs regarding areas of general concern to the patient as well as feelings about illness, terminal illness, and social factors surrounding such circumstances. The goal of this document is to provide a decision maker some guidance to make treatment decision for the patient if he or she becomes incapacitated. The values history differs from basic living wills and durable powers of attorney because it is not necessarily determining what care will be given and who shall decide such care if the patient lacks capacity. Instead, the values history attempts to provide the patient with an opportunity to be introspective about his or her desires, beliefs, and goals in life, which then may provide insight into what kinds of care are appropriate. The values history, of course, may be made a part of a living will and durable power of attorney document.

Additional Reading.   B. A. Rich, "The Values History: A New Standard of Care," *Emory Law Journal* 40 (1991), pp. 1109–81.

Further Reading

Durable Power of Attorney

Apfel JB. Living Wills versus Durable Health Care Powers of Attorney After Cruzan. *Pa Law* 1991;13:10.
Mayer E, Waldman MJ. Durable Power of Attorney for Health Care. In: *American Jurisprudence,* 2d ed. Rochester, NY: Lawyers Cooperative Publishing Co., 1998;§577.
Schmitt MN. The Durable Power of Attorney: Applications and Limitations. *Mil L Rev* 1991;132:203–30.
Stiefel LS. A Time to Live, a Time to Die. *Akron L Rev* 1991;24:699–740.
Wagley SM. After Cruzan: The Changing Art of Drafting Living Wills and Durable Powers of Attorney. *Me B J* 1992;7:160–66.

Living Will

Baptiste KE. *Living Wills.* Pub. no. D4-5221. New York: Practising Law Institute — Tax Law and Estate Planning, May 1991.

Goldberg IV. Supreme Court Case Shows When Living Wills Can Be Used to Carry Out a Client's Wishes. *Est Plan* 1990;17:328–31.
Nonovic SJ. The Living Will: Preservation of the Right-to-Die Demands Clarity and Consistency. *Dick L Rev* 1990;95:209–34.
Shepherd S. Living Wills: Why a Patient's Last Wishes Are Not Always Respected. *How L J* 1991;34:229–41.
Tillman B. Exercising the Right to Die: North Carolina's Amended Natural Death Act and the 1991 Health Care Power of Attorney Act. *N C L Rev* 1992;70:2108–24.
Van Ess CK. Living Wills and Alternatives to Living Wills: A Proposal — The Supreme Trust. *Val U L Rev* 1992;26:567–93.

Objections to the Use of Advance Directives

Larson EJ, Eaton TA. The Limits of Advance Directives: A History and Assessment of the Patient Self-Determination Act. *Wake Forest L Rev* 1997;32:249–93.
Peters PG. The State's Interest in the Preservation of Life: From Quinlan to Cruzan. *Ohio St L J* 1989;50:891-977.

Oral Directives

Bowers VJ. Advance Directives: Peace of Mind or False Security? *Stetson L Rev* 1996;26:677–723.
Rich BA. Advance Directives. *J Legal Med* 1998;19:63–97.
Rich BA. The Values History: A New Standard of Care. *Emory L J* 1991;40:1109–81.
Rosnack RL. Termination of Life-Sustaining Treatment: The Decision-Making Process After Cruzan v. Missouri Department of Health. *Baylor L Rev* 1991;43:841–71.

See Also

Meisel A. The Right to Die. *Pa Law* 1990;12:8–13.

Patient Self-Determination Act

Cate FH. Implementing the Education Mandate of the Patient Self-Determination Act. *Health Law* 1993;7:11–13.
Cate FH, Gill BA. The Patient Self-Determination Act: Implementation Issues and Opportunities. *Health Law* 1992;6:1–8.
Larson EJ, Eaton TA. The Limits of Advance Directives: A History and Assessment of the Patient Self-Determination Act. *Wake Forest L Rev* 1997;32:249–93.
Mulholland KC. Protecting the Right to Die: The Patient Self-Determination Act of 1990. *Harv J on Legis* 1990;28:609–30.
Obade CC. Advance Healthcare Planning Under the New Federal Patient Self-Determination Act. *Prac Law* 1992;38(3):11.

Refolo MA. The Patient Self-Determination Act of 1990: Health Care's Own Miranda. *J Contemp Health L & Pol'y* 1992;8:455–71.

Salatka MA. The Patient Self-Determination Act of 1990: Issues Regarding the Facilitation of Advance Directives, Patient Autonomy, Assisted Suicide, and Euthanasia. *J Pharmacy & L* 1993;1:155–76.

Shugrue RE. The Patient Self-Determination Act. *Creighton L Rev* 1993;26:751–83.

Potential Reasons for Limited Advance Directive Use

Canton NL. Prospective Autonomy: On the Limits of Shaping One's Post-Competence Medical Fate. *J Contemp Health L & Pol'y* 1992;8:13–48.

Larson EJ, Eaton TA. The Limits of Advance Directives: A History and Assessment of the Patient Self-Determination Act. *Wake Forest L Rev* 1997;32:249–93.

Refolo MA. The Patient Self-Determination Act of 1990: Health Care's Own Miranda. *J Contemp Health L & Pol'y* 1992;8:455–71.

Wrongful Living and Other Causes of Action Involving Advance Directives

Donuhue J. "Wrongful Living": Recovery for a Physician's Infringement on an Individual's Right to Die. *J Contemp Health L & Pol'y* 1998;14:391–419.

Hackleman TJ. Violation of an Individual's Right to Die: The Need for a Wrongful Living Cause of Action. *U Cin L Rev* 1996;64:1355–81.

Jeffreys JH. Advance Directives: Are They Worth the Paper They're Written On? *N J Law* 1998;190:17–39,18–19.

Knapp WC, Hamilton F. "Wrongful Living": Resuscitation as Tortious Interference with a Patient's Right to Give Informed Refusal. *N Ky L Rev* 1992;19:253–76.

Milani AA. Better Off Dead Than Disabled?: Should Courts Recognize a "Wrongful Living" Cause of Action When Doctors Fail to Honor Patients' Advance Directives? *Wash & Lee L Rev* 1997;54:149–228.

Other Reading

Aikman PJ, Thiel EC, Martin DK, Singer PA. Proxy, Health, and Personal Care Preferences: Implications for End-of-Life Care. *Cambridge Q J Healthcare Ethics* 1999;8:200–10.

American Medical Association. *Elements of Quality of Care for Patients in the Last Phase of Life.* Chicago: American Medical Association, 1997.

Bateman RB. Attorneys on Bioethics Committees: Unwelcome Menace or Valuable Asset? *J L & Health* 1994–1995;9:247–72.

Bowers VJ. Advance Directives: Peace of Mind or False Security? *Stetson L Rev* 1996;26:677–723.

Colen BD. *The Essential Guide to a Living Will: How to Protect Your Right to Refuse Medical Treatment.* New York: Prentice-Hall, 1991.

Freeman B. Competence, Marginal and Otherwise: Concepts and Ethics. *Int'l J L & Psych* 1981;4:53–72.

Garwin M. The Duty to Care — The Right to Refuse: Changing Roles of Patients and Physicians in End-of-Life Decision-Making. *J Legal Med* 1998;19:99–125.

Gibson J. Reflecting on Values. *Ohio St L J* 1990;51:451–71.

Harmon L. Falling Off the Vine: Legal Fictions and the Doctrine of Substituted Judgment. *Yale L J* 1990;100:1–71.

Harrison P. Advance Health Care Directors. *S C Law* 1991;3:29–31.

Kapp MB. Advance Health Care Planning: Taking a "Medical Future." *S Med J* 1988;81:221–24.

Lo B. Unanswered Questions About DNR Orders. *JAMA* 1991;265:1874–75.

Margolis W. The Doctor Knows Best? Patient Capacity for Health Care Decision-Making. *Or L Rev* 1992;71:909–37.

Meisel A. *The Right to Die.* New York: Wiley Law Publications, 1989.

Richard SM. Someone Make Up My Mind: The Troubling Right to Die Issues Presented by Incompetent Patients with No Prior Expression of a Treatment Preference. *Notre Dame L Rev* 1989;64:394–421.

Saks ER. Competency to Refuse Treatment. *N C L Rev* 1991;69:945–99.

Shugrue RA. The Patient Self-Determination Act. *Creighton L Rev* 1993;26:751–83.

Snyder JW. A Systematic Approach to the Decision to Terminate Treatment. *Hosp Phys* 1995;31(5):25–31.

Sulmasy DP, Terry PB, Weisman CS, Miller DJ. The Accuracy of Substituted Judgments in Patients with Terminal Diagnoses. *Annals Int Med* 1998;128:621–29.

Williams P. *The Living Will and the Durable Power of Attorney for Health Care Book.* Oak Park, IL: P. Gaines Co., 1991.

Wolff KR. Determining Patient Competency in Treatment Refusal Cases. *Ga L Rev* 1990;24:733–57.

Web Sites

Advance directives information/choices in dying: *http://www.choices.org*

Choice in dying: *http://www.echonyc.com/~choice/*

DeathNET: *http://www.rights.org/deathnet/open.html*

Deliverance: *http://www.euthanasia.net/*

Durable power of attorney: *http://www.cc.hih.gov/*

Dying with dignity: *http://www.web.apc.org/dwd/index.html*

End of life, exploring death in America: *http://www.npr.org/programs/death*

End-of-life resources: *http://ccme-mac4.bsd.uchicago.edu/ccmedocs/death*

Fosmire Station — Medical ethics: *http://www.afss.com/*

Growth House: *http://www.growthhouse.org/*

Health at home: *http://www.wjhs.org/*
The Hemlock Society USA: *http://www.irsociety.com/*
HIV in site: *http://hivinsite.ucsf.edu/topics/end_of_life/advance_directives/*
Last acts: *http://lastacts.rwif.org/*
Links to death and dying related sites: *http://www.euthanasia.org/links.html*
Living will site: *http://www.agingwithdignity.org*

Other legislation: *http://cdllhc.sph.unc/courses/hpaa70/lectures/lec9/tsldo25.htm*
Project on death in America: *http://www.soros.org/death.html*
Ten legal myths about advance medical directives: *http://www.abaret.org/elderly/myths.html*
The Webster death and dying page: *http://www.kalsden.com/death/index.html*

16
Definitions of Death

Anna V. Schlotzhauer and Bryan A. Liang

Important legal and policy issues arise in clinical circumstances that implicate the definition of *death* (see Table 16–1).[1] Once a determination of death is made according to accepted legal and medical standards, organs can be harvested for transplantation and life-support measures can be removed. In addition, the assets under the deceased's will can be transferred, life insurance policies become collectable, and several other legal and financial changes go into effect.

Death was once a simple determination made by family members in the home upon the cessation of heart and lung function.[2] With the development of respirators and other life-support measures that replace the functions of the heart and lungs, defining and diagnosing death became increasingly difficult. After much passionate debate, the Uniform Determination of Death Act,[3] which recognizes whole brain death as equivalent to traditional cardiopulmonary death, emerged and was adopted by all states. However, because a determination of death is an emotional subject that necessitates consideration of the patient's religious and personal beliefs as well as the futility and expense involved with prolonged life support, the debate continues. This chapter presents the existing legal definitions of death and examines the benefits, concerns, and issues related to these standards.

Cardiopulmonary Death

Traditionally, both legal and medical death were defined as the irreversible cessation of respiration and circulation. Cardiopulmonary death was easily diagnosed since the absence of breathing and blood flow meant certain death to all organs, including the brain, within a short period of time due to oxygen depletion. In the late 1950s, technological advances permitted cardiopulmonary function to be maintained artificially. While this life-sustaining technology could keep existing, uncompromised organs functional by maintaining blood flow and oxygen supply, it could not undo damage to the brain. Ethical and legal problems arose when patients with no chance of recovery, specifically those with a total loss of brain function, were being maintained for long periods of time. Based on the traditional cardiopulmonary definition of death, such patients were still deemed to be alive; however, continued "life support" was of no real benefit.[4]

The increasing use and sophistication of life-supportive and resuscitative measures made it clear that the existing definition of *death* had to be reevaluated.[5] Before discarding the cardiopulmonary criteria that had served as a bright line division between life and death for centuries, ethicists and physicians had to take the precursor step of redefining

---

[1]See, generally, People v. Eulo, 472 N.E.2d 286 (N.Y. 1984); People v. Mitchell, 183 Cal.Rptr. 166 (Ct. App. 1982) (providing a history of the evolution and adoption of the brain death standard).

[2]See, e.g., L. M. Tarantino, "Withdrawal of Life Support: Conflict Among Patient Wishes, Family, Physicians, Courts and Statutes, and the Law," *Buffalo Law Review* 42 (1994), pp. 623–52.

[3]Uniform Determination of Death Act §1 (1981).

[4]President's Commission for the Study of Ethical Problems in Medicine and Biomedical and Behavioral Research, *Defining Death: A Report on the Medical, Legal and Ethical Issues in the Determination of Death* (Washington, DC: Government Printing Office, 1981).

[5]See, e.g., J. Humber, "Statutory Criteria for Determining Human Death," *Mercer Law Review* 42 (1991), pp. 1069–85.

Table 16–1. Criteria for Defining Death

	Cardiopulmonary Death[*]	Whole Brain Death[**]	Higher Brain Death[***]
Diagnosis	Cessation of respiration and circulation; death to other organ systems will inevitably follow within minutes.	Cessation of functions of the entire brain, including brain stem; often confirmed by EEG.	Loss of cerebral and cerebellum function; brain stem still functional.
Can body function be maintained artificially?	Not after 10- to 15-minute window in which organs and brain die; patient sometimes can be resuscitated and placed on life support if cessation of cardiopulmonary function is immediately discovered.	Yes, using ventilators and other artificial supportive means.	Body often can continue vital functions but needs continued support in the form of hydration and nutrition.
Problems with diagnosis	None.	Initial concern re: possible overdiagnosis, with modern safety measures, not a relevant risk.	Opponents fear slippery slope as to how much brain death is enough; also some cases of recovery after periods of prolonged diagnosed PVS/coma.
Patient legal status	Dead, equivalent to whole brain death under the law.	Dead, equivalent to "cardiopulmonary death" under the law.	Alive.
Can organs legally be removed?	Yes, although heart, liver, and kidneys no longer will be useable and other organs may be compromised.	Yes, after death is pronounced according to accepted criteria for diagnosis by a physician not involved with organ recipient.	No, not even with consent. Removal of organs will be deemed a homicide.

[*]See, e.g., H. Beecher, "A Definition of Irreversible Coma. Special Communication: Report of the Ad Hoc Committee of the Harvard Medical School to Examine the Definition of Death," *JAMA* 205 (1968), pp. 337–40.

[**]See, e.g., President's Commission for the Study of Ethical Problems in Medicine and Biomedical and Behavioral Research, *Defining Death: A Report on the Medical, Legal and Ethical Issues in the Determination of Death.* Washington, DC: Government Printing Office, 1981.

[***]See, e.g., J. B. Oldershaw, J. Atkinson, and L. D. Boshes, "Persistent Vegetative State: Medical, Ethical, Religious, Economic and Legal Perspectives," *DePaul Journal of Health Care Law* 1 (1997), pp. 495–536.

life.[6] Life no longer could be equated solely with the traditional vital signs of circulation and respiration, since machines could replace these functions. As the understanding of human physiology continued to expand and the controlling role of the brain was elucidated, it became apparent that human life was inextricably linked to brain function.[7]

Whole Brain Death

In 1968, the Ad Hoc Committee of the Harvard Medical School was one of the first to formally advocate a new definition of *death* based on neurological criteria. The committee recommended that death be declared before life-support measures are turned off where the patient is in an "irreversible coma." An "irreversible coma" was described as a state of unreceptivity and unresponsitivity with no movement, breathing, or reflexes, accompanied by a flat electroencephalogram.[8] This new definition was intended to address the problem of keeping alive indefinitely patients who could not survive without any medical support and to prevent controversy in obtaining organs for transplantation.[9]

In 1970, the state of Kansas was the first to act on the ad hoc committee's recommendation and legally recognize the "absence of spontaneous brain function" as equivalent to cardiopulmonary death.[10] The state's lengthy statute met with much criticism but was a bold

[6]H. Beecher, "A Definition of Irreversible Coma. Special Communication: Report of the Ad Hoc Committee of the Harvard Medical School to Examine the Definition of Death," *JAMA* 205 (1968), pp. 337–40.

[7]President's Commission, *Defining Death.*

[8]See Beecher, "A Definition of Irreversible Coma."

[9]See ibid.

[10]See, e.g., L 1970, ch 348, Kan Laws 994, codified at *Kansas Statutes Annotated* §77-202.

first step toward addressing the growing unsuitability of the cardiovascular criteria for defining death. Meanwhile, courts struggled to reconcile the committee's proposal and new medical advances with their own conflicting statutory and common law definitions, which recognized only traditional cardiopulmonary death.[11]

After much debate and several other proposals,[12] the 1980 Uniform Determination of Death Act (UDDA) was put forth by the president's commission.[13] The UDDA simply provided that "an individual who has sustained either (1) irreversible cessation of circulatory and respiratory functions or (2) irreversible cessation of all functions of the entire brain, including the brain stem, is dead."[14] Critics disapproved of the alternative yet equal criteria of whole brain death and cardiopulmonary death, insisting that cessation of cardiopulmonary function was merely one test for brain death in the absence of artificial life-support measures.[15] However, this distinction was perceived as relatively minor, and despite initial efforts to limit the UDDA to only the whole brain death criteria, the proposed definition has been adopted, in some form, by most states.[16]

With the adoption of the brain death criteria came the concerns that patients who were merely in a temporary state of unconsciousness might be misdiagnosed as dead, making their organs inappropriately subject to transplant harvesting. For this reason, many modern statutes impose precautionary measures for diagnosing brain death to avoid any possibility or appearance of impropri-

ety in transplant efforts. Prior to pronouncing brain death, a physician who is not associated with any transplant effort must document his or her findings and a second disinterested physician must confirm the diagnosis.[17] In addition, detailed guidelines for diagnosing brain death must be followed. A typical set of brain death diagnostic guidelines is exemplified by the following used by surgeons at the University of Southern California Medical Center:

The clinical diagnosis of brain death. (An EEG is not required):

1. The cause of brain death must be specifiable and irreversible.
2. Exclude the effects of CNS depressing drugs and muscle relaxants as verified by "Tox Screen" (SMAC).
3. There must be no spontaneous respiration.
   a. Pre-oxygenate with 100% O_2 for 10 minutes
   b. Ensure that the pCO_2 is more than 5.3kPa (40 mmHg)
   c. Disconnect ventilator
   d. Administer O_2 at 6 minutes
   e. Observe for any spontaneous respiration for 10 minutes
4. The rectal temperature must be above 35° C.
5. All the brain stem reflexes must be absent.
   a. Pupils fixed and usually dilated
   b. Absent corneal reflex
   c. No gag reflex or response to tracheal suctioning
   d. Absent vestibulo-ocular reflex (cold caloric test). Check that tympanic membranes are intact. Inject 30 ml ice-cold water into each ear. There should be no eye movement of any kind
   e. Absent oculo-cephalic reflex (doll's eye movement)
   f. No motor response within the cranial nerve distribution to stimulation of any somatic area, e.g., grimacing
   g. Spinal and tendon reflexes may be present.
6. Two licensed physicians who are not members of the transplant team must write a note in the progress notes stating that the patient has irreversible and total cessation of brain function. The note should give findings which led to this conclusion.[18]

If physicians comply with accepted medical practices for diagnosing brain death and follow the statutory safeguard measures in reaching such a diagnosis, courts have been hesitant to hold them liable for removal of life support, even if done without clear consent of the patient's family mem-

[11]See, e.g., State v. Fierro, 603 P.2d 74, 77 (Ariz. 1979) (finding that it was acceptable to remove life support from a brain-dead patient because this was merely stepping aside and letting the natural course of events lead from brain death to common law death).

[12]See, e.g., Uniform Brain Death Act §1 (1978); A. Capron and L. Kass, "A Statutory Definition of the Standards for Determining Human Death: An Appraisal and Proposal," *University of Pennsylvania Law Review* 121 (1972), pp. 87–118.

[13]President's Commission, *Defining Death.*

[14]Uniform Determination of Death Act §1 (1980).

[15]See, e.g., J. Bernat, C. Culver, and B. Gert, "Defining Death in Theory and Practice," *Hastings Center Report* 12 (1982), pp. 5–9.

[16]See, e.g., *Alabama Code* §22-31-1 (1998); *California Health and Safety Code* (St. Paul, MN: West, 1997), section 7180(a); *Florida Statutes Annotated* (St. Paul, MN: West, 1993), section 382.009(1); *Michigan Compiled Laws Annotated* (St. Paul, MN: West, 1992), section 333.1033; *Montana Code Annotated* §50-22-101 (1995); *North Carolina General Statutes* §90-323 (1993); *Ohio Revised Code Annotated* (Cincinnati: Anderson, 1994), section 2108.30; 1999 Bill Text IA S.B. 12 (Iowa's proposal to adopt the UDDA for all circumstances in which a determination of death must be made).

[17]See, e.g., *Virginia Code Annotated* (Charlottesville, VA: Michie 1998), section 54.1-2972(c); *California Health and Safety Code* §7181 (1999).

[18]Guidelines for Certification of Brain Death, available at http://www.usc.edu/hsc/medicine/surgery/trauma/Trauma_Protocols/15BRAIN.html.

bers.[19] Similarly, where there is even a minimal amount of brain stem activity, doctors are justified in refusing to remove life support in the absence of clear and convincing proof that this is what the patient would have wanted.[20]

Higher Brain Death

The expansion of the legal definition of *death* to include "whole brain death" has overcome many ethical problems associated with using the cardiopulmonary definition of death to justify "keeping corpses ventilated" but does not address those patients with irreversible brain damage who can breathe by themselves. These patients, who are often diagnosed as being in a persistent vegetative state (PVS), lack higher brain function, which controls emotion, consciousness, and cognition, yet continue to maintain at least partial brain stem function. This can occur because the brain stem is more resilient to damage resulting from oxygen deprivation and so can survive insults that will completely damage the higher brain. Because the brain stem supports involuntary functions such as breathing, heart activity, and reflexes, these patients may often appear to grimace and yawn despite their lack of any higher brain function. At any given time, as many as 10,000–25,000 adult patients and 4,000–10,000 children fall into this category.[21]

Because PVS patients fall short of the legal whole brain death standard, they create a questionable middle ground between life and death that medical professionals and ethicists are struggling to address.[22] Much of this debate involves a further determination of what "person-hood" really is, since only "persons" have a right to life, liberty, and justice under the Constitution. Therefore, only when *personhood* is fully defined can a corresponding definition of *death* be properly constructed.[23] Proponents of using the higher brain death criteria to determine death argue that life, legal personhood, and consciousness are synonymous, since without consciousness, all that makes us individual human beings is lost.[24]

Courts and state legislatures are hesitant to adopt a "higher brain" or neocortical standard for defining death, simply because such a standard cannot be ascertained with the same level of certainty as "whole brain death." Technologies such as the electroencephalogram (EEG), positron emission tomography (PET), computerized axial tomography (CT), and magnetic resonance imaging (MRI) can be used to confirm lack of spontaneous brain activity in the cerebrum.[25] However, only after the lapse of a substantial period of time, when the hemispheres of the higher brain show clear degeneration, can an irreversible vegetative condition be confirmed.[26] Indeed, another recently reported case of a PVS patient recovering cognition after a prolonged coma emphasizes the difficulty in achieving a concrete diagnosis of "neocortical" or higher brain death.[27]

Many high-profile "right to die" cases involving PVS patients demonstrate the difficult legal and ethical issues that can arise for those patients who have "higher brain

[19]See, e.g., Gallups v. Cotter, 534 So.2d 585, 588–89 (Ala. 1988); Lovato v. District Court of the Tenth Judicial Dist., 601 P.2d 1072 (Colo. 1979) (authorizing removal of life support of brain dead child over objection of parents); Petition of Jones, 433 N.Y.S.2d 984 (Sup. Ct. 1980) (finding that where the brain death standard has been accepted, if brain death is determined according to accepted guidelines, there is no need for any court authorization prior to removal of life support); *Ohio Revised Code Annotated* (Cincinnati: Anderson, 1998), section 2108.30 (stating that physicians who make a determination of death in accordance with state brain death statute will not be held civilly liable or prosecuted criminally for acts based on that determination).

[20]See, e.g., McVey v. Englewood Hosp. Ass'n., 542 A.2d 450 (N.J. 1987).

[21]Multi-Society Task Force on PVS, "Medical Aspects of the Persistent Vegetative State," *New England Journal of Medicine* 330 (1994), pp. 1499–1508.

[22]See, e.g., R. Veatch, "Correspondence," *Hastings Center Report* 12 (1982), p. 45; D. R. Smith, "Legal Recognition of Neocortical Death," *Cornell Law Review* 71 (1986), pp. 850–88. See also D. O. Linder, "The Other Right to Life Debate: When Does Fourteenth Amendment 'Life' End?" *Arizona Law Review* 37 (1995), pp. 1183–1207 (arguing that states should be free to define *death* so as to exclude PVS patients from the constitutional class of "persons" entitled to medical care).

[23]See, e.g., Roe v. Wade, 410 U.S. 113, 156–157 (1973) (finding that fetuses are not persons under the Constitution); R. E. Cranford and D. R. Smith, "Consciousness: The Most Critical Moral (Constitutional) Standard for Human Personhood," *American Journal of Law and Medicine* 13 (1987), pp. 233–48.

[24]See Cranford and Smith, ibid.; C. M. Kester, "Is There a Person in That Body? An Argument for the Priority of Persons and the Need for a New Legal Paradigm," *Georgia Law Journal* 82 (1994), pp. 1643–87; R. M. Veatch, "The Impending Collapse of the Whole-Brain Death Definition of Death," *Hastings Center Report* 23 (1993), pp. 18–24.

[25]See, e.g., J. P. Richardson and T. J. Keay, "Practical Problems in the Withdrawal of Nutrition and Hydration from Two Patients in a Persistent Vegetative State," *Archives of Family Medicine* 2 (1993), pp. 981–86.

[26]"Position of the American Academy of Neurology on Certain Aspects of the Care and Management of the Persistent Vegetative State Patient: Adopted by the Executive Board, American Academy of Neurology, April 21, 1988, Cincinnati, Ohio," *Neurology* 39 (1989), pp. 125–26 (recommending a three-month evaluation period before diagnosing a patient as PVS); Council of Scientific Affairs and Council on Ethical and Judicial Affairs, "Persistent Vegetative State and the Decision to Withdraw or Withhold Life Support," *JAMA* 263 (1990), pp. 426–30 (recommending a 12-month evaluation period before diagnosis of PVS).

[27]See, e.g., N. L. Childs and W. N. Mercer, "Late Improvement in Consciousness After Post-Traumatic Vegetative State," *New England Journal of Medicine* 334 (1996), pp. 24–25.

death" but fall short of the legal whole brain death standard.[28] In the case of *In re Quinlan*, Karen Ann Quinlan became permanently unconscious after a drug overdose. Her father was appointed her legal guardian and wanted to have her life support removed, but the hospital physicians refused. After a long court battle, the New Jersey Supreme Court held that as her legal guardian, her father could order withdrawal of life support on the basis of Quinlan's right to refuse treatment. After her ventilator was removed, Quinlan's body continued to function for an additional nine years with artificial hydration and nutrition. The more recent case of *Cruzan v. Director, Missouri Dept. of Health* involved similar circumstances, but in this case, Cruzan's father struggled to have her artificial hydration and nutrition removed after it became apparent that she would never regain consciousness.[29]

In both of these cases, the courts resolved the issues based on the patients' rights to refuse treatment.[30] In holding that individuals can refuse treatment in the form of hydration and nutrition, the Supreme Court in *Cruzan* clearly operated under the assumption that Cruzan was alive, since she had suffered irreversible brain damage to only the upper portion of her brain and therefore did not meet the legal whole brain death criteria. Yet, the question of whether patients in Cruzan's condition should be considered alive was apparent when Justice Stevens, in his dissent, contemplated that Nancy Cruzan's life might have "expired when her biological existence ceased serving any of her own interests."[31]

Since these first difficult cases, courts generally have concluded that not every life is worth sustaining medically and now permit the removal of life-sustaining treatment for patients deemed to be in a persistent vegetative state according to patient and family wishes.[32] While the right to refuse treatment rationale solves the problem of

forcing treatment on patients with higher brain death, it does not alter, and in fact relies on, the legal conclusion that these patients still are alive. Therefore, nothing can be done in cases where families of PVS patients seek to continue treatment indefinitely, where medical professionals have determined that treatment is futile and arguably abusive.[33] Proponents of expanding the legal definition of *death* to encompass those with higher brain death believe that such expansion will address both of these issues. Nonetheless, regardless of how *death* is defined legally, conflicts will remain that arise out of personal definitions of *death* held by physicians, patients, and family members.

Patient-Determined Definition of Death

In the midst of the ongoing debate on how ethical and acceptable it is to expand the definition of *death*, some states have begun considering an additional factor: the moral and religious beliefs of their patients.[34] In 1991, New Jersey state law was changed to read:

> The death of an individual shall not be declared upon the basis of neurological criteria pursuant to sections of this act when the licensed physician authorized to declare death has reason to believe . . . that such a declaration would violate the personal religious beliefs of the individual. In these cases, death shall be declared, and the time of death fixed, solely upon the basis of cardiopulmonary criteria.[35]

This modification in the law permitted religious individuals to opt for the more narrowly defined cardiopulmonary criteria for death. However, in granting such religious exceptions to the broader statutory "whole brain death" definitions, situations identical to those that prompted the adoption of the whole brain death standard have arisen.

One such example is the case of Mariah Scoon.[36] Mariah, a five-month-old baby, was declared brain dead. Her parents, who had recently become born-again Chris-

---

[28]See, e.g., In re Quinlan, 355 A.2d 647 (N.J. 1976); In re Jobes, 510 A.2d 133 (N.J. Super. Ct. Ch. Div. 1986); Brophy v. New England Sinai Hosp., 497 N.E.2d 626, 628 (Mass. 1986); Cruzan v. Director, Missouri Dept. of Health, 497 U.S. 261, 266 (1990); In re Eichner, 426 N.Y.S.2d 517 (App. Div. 1990).

[29]Cruzan v. Director, Missouri Dept. of Health, 497 U.S. 261, 110 S.Ct. 2841 (1990).

[30]J. B. Oldershaw, J. Atkinson, and L. D. Boshes, "Persistent Vegetative State: Medical, Ethical, Religious, Economic and Legal Perspectives," *DePaul Journal of Health Care Law* 1 (1997), pp. 495–536.

[31]Cruzan v. Director, Missouri Dept. of Health, 497 U.S. 261, 351 (1989) (Stevens, J., dissenting).

[32]In re Estate of Longeway, 549 N.E.2d 292 (Ill. 1989); McConnell v. Beverly Enterprises-Connecticut, Inc., 553 A.2d 596, 603 (Conn. 1989); Gray v. Romero, 697 F.Supp. 580 (R.I. 1988); Rasmussen v. Fleming, 741 P.2d 674 (Ariz. 1987); In re Gardner 534 A.2d 947 (Me. 1987); Delio v. Akron General Medical Ctr., 426 N.E.2d 809 (Ohio 1980); In re L.H.R., 321 S.E.2d 716 (Ga. 1984).

[33]See, e.g., M. Angell, "The Case of Helga Wanglie: A New Kind of Right to Die Case," *New England Journal of Medicine* 325 (1991), pp. 511–12.

[34]For a thorough discussion on different religious views of death and dying, see, generally, Oldershaw et al., "Persistent Vegetative State"; T. Stacy, "Death, Privacy, and the Free Exercise of Religion," *Cornell Law Review* 77 (1992), pp. 490–595.

[35]*New Jersey Statutes Annotated* (St. Paul, MN: West, 1998), section 26:6A-5; P. Armstrong and R. Olick, "Innovative Legislature Initiatives: The New Jersey Declaration of Death and Advance Directives for Health Care Acts," *Seton Hall Legislative Journal* 16 (1992), pp. 177–97.

[36]G. J. Annas, "When Death Is Not the End," *New York Times* (March 2, 1996), p. A2.

tians, petitioned to prevent the declaration of death based on the New Jersey Religious Freedom Law and wanted to take drastic measures to keep her alive. The prospect of using modern medical advances to maintain Mariah's body when there was no chance of recovery prompted one well-known ethicist to pronounce that "Maintaining a corpse in an intensive care unit for a few days may be reasonable as a matter of sensitivity to religious or moral beliefs, but treating a dead body as if it were alive for a long period is bizarre and arguably a violation of basic human dignity."[37] His opinion highlights the clear clash between religious beliefs, which often require aggressive life-sustaining treatments at any cost, and medical prudence, which considers the effectiveness of treatment and the likelihood of recovery.[38]

The federal Religious Freedom Restoration Act of 1993 (RFRA) states that the free exercise clause of the First Amendment permits the government to burden religious beliefs only if there is a compelling state interest.[39] There is some debate as to whether RFRA can be interpreted to have the same effect as the New Jersey law in permitting individuals to opt for a declaration of death based on the cardiovascular criteria. Such an interpretation of RFRA would require that the government provide medical care for brain-dead religious individuals in excess of the care that is provided for nonreligious patients on the basis of the UDDA. Because this might appear to be preferential treatment on the basis of religion, such an interpretation might be difficult to establish.[40]

On the other hand, RFRA and the Free Exercise Clause do provide an established basis for individuals seeking to refuse additional treatment.[41] In refusing additional treatment on the basis of religious beliefs, the high medical costs associated with aggressively maintaining a brain-dead patient until cardiovascular death occurs are not required. For this reason, it is conceivable that RFRA might be interpreted to permit individuals to expand the definition of *death* beyond the current statutory definition

on the basis of religion.[42] While several ethicists support permitting patients to select from the traditional cardiovascular definition of death, the current legal whole brain death standard, or the broader higher brain death definition, regardless of religious belief,[43] such an interpretation of RFRA may create more problems than it would solve. If RFRA is interpreted to permit a diagnosis of death, for example, for a PVS patient, and active measures are taken at that point to terminate bodily functions, there would be a conflict with existing homicide laws.[44]

Anencephalic Infants

Anencephaly is a developmental disorder that results in infants being born with major portions of the brain, skull, and scalp missing. These neonates are not conscious and cannot experience any thoughts or emotions but can be born with partially developed brain stems that permit them to maintain autonomic functions of organs such as the heart, lungs, and kidneys.[45] Nonetheless, without aggressive life-saving measures, most anencephalic infants will die within a few days of birth. Like PVS patients, anencephalic infants cannot be considered legally dead under the current whole brain death law. However, the medical community has distinguished these infants from PVS patients because not only are they not presently conscious and unable to ever become conscious, anencephalic infants have never been conscious.[46]

In the 1992 case of *In re T.A.C.P.*, the parents of an infant diagnosed as anencephalic prior to birth decided to carry the baby to term so that its organs could be used for transplantation.[47] When T.A.C.P. was born, the hospital refused to harvest the organs prior to cardiovascular death for fear that they might incur civil or criminal liability, even though waiting for the infant to be considered dead under the UDDA would reduce the chance of the organs being viable for transplantation.[48] T.A.C.P.'s parents filed

---

[37]Ibid.

[38]See., e.g., M. D. Stern, "'And You Shall Choose Life' — Futility and the Religious Duty to Preserve Life," *Seton Hall Law Review* 25 (1995), pp. 997–1014; A. D. Shewmon, "'Brainstem Death,' 'Brain Death' and Death: A Critical Re-Evaluation of the Purported Equivalence," *Issues in Law and Medicine* 14 (1998), pp. 125–45; P. A. Byrne, "Understanding Brain Death," a presentation at the Institute of Human Values and Medical Ethics, New York Medical College, New York (transcript available at http://www.top.net/vitalsigns/vsmbraindeath.html).

[39]42 U.S.C.A. §§2000bb-1–2000bb-4 (West, 1993).

[40]D. M. Smolin, "Praying for Baby Rena: Religious Liberty, Medical Futility, and Miracles," *Seton Hall Law Review* 25 (1995), pp. 960–96.

[41]See, e.g., D, M. Smolin, "The Free Exercise Clause, the Religious Restoration Act, and the Right to Active and Passive Euthanasia," *Issues in Law and Medicine* 10 (1994), pp. 3–54.

[42]Religious Freedom Restoration Act, 42 U.S.C.A. §§2000bb-1–2000bb-4 (West, 1993).

[43]See Veatch, "The Impending Collapse"; K. G. Gervais, *Redefining Death* (New Haven, CT: Yale University Press, 1986), pp. 183–216.

[44]See, e.g., Smolin, "The Free Exercise Clause."

[45]See, e.g., In re T.A.C.P., 609 So.2d 588, 590 (Fla. 1992).

[46]See, e.g., J. A. Friedman, "Taking the Camel by the Nose: The Anencephalic as a Source for Pediatric Organ Transplants," *Columbia Law Review* 90 (1990), pp. 917–78.

[47]In re T.A.C.P., 609 So.2d 588 (Fla. 1992).

[48]R. LaFreniere, "End-of Life Issues: Anencephalic Infants as Organ Donors," *Journal of the American College of Surgeons* 187 (1998), pp. 443–47 (describing the Loma Linda transplant program, in which organs from anencephalic infants harvested postmortem yielded only a one-in-nine chance of success in transplantation).

suit and the court ultimately refused to expand the common law of the state of Florida to equate anencephaly with death. The basis for the court's decision in part was a lack of consensus in the medical community that the organs of anencephalics should be used for transplantation.[49]

Soon after the decision of *In re T.A.C.P.*, the Council of Ethical and Judicial Affairs of the American Medical Association put forth an opinion stating that it should be permissible to consider an anencephalic infant as an organ donor even though the infant still legally is deemed to be alive.[50] The committee considered the grave need for pediatric organs for transplantation versus the very limited expected life span of an anencephalic infant and concluded that both the lifesaving benefit to the donor children and the psychological benefit to the parents of the anencephalic infant justified this exception. The opinion required (1) two physicians with special expertise who were not affiliated with the transplant team to diagnose the anencephaly, (2) the parents had to initiate any discussion of organ donation, and (3) the Council Guidelines for the Transplantation of Organs had to be followed. Only a few months after this opinion was published, a great deal of criticism and controversy led the American Medical Association to reverse its stance and condone organ retrieval from anencephalic infants only after a whole brain death diagnosis is made.[51]

Alternatives to the AMA's attempt to exempt this class of patients from the Uniform Anatomical Gift Act (discussed next), which requires the donor to be dead, have been proposed. In Europe, physicians consider anencephalic infants as "brain absent"; therefore, a formal diagnosis of brain death is moot and organs can be removed for transplantation without extensive examination.[52] Others continue to argue that permitting such patients to be examined under the higher brain death criteria would be best. However, under the current law, hospitals must wait for anencephalic infants to experience either cardiopulmonary or whole brain death before legally harvesting their organs.[53]

Organ Donation

The 1968 Uniform Anatomical Gift Act (UAGA) mandates that an individual must be dead ("dead donor rule")

before his or her organs may be removed for use in transplantation.[54] As discussed, a finding of death according to the widely adopted UDDA requires either irreversible cessation of circulatory and respiratory functions or irreversible cessation of all functions of the entire brain, including the brain stem.[55] Prior to removing organs from a brain-dead patient, two physicians who are unaffiliated with the organ recipient or the transplant process must confirm the brain death diagnosis according to accepted medical guidelines as well as document those findings.[56]

The UAGA permitted individuals over the age of 18 to decide if they wanted to donate organs at death.[57] Where there was no evidence of such a decision, the UAGA permitted family members to step in and authorize or refuse such a donation.[58] The 1987 revision of the UAGA required hospital personnel to ask patients if they are organ donors, discuss organ donation with the patients if they are not currently donors, and obtain a copy of the document specifying their intent.[59] The provisions of the UAGA and its 1987 revision have been adopted in a significant number of states.[60]

Despite the measures provided in the 1968 Uniform Anatomical Gift Act, its 1987 amendment, and several other legislative attempts to structure and improve the system of organ donation in this country, there is still a grave shortage of organs available for transplantation purposes.[61] At any given time, approximately 38,000 patients are waiting for a suitable organ donor while there are only 4,000 donors annually.[62] Numerous proposals have been

[49]In re T.A.C.P., 609 So.2d 588, 594 (Fla. 1992).

[50]Council on Ethical and Judicial Affairs, American Medical Association, "The Use of Anencephalic Neonates as Organ Donors," *JAMA* 273 (1995), pp. 1614–18.

[51]J. Firshein, "American Medical Association Reinstates Restrictive Infant Donor Policy," *Lancet* 346 (1995), p. 1618.

[52]W. Holzgreve, F. K. Beller, and B. Buchholz, "Kidney Transplantation from Anencephalic Donors," *New England Journal of Medicine* 316 (1987), pp. 1069–70.

[53]Uniform Determination of Death Act §1 (1980).

[54]Uniform Anatomical Gift Act §8(b) (1968).

[55]Uniform Determination of Death Act §1 (1980).

[56]See, e.g., *Virginia Code Annotated* (Charlottesville, VA: Michie, 1998), section 54.1-2972(c).

[57]Uniform Anatomical Gift Act §2(a) (1968).

[58]Uniform Anatomical Gift Act §3(a) (1968).

[59]Uniform Anatomical Gift Act §5(a) (1987).

[60]M. C. Gorsline and R. L. K. Johnson, "The United States System of Organ Donation, the International Solution, and the Cadaveric Organ Donor Act: 'And the Winner Is . . . ,'" *Journal of Corporate Law* 20 (1994), pp. 5–50 (stating that, by 1972, all states had adopted the 1968 UAGA and, by 1994, 13 states had adopted the 1987 UAGA revision).

[61]See, e.g., A. C. MacDonald, "Organ Donation: The Time Has Come to Refocus the Ethical Spotlight," *Stanford Law and Policy Review* 8 (1997), pp. 177–84 (listing the reasons for the failure of the current organ donation system as a failure of potential donors to sign written directives, existing donor cards not being located, failure of medical personnel to recover organs based solely on written directives, failure of hospital personnel to approach families to request donation when decedent has no donor card, families' refusal to consent, and failure of medical examiners to release bodies for organ recovery).

[62]A.C. MacDonald, Organ Donation: The Time Has Come to Refocus the Ethical Spotlight. *Stanford Law and Policy Review* 8 (1997), pp. 177–84.

put forth to address the shortage of organs by increasing the pool of donors. One feasible proposal is a system of mandated choice in which individuals would be required to state whether they would like to be an organ donor at regular intervals such as during the filing of taxes or the renewal of a driver's license. Another possible yet more drastic proposal is to change the system of donation from one of voluntarism to one of presumed consent in which physicians may remove organs for transplantation without consent unless there is an express objection by the patient or his or her family.[63]

Until the system of organ donation is improved and more donors are secured, solutions to the problem of organ shortage will be sought out on other fronts. Improved efficiency in cadaveric organ retrieval that permits physicians to use hearts and livers from legally dead patients has provided a small increase in organ supply.[64] In addition, ethicists are scrutinizing the legal line between life and death to determine if organs from near death patients with no hope of recovery can be salvaged.

The University of Pittsburgh Medical Center recently adopted a new protocol that permits the retrieval of organs from hopeless patients who may or may not fit the whole brain death criteria yet are dependent on respirators for cardiovascular function. Respirator-dependent patients do not experience full brain death after removal of life support until the brain and brain stem have ceased functioning due to lack of blood flow and oxygenation. During that time, all organs that might be useable for transplantation are significantly compromised as well. The Pittsburgh protocol takes advantage of the fact that the UDDA considers both the whole brain death and the cardiovascular criteria as equivalent for a legal determination of death and calls for a declaration of death two minutes after cardiac function has ceased.[65]

For other hopeless patients who are not respirator dependent, for example, PVS patients, such an approach is no option. Despite emphasis on exempting anencephalic infants from the "dead donor rule" of the UAGA because they have no chance of ever gaining consciousness, the discourse on similarly exempting patients in a persistent vegetative state has been fairly limited. It has

been deemed ethically and morally acceptable to let long-term PVS patients die after withdrawal of life-supportive hydration and nutrition because they are presumed to be nonsentient. Such termination of life-support measures is legally acceptable because the courts have recognized the patient's right to refuse treatment.[66] Unfortunately, the removal of nutrition and hydration from PVS patients causes a slow death from eventual electrolyte imbalance or dehydration that may take 10–12 days. In the process, all the patients' transplantable organs are destroyed.[67]

Some ethicists concerned with reducing the organ shortage have proposed an exception to the "dead donor rule" of the UAGA for PVS patients in cases where physicians and family already have decided to withdraw life-supportive measures. Like the exception to the "dead donor rule" proposed and temporarily implemented for anencephalic infants, this exception would permit removal of organs from PVS patients before the patient is legally dead according to the UDDA.[68]

Financial Considerations

One of the Harvard ad hoc committee's stated reasons for putting forth criteria for a uniform definition of *brain death* was to prevent the expenses associated with keeping brain-dead patients alive.[69] Each year, billions of dollars are spent maintaining partially or totally brain-dead patients on life support, with the average cost running about $45,000 per month for each patient.[70] The tragic circumstances surrounding a diagnosis of brain death or brain damage usually preclude family members from

[63]See, generally, Council on Medical and Judicial Affairs, American Medical Association, "Strategies for Cadaveric Organ Procurement: Mandated Choice and Presumed Consent," *JAMA* 272 (1994), pp. 809–12.

[64]S. J. Youngner and R. M. Arnold, "Ethical, Psychological and Public Policy Implications of Procuring Organs from Non-Heart-Beating Cadaver Organs," *JAMA* 269 (1993), pp. 2769–74.

[65]See, e.g., M. F. Anderson, "The Future of Organ Transplantation: From Where Will New Donors Come, to Whom Will Their Organs Go?" *Health Matrix* 5 (1995), pp. 249–310 (describing the Pittsburgh protocol and pointing out the many problems associated with this approach).

[66]See, e.g., In re Quinlan, 355 A.2d 647 (N.J. 1976); In re Jobes, 510 A.2d 133 (N.J. Super. Ct. Ch. Div. 1986); Brophy v. New England Sinai Hosp., 497 N.E.2d 626, 628 (Mass. 1986); Cruzan v. Director, Missouri Dept. of Health, 497 U.S. 261, 266 (1990). See also *Arizona Revised Statutes Annotated* §§36-3201–3204 (1993); *Connecticut General Statutes Annotated* (St. Paul, MN: West, 1992), section 19a-570(1); *Florida Statutes Annotated* (St. Paul, MN: West, 1993), section 765.101; *Iowa Code Annotated* (St. Paul, MN: West, 1993), sections 144A.2, 144B.6; *Louisiana Revised Statutes Annotated* (St. Paul, MN: West, 1992), section 40:1299.58.2; *New York Public Health Law* (St. Paul, MN: West, 1993), section 2984; *North Carolina General Statutes* §90-322(a) (1992).

[67]R. Hoffenberg, M. Lock, and N. Tilney, "Should Organs from Patients in a Permanent Vegetative State Be Used for Transplantation?" *Lancet* 350 (1997), pp. 1320–21.

[68]Ibid.

[69]Beecher, "A Definition of Irreversible Coma."

[70]See, e.g., Tarantino, "Withdrawal of Life Support" (citing the case of In re Wanglie in which Ms. Wanglie was a PVS patient requiring a respirator); Multi-Society Task Force on PVS, "Medical Aspects of the Persistent Vegetative State" (cost of maintaining patients in a persistent vegetative state in the United States is between $1 and $8 billion annually).

focusing on financial considerations; however, these expenses and the related costs associated with organ transplantation must be allocated.

A typical insurance contract will cover treatment that is medically necessary.[71] Treatment is considered medically necessary when it is ordered by a physician, is commonly and customarily recognized throughout the doctor's profession as appropriate in the treatment of the existing sickness or injury, and is neither educational nor experimental in nature.[72] When a patient is diagnosed as legally dead based on the accepted criteria, life support may be immediately removed. The cost of emergency care and the related medical expenses necessary for a diagnosis of death usually are covered by insurance, but after a diagnosis of death is made, the continued treatment ceases to be medically necessary.[73]

In the case of *Cavagnaro v. Hanover Insurance Company, Inc.*, the state of New Jersey refused to hold an automobile insurance company responsible for the medical expenses of Michael, a 14-year-old brain-dead patient who was maintained for 12 days so that family members could decide if organ donation was appropriate. The court based its decision on the state's "no fault act," which required insurance companies to cover only medical expenses for necessary medical treatment. *Medical treatment* in this case was defined to be that treatment that is for the purpose of preserving life and relieving the patient from pain and disability. Because sustaining a brain-dead patient to maintain his organs for transplantation accomplishes neither of these goals, the insurance company was not liable for those expenses incurred after the diagnosis of Michael's brain death.[74] Had Michael's family ultimately decided to donate his organs, many states would shift the expense of maintaining his body after brain death to the organ-procuring agency.[75]

In cases where there is no clear finding of whole brain death and the patient retains even a minimal amount of brain function, hospitals will be required to "determine the existence, veracity, and effect of an incompetent's orally expressed wishes" prior to removing life support.[76]

During the time that it takes for family members and courts to determine the patient's wishes or appoint a guardian to make decisions on behalf of the patient, the hospital is obligated to maintain the patient on life support and the medical expenses incurred are the responsibility of the patient. This holds true even where family members insist that life support be removed from the initial determination of irreversible brain damage.[77]

Once death is confirmed, the surviving spouse and family members have numerous other financial considerations. Life insurance policies of the deceased become payable, estates must be distributed, marriage ends, business partnerships terminate, and disability benefits cease.[78] All these legal processes begin on a formal determination of death, and at times, the exact time of death is a critical factor. For example, in cases where two spouses are fatally injured simultaneously, the time between their actual deaths determines survivorship and the distribution of their estates.[79]

The expansion of the legal definition of *death* to encompass whole brain death eliminated the ability of health care agents and designated decision makers who have an interest in the distribution of assets to prolong the use of life support of a brain-dead patient to prolong the time of death. For instance, it is easy to understand why the family of a patient receiving disability and health care benefits would want to maintain the brain-dead patient long enough to collect a final payment. The moment of a diagnosis of brain death is the time of death for legal purposes and continued life support will not alter this determination.[80] However, under the current law, even a minimal amount of brain death function will revert the time of death to the moment of cessation of cardiovascular function, and the time of death will be dependent on the moment at which life support is removed.

Notes on Definitions of Death

Beyond Higher Brain Death

Proponents of the higher brain death criteria for defining *death* argue that when consciousness is lost, personhood is lost. Those who oppose expanding the brain death criteria

[71]See Pirozzi v. Blue Cross-Blue Shield, 741 F.Supp. 586, 589 n.5 (E.D. Va. 1990). See, generally, M. A. Hall and G. F. Anderson, "Models of Rationing: Health Insurers' Assessment of Medical Necessity," *University of Pennsylvania Law Review* 140 (1992), pp. 1637–1712.

[72]See, e.g., Doza v. Crum & Forster Ins. Co, 716 F.Supp. 131, 134 (D.N.J. 1989) (referring to the policy at issue).

[73]Cavagnaro v. Hanover Insurance Co., 565 A.2d 728, 730 (N.J. Super. 1989).

[74]Cavagnaro v. Hanover Insurance Co., 565 A.2d 728, 730–31 (N.J. Super. 1989).

[75]See, e.g., *South Carolina Code Annotated* (New York: Lawyers Cooperative Publishing Co., 1998), section 44-43-1010.

[76]See, e.g., McVey v. Englewood Hosp. Ass'n, 524 A.2d 450, 451 (N.J. 1987).

[77]See, e.g., McVey v. Englewood Hosp. Ass'n, 524 A.2d 450, 451 (N.J. 1987).

[78]See, e.g., *Texas Probate Code Annotated* (St. Paul, MN: West, 1997), section 47. See also Cranford and Smith, "Consciousness."

[79]See, e.g., J. C. Benson and R. Austin, "The Impact of Advance Medical Directives on Distribution of Estate and Assets Under the Simultaneous Death Act," *Elder Law Journal* 5 (1997), pp. 1–15.

[80]See, e.g., *New Jersey Statutes* (St. Paul, MN: West, 1998), section 26:6A-5(d).

object primarily because higher brain death is much more difficult to diagnose with certainty than lower brain death. However, acknowledging upper brain function or consciousness as equivalent to life presents many additional concerns. One of these concerns is how will patients suffering from severe dementia be classified. Such patients are conscious in that they can react to some stimuli in their environment, but those with advanced Alzheimer's disease or profound retardation often are not self-aware and thus lack any identity. Many philosophers argue that the death of the essence or identity, in a sense, is equivalent to the death of that person.

Additional Reading.   J. Areen et al., "Defining Death," in *Law, Science and Medicine* (Westbury, NY: Foundation Press, 1996), pp. 1097–1114; K. G. Gervais, *Redefining Death* (New Haven, CT: Yale University Press, 1986), pp. 183–216.

Death Certificates

Once death has been diagnosed according to legal and medical standards, it is documented and reported to the appropriate state and federal agencies. Death certificates typically contain the name of the decedent, place of birth, date and time of death, names of parents, race, decedent's occupation, location of death, and cause of death. In addition, most death certificates have space for comments of the attending physician regarding the condition of the patient just prior to death. Death certificates generally are accessible to the public; however, in cases where there is information regarding communicable diseases or other information protected under confidentiality laws, the death certificates are issued without the confidential information. Full death certificates, including information deemed to be confidential, usually are disclosed only to immediate family and their representatives, to government agencies, and when ordered by a court.[81]

Additional Reading.   A. S. Leonard, M. A. Bobinski, and M. L. Closen, "The Legal Issues of Death and Dying," in *AIDS Law and Policy* (Houston: John Marshall Publishing Co., 1995), pp. 467–513; S. S. Sanbar et al., "The Process of Dying," in *Legal Medicine* (St. Louis: Mosby, 1998), pp. 353–64.

Fetuses

Under the current legal and medical standard of whole brain death, it is clear that traditional patient viability no longer is the bright line between life and death at the end

of life. Nonetheless, in *Roe v. Wade*, the Supreme Court stated that viability is the standard for determining the beginning of life.[82] This finding by the court permits pregnant women to place their own privacy interests above the life of the fetus prior to fetus viability and is the basis for legal abortion.[83] The higher brain, consciousness, or psychological criteria for brain death as opposed to the current biological whole brain death criteria provide a means for reconciling these conflicting views as to when life and personhood truly exist.[84]

Fetuses do not develop brain stem function until about 8 weeks' gestation and do not develop any of the cortical structures necessary for consciousness until 20–24 weeks' gestation.[85] If applying the current biologically based whole brain death criteria, fetuses would be considered brain dead or nonpersons up until the point at which they develop some brain stem function. Since traditional legal viability and the development of the higher brain both occur during the same stage of pregnancy, between 20 and 24 weeks, applying the consciousness-based definition of *personhood* would be reasonable and not unduly burdensome to the legal machinery currently in place.[86]

Additional Reading.   C. M. Kester, "Is There a Person in That Body?: An Argument for the Priority of Persons and the Need for a New Legal Paradigm," *Georgia Law Journal* 82 (1994), pp. 1643–87; B. Steinbock. *Life Before Birth: The Moral and Legal Status of Embryos and Fetuses* (New York: Oxford University Press, 1992).

Homicide

Whether by independent reasoning or through adoption of statutory definitions, the courts of all states recognize brain death as legally equivalent to traditional cardiovascular death for purposes of homicide.[87] The notion that

---

[81]See, e.g., *Florida Statutes* ch. 382.025 (1998).

[82]Roe v. Wade, 410 U.S. 113, 160 (1973).

[83]Roe v. Wade, 410 U.S. 113, 160 (1973).

[84]See, e.g., Kester, "Is There a Person in That Body?"

[85]See, e.g., N. K. Rhoden, "Trimesters and Technology: Revamping *Roe v. Wade*," *Yale Law Journal* 95 (1986), pp. 639–63; D. G. Jones, "Brain Birth and Personal Identity," *Journal of Medical Ethics* 15 (1989), pp. 173–77.

[86]See, generally, Stacy, "Death, Privacy, and the Free Exercise of Religion"; L. H. Glantz, "Abortion and the Supreme Court: Why Legislative Motive Matters," *American Journal of Public Health* 76 (1986), pp. 1452–55; Thornburgh v. Am College of Obs & Gyn, 476 U.S. 747 (1986).

[87]See, e.g., Cowan v. State, 399 So.2d 1346 (Miss. 1981) (applying traditional Mississippi causation principles to establish legal death of a brain-dead patient to support a manslaughter charge); State v. Fierro, 603 P.2d 74, 77 (Ariz. 1979); State v. Shaffer, 574 P.2d 205 (Kan. 1977); Commonwealth v. Golston, 366 N.E.2d 744 (Mass. 1977), *cert. denied* 434 U.S. 1039 (1978).

the removal of life-supportive measures from a legally brain-dead victim is an intervening cause that breaks the chain of causation was uniformly discarded by the courts.[88] In the same vein, the argument made by several defendants that the removal of organs for donation after a determination of legal brain death likewise has been rejected as an intervening cause of death.[89]

In homicide cases, as in all other cases where a legal determination of death guides the appropriate course of action, the current "whole brain death" standard leaves those victims who suffer higher brain death, but not brain stem death as well, unaccounted for. Just as a killer whose victim dies one year and one week after being brutally beaten may not be charged with a homicide in some jurisdictions,[90] so can a killer whose victim retains lower brain stem function avoid the charge. The highly publicized case of Claus Von Bulow demonstrates this point. Claus Von Bulow allegedly injected his wife with insulin in an attempt to kill her so that he could marry his mistress. Mrs. Von Bulow was found to be in an irreversible coma yet her body remained capable of functioning and appeared intact. Mr. Von Bulow could be charged only with attempted murder, regardless of his intentions, even though Mrs. Von Bulow would never recover consciousness.[91]

Homicide law uniformly applies the whole brain death criteria as the basis for determining when a life has been taken. However, the standard for determining death does not change based on the intent of the party directly responsible for death. Homicide may just as readily be charged when organs from a patient with only higher brain death are removed for altruistic purposes or when family and physicians seek to actively terminate a PVS patient's life in order to honor that person's wishes. In such cases, the courts permit the removal of life-support measures but make it clear that any affirmative action to hasten death or remove organs from such "living" patients will support a homicide charge.[92]

Homicide and AIDS

The adoption of the UDDA whole brain definition of *death* ensures that parties responsible for the brain death of an individual, even one maintained artificially after the maximum statutorily required time for death, can be charged for murder. When an HIV-infected person intentionally or recklessly transmits HIV to an uninfected individual, death is fairly certain, but not likely to occur before the expiration of the maximum time frames permitted under statute. Under traditional criminal theories, even though a person intentionally transmits the deadly HIV virus, he or she is likely to be prosecuted under on a charge of only assault or reckless endangerment. The opposition to expanding the definition of death to apply even to PVS patients and anencephalic infants makes it implausible that it will ever be extended to persons infected with HIV. Therefore, the approach taken by many states has been to make intentional transmission of the HIV virus a separate felony.[93]

Additional Reading. M. E. Schecter, "AIDS: How the Disease Is Being Criminalized," *Criminal Justice* 3 (1988), pp. 6–41.

International Standards of Death

In the United States, the definition of death relies alternatively on the cardiopulmonary death and whole brain death criteria and a great deal of debate concerns whether the definition should be expanded to recognize the higher brain death criteria. Many countries also are debating the definition of *death* and the corresponding legal and ethical ramifications. Japan, for example, currently does not recognize whole brain death as equivalent to cardiovascular death. For this reason, organ transplants are not performed and Japanese patients in need of organs must go overseas and pay exorbitant prices.[94] In Germany, the whole brain definition of *death* is used; however, an exception is made for anencephalic infants, whose organs may be removed for transplantation prior to death.[95] In

[88]State v. Watson, 467 A.2d 590 (N.J. Super. 1983); State v. Meints, 322 N.W.2d 809 (Neb. 1982); Swafford v. State, 421 N.E.2d 596 (Ind. 1981); State v. Inger, 292 N.W.2d 119 (Iowa 1980).

[89]People v. Eulo, 472 N.E.2d 286 (N.Y. 1984); People v. Bonilla, 472 N.E.2d 286 (N.Y. 1984); State v. Shaffer, 574 P.2d 205 (Kan. 1977).

[90]See, e.g., D. E. Walther, "Taming a Phoenix: The Year-and-a-Day Rule in Federal Prosecutions for Murder," *University of Chicago Law Review* 59 (1992), pp. 1337–61 (discussing current status of the one year and one day rule, which is still in effect in federal courts and some state courts); "Homicide III. Causal Connection Between Act and Death," in *American Jurisprudence,* 2d ed. (Rochester, NY: Lawyers Cooperative Publishing, 1998), vol. 40, p. 14 (listing which states follow year and a day rule and which states have abolished or amended the rule).

[91]See Martha Von Bulow v. Claus Von Bulow, 657 F.Supp. 1134 (S.D. N.Y. 1987); State v. Claus von Bulow, 475 A.2d 995 (R.I. 1984).

[92]See, e.g., Cranford and Smith, "Consciousness."

[93]See, e.g., A. S. Leonard, M. A. Bobinski, and M. L. Closen, "The Legal Issues of Death and Dying," in *AIDS Law and Policy* (Houston: John Marshall Publishing Co., 1995), pp. 467–513 (describes case of Eva Marie Kearns, a prostitute in Carson City, Nevada, sentenced to 20 years in prison for solicitation after testing positive for HIV); *California Health and Safety Code* (St. Paul, MN: West, 1999), section 120291; *Florida Statutes* ch. 775.0877 (1998).

[94]R. B. Leflar, "Informed Consent and Patients' Rights in Japan," *Houston Law Review* 33 (1996), pp. 1–60.

[95]B. Brandon, "Anencephalic Infants as Organ Donors: A Question of Life or Death," *Case Western Reserve* 40 (1990), pp. 781–824.

France, the whole brain death definition of *death* was adopted only recently.

Additional Reading.   R. B. Leflar, "Informed Consent and Patients' Rights in Japan," *Houston Law Review* 33 (1996), pp. 1–60; N. Lenoir, "International Symposium on Law and Science at the Crossroads: Biomedical Technology, Ethics, Public Policy, and the Law: French, European, and International Legislation on Bioethics," *Suffolk University Law Review* 27 (1993), pp. 1249–70.

Further Reading

Anencephalic Infants

Friedman JA. Taking the Camel by the Nose: The Anencephalic as a Source for Pediatric Organ Transplants. *Columb L Rev* 1990;90:917–78.

Harden JN. The "Gift" of Life: Should Anencephalic Infants Die to Serve Noble Goals? *Cumb L Rev* 1997;27:1279–1310.

Justice JS. Personhood and Death — The Proper Treatment of Anencephalic Organ Donors Under the Law. *In re T.A.C.P.*, 609 So.2d 588 (Fla. 1992). *U Cin L Rev* 1994;62:1227–79.

Kaufman EH. *Pediatric Brain Death and Organ/Tissue Retrieval: Medical, Ethical and Legal Aspects.* New York: Plenum Publishing Corp., 1989.

McCullagh PJ. *Brain Dead, Brain Absent, Brain Donors: Human Subjects or Human Objects?* Somerset, NJ. John Wiley & Sons, 1993.

Financial Considerations

Tarantino LM. Withdrawal of Life Support: Conflict Among Patient Wishes, Family, Physicians, Courts and Statutes, and the Law. *Buffalo L Rev* 1994;42:623–52.

Higher Brain Death

Cranford RE, Smith DR. Consciousness: The Most Critical Moral (Constitutional) Standard for Human Personhood. *Am J L and Med* 1987;13:233–48.

Linder DO. The Other Right to Life Debate: When Does Fourteenth Amendment "Life" End? *Ariz L Rev* 1995;37:1183–1207.

Oldershaw JB, Atkinson J, Boshes LD. Persistent Vegetative State: Medical, Ethical, Religious, Economic and Legal Perspectives. *DePaul J Health Care L* 1997;1:495–536.

Smith DR. Legal Recognition of Neocortical Death. *Cornell L Rev* 1986;71:850–88.

Zaner RM. *Death: Beyond Whole-Brain Criteria (Philosophy and Medicine, Vol 31).* Hingham, MA: D. Reidel Publishing Co., 1988.

Organ Transplantation

Anderson MF. The Future of Organ Transplantation: From Where Will New Organs Come, to Whom Will Their Organs Go? *Health Matrix* 1995;5:249–310.

Chapman JR. *Organ and Tissue Donation for Transplantation.* New York: Oxford University Press, 1997.

Gorsline MC, Johnson RLK. The United States System of Organ Donation, the International Solution, and the Cadaveric Organ Donor Act: "And the Winner Is . . ." *J Corp L* 1994;20:5–50.

Schwindt R, Vining A. Proposal for a Mutual Insurance Pool for Transplant Organs. *J Health Politics, Pol'y & Law* 1998;23:725–41.

Patient–Determined Definition of Death

Boozang KM. An Intimate Passing: Restoring the Role of the Family and Religion in Dying. *U Pitt L Rev* 1997;58:549–617.

Oldershaw JB, Atkinson J, Boshes LD. Persistent Vegetative State: Medical, Ethical, Religious, Economic and Legal Perspectives. *DePaul J Health Care L* 1997;1:495–536.

Stacy T. Death Privacy, and the Free Exercise of Religion. *Cornell L Rev* 1992;77:490–595.

Whole Brain Death

Beauchamp TL, Veatch RM. *Ethical Issues in Death and Dying.* Old Tuppan, NJ: Prentice-Hall, 1995.

Beecher H. A Definition of Irreversible Coma. Special Communication: Report of the Ad Hoc Committee of the Harvard Medical School to Examine the Definition of Death. *JAMA* 1968;205:337–40.

Cantor NL. Philosophy and the Law: The Real Ethic of Death and Dying. *Mich L Rev* 1996;94:1718–38.

Furrow BR, Greaney TL, Johnson SH, Jost TS, Schwartz RL. Defining Death. In: *Bioethics: Healthcare Law and Ethics.* St. Paul, MN: West Publishing Co., 1997;179–207.

Lamb D. *Death, Brain Death and Ethics.* Brookfield, VT: Ashgate Publishing Co., 1996.

Machado C. *Proceedings of the Second International Symposium on Brain Death, Havana, Cuba, 27 February–1 March 1996.* New York: Elsevier Science, 1995.

President's Commission for the Study of Ethical Problems in Medicine and Biomedical and Behavioral Research. *Defining Death: A Report on the Medical, Legal and Ethical Issues in the Determination of Death.* Washington, DC: Government Printing Office, 1981.

Sanbar SS, Gibofsky A, Firestone MH, LeBlang TR. The Process of Dying. In: *Legal Medicine.* St. Louis: Mosby, 1998;353–64.

Singer P. *Rethinking Life and Death.* New York: St. Martin's Press, 1994.

Walton DN. *Brain Death*. Indianapolis: Purdue University Press, 1995.

Web Sites

American Share Foundation: *http://www.asf.org*

Brain death: Is that dead enough?: *http://www-hsc. usc.edu/~mbernste/ethics.braindeath.html*

Brain death criteria: Neurology: *http://www.medstudents. com.br/neuro/neuro5.htm*

Brain injury and brain death resources: *http://www. changesurfer.com/BD/Brain.html*

Death and dying — Legal links: *http://dying.miningco. com/msub2.htm*

Life source — Organ donation: *http://www.lifesource.org*

Medical Futility Journal article list: *http://www.okstate.edu/ artsci/philosophy/futility/artautho.htm*

Organ donation — Government site: *http://www.organ donor.gov*

United Network for Organ Sharing (UNOS): *http://www. unos.org*

Index